Pediatric Rheumatology for the Practitioner

Second Edition

Jerry C. Jacobs

Pediatric Rheumatology for the Practitioner

Second Edition

With 330 Illustrations in 422 Pieces

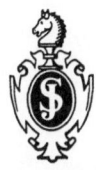

Springer Science+Business Media, LLC

Jerry C. Jacobs, M.D.
Professor of Clinical Pediatrics
Director, Section of Pediatric Rheumatology
  and the Regional Arthritis Program
  (RAP-4-Kids) at the
Columbia-Presbyterian Medical Center
New York, NY 10032 USA

Library of Congress Cataloging-in-Publication Data
Jacobs, Jerry C.
    Pediatric rheumatology for the practitioner / Jerry C. Jacobs.—
2nd ed.
      p. cm.
    Includes bibliographical references and index.
    ISBN 978-1-4757-6152-8   ISBN 978-1-4757-6150-4 (eBook)
    DOI 10.1007/978-1-4757-6150-4

    1. Pediatric rheumatology. I. Title.
    [DNLM: 1. Collagen Diseases—in infancy & childhood.   WD 375
J17p]
    RJ482.R48J3   1992
    618.92'723—dc20
    DNLM/DLC
    for Library of Congress   91-5210

Printed on acid-free paper.

Production managed by Ellen Seham; Manufacturing supervised by Rhea Talbert.
Typeset by Asco Trade Typesetting Ltd., Hong Kong.

9 8 7 6 5 4 3 2 1

ISBN 978-1-4757-6152-8

To my wife Isabel, who has provided very special inspiration for 42 years; and to Deborah, Daniel, and Paul, who added another dimension to my life and sometimes sacrificed their own needs to those of other children.

To all my teachers, but especially to Gilbert Hiatt and Charles Frankel, who taught a generation of Columbia College students about life; to Robert Loeb, Dana Atchley, and Rustin McIntosh, who taught a generation of physicians about devotion to the care of the sick; to Charles Ragan, who convinced me to study rheumatic disease; and to Charles Christian who provided my training and inspiration.

To all the sick children and their families, who are the substance of this book and for whom we hope to do more.

"To study the phenomena of disease without books is to sail an uncharted sea, while to study books without patients is not to go to sea at all."

—W. Osler ("Books and Men," *Boston Medical and Surgical Journal*, 144:60–61, 1901)

Contents

6   Dermatomyositis

9   The Power of Positive Thinking

Index

Preface to the Second Edition

Exactly ten years have elapsed since I wrote the preface to the first edition; pediatric rheumatology has grown into an accepted specialty and this year 103 physicians applied to take the first sub-Board examination. The extensive discussion of differential diagnosis required even further expansion: post-streptococcal arthritis, thrombotic thrombocytopenic purpura, Parvo 19, Muckle-Wells syndrome, Weber-Christian disease, transient hyperphosphatasemia of infancy, erythromelalgia, primary hyperoxaluria, fibromyalgia, sito-sterolemia, AIDS, arthritis as a manifestation of substance abuse, HLA-B27 associated familial thrombocytopenia with spondyloarthritis, Schmidt's syndrome, the anticardiolipin syndrome, inclusion body myositis and the toxic oil and L-tryptophan induced eosinophilia-myalgia and Parry-Romberg syndromes are only some of the added sections. The discussion of Lyme disease, the most common identifiable cause of arthritis in the United States, has been greatly expanded.

What has changed most in ten years, however, is drug treatment of the rheumatic disorders. Non-steroidal antiinflammatory drugs (NSAIDs) have replaced aspirin as the standard treatment of childhood arthritis, and methotrexate, not previously used at all, has become the drug of choice for the most severely ill children. Sulfasalazine, also not previously used at all, is now the most commonly used "disease modifying" agent in our clinic, and the last gold shot given to a child here was in 1986. Sections on preventing death from disseminated intravascular coagulation (DIC) and on how to better control fever in systemic JRA have been added. The severe cardiac sequelae of Kawasaki disease, the most common cause of acquired heart disease in U.S. children 10 years ago, have been almost totally prevented by early diagnosis and prompt administration of gamma globulin. And we have learned that severe lupus nephritis needs even more aggressive treatment than we previously offered if renal function and life are to be preserved. We've failed only once in preventing a child from becoming wheelchair bound from arthritis in this decade, and I believe we could have done better for him too, and we've had no deaths in JRA or dermatomyositis or renal failure or deaths in Caucasian children with lupus. Until I had completed writing this edition I did not realize how much had changed.

Jerry C. Jacobs

Preface to the First Edition

Definition of the Rheumatic Disorders: "A typical hippie commune, a hitherto forbidden clone, sharing a mystery of origin, living together but unrelated, widely misunderstood, difficult to control or to treat, error-prone, over-reactive sometimes to familiar antigens, to parental influence and to medical authority, given to strange drugs, difficult to recognize from each other and adding a few more mixed-up syndromes to their number from time to time . . ."*

This book complements the authoritative multiauthored texts on rheumatic disease by providing special insight into the care of children with rheumatic disease. Rheumatologists, orthopedists, and physiatrists are familiar with the principles of diagnosis and management of rheumatic diseases in adults, and they are called upon to apply their special knowledge to the care of children. Their devotion to young patients is evidenced by their attendance in overwhelming numbers at the relatively few seminars pediatric rheumatologists have been able to provide. My goal is to help them sharpen their diagnostic and therapeutic strategies. If each gains even a little from reading this book, the children will benefit, and I know that their doctors will obtain greater satisfaction from caring for them.

Inevitably in a one-author text whose primary purpose is to provide information to family practitioners and pediatricians, opinions will be expressed which may seem arbitrary to specialized physicians. In some instances my knowledge of orthopedics, internal medicine, and physiatry must seem a bit primitive to real experts in these individual disciplines. It is not necessary, however, that we always agree. What I have written is based

* Paraphrased from Eric Bywaters, at the VIIIth European Congress of Rheumatology, Helsinki, Finland, June 1, 1975. *See* Bywaters EGL: The historical evolution of the concept of connective tissue disease. Scandinavian Journal of Rheumatology. Supplement 12:11–29, 1976.

largely on personal experience, and where the knowledgeable physician disagrees, it is hoped he will find our private debate stimulating.

For those whose primary mission is the care of children, my purposes are quite different. When invited by the Editors to contribute this volume to a new series of monographs entitled "Comprehensive Manuals in Pediatrics," I made a firm commitment to provide primary care physicians with the multiple perceptions which are part of my clinical judgment in the diagnosis and care of children with musculoskeletal disorders. It is not my intention to provide an encyclopedic text. The reader is encouraged, whenever the opportunity presents, to consult the many outstanding sources of rheumatologic information.

In the aggregate, the disorders discussed in this book inflict a considerable burden on children. Musculoskeletal disease accounts for nearly 2 percent of all visits to pediatricians and is one of the most common causes of chronic disability. Despite the evident need, relatively few medical schools have divisions of pediatric rheumatology. As a result, most pediatricians in practice today have had scanty training in the diagnosis and management of rheumatic disorders, or even in physical examination of the joints. The differential diagnosis of musculoskeletal pain in childhood is among the most complex of any in medicine. More than one hundred entities must be considered. For this reason, fully one-third of this book is devoted to differential diagnosis. The "nonrheumatic disorders," traditionally relegated to the back of encyclopedic texts, have been brought "up front." With only a little help, every primary care physician for children can become more expert in differential diagnosis and can obtain great satisfaction from having developed these skills.

Diagnosis and treatment are the focus of the chapters on the specific rheumatic diseases. Theories about disease causation are presented only to whet the appetite. The principles of treatment have been emphasized, and in every instance I have tried to provide the physician with a plan of therapy which is acceptable, albeit at times controversial. In the ideal world, every child with rheumatic disease would have the benefit of the care of a full-time pediatric rheumatologist. Such a world does not now and will not soon exist. Pediatricians find it hard enough to work out a therapeutic strategy for these children without becoming embroiled in all the controversy on which rheumatologists thrive. It is well known that on rheumatology rounds expert physicians rarely advocate an identical plan of therapy for a given patient. A dialogue takes place from which the responsible individual must synthesize his plan of action. I have tried to provide an acceptable plan for primary physicians who do not have the opportunity to participate in this dialogue but are faced with the responsibility of caring for the patient.

Most pediatric rheumatologists already know much of the material in this book. We are a small group and exchange ideas frequently. I hope they find a few tidbits, but one can hardly justify writing a book for pediatric rheumatologists. For the pediatric rheumatologist, perhaps the most controversial of all the concepts contained in this book is my suggestion that Reiter's syndrome and ankylosing spondylitis are prototype descriptions of different stages of a single disease, which might best be called spondyloarthritis and which in many or most individuals does not affect the spine. This formulation greatly simplifies the nomenclature, since, otherwise, new names must be created for the majority of patients with this form of arthritis who have neither the Reiter's triad nor ankylosis of the spine, and are unlikely to develop either despite their increased susceptibility to both. The historical terms Reiter's syndrome and ankylosing spondylitis may be retained for what they originally meant, without endless modification, and the same term may be used for the same disorder in both children and adults. An entire chapter is devoted to this relatively unstudied childhood disorder, which affects five times as many children as SLE, dermatomyositis, and scleroderma combined.

I cannot emphasize enough the importance of positive physician attitudes in minimizing rather than creating dysfunction. Over the past twenty years we have made relatively little progress in terms of new "curative" drugs or techniques or in the final understanding of the pathogenesis of any of these diseases. Yet any comparative study of the function of these children and their families in society shows dramatic advances. This is the triumph of pediatric rheumatology. Reduced hospitalization, little school absence, no special (but unequal) classes, less destruction of the family—these are our achievements. All have been accomplished primarily with the same old tools that were available before. The commitment to function, coupled with early skillful diagnosis and intervention, has enabled us to use both new and old drugs more effectively and to avoid modes of therapy which enhance dysfunction. Pediatric rheumatologists didn't invent functional attitudes, but perhaps nowhere are they more crucial than in the care of visibly crippled children, and so perhaps their significance is most dramatically demonstrated in our patients.

Rheumatology has been largely a stepchild of medicine, devoid of great discoveries. The study of rheumatic diseases is fascinating but frustrating. We have had to settle for stimulating immunologic research, identifying and describing subsets of disease, establishing diagnostic criteria, designing therapeutic trials, and setting standards for exemplary care of patients. Prevention and cure remain as challenges for those who now choose pediatric rheumatology for their career. Hopefully, medical students and house officers who use this book will be encouraged to consider pediatric rheumatology as a potential career. If this book stimulates young doctors to study and improve the care of children with rheumatic diseases, it will have more than served its purpose.

Jerry C. Jacobs

Acknowledgments

It is not possible to thank individually everyone who has contributed to the preparation of this book. Much has been learned from the children who suffer with these diseases and from their parents. Medical students, house officers, nurses, social workers, therapists, and clinic personnel, together with all of my physician colleagues at the Columbia-Presbyterian Medical Center, make up the team for the care of these patients and I welcome this opportunity to express my admiration and appreciation to all of them.

Dr. Walter Berdon contributed many, many hours to the selection and interpretation of the radiographs; most of these were photographed for publication by Michael Carlin; almost all in Chapter 5 were photographed by Edward R. Hajjar. Drs. H. Joachim Wigger, Austin D. Johnston, David N. Silvers, Conrad L. Pirani and William A. Blanc provided the pathologic photomicrographs and their interpretation. Many of the clinical photographs were taken by the late Harry Preston and Grace MacMullen and by Bill Kramer. Bob Masini took some of the recent photographs. John W. Karapelou drew all of the wonderful figures.

The first edition manuscript was typed by Loretta Henke, one of the world's leading experts in interpreting poor handwriting.

I would like to thank, in particular, the late Larry Carter for his continuous encouragement, which was badly needed. I am grateful to all of these individuals and to many others for their help and for their friendship.

Pediatric Rheumatology for the Practitioner

Second Edition

1

Clinical Techniques in Pediatric Rheumatology

Taking the History

Therapy begins when the doctor greets the patient at the doorstep and continues as the history is taken. The interview should be a constructive experience for the patient and the family, clearly indicating the physician's compassionate interest in them and in the details of the problem that has brought them. The parents and older child are the physician's allies in working out the problem; it is a joint undertaking. Skillful interviewing with a thorough approach to organization and analysis of detail in the effort to ascertain just what is wrong and what steps are needed to further define or treat the problem convinces the family they are in good hands and encourages cooperation.

The initial consultation visit sets the stage for the future care of the patient. The physician should be unhurried and undisturbed. Extra time spent at the first visit often reduces the number of subsequent visits required and the time necessary for the future care of the patient. During this visit, the doctor has an opportunity to observe the patient and his family and to note their interaction.

When the appointment is scheduled, the receptionist asks about the nature of the problem and what care has already been obtained. If the child is in pain, acutely ill, or missing school, a prompt appointment is arranged. The family is asked to bring along copies of prior evaluations and test reports and any radiographs that have been obtained. To that extent, then, the "chief complaint" is presented at the time the appointment is scheduled.

The history of the child's illness can then begin with a family history. Care is taken to establish the family constellation and any history of prior marriages of the parents. The usual family history of disease is embellished with specific questions about rheumatic disease, including, in addition to arthritis and other rheumatic diseases, low back pain worse on arising, psoriasis, colitis, ileitis, iritis, prostatitis, heel pain, and any symptoms similar to those of

1

Table 1.1. Rheumatologic Disease: Checklist Evaluation Form

	Present on	
	History	*Physical Examination*
Joints		
Pain on motion or tenderness		
Swelling		
Limitation of motion		
Jelling or morning stiffness		
Muscles		
Proximal muscle weakness		
Atrophy		
Skin		
Rash or fingernail abnormalities		
Nodules		
Alopecia		
Scleroderma		
Raynaud's phenomenon		
Edema		
Hyperpigmentation		
Fingertip (toe) ulcers		
Telangiectasia		
Calcinosis		
Gastrointestinal		
Dysphagia		
Reflux (symptoms)		
Bloating		
Abdominal pain		
Diarrhea		
Constipation		
Dry mouth, mouth sores		
Salivary gland enlargement		
Hepatosplenomegaly		

the youngster. In childhood rheumatic disease, the family history often provides significant relevant information. A checklist may help in summarizing and recording the information obtained (Table 1.1).

The social history includes the occupations of the parents and what effect the illness is having on their family life. Occupants of the home are determined, and sleeping arrangements are established. The child's school grades, performance, and attendance are noted, and inquiry is made about any recent change in school. The child's attitude toward the symptoms and any alteration in his life-style caused by or attributed to them is evaluated.

Table 1.1. (*Continued*)

	History	Present on Physical Examination

Ocular
Dry eyes
Blurred vision/uveitis
Conjunctivitis
Blepharitis

Urinary
Dysuria
Genital ulcers

Cardiopulmonary
Pericardial or pleuritic pain
Dyspnea
Orthopnea

Family History
Inflammatory low back pain
Heel pain
Knee problems
Arthritis or other rheumatic disease
Inflammatory bowel disease (colitis/
  ileitis)
Prostatitis/urethritis/cervicitis
Uveitis/iritis/conjunctivitis/blepharitis
Psoriasis

While the routine history of pregnancy, birth, the neonatal period, development, immunizations, allergies, infectious diseases, operations, injuries, and prior illness is elicited, special attention is paid to any unusual illnesses and to all prior hospitalizations.

The history of the present illness begins with the invitation "Tell me why you came to see me" and continues with "Can you remember exactly how it all began?" It is sometimes important to know whether the pain first appeared on arising or during a mathematics examination. The family is encouraged to provide every bit of information; nothing is considered irrelevant. The doctor listens attentively, not without diagnostic hypotheses to be explored but without firmly preconceived diagnostic notions.

The importance of creative analytic listening by a physician who is intrigued and challenged by the problem and uses reason and imagination in his effort to solve it cannot be overestimated. An effort is made not to interrupt, but many opportunities arise where the physician can spontaneously inter-

ject needed questions to obtain additional information and help in organization of the information. If the patient rambles too much, it is helpful to
summarize what has been detailed so far so as to indicate how you are orga-
nizing the material provided.

Special attention is paid to the signs and symptoms of rheumatic disease,
including pain, swelling, limitation of motion, stiffness and gelling after in-
activity, and weakness. Skin rashes, eye manifestations, and genitourinary
and bowel symptoms are specifically inquired about (Table 1.2). Special
inquiry is made about any injury or illness during the months prior to the onset of the present problem, especially diarrheal illness or change in bowel
frequency.

After eliciting all of the details of the patient's current illness and the effect
it is having on each member of the family, the response to whatever therapy
has been provided, the family history, and the history of prior illness, the
physician generally has an excellent grasp of the problem. An optimal

Table 1.2. Skin and Mucous Membrane Signs of Connective Tissue Disease

Rash
   1. Butterfly
   2. Vasculitic
   3. Purpura
   4. Evanescent salmon-pink rash typical of juvenile rheumatoid arthritis (JRA)
   5. Dermatographia
   6. Psoriasis
   7. Dermal edema
   8. Livedo reticularis
   9. Keratoderma blennorrhagicum
  10. Heliotrope of eyelids
  11. Gottron's sign over extensor surfaces of joints
  12. Rheumatoid nodules
  13. Nodular panniculitis
  14. Fingertip ulcers or pitting scars
  15. Telangiectasias
  16. Discoid lesions of skin or ear pinnae

Skin thickening, tightening, contractures, calcinosis
Alopecia and frontal hair fracturing
Mouth and genital ulcers, balanitis of penis, tongue lesions
Dryness of the eyes and mouth
Raynaud's phenomenon
Fingernail abnormalities
Psoriatic pitting
Onycholysis
Ungual telangiectasias

history-taking interview generally provides the diagnostic hypothesis, which is confirmed by the physical examination and laboratory studies.

The importance of the history and submitted primary source data in diagnosis depends on the clinical situation. If physical features visible from a distance provide an obvious diagnosis, the history is taken as an aid to the care of the patient rather than for its diagnostic potency. However, a large number of patients who are brought to the pediatric rheumatologist have mysterious symptoms that have not led to a diagnosis on visits to other physicians. These patients have usually been subjected to repeated physical examinations and laboratory studies; it is unlikely that an additional physical examination or laboratory studies will provide the diagnosis. In these cases, the history often provides the diagnosis through a process called pattern recognition. This is a somewhat intuitive recognition of the pattern of illness, analogous to recognizing the species of birds in flight. Pattern recognition is an important diagnostic skill in rheumatology.

The history-taking interview provides the physician with more than just an answer to the question: "What is wrong with this patient?" It sets the stage for special emphasis on the physical examination and for laboratory and radiographic studies that may be required. In addition, during this interview, one can get an idea of what goals are appropriate for the patient; what joint is affected is not as important as how the child and the family are functioning with the problem. In rheumatologic disease, maintenance of function is an important goal, and the interview provides clues as to the strategy that may be adopted by the physician to best achieve that goal.

The interested reader is referred to: Smith RC, Hoppe RB. The patient's story: Integrating patient- and physician-centered approaches to interviewing. Ann Intern Med 115:470–477, 1991 and: Cohen-Cole SA. The medical interview: The three-function approach. Mosby Year Book, St. Louis, 1991.

Physical Examination

Rheumatologic diagnosis requires a thorough general physical examination with additional emphasis on the skin and musculoskeletal systems (see Table 1.1). Special attention is paid to the general appearance of the patient, emotional responses, nutrition, and an incremental graph of height and weight. In addition to evaluating any evident rashes, the skin is examined for dermatographia, livedo reticularis, nodules, edema, changes in dermal thickness, tightening, contractures, pigmentation, ungual or dermal telangiectasias, nail changes, and alopecia or frontal hair fracturing (Table 1.2). Raynaud's phenomenon may be elicited and fingertip circulation, ulceration, or pitted scars are noted. Ulceration is also sought in the mucous membranes of the mouth or genital region, and the eyes and mouth are examined for unusual dryness. Muscle strength is ascertained by having the child climb up

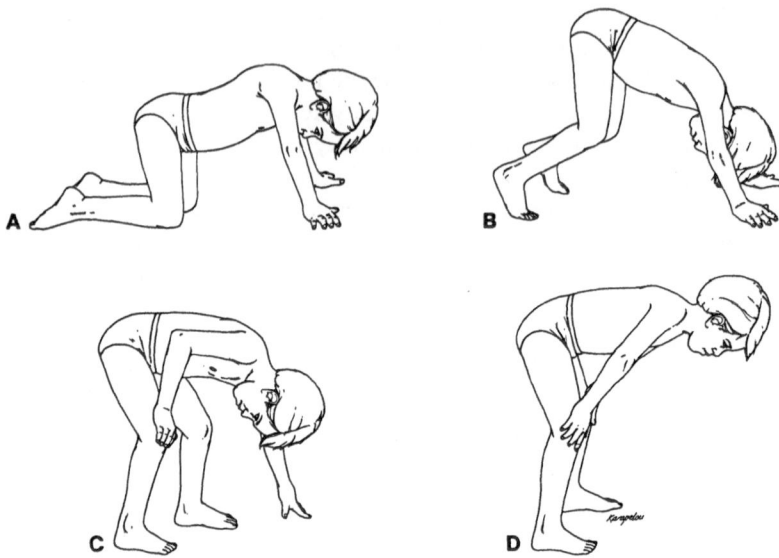

Figure 1.1. Test of muscle strength to elicit Gowers' sign. Child is placed supine on the floor and directed to rise. He is unable to rise without first rolling over to the prone position and then gradually pushing himself up, first onto his knees (**A**), then walking along the floor with his hands (**B**), then gradually using first one knee (**C**) and ultimately both knees (**D**) as aids to hold on to while he pushes himself erect. While initially described as a classic sign of children with muscular dystrophy, this sign is very useful in evaluating truncal weakness in general and is of special value in rheumatology in children with dermatomyositis or with steroid myopathy.

on to the table and rise from a supine position and by testing the resistance capacity of individual muscle groups (Fig. 1.1). Loss of muscle strength may be graded in accordance with the commonly used system depicted in Table 1.3. Testing of muscle strength only takes a minute.

Physical Examination of the Joints

Examination of the joints is of particular importance in the diagnosis and management of patients with rheumatic disease. There can be no substitute for experience in examining the joints. The pediatrician has relatively little opportunity to perform such examinations with expert guidance. As a result of a heavy caseload, limited anatomic expertise, the multiplicity of joints with differing standards of normalcy, and a minimum of supervised experience during residency training, the pediatrician is unlikely to ever become an expert in joint pathology and examination.

The purpose in including a discussion of physical examination of the joints in this book is not to try to make experts of pediatricians. I do hope that after

Table 1.3. Muscle-Strength Grading Chart

Muscle Gradations	Description
5—normal	Complete range of motion against gravity with full resistance
4—good	Complete range of motion against gravity with some resistance
3—fair	Complete range of motion against gravity
2—poor	Complete range of motion with gravity eliminated
1—trace	Evidence of slight contractility. No joint motion
0—zero	No evidence of contractility

reading this oversimplified discussion the pediatrician will feel more comfortable about beginning to examine joints. The best way to start is with oneself, studying the normal appearance and range of motion of each joint when one is at leisure. Then, while examining normal children, when the office schedule is not too hectic, just for fun, begin to examine the joints, testing their range of motion. In this fashion, the reader can expect to develop sufficient expertise in joint examination to distinguish normal from abnormal and, to a certain extent, to quantify any functional loss.

If after doing these exercises the pediatrician wishes to further improve his examining skills, he may enjoy reading two outstanding books devoted entirely to this subject: (1) Howard F. Polley and Gene G. Hunder, *Rheumatologic Interviewing and Physical Examination of the Joints*, 2nd ed. Saunders, Philadelphia, 1978, and (2) Stanley Hoppenfeld, *Physical Examination of the Spine and Extremities*. Appleton-Century-Crofts, New York, 1976.

Inspection, Palpation, Range of Motion, and Strength

Examination of the joints consists of inspection, palpation, and determining the range of motion possible in the joint (Table 1.4). The examination begins with inspection, observing symmetry, loss of normal contour and landmarks, distension and fullness, erythema, atrophy, angulation, and deformity.

The joint and periarticular areas are then palpated, noting pain, tenderness, warmth, and swelling. Effusions are generally easily felt and may be ballotted. Synovial hypertrophy often extends outside and around the joint and has a doughy (boggy) feel accounting for periarticular thickening and loss of normal landmarks. Bursae and synovial outpocketings are commonly swollen with fluid in arthritic children and generally have well-defined margins. Fluid in the joint may be ballotted, whereas synovial thickening and induration are palpable but do not feel like fluid. In the chronically inflamed joint, one often feels both boggy thickening of the synovium and fluid.

Bony palpation may be performed with the joint in several positions. If bony tenderness is present, it is often possible to distinguish the point tenderness of metaphyseal infection from the more generalized but exquisite tender-

Table 1.4. Examination of the Joints

Inspection
Gait
Loss of normal contour and landmarks
Distension and fullness
Angulation and deformity

Palpation
Pain, tenderness, warmth
Effusion and distension
Induration—"boggy" swelling
Nodules

Movement
Range of motion
Stability

Strength
Muscle-strength grading

ness of periostitis, sometimes which is so severe that fine touch of the skin is painful. Inconsistent findings are characteristic of hysterics, who sometimes also complain of pain on light touch.

The range of motion is then determined. Normal range of motion for most important joints is described in Table 1.5. Flexion contractures are the hall-

Table 1.5. Range of Motion of Various Joints

	Flexion	*Extension*	*Internal Rotation*	*External Rotation*	*Abduction*	*Adduction*
Hip	120°	30°	35°	45°	45–50°	20–30°
Knee	135°	2–10°	10°	10°	0	0
Ankle	50°	20°	5° inversion	5° eversion	10° forefoot	20°
First MTP	45°	70–90°				
Wrist	80°	70°			20° radial deviation	30° ulnar deviation
Elbow	135°	0–5°	90° supination	90° pronation		
Shoulder	90°	45°	55°	40–45°	180°	45°
MCPs	90°	30–45°			20°	0°
Thumb	70° palmar	0				
Neck	45°	50°	80° right	80° left	40° lateral bend	40° lateral bend

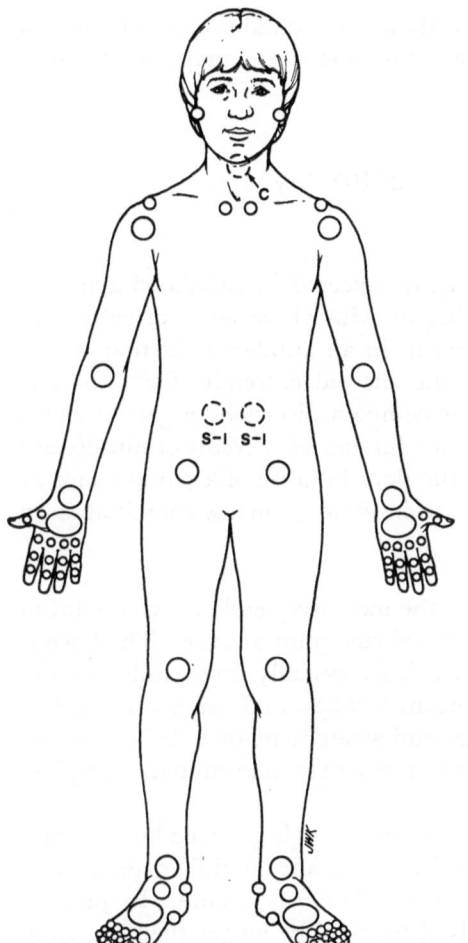

Figure 1.2. Joint mannequin used for charting. Marked circle indicates affected joint or enthesis.

mark of childhood arthritis. Motion is tested in all the planes of motion possible for a given joint. Stability and strength can be evaluated at the same time. A joint chart or mannequin is helpful for notation of degrees of lost motion if many joints are affected (Fig. 1.2). If active range of motion is limited, passive range of motion can be determined and expressed as the number of degrees of motion lost from normal. Normal can be established by testing one's own joint. Muscle strength can be graded in accordance with a standard grading system (Table 1.3).

It is extremely important to do a general examination of all joints and not limit oneself solely to the area of complaint. It is common in examining arthritic children to discover significantly reduced range of motion, especially in the wrists, elbows, and hips, even though the child has no complaints referrable to those areas. Testing range of motion in the major joints takes less then 1 min of examining time.

Physical Examination of the Lower Extremity and Lumbar Spine

Lower-extremity joints are most frequently affected in childhood arthritis. Examination of the lower extremity begins with observation of gait. Pain anywhere in the low extremity may result in an antalgic gait; that is, the child, when walking, puts weight on the affected extremity for a shorter-than-normal time to avoid pain. Other common disorders of gait in childhood arthritis include lateral or posterior lurches as a result of hip disease and avoidance of placing the heel on the floor because of a painful spur or Achilles tendon. With increasing disease in many joints, a combination of abnormalities may occur.

Examination of the Knee. The knee is the most frequently affected joint in childhood arthritis and is often the only affected joint at onset. The knee is also the most frequently injured joint, being especially susceptible because of its unprotected exposure and important location and the great stress to which it is subjected. The knee bends and straightens over 100 times per minute during walking and is subjected to greater stress in running, jumping, and twisting.

Patients with affected knees often stand with a slightly flexed knee. Weakness of the quadriceps muscle and inability of the knee to fully extend result in an unstable knee at the time the heel strikes the ground. In juvenile rheumatoid arthritis (JRA), the involved leg may be longer than the uninvolved or less involved as a result of accelerated maturation and growth from hyperemia of the epiphysis. This may result in an increased flexion contracture or valgus of the more involved knee to compensate for the extra length when walking. This may be combated by a heel lift on the uninvolved (opposite) shoe. Excessive valgus angulation of the knee may also result from disease at the hip that, by causing limitation of external rotation, requires valgus positioning of the knee for balance.

Swelling of the knee may be either localized, a result of fluid in one of the bursae about the knee [prepatellar, suprapatellar, infrapatellar, pes anserine, or gastrocnemius-semimembranous (Baker's cyst)], or may be generalized due to fluid in the joint itself or a combination of fluid in the joint and inflammation in the bursae and soft tissues around the joint.

The suprapatellar bursa usually communicates with the articular synovial space and is generally thought of as a pouch of the knee rather than a bursa. However, in childhood arthritis, a ball-valve mechanism sometimes seems to result in more fluid in the pouch than in the knee itself. An analogous swelling occurs in some cases of "Baker's cyst," where the cyst communicates directly with the joint, really representing an outpocketing of synovial membrane that creates a synovial pouch behind the knee. Examination of the knee generally begins with palpation of these bursae and outpocketings and then proceeds to palpation of the synovial membrane. The suprapatellar pouch first is compressed, and the joint may then be lightly palpated with the thumb and forefinger of the other hand for fluid and for synovial thickening. It is often difficult to distinguish fluid from synovial thickening, and both are often present simultaneously. When there is sufficient fluid, the patella is ballottable (i.e., rebounds after being pushed down as a result of fluid being first pushed to the side and then flowing back under the patella).

The patella must be separately evaluated when examining the knee. It plays an important role in knee function. If infected, it may be the primary cause of a knee effusion. Prepatellar bursitis and patella osteomyelitis can usually be distinguished from pathology in this joint by careful palpation. Chondromalacia (roughening of the undersurface of the patella) is common in athletic teenagers. If the undersurface of the patella grates when the knee is flexed and extended or when the patella is pushed against the femur, chondromalacia may be present. The undersurface of the edges of the patella may be palpated by pushing the patella to first one and then the other side and feeling under the edges.

Range of motion of the knee is then tested (Fig. 1.3). The knee may normally be flexed so the heel touches the buttock in a child and may be extended a little beyond neutral. There is also about 10° of internal or external rotation possible with the femur held in a fixed position. Special examinations for torn ligaments are beyond the scope of this discussion and are best performed by orthopedic surgeons.

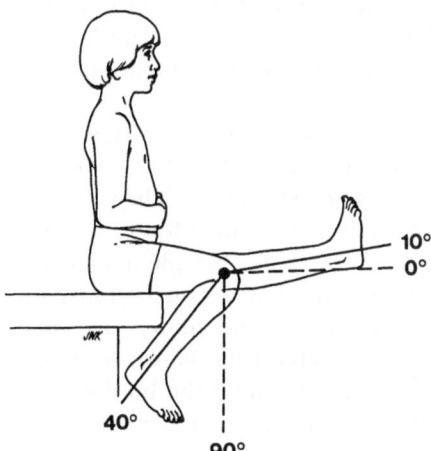

Figure 1.3. The knee should be able to hyperextend about 10° and to flex 40°.

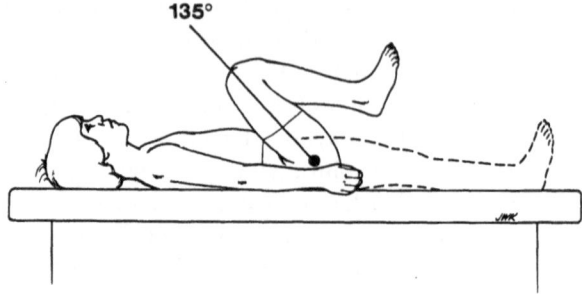

Figure 1.4. Children usually can flex their hips so as to draw their knees right up to the chest, or at least 135°.

Examination of the Hip. The lumbar spine normally curves anteriorly (lumbar lordosis): Flexion deformities of the hip result in increased lumbar lordosis as a substitute for hip extension. As a result, increased lumbar lordosis with exaggerated protrusion of the buttocks may be the first sign of unrecognized arthritis in the hips (see Figs. 3.6 and 9.5).

Bony palpation about the hip includes discriminating the iliac crest, iliac tubercle, pubic tubercles, greater trochanter, ischial tuberosity, posterior iliac spine, vertebral spinous processes, and the sacroiliac joint. Soft-tissue palpation includes flexor, extensor, adductor, and abductor muscle groups.

The most important part of the examination of the hip for the pediatrician is evaluation of the range of motion (Fig. 1.4). Pediatricians are generally experienced in this area from examination of the newborn for hip dysplasia. The child should be able to abduct the hip at least 45° and to bring it across the midline (adduct) 20° with the knee bent (Fig. 1.5). Most children can flex their hips to their chests (at least 135°) and extend the hip at least 30° (Fig. 1.6). With the child supine on the table, the leg should be able to be externally rotated at the hip by 45° and internally rotated 35°. Muscle strength of hip flexors, extensors, abductors, and adductors is tested at the same time.

Examination of the Lumbar Spine. Paravertebral muscle spasm results in awkward or unnatural movements during undressing and bending. Paravertebral muscles in spasm and a pelvic tilt may be grossly visible. The vertebral bodies should be palpated. Pain from diskitis or tumors invading the spinal cord may be referred to the hip, thigh, or even the knee. Simple maneuvers such as deep-knee bends and touching the toes provide an opportunity for the examiner to observe evidence of abnormality in the spine, hips, and knees. Normally, the child can touch his toes, extend his back 30° at the lumbar area, move it laterally 50° to each side, and rotate the lumbar area 30° to each side (Fig. 1.7). When paravertebral muscle spasm is present, the

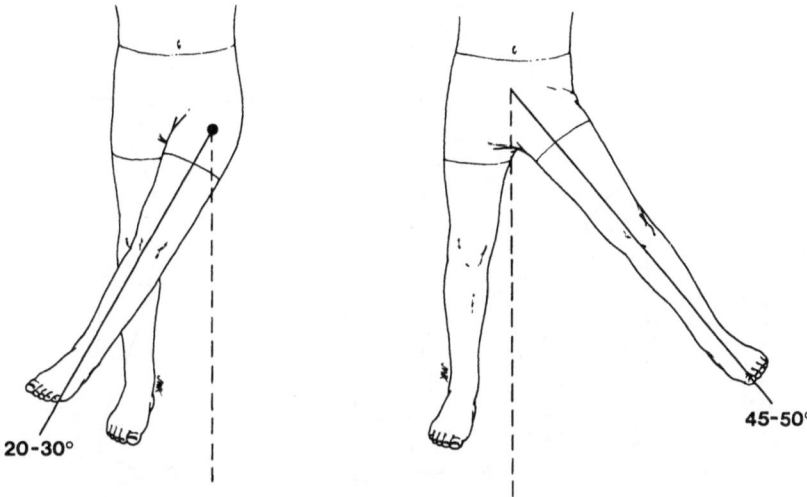

Figure 1.5. Each leg should be able to be abducted laterally from the midline about 45° and adducted across the opposite leg at least 20°.

patient may bend solely at the hips, maintaining lumbar lordosis instead of the smooth curve that is normally seen on bending forward (Fig. 1.7A).

The sacroiliac joint is the articulation of the bony pelvis with the sacrum and transmits the weight from the entire upper body to the pelvis and lower extremities. Some motion exists in these joints in children and young adults. Palpation of the sacroiliac joint is important since it is sometimes tender in childhood spondyloarthritis. Septic sacroiliitis also occurs in childhood; the exquisite tenderness of osteomyelitis about the sacroiliac joint is easily differentiated from the more subtle pain of spondyloarthritis. Pain in the sacroiliac joint can also be elicited by pressing the pelvis from both sides toward

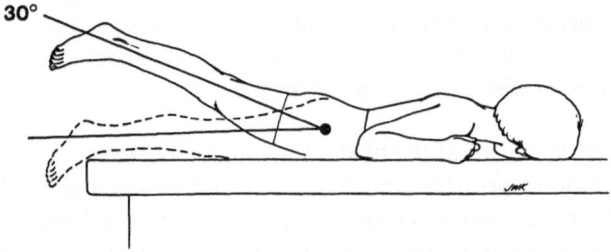

Figure 1.6. With the knee bent and the child in the prone position, the hip should be able to extend about 30°.

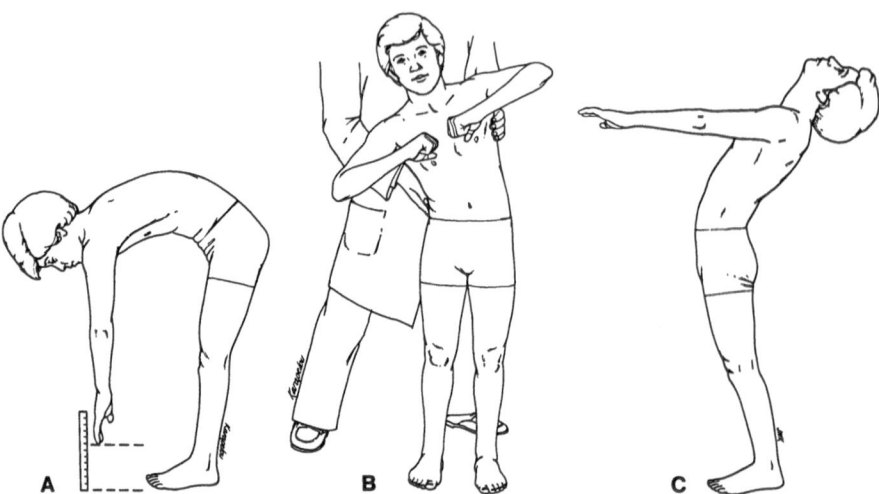

Figure 1.7. Most children can bend to touch their toes without bending their knees. (**A**) The measurement of flexion of the lumbar spine is most important in children with spondyloarthritis and has been undervalued as part of the pediatric physical examination. The fingertip-to-floor distance should be measured and recorded in children who cannot perform this maneuver. This measurement is useful for evaluating progression or remission of disease, and may be used as a measure of drug efficacy. More elaborate tests are standardized for adults and may be useful in teenagers (see Merritt, JL et al.: "Measurement of Trunk Flexibility in Normal Subjects: Reproducibility of Three Clinical Methods. *Mayo Clin Proc* 61:192–197, 1986). (**B**) Lateral bending of the lumbar spine should be equal on both sides; gross abnormalities or pain should be noted. (**C**) Extension of the lumbar spine is usually normal in children with spondyloarthritis but may be painful in those with spondylolisthesis.

the midline (pelvic work test) or by hanging the leg of the supinely placed patient off the examining table while he holds the opposite leg fully flexed against his chest (Gaenslen's sign). Raising the straight leg with the patient supine may produce pain in the back and all along the course of the sciatic nerve if there is disk or sciatic nerve disease. If the leg is lowered to where pain disappears and the foot is then dorsiflexed, reproducing the sciatic pain, this confirms disease along the course of the sciatic nerve. Pain in the opposite leg with the straight-leg-raising test indicates a space-occupying lesion such as a herniated disk in the lumbar region.

Examination of the Foot and Ankle. The ankle and foot are commonly involved in childhood arthritis and have received increasing attention since spondyloarthritis has been recognized in children. Swelling of the ankle joints or of joints in the foot may be visible to inspection, and synovial pouches (outpocketings) may be seen. Palpation may reveal bony tenderness in the calcaneus, especially near the sites of insertion of the Achilles tendon or the plantar fascia. Pain and crepitus on motion of the first metatarsal

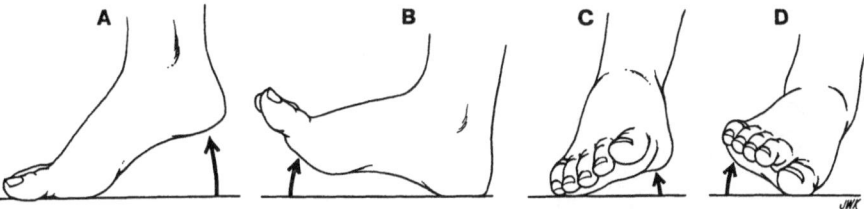

Figure 1.8. The range of motion of the ankle can be evaluated quickly by having the youngster (**A**) push up on his toes to test plantar flexion (50°); (**B**) raise his toes off the ground to test dorsiflexion (20°); (**C**) invert the foot (5°); and (**D**) evert the foot (5°). The forefoot should also be able to be abducted 10° and adducted 20° by the examiner.

should be especially evaluated, as this joint is selectively affected in spondyloarthritis and, on occasion, is the only affected joint at the time of presentation of childhood spondyloarthritis. The Achilles tendon may also be tender and thickened in spondyloarthritis, and the retrocalcaneal bursa, palpated under the Achilles tendon, may also become inflamed. Spurs may form at the inflamed attachments (entheses) of the Achilles tendon and plantar fascia to the calcaneus.

The heel is the ideal place to become familiar with the concept of an enthesopathy, long neglected in rheumatology and especially neglected in children. Inflammation at the enthesis is the hallmark of the spondyloarthropathies. Periosteal pain, bone pain from erosions, and pain in the tendons and fascia can all be demonstrated at the insertions of the Achilles tendon and the plantar fascia into the calcaneus. These signs are rare in childhood arthritis other than in spondyloarthropathy (see Chapter 4).

The range of motion of the ankle involves dorsiflexion (20°) and plantar flexion (50°) at the ankle mortise (articulation of the tibia and fibula with the talus), and inversion (5°) and eversion (5°) at the subtalar joint (Fig. 1.8). Forefoot abduction (10°) and adduction (20°) take place at the midtarsal (talonavicular and calcaneocuboid) joints. The first metatarsal joint normally flexes 45° and extends 70–90° (Fig. 1.9); normal toe-off for proper walking requires a minimum of 35° extension. Pain in the first metatarsophalangeal (MTP) joint results in abnormal gait and may result in additional pain as a result of abnormal pressure being applied to other toes. Unlike the other toes, there is normally no extension at the proximal interphalangeal (PIP) joint of the great toe.

Examination of the Upper Extremity

Examination of the Wrist and Hand. The wrist is the most frequently affected upper-extremity joint in childhood arthritis and may have considerable hidden deformity. This is because the wrist is normally positioned in

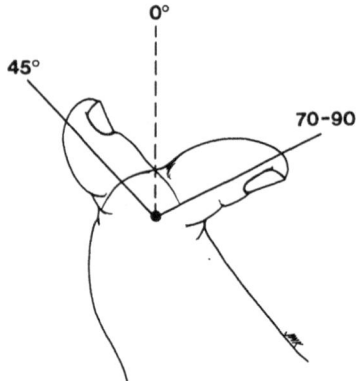

Figure 1.9. Motion at the first metatarsophalangeal joint is an important part of the examination, since this joint is frequently affected in childhood spondylorathritis and sometimes is the sole affected joint at the time the patient is first seen. The joint should be able to flex 45° and extend at least 70°.

only mild extension, so in a child considerable loss of extension is possible without attracting the attention of surrounding adults. Children do not realize that they are losing strength in the wrist as, a result of the inability to extend. Even synovial outpocketings at the wrists are commonly ignored or referred to as "ganglions." When the examiner presumes a swelling to be a ganglion, it is incumbent upon him to demonstrate a normal range of motion; synovial outpocketings associated with loss of motion are characteristic and diagnostic of arthritis. In addition to 70° extension, the wrist normally can flex 80° and can deviate 20° to the radial side and 30° to the ulnar side (Fig. 1.10).

Range of motion at the metacarpophalangeal joints includes 30° of extension and 90° of flexion. Proximal interphalangeal joints normally flex 100°,

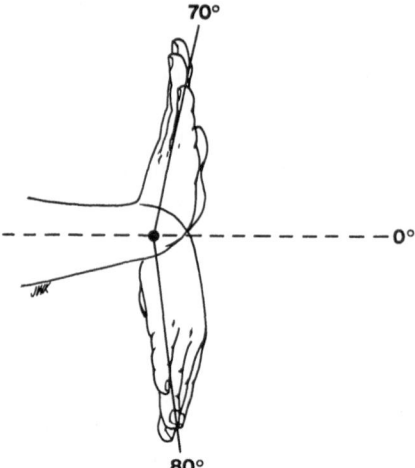

Figure 1.10. In polyarticular JRA, the wrist is frequently affected, and a flexion contracture at the wrist is common in polyarticular disease. This is an area for major physiotherapy effort, as wrists that have no extension have great weakness. Measurement of the number of degrees of wrist extension lost is performed at each examination and recorded. Limitation of full flexion occurs only in severe disease.

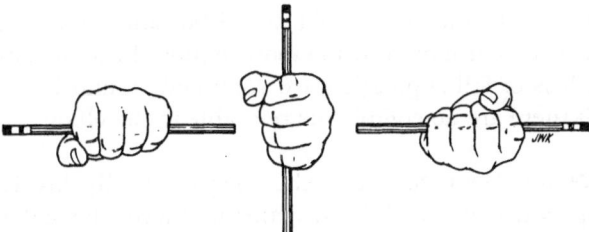

Figure 1.11. The elbow is frequently affected in all forms of childhood arthritis and is the commonest upper-extremity joint affected in spondyloarthritis. In cases of what appears to be monoarticular arthritis, evidence of JRA rather than infection, trauma, a foreign body, or orthopedic pathology can often be obtained by examining the "asymptomatic" elbow. The most common limitation in childhood arthritis is a loss of full supination. Tests of pronation and supination are performed with the elbow flexed at 90° and held against the body; a pencil is held in the hand to evaluate the position. Any loss of supination is noted.

and distal interphalangeal joints extend 10° and flex 90°. The thumb can flex to touch the tips of each finger and the pad at the base of the fifth finger and can abduct away from the index finger by 50°.

Examination of the Elbow. Swelling may be apparent on inspection, especially if unilateral so one elbow can be compared to the other. The localized swelling of olecranon bursitis is easily distinguished from diffuse swelling of the elbow. Warmth and tenderness are evaluated and rheumatoid nodules are felt for at the extensor surface where, if present at all, they are most commonly found. The elbow supinates and pronates 90° (Fig. 1.11), extends to a straight position, and flexes 135° (Fig. 1.12). The test for supination and

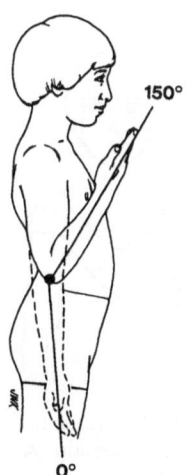

150°

0°

Figure 1.12. As elbow disease progresses in arthritic children, they lose full extension; the elbow should be able to bend from 0 to 150° (i.e., to be fully extended). Any limitation of extension should be recorded.

pronation is done with the elbow held flexed 90° and against the chest to avoid confusing shoulder motion with elbow motion. Flexion contractures at the elbow and loss of full supination are commonly found in children with arthritis even if there are no complaints referable to the elbow.

Examination of the Shoulder. The shoulder is usually involved only in rather severe polyarticular childhood arthritis. Sternoclavicular and acromioclavicular joints may be affected in addition to the glenohumeral (shoulder) joint. Synovial outpocketings and cystic swellings are sometimes seen in severely affected youngsters. Range of active motion may be conveniently tested by having the child perform three maneuvers: (1) place his hand on the opposite shoulder, (2) place his hand behind his head on the opposite shoulder, and (3) place the back of his hand behind his back so his fingers touch the opposite acromium (Fig. 1.13). These maneuvers require 180° of abduction and 45° of adduction, 90° of flexion and 45° of extension, and 55° of internal rotation and 40° of external rotation, and test motion at the glenohumeral and scapulothoracic articulations and motions requiring a combination of both. Movement at the sternoclavicular and acromioclavicular joints also takes place during shoulder motion.

Examination of the Temporomandibular Joint (TMJ)

The TMJ opens and closes between 1500 and 2000 times daily and is frequently affected in polyarticular childhood arthritis. The joint may be palpated with the mouth closed and during opening and closing. Pain and crepitus may be apparent. The mouth span and any hypoplasia of the chin can be noted at the same time.

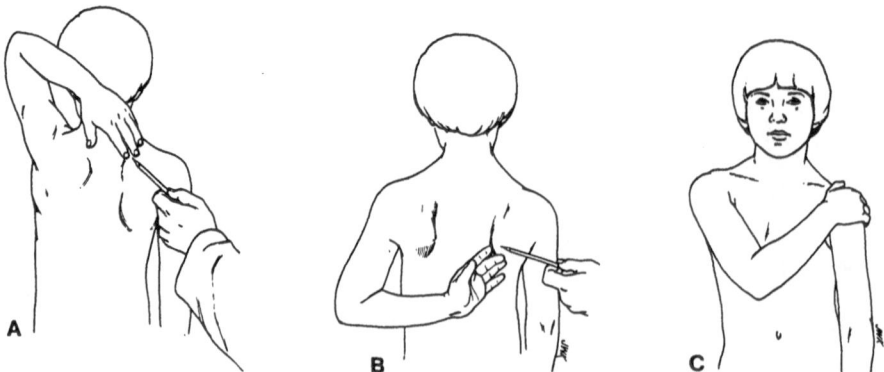

Figure 1.13. Shoulder limitation is not common in JRA but, when present, often goes unnoticed. The Apley scratch test is an easy way to evaluate shoulder motion, testing (**A**) external rotation and abduction and (**B** and **C**) internal rotation and adduction.

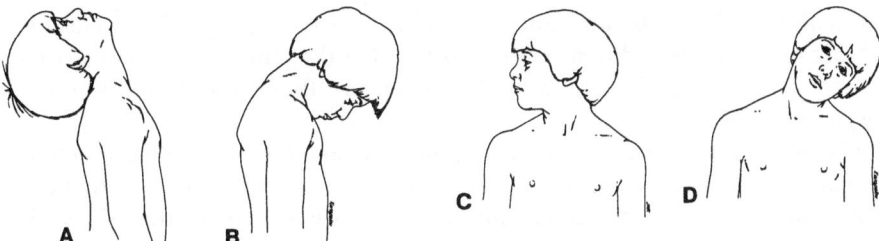

Figure 1.14. (**A**) Neck extension, (**B**) flexion, (**C**) rotation, and (**D**) lateral bending are evaluated. Limitations of extension and of lateral bending and rotation are common in polyarticular JRA and in ankylosing spondylitis.

Examination of the Cervical Spine

Pediatricians are accustomed to examining the neck for meningeal signs and are aware that the neck should be able to flex so that the chin touches the chest and that it can extend so that the head can touch the back (Fig. 1.14A and B). In the examination for arthritis, it can be noted that the neck rotates to either side so that the chin is in line with the shoulder and that the neck can bend laterally 45° toward each shoulder (Fig. 1.14C and D).

Posture

The child should be observed in the lateral position for any forward tilting of the head which, with flattening of the anterior chest wall, thoracic kyphosis, and loss of lumbar lordosis, is characteristic of the posture of ankylosing spondylitis. These patients also frequently have hip disease and stand with flexed hips. Chest expansion may be limited. Although standards do not exist for children, chest expansion can be evaluated and measured with a tape in teenagers and compared at repeated visits. The measurement is performed at the nipple line after instructing the patient to breathe out fully and then take a maximum breath.

Evaluation of the Functional State of the Patient

Once the history is taken and the physical examination has been performed, the physician can make a determination about the functional state of the patient. Is the youngster functioning normally despite the disease? If not, is the loss of function proportional to visible disability? How does this child function in comparison to other children with the same evidences of physical disease?

When organic disease is obvious, such an evaluation leads to setting up reasonable goals of therapy and helps the physician judge the needs for specific medications and treatments and whether the child or family is so distressed that psychiatric help is needed to restore them to optimal function despite the illness.

The physician must guard against his natural concern only with *disease* and his tendency to reject patients who are *ill* but do not have disease. The nonfunctioning child is ill; if one cannot find a disease to explain this illness, it does not mean there is nothing wrong or that the child does not require treatment for his illness. Physicians have the responsibility to heal the sick, whether they have a disease or not.

Some children who are ill with musculoskeletal complaints have no evidence of organic disease on physical examination or on laboratory study. Their limited function is clearly out of proportion to the limitations imposed even by severe dermatomyositis, scleroderma, lupus, or rheumatoid arthritis. A physician accustomed to caring for chronically sick children who are attending school each day and enjoying reasonable life-styles may find himself confronted with a home-bound child who has no certain abnormalities on physical examination or in the laboratory. These children then have disability far in excess of any visible signs of disease. That should be dealt with promptly at the first visit (see Chapter 2, under Psychiatric Disorders). The problem of children out of school for months or in bed with withdrawal and depression is accentuated by the physician who has to be certain there is *no* physical illness present *at all* before he decides to deal with disability or sends the patient somewhere where the disability can be dealt with. This error is avoided by making separate judgments about the course of action to be followed to continue to explore the possibility of physical illness and the course of action to be taken to get the patient back in the mainstream whether or not he has any physical illness. Since both of these courses of action should be pursued simultaneously, it is just after the physical examination is completed that the physician must "bite the bullet" on this issue.

While this problem exists in rheumatology with patients of any age, the problem of recognizing disability out of proportion to visible evidences of disease is accentuated in youth since others are not dependent on the "sick" individual for support. Physicians forget that a youngster not attending school daily is the equivalent of an adult not going to work. Families often state that nonfunction is the result of physician instruction not to function; this usually means some physician has "read the child's mind" or the parent's and prescribed what was sought as the prescription. Nonfunction is accepted at face value and dealt with directly; if the youngster can return to school the next day and live a normal life, then no psychiatric help may be necessary. If there is obviously no chance of the child returning to a life-style appropriate for visible and comprehensible disability, then the synthesis of that problem should be achieved at the time of this first visit and appropriate action taken to find the help needed to get the child functioning again.

Laboratory Procedures

Synovial Fluid Analysis

Examination of the joint fluid is essential when monarticular arthritis suggests the possibility of infection. Arthrocentesis should generally be performed by the orthopedic surgeon, who has the most experience in that procedure. The fluid will be examined for volume, viscosity, color, clarity, a cell count, protein, and sugar; a smear is made for staining, and fluid is planted for culture in all appropriate media. The mucin clot test has not been found useful in pediatrics, and since gout is not seen in children, tests for uric acid crystals are not usually necessary. Tests for complement, immune complexes, antinuclear factors, and rheumatoid factors are hard to interpret and are considered research procedures.

The primary purpose of arthrocentesis is to exclude septic infection. While any generalization about white cell counts in septic joint fluid is subject to exception, fluid with a white blood count over 100,000/mm^3 (mostly polymorphonuclears) is usually septic and should be considered so until proved otherwise. Lower synovial fluid cell counts do not exclude the possibility of sepsis. Septic fluid usually has a very high protein and a sugar more than 25% below simultaneously obtained blood sugar. The specimen obtained for cell count should be obtained in a heparinized syringe so it will not clot. No procaine-containing preservative that may sterilize the culture artificially should be injected into the joint or area to be aspirated until after the specimen for culture is obtained.

Sterile joint fluid does not assure the physician that the patient does not have osteomyelitis in bone where the infected metaphysis is outside of the joint, such as at the knee (Fig. 2.11). Septic infection may be proved by examination of joint fluid but is never excluded on the basis of sterile joint fluid.

Laboratory Evaluation for Rheumatic Disease

Laboratory tests are not helpful in establishing the diagnosis of JRA (see Chapter 3), but they are helpful in excluding or providing evidence of dermatomyositis, systemic lupus erythematosus (SLE), or other disorders that may be confused with rheumatic disease (see Chapter 2). In childhood arthritis, laboratory studies may help in determining the subset of the patient, i.e., is the patient rheumatoid factor or ANA positive, does he carry HLA-B27, DR4, or DR5, and is she hypogammaglobulinemic?

Reasonable laboratory studies to be performed in patients being evaluated for rheumatic disease are listed in Table 1.6. The significance of the laboratory studies is discussed in the sections on the individual diseases. The

Table 1.6. Laboratory and Radiographic Studies in Pediatric Rheumatology

CBC with differential count
ESR
Rheumatoid factor
Antinuclear factor
SMAC (20 chemistries including CPK)
Urinalysis
Quantitative immunoglobulins G, M, A*
Lyme antibodies
Antistreptococcal antibodies[†]
Tuberculin skin test**

For SLE
Coombs' test
Platelet count and reticulocyte count
Serologic test for syphilis
Total hemolytic complement and complement components*
Farr test (DNA binding)
Coagulation profile, anticoagulant antibody, anticardiolipin
Anti-Sm, RNP, Ro, La
24-h urine creatinine and protein with computation of creatinine clearance
Chest x-ray

For Dermatomyositis
Electromyogram
ENA with Sm and RNP
Toxoplasmosis FA test
Chest x-ray
Muscle biopsy[†]
T-3, T-4

For Pauciarticular and Polyarticular JRA
HLA-B27*
T-3, T-4[†]
Slit-lamp examination of the eye

laboratory studies ordered must be individualized for a given patient; no schema may be applied to every patient.

Radiographic Techniques in Childhood Rheumatic Disease

Radiographs are not useful in making an early diagnosis of any of the child-hood rheumatic diseases, but they may be helpful in providing clues favoring another diagnosis. Thus, x-rays of a single involved joint should always be obtained. In all cases of unexplained knee pain, films of the hips and lower spine are also obtained. The roles of ultrasonography and MRI studies in

Table 1.6. (*Continued*)

For Kawasaki Disease
EKG, chest x-ray
Two-dimensional echocardiogram
Leptospira agglutinins

For Scleroderma
Esophogram, chest x-ray
ENA with Sm and RNP, antitopoisomerase (Scl 70), anticentromere

For Systemic JRA
Chest x-ray, EKG, echocardiogram, HLA-B27,* urinary catecholamines[†]
Abdominal ultrasound[†]
Slit-lamp examination of the eye
Technetium bone scan[†]
Gallium scan[†]
Bone marrow examination[†]
Small-intestinal series[†]
CT and MRI studies[†]
Ferritin (older patients)

For Systemic Vasculitis
Electromyogram and nerve conduction studies
All tests done for SLE
Hepatitis antigens and antibodies, cryoglobulins
Antineutrophil cytoplamic antibody (ANCA)
Aortogram, vessel MRI[†]
Muscle biopsy, sural nerve biopsy, skin lesion biopsy[†]

* Identifies some populations especially susceptible to rheumatic disease.
** Monarticular arthritis with a positive tuberculin skin test requires synovial biopsy.
[†] In selected cases only.

early disease are not yet well defined. In more advanced disease, radiographs may serve to provide an objective measure of severity; they should be taken infrequently to avoid unnecessary radiation. Radiographs are interesting, but they do not contribute substantially to the management of JRA except in advanced cases.

A chest x-ray is obtained in systemic JRA, SLE, dermatomyositis, and scleroderma; where sarcoidosis is a consideration; when the tuberculin test is positive; or if otherwise clinically required.

Small-bowel and colon x-rays are obtained when inflammatory bowel disease (IBD) is a possibility; colonoscopy with intestinal biopsy is sometimes diagnostic of IBD where other studies are negative. An abdominal ultrasound is obtained if neuroblastoma is a consideration.

Ultrasound is useful in demonstrating hidden pelvic and abdominal abscess, pyomyositis, coronary aneurysms in Kawasaki disease, small amounts of pericardial fluid in systemic JRA, and a cardiac myxoma. Radionucleotide scanning may be helpful in identifying hidden abscess, malignancy, bone infection, or an osteoid osteoma. Computerized axial tomography and magnetic resonance imaging are aids to the exclusion or localization of hidden infection or tumor that might otherwise be mistaken for JRA.

2

The Differential Diagnosis of Arthritis in Childhood

The differential diagnosis of arthritis is exhaustive (see table of contents; Chapter 2). The 1988 edition of the *Primer on the Rheumatic Diseases*,[1] prepared by a committee of the American College of Rheumatology (ACR), lists over 100 disorders in which arthritis may be a significant manifestation. A few of these conditions have not yet been reported in children. We have also found it necessary to add to this exhaustive list. Several additional disorders were recently first seen in children in our own clinic, and there continue to be new additions to this list each year.

As a preliminary diagnostic approach, trouble in and around the joints may be thought of as infectious, inflammatory, traumatic, biochemical, neo-plastic, or degenerative. In the final analysis, the pattern of the patient's symptoms, the findings on the examination, and the results of the appropri-ate laboratory and radiographic determinations usually enable a specific diagnosis. A good deal of clinical sleuthing is frequently necessary. The ability to make the diagnosis may depend on some familiarity with each of the entities discussed in this chapter. It's hard to make a diagnosis you don't think of and consider. For organizational purposes, the classification prop-osed by the ACR has been modified as shown in Table 2.1. As new know-

Table 2.1. Classification of Musculoskeletal Disorders of Childhood

I. Chronic arthritis of unknown origin
II. Chronic connective-tissue syndromes
III. Acute rheumatic and inflammatory conditions
IV. Acute and chronic infections of the bones and joints
V. Traumatic and degenerative disorders
VI. Biochemical disorders: acquired, congenital, and familial
VII. Neoplasms
VIII. Psychiatric disorders

ledge is acquired, categories may change, and items will be changed from one category to another. The disorders listed under the headings Chronic Arthritis of Unknown Origin and Chronic Connective-Tissue Syndromes will be discussed in Chapter 3–8. The differential diagnosis of the other disorders that may be associated with musculoskeletal pain in children is reviewed in this chapter. These are the disorders that must be "excluded" in order to make a diagnosis of juvenile rheumatoid arthritis (JRA) or of spondyloarthritis (see Chapter 3 under Differential Diagnosis).

Acute Rheumatic Conditions

The acute rheumatic conditions (Table 2.2), with the exception of acute rheumatic fever and poststreptococcal reactive arthritis are always characterized by the presence of arthritis and rash. Most of these conditions are not rare, and with the exception of Mucha-Habermann disease, Sweet's syndrome and thrombotic thrombocytopenic purpura every pediatrician can expect to see patients with these disorders from time to time in his practice.

Table 2.2. Clinical Features of Acute Rheumatic Syndromes*

Erythema Nodosum	*Kawasaki Disease*
Nodular panniculitis on extensor surfaces of the legs	Polymorphous rash
	Cervical lymphadenopathy
Arthritis	Conjunctival hyperemia
R/O tuberculosis, streptococcal infection, inflammatory bowel disease, sarcoid, fungi, drug reaction (birth-control pills, propylthiouracil, others)	Cracked lips
	Erythematous palms and soles
	Edema of the dorsum of the palms and soles
Henoch-Schönlein Purpura	*Serum-sickness-like Reactions*
Purpuric rash on lower extremities	Migratory polyarthritis
Abdominal colic	Erythema multiforme
Arthritis	Angioneurotic edema
Mucha-Habermann Disease (acute parapsoriasis)	*Sweet's Syndrome*
Episodic chickenpox-like rash	Rash (painful plaques)
↑ ESR	Arthralgia/arthritis
	↑ ESR
	Also seen after intestinal bypass surgery
Acute Rheumatic Fever	
Migratory polyarthritis	*Thrombotic Thrombocytopenic Purpura*
Acute carditis	Thrombocytopenic purpura
Chorea	Microangiopathic hemolytic anemia
Erythema marginatum	Renal disease; Neurologic signs
Rising antistreptococcal antibody titers	

* In addition to fever.

Acute Rheumatic Fever

Improved socioeconomic conditions, prompt diagnosis, the prevention of recurrent attacks by "prophylactic" penicillin, and adequate treatment of streptococcal sore throat resulted in a greatly lowered incidence of acute rheumatic fever (ARF) from 1970 to 1984.[2] Since 1985 there has been a resurgence of epidemic rheumatic fever in the continental United States.[3-5] Many pediatricians complete training without ever having cared for a child with ARF. As a result, pediatricians often seem surprised, confused, and upset when confronted with a child with ARF. They may resist making the presumptive diagnosis and so do not institute or maintain an appropriate therapeutic regimen. The following Case Report from our own hospital illustrates this problem.

Case Report

This 9-year-old boy presented with a 12-day history of intermittent rash and migratory polyarthritis. Physical examination was normal except for mild tenderness of an ankle. The erythrocyte sedimentation rate was 95 mm/h. A presumptive diagnosis of JRA was made, and he was begun on aspirin, 110 mg/kg/day. The symptoms disappeared promptly. A throat culture was subsequently reported to demonstrate group-A beta-hemolytic streptococci, and treatment with oral penicillin was begun. The antistreptolysin titer rose from 1:340 to 1:680 Todd units. Because of vomiting associated with what was thought to be an intercurrent illness, the salicylate was totally discontinued. Rash and arthritis promptly recurred (Fig. 2.1), and nodules were now noted at the occiput, elbow, and sole of the foot (Fig. 2.2). The physician interpreted the rash as "angioneurotic edema" due to the penicillin. Four days later, the boy was admitted to the hospital in profound congestive heart failure with pulmonary edema. A gallop rhythm was noted, and the heart tones were muffled. A pericardial friction rub and grade III mitral systolic and diastolic murmurs were heard. There was obvious erythema marginatum and a knee effusion. His physicians now realized that he had ARF. Treatment with prednisone and diuretics was successful, and he was dramatically improved within 24 h and was no longer in congestive heart failure within 48 h. Aspirin was then begun, and the steroids were weaned over a 10-day period without adverse effect. Aspirin was inadvertently abruptly discontinued 4 weeks later at the time of hospital discharge. Although erythema marginatum then promptly recurred and persisted for 2 months, fortunately no other signs of rheumatic activity were apparent. A grade II mitral systolic murmur persists. The child continues to receive rheumatic prophylaxis with L-A Bicillin, 1.2 million units IM every 21 days.

As illustrated by this patient, the physician today has little difficulty in making a diagnosis of ARF when obvious valvular carditis follows a known streptococcal sore throat. This is not the usual situation, however. Erythema marginatum, chorea, and rheumatic nodules are also definitive diagnostic

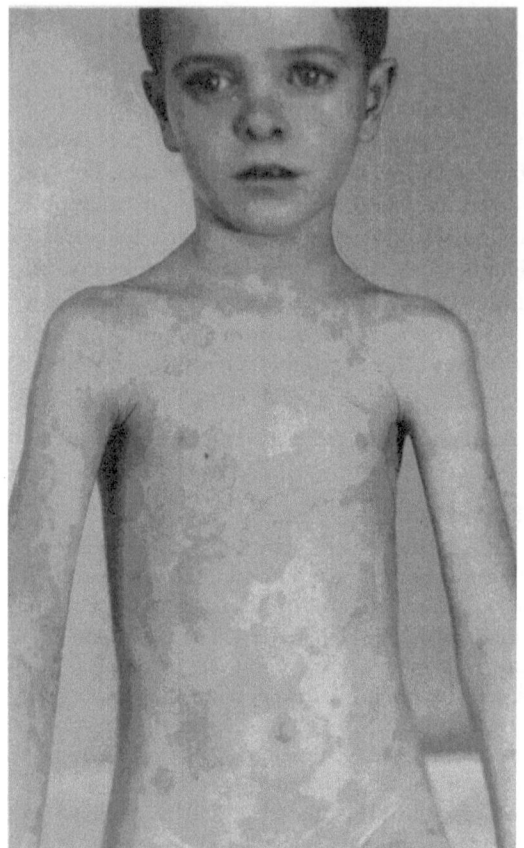

Figure 2.1. Typical erythema marginatum rash in a 9-year-old boy with acute rheumatic fever.

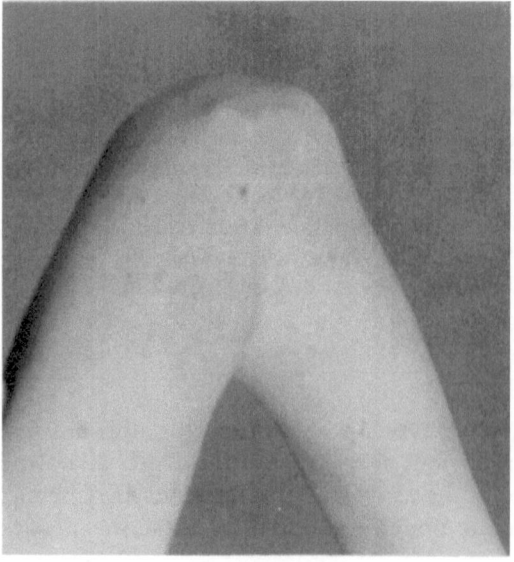

Figure 2.2. Rheumatic nodules were found on many extensor surfaces and on the occiput (same patient as in Fig. 2.1).

Table 2.3. Revised Jones Criteria for Guidance in the Diagnosis of Rheumatic Fever

Major	*Minor*
Carditis	Fever
New or changing murmurs	Arthralgia
Cardiomegaly, congestive heart failure	History of prior attack of rheumatic fever
Pericarditis	Elevated ESR, CRP
Migratory polyarthritis	Prolonged P-R interval on ECG
Chorea	Rising titer of antistreptococcal
Erythema margination	antibodies
Subcutaneous nodules	

Diagnosis is likely with two major criteria or one major and two minor.
Diagnosis is doubtful when evidence of recent streptococcal illness cannot be documented
by history of scarlet fever, isolation of Group A streptococcus from throat culture, or rising
titer of antistreptococcal antibodies.

(Modified with permission from "Report of the ad hoc Committee of the American Heart Association Council on Rheumatic Fever and Congenital Heart Disease." *Circulation* 69:204A–208A, 1984. Copyright by the American Heart Association.)

findings, but they are seen so infrequently now that they may not be recognized even when they are present. The more frequent diagnostic problem initially confronting the pediatrician is a youngster with polyarthralgias and an elevated erythrocyte sedimentation rate (ESR) who does not (yet) fulfill the modified Jones diagnostic criteria promulgated by the American Heart Association as a useful guide to the diagnosis of ARF (Table 2.3).

When examining a child with joint pain, it is often helpful to remember that a diagnosis of arthritis does not require swelling. Pain or tenderness *plus limitation of motion* of a joint, even without swelling, constitutes evidence of arthritis. In some joints such as the hips, swelling can almost never be seen on physical examination. The differentiation of arthralgia from arthritis is often solely dependent on demonstrating a range of motion limited by pain. In my experience, many children said to have polyarthralgia can be demonstrated to have arthritis provided *all* of the joints are carefully subjected to range-of-motion examination. Any joint may be affected in ARF, although the most frequently involved are the knees, ankles, elbows, and wrists.

The migratory quality of the arthritis in ARF helps to differentiate ARF from JRA. The joint that was so exquisitely painful yesterday in children with ARF is often painless today, even though some swelling may persist. Yesterday's painful joint is likely to be better today even without any therapy and even though another joint has now become tender and has limited motion. This migratory quality contributes to the dramatic efficacy of aspirin in ARF since aspirin in adequate doses usually prevents new joint involvement. In questionable cases, a day or 2 of observation without any therapy is often helpful in demonstrating the typical migratory quality of the arthritis.

In older children additive rather than migratory arthritis may cause confusion.[6,7]

In some children with polyarthritis, JRA is a more reasonable early diagnostic consideration than it was in the boy described above. In children under age 4, for example, rheumatic fever is very rare, so most very young children with persistent polyarthritis in this age group do turn out to have JRA. This is even more likely if they also have pericarditis without mitral valvulitis. Pericardial effusions are almost never seen as an isolated cardiac manifestation of ARF but are a common feature of early systemic JRA. The typical JRA rash (provided it can be differentiated from the erythema marginatum of ARF) and uveitis in those rare systemic JRA patients who have eye involvement may also be helpful in differential diagnosis. Nodules that appear soon after the onset of polyarthritis, as in this patient, always indicate ARF in our experience. In JRA, nodules are a late manifestation and are seen only in patients in whom the diagnosis of chronic rather than acute disease is obvious.

Children over the age of 4 who have polyarthritis, however, should initially be considered to have ARF; the diagnosis of a more chronic disease should be postponed until evidence of chronicity is apparent or the course and manifestations are inconsistent with ARF. After adequate blood cultures have been obtained, children thought to have ARF are started on aspirin and full doses of penicillin. "Prophylactic" doses are initiated only after completion of a full 10-day course of penicillin aimed at eradicating streptococci from the nasopharynx. Prednisone is reserved for patients whose rheumatic carditis is accompanied by congestive heart failure or pericarditis, as in the child cited above.

The commitment to rheumatic "prophylaxis" can always be changed if it becomes apparent that a presumptive diagnosis of ARF was erroneous. The old idea of being afraid to "label" a patient or treat a patient with a presumptive diagnosis led to unnecessary and harmful long hospitalizations and sometimes resulted in recurrent attacks of rheumatic carditis. Labels may easily be changed as often as necessary.

The arthritis of ARF rarely continues for more than 3 weeks when untreated; the elevated ESR rarely persists for more than 6 weeks. However, in recent years, we have seen patients in whom recrudescences of rheumatic fever were produced by intermittent aspirin treatment or premature or abrupt aspirin withdrawal. These children were then thought, in error, to have JRA. With consistent aspirin treatment (100 mg/kg/day), the arthritis promptly disappeared. In children with ARF, after the ESR has returned to normal, the aspirin should be reduced gradually over a period of a few weeks in order to avoid a rebound of arthritis and/or carditis. Abrupt withdrawal of aspirin in children with subclinical rheumatic carditis may precipitate overwhelming life-threatening pancarditis, as it did in the patient described above.

Rheumatic fever may occur with acute glomerulonephritis in the same patient at the same time.[8] Second attacks of rheumatic fever, now being seen in inner-city immigrant populations in which the initial attack was unrecognized, often have a more fulminant presentation, sometimes with rheumatic pneumonia and/or "galloping" carditis.[9]

Poststreptococcal Reactive Arthritis

Patients who develop prolonged polyarthritis after Group A beta-hemolytic streptococcal infection and who do not fulfill modified Jones criteria for a diagnosis of acute rheumatic fever have been classified as poststreptococcal arthritis.[10] All published series of such patients report a relatively high risk (8%) of subsequent second-attack rheumatic fever with carditis in this population. It was recognized by clinicians a generation ago that rheumatic fever could be occasionally followed by prolonged arthritis or arthralgia.[11] Just as patients with what was once thought to be rheumatic chorea or scarlatinal arthritis[12] bear a significant risk of subsequent rheumatic heart disease, so do those children who have what has been called poststreptococcal reactive arthritis.[7] It is probably best to provide "lifetime" penicillin prophylaxis for such patients to prevent streptococcal sore throats and recurrent attacks of rheumatic fever.

Case Report

A $10\frac{1}{2}$-year-old girl was seen in April 1983 because of 1 week of migratory polyarthritis in one ankle, then the other, and then finger and toe pain. Three years before she had been hospitalized with a 3-month arthritic illness called "poststreptococcal arthralgia." Her twin sister also has had prolonged episodes of arthritis. Physical examination revealed left ankle and tarsal effusions with considerable tenosynovitis; ESR 67, ASO 120, ADB 2720. The patient was treated with aspirin but had persistent elevation of the ESR and arthritis in the ankles and feet for 2 months. Oral penicillin "prophylaxis" was given to prevent streptococcal sore throats. The mother was not faithful in providing penicillin and $1\frac{1}{2}$ years later the girl was readmitted with rheumatic carditis associated with polyarthritis. Despite aspirin therapy (salicylate level 33 mg/dl) arthritis persisted for several months. She was maintained on penicillin prophylaxis but again the mother was not faithful and $1\frac{1}{2}$ years later (age $13\frac{1}{2}$) she was admitted again—this time with life-threatening rheumatic carditis which required treatment with prednisone. With intramuscular bicillin prophylaxis she has remained well ever since without either arthritis or evidence of rheumatic activity, but with permanent mitral insufficiency.

As a result of this experience and the experiences of many others we recommend that so-called poststreptococcal arthritis be considered a variant of acute rheumatic fever and that these children remain on penicillin "forever." There is some evidence that prolonged arthritis is now more commonly a feature of acute rheumatic fever (20%) than it was in the past.[6,7]

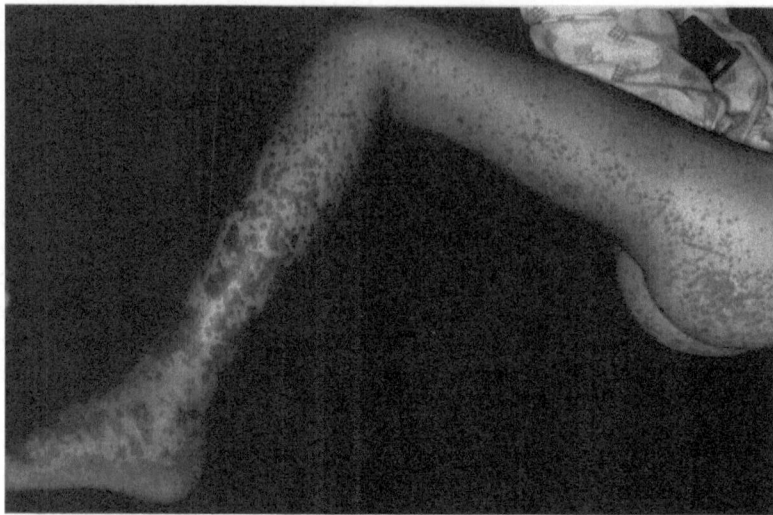

Figure 2.3. Extensive rash of Henoch-Schönlein purpura. The severe edema of the feet extends up to the lower legs.

Henoch-Schönlein Purpura

Arthritis, colicky abdominal pain, and a characteristic lower-extremity and buttock papular (palpable) purpuric rash (Fig. 2.3) constitute the diagnostic triad of Henoch-Schönlein purpura (H-S purpura).[13] Abdominal colic often precedes the rash and arthritis. When H-S purpura is suspected as the cause of colicky abdominal pain in a child who has no other manifestations, a slap on the buttocks sometimes resolves the diagnostic dilemma by eliciting the purpura. Young children, especially boys, are most frequently affected.

H-S purpura seems to be a small-vessel-IgA-and-alternate-complement-pathway-mediated immune-complex vasculitis that can be set off by a variety of infectious and noninfectious stimuli. When the dermal vasculitis is severe, there may be considerable edema, especially of the dorsum of the hands and feet or in the scrotum, forehead, and periorbital areas (Fig. 2.3). Hematuria and mild gastrointestinal bleeding are also common. Rarely, life-threatening pulmonary hemorrhage may occur.[13a] Ninety-seven percent of affected children completely recover.[14]

The diagnosis of H-S purpura is not difficult when the rash is apparent. However, in those few cases in which arthritis precedes the rash, sometimes for weeks, it is impossible to recognize that the arthritis is a feature of this syndrome, as is illustrated by a recent patient.

Case Report

An 8-year-old boy became ill with fever, sore throat, and cervical lymphadenopathy for which he was given 10 days of oral penicillin treatment. Three weeks later, he developed fever and polyarthritis, which responded to aspirin, recurred when aspirin was withdrawn, and was again controlled with aspirin therapy. The rash of H-S purpura first appeared 3 weeks later and was accompanied by severe abdominal cramps and cutaneous edema (Fig. 2.3). The aspirin was discontinued and prednisone was administered; he required a dose of 30 mg daily for 3 weeks to prevent symptoms, which was then successfully changed to 75 mg every second morning, which could be weaned away over a 10-week period. There was no evidence of renal disease, and he has been well since.

Arthritis in H-S purpura is usually transient and characterized by pain, stiffness, and effusion in the large joints of the lower extremities and sometimes in the wrists and elbows. Without treatment, it may come and go over a period of weeks, and recurrences of the whole syndrome are common within a period of 6 months after onset; occasional patients have recurrences as late as 2 years after the initial episode.

When arthritis is present alone, it is usually easily controlled with aspirin. We use prednisone only for those children who have severe abdominal colic, but we do not hesitate to use corticosteroids in that group since 8% of children with severe colic with H-S purpura may have massive gastrointestinal hemorrhage or intussusception. The abdominal pain usually subsides soon after the prednisone is begun, and intussusception and hemorrhage do not then occur. If arthritis is present with abdominal colic, it also subsides promptly with the steroid therapy.

Chronic renal sequelae are frequently reported in older children and adults with H-S purpura but are rare in young children in the United States. When renal disease does occur, it does not seem to respond to corticosteroid treatment.

Kawasaki Disease
(Mucocutaneous Lymph Node Syndrome)

This is probably the most common acute rheumatic condition of childhood. The reader is referred to Chapter 7 for a detailed discussion.

Erythema Nodosum

Erythema nodosum is a dramatic clinical syndrome characterized by the sudden appearance of fever and a crop of typical warm, red, tender cutaneous nodules on the extensor surfaces of the anterior tibiae (Fig. 2.4).[15] In severe cases, lesions may extend up both the arms and legs. The skin lesions are frequently associated with arthralgia and joint effusions. The pathologic finding, perivascular granulomatous septal panniculitis, is consistent with a delayed hypersensitivity reaction.

Erythema nodosum may be a reaction to many specific infectious agents, including the *Streptococcus*, tubercle, or leprous bacillus; *Leptospira*; psittacosis;

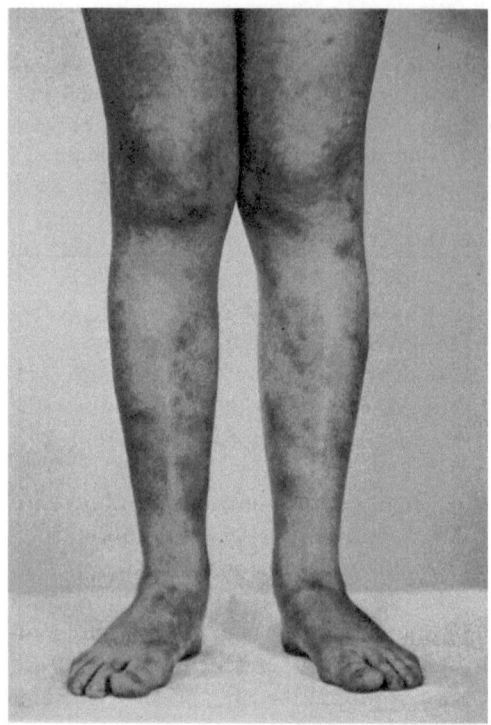

Figure 2.4. Nodular panniculitis of the pretibial surfaces (erythema nodosum) may be a reaction to many infectious agents or a sign of inflammatory bowel disease. This patient has a right knee effusion, a common finding in patients with erythema nodosum.

Yersinia; cytomegalovirus;[16] and fungal agents, including those causing coccidioidomycosis, blastomycosis, and histoplasmosis. In the San Juaquin Valley, 80% of cases are due to coccidiodomycosis. In most cases in children in New York, no underlying inciting disease is found. However, in our experience, when an etiology can be established, the single most frequent primary diagnosis in children is inflammatory bowel disease (IBD), and this diagnosis must be considered in every patient. Sarcoidosis is the most common single etiology in young adults followed in frequency by IBD and drug allergy, especially allergy to oral contraceptives.

Although new crops of lesions appear and the "attack" usually lasts for a few weeks, the lesions very rarely ulcerate, and the process is self-limited. Aspirin therapy is adequate for most cases, but corticosteroids may be used in the most severe cases after the tuberculin skin test is proved to be negative.

Serum Sickness and Drug Reactions

Most mild cases of erythema multiforme are precipitated by herpes simplex virus infection.[17] Serum sickness, the classic form of antigen-antibody (immune) complex disease, which results from the injection of heterologous serum is rarely seen today. However, similar allergic reactions for which serum sickness is the model are common.[18] With the recent increase in use of sulfa drugs and cefaclor, which are frequent inducers of serum-sickness-like reactions, we are seeing many more cases.[18a] Most are mild, with hives and few other symptoms, and disappear promptly following withdrawal of the drug or other allergen. Some more closely resemble true serum sickness with the sudden onset of urticarial or erythema multiforme skin lesions, angioneurotic edema, lymphadenopathy, arthritis, and polyserositis. In addition to the swelling of the fingers, which is associated with angioneurotic edema, the large joints are frequently effused, stiff, and painful, usually without heat or redness. The ESR is usually normal, but the total hemolytic complement is sometimes low due to binding in immune complexes; these laboratory determinations may be helpful in differential diagnosis.

Most of these reactions are mild and are easily controlled with antihistamines and aspirin after the offending agent has been withdrawn. Corticosteroids are reserved for use in only the most severe cases. A few children, however, develop the more serious drug- or infection-induced vasculitis termed Stevens-Johnson syndrome, which is characterized by bullae and mucocutaneous lesions (Fig. 2.5).[19–21]

Occasionally, children seem to go through a "stage" in which erythema multiforme with arthralgias or arthritis follows each presumed viral illness. Sometimes the offending agent is something special given to the child only when he is ill. In one such patient, we discovered that the ingestion of certain brands of cherry soda or cherry-flavored medications produced the reaction. Extensive detective work established that almond extract, often used in cherry flavors, was the culprit.[22]

Lyme disease is a rare cause of urticaria.[22a]

Symmetric inflammatory drug-induced arthritis (as well as other autoimmune diseases such as thyroiditis, pemphigus, vitiligo, and vasculitis) may be induced by Interleukin-2 (IL-2) treatment of malignancy.[22b]

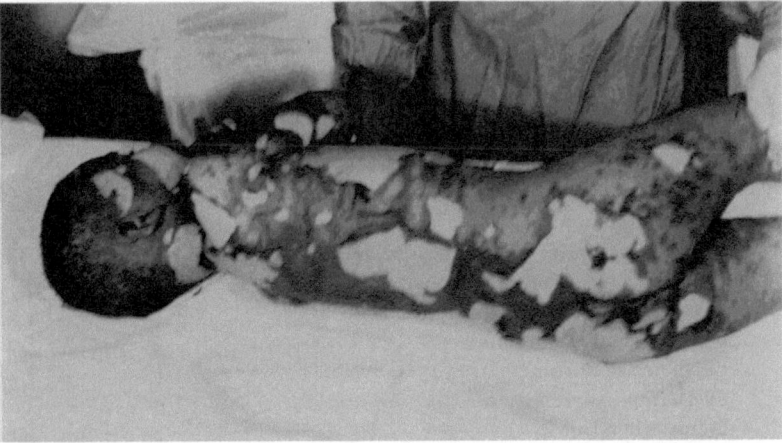

Figure 2.5. Stevens-Johnson syndrome (erythema multiforme with bullae and mucocutaneous lesions). In the fully expressed form pictured, this condition is easily distinguished from Kawasaki disease, the most common mucocutaneous disorder now seen in our clinic (see Chapter 7).

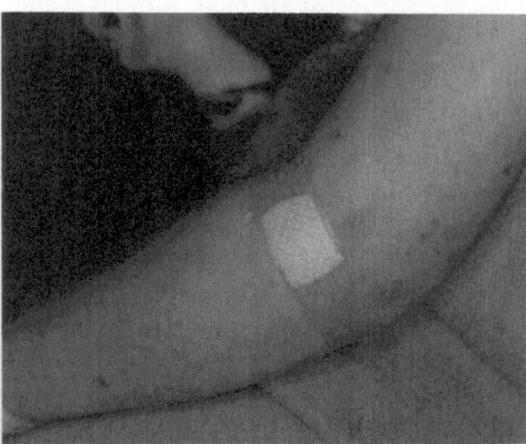

Figure 2.6. The rash of Mucha-Habermann disease (acute parapsoriasis) resembles that of varicella but also has vasculitic features. Recurrent crops of lesions were associated with arthralgias and an elbow effusion in this patient. Recurrent episodes of arthritis and rash may continue for up to 2 years in these children. A severe form occurs rarely (see Luberti et al. Pediatr Derm 8:151–157, 1991).

Mucha-Habermann Disease (PLEVA)

A little-recognized but not rare cutaneous perivasculitis, Mucha-Habermann disease (acute parapsoriasis), is characterized by the development of recurrent crops of vesicular lesions resembling pox, associated with pain and effusions in large joints and a slightly elevated ESR (Fig. 2.6).[23,24] The diagnosis is established by punch biopsy of the lesions; histopathologic examination shows a V-shaped perivascular *lymphocytic* infiltration about normal blood vessels (Fig. 2.7). The etiology is unknown. Mucha-Habermann disease is one of a group of arthritic syndromes that may be associated with inflammatory dermatoses (Table 2.4).

The arthritis associated with Mucha-Habermann disease is mild and transient and responds well to aspirin but may recur with each recurrent crop of

Table 2.4. Disorders in Which Arthritis May Be Associated with Inflammatory Dermatoses

Mucha-Habermann disease
Sweet's syndrome, inflammatory bowel disease and intestinal
    bypass syndrome
Erythema elevatum diutinum
Leukocytoclastic angiitis
Erythema nodosum
Pyoderma gangrenosum
Behcet's syndrome
Keratoderma blennorrhagicum (Reiter's syndrome)
Pancreatitis
Acne fulminans

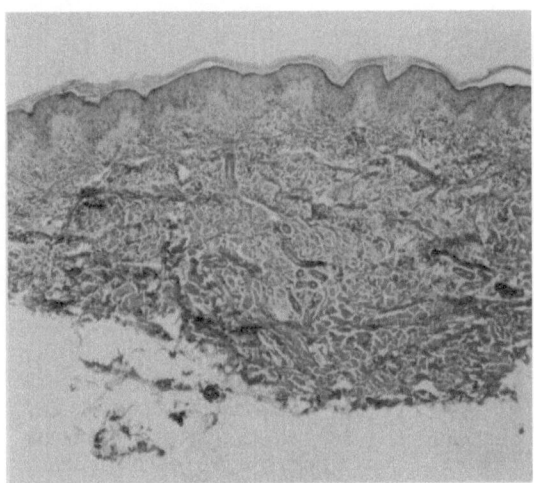

Figure 2.7. Histologic section from lesion shown in Fig. 2.6. Early epidermal necrosis with a perivascular lymphocytic infiltrate and extravasated erythrocytes is characteristic of Mucha-Habermann disease. (**A**) Low-power X40; (**B**) X250.

A

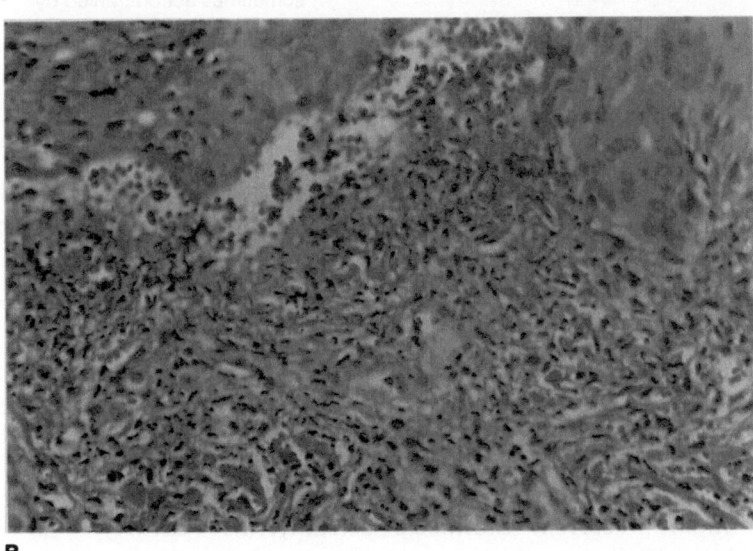

B

skin lesions. Although the illness usually subsides in a few months, we have seen one child who continued to have episodes for 2 years, the maximum previously reported by others.

Sweet's Syndrome

Acute febrile neutrophilic dermatosis (Sweet's syndrome) is another disorder characterized by crops of skin lesions associated with fever, myalgias,

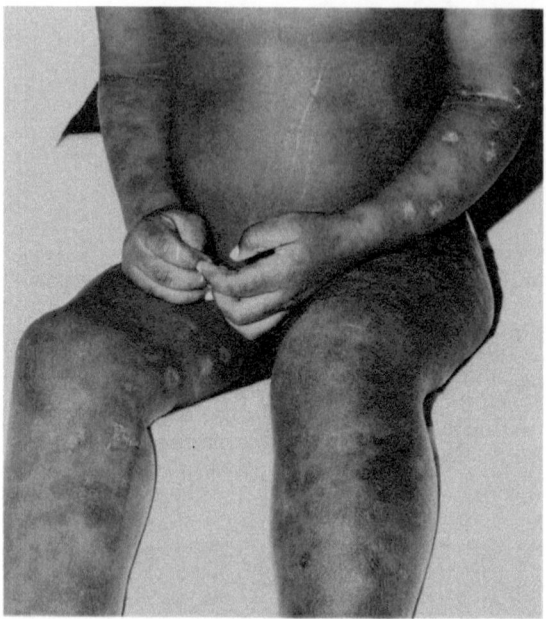

Figure 2.8. Sweet's syndrome (acute febrile neutrophilic dermatosis; onset age: 10 months; photo: age 5 years) was characterized by recurrent episodes of high fever and skin rash, sometimes accompanied by arthritis. The episodes stopped following a single course of corticosteroid therapy.

arthralgias, and, occasionally, arthritis.[25–27] The skin lesion is clinically distinctive and consists of raised *painful* plaques (Fig. 2.8) that, on histologic examination, show a dense, neutrophilic, small-vessel perivascular infiltrate in the mid- and upper dermis. Polymorphs generally predominate, and some are disrupted, creating nuclear fragments and "dust" about the vessel (Fig. 2.9). There are no changes in the blood vessels themselves. The whole syndrome is responsive to a brief course of corticosteroid therapy. In some cases, a single brief course of treatment is "curative," but there may be recurrent episodes over a period of years. Untreated episodes often last for 2 months. Similar or identical syndromes occur following ileojejunal bypass surgery and in association with malignancy, Fanconi and dyserythropoetic anemias,[28] chronic recurrent multifocal osteomyelitis (CRMO)[29] and Behçet's syndrome.[30]

Case Report

A black female developed the first of many recurrent episodes of rash, fever to 106°, and ankle effusions at the age of 10 months. Except for a very high ESR and leukocytosis with each episode, there were no abnormal findings on many studies performed during several long hospitalizations. A biopsy of the rash, when we first saw the patient at age 5, was suggestive of Sweet's syndrome (Fig. 2.9). She was treated with a brief course of prednisone, had a prompt and complete subsidence of symptoms, and has remained well without recurrence for many years.

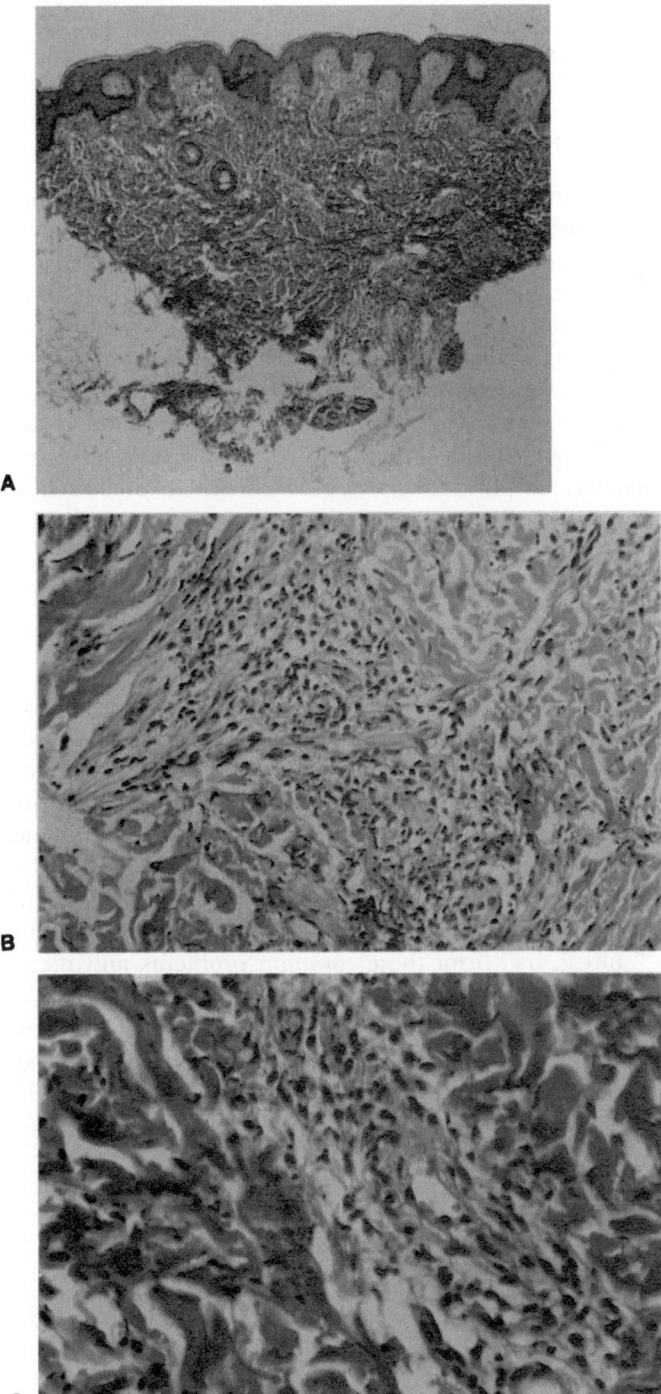

Figure 2.9. Skin biopsy of patient shown in Fig. 2.8. A heavy inflammatory reaction, largely but not exclusively perivascular, is seen in the upper half of the cutis and extending into the superficial subcutis (**A**). The cell population includes a mixture of mononuclear and poly-morphonuclear neutrophils; many of the latter are disrupted creating nuclear debris (**B**). Lateral to the area of major involvement are perivascular collections of inflammatory cells in which mononuclear cells predominate, but neutrophils are also present (**C**). Despite the unusual numbers of mononuclear cells, this biopsy was interpreted by Lewis Shapiro as representing Sweet's syndrome, which led to appropriate treatment of the child. (**A**) ×40; (**B**) ×250; (**C**) ×400.

Thrombotic Thrombocytopenic Purpura (TTP)

Although TTP is rare, the occurrence of the clinical pentad of thrombocytopenic purpura, microangiopathic hemolytic anemia, fever, renal disease, and varying neurologic signs or symptoms was first recognized in a child and is part of the differential diagnosis of multisystem diseases. Fatal myocarditis and myocardial hemorrhage may occur.[31] Although the etiology remains unknown, prompt recognition of this now-treatable disorder is essential. Formerly universally fatal, 90% of patients treated with fresh-frozen plasma and plasma exchange now survive. High-dose intravenous gamma globulin induced remission in one patient resistant to plasmapheresis, exchange transfusion, splenectomy, antiplatelet agents, glucocorticoids, and vincristine.[32,33]

Acute and Chronic Infections of the Bones and Joints

Acute Hematogenous Osteomyelitis

General Considerations. Fever and limp or disuse of an extremity require that the physician consider osteomyelitis as a possible diagnosis (Tables 2.5 and 2.6). Although osteomyelitis is not uncommon in a large pediatric center, it is a rarity in any individual pediatrician's office. However, our studies show that pediatricians have even more difficulty with this diagnosis than with other equally rare or even rarer conditions (Tables 2.7 and 2.8). This is not surprising since the frequency with which children limp with minor trauma or have fever as a result of viral illness makes it difficult for the physician to "shift gears" from these common problems and recognize the serious potential of this combination of symptoms in this one patient. This problem is further accentuated by the need for immediate diagnosis and emergency care. Late diagnosis has been the rule in all published series and is often associated with greatly increased morbidity for the patient.[34–37] With

Table 2.5. Presenting Complaints in 79 Children with Osteomyelitis*

Data	Number of Patients
Bone pain and limp or disuse	79
Fever (average 102.3°F)	68
Joint pain	51
History of injury prior to 24 h	26
History of injury over 24 h	10

Source: Jacobs, ref. 34.
*Excluding children under 1 month of age, postoperative infections, and children with sickle-cell anemia.

Acute and Chronic Infections of the Bones and Joints **41**

Table 2.6. Bones Affected in Childhood Osteomyelitis

Bone	Number of Cases
Femur	16 (6 with septic hip, 1 with knee)
Tibia	17 (1 with septic knee, 2 with ankle)
Fibula	9
Pelvics	11 (2 with septic hip)
Patella	3 (3 with septic knee)
Os calcis	3
Metatarsal	3
Tarsal	1
Toe	1
Vertebra-disk	3
Humerus	6 (2 with septic elbow, 1 with shoulder)
Radius	4 (1 with septic wrist)
Ulna	1
Hand-rib	4

Source: Jacobs, ref. 34.

Table 2.7. Columbia-Presbyterian Medical Center, 1965–1974, Primary Diagnosis Made in 79 Patients with Osteomyelitis

Diagnosis	Number of Patients
Osteomyelitis	13
Cellulitis	14
Trauma	24
"Virus," upper respiratory infection	19
Rheumatoid arthritis	2
Acute rheumatic fever	3
Other	4
Osteomyelitis considered at first visit but rejected	18

Source: Jacobs, ref. 34.

Table 2.8. Difficulty Making Diagnosis of Osteomyelitis, Contrasted with Septic Arthritis

Data	Osteomyelitis (%)	Septic Arthritis (%)
Seen by physician before 48 h	82	94
Diagnosed at first visit	37	70
Diagnosis within 48 h	20	65

Source: Jacobs, ref. 34.

a better understanding of the special problems associated with making a diagnosis of osteomyelitis, early diagnosis can be achieved.

Presentation. The usual and repetitive presentation is the sudden onset of fever and limb pain, often after an inconsequential injury, rarely as a result of spread of infection directly through a surgical site or open wound. We find it most helpful to think of the diagnostic situation as analogous to that of acute appendicitis:

Fever and bone pain (limp, disuse of extremity)	Right lower quadrant abdominal pain and vomiting
Osteomyelitis	Acute appendicitis

A careful examination is then performed seeking specific evidence for or against this diagnostic hypothesis.

Examining the Bone. Point tenderness of bone is always present and diagnostic but, as in a toothache, may be hard to localize. As the infection spreads to the surface, cellulitis may become obvious, make examination difficult, and distract the physician from the underlying pathology. A slow and thorough examination, starting at a great distance from the affected area, helps to reassure the patient and secure his cooperation. It may be possible to elicit periosteal rebound tenderness by pressing and releasing pressure on the bone at a distance from the affected area, using techniques familiar to all physicians from examination of the abdomen. This may indicate the point of maximal tenderness that can then be avoided until the last part of the examination. When point tenderness of bone is documented in a febrile patient, the presumptive diagnosis is osteomyelitis and the physician proceeds with a management plan appropriate for that diagnosis (Fig. 2.10).

Significance of Adjacent Joint Effusions. Since osteomyelitis most commonly starts at the metaphysis of bone, the nearby joint is often swollen. When the metaphysis is outside the joint capsule, as at the knee, the effusion is "sympathetic" and does not suggest septic infection (Fig. 2.11). The aspiration of sterile "reactive" joint fluid from the knee is what should be expected in osteomyelitis in the distal femur or proximal tibia and cannot be used as evidence against the diagnosis of bone infection. Careful palpation of the adjacent bones is performed when the knee is examined and reveals point tenderness when the bone is infected.

The situation is totally different when the metaphysis is inside the joint, as at the hip. There the effusion is often infected, and one must remember that the demonstration of sepsis in the hip joint does not exclude the possibility of osteomyelitis. On the contrary, the possibility of osteomyelitis of the femur must be considered whenever there is sepsis in the hip joint. Osteomyelitis of

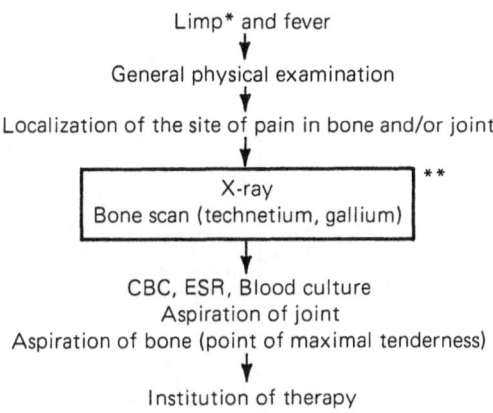

Figure 2.10. Module for diagnosis and management of osteomyelitis.

the femur or the tibia constitutes 40% of childhood osteomyelitis, accentuating the importance of these anatomic considerations. Hip, groin, buttock, and abdominal pain may also be manifestations of pelvic-bone osteomyelitis, including sacroiliac osteomyelitis, another frequent site of bone infection in childhood (Table 2.6).[38]

Systemic Manifestations. If the infection spreads systemically, more than one bone and/or joint may be infected, and the illness may then be mistaken for rheumatic fever or rheumatoid arthritis. Teenagers, particularly boys, seem especially susceptible to this form of staphylococcal septicemia. When the infection becomes life-threatening as a result of septic embolization to lung, heart, and kidney, the primary focus in bone may not be noticed at all, and appropriate therapy may be delayed.[35,36]

Laboratory Studies. Blood is obtained for a complete blood count and ESR, both of which are sometimes surprisingly normal (Table 2.9). A blood culture is also obtained; in 20% of cases in which a pathologic organism is demonstrated, it is found in the blood culture alone and not in the bone or joint aspirants (Table 2.10). If there is a joint effusion, fluid is aspirated in a heparinized syringe for cell count, and specimens are obtained for culture and smear and for joint-fluid sugar determination. Following adequate sedation and after the bone scan is completed (if a scan can be obtained immediately), the bone itself is aspirated at the point of maximal tenderness for smear and culture. While laboratory studies may confirm the clinical diagnosis, they are sometimes misleadingly reassuring, and the immediate diagnosis

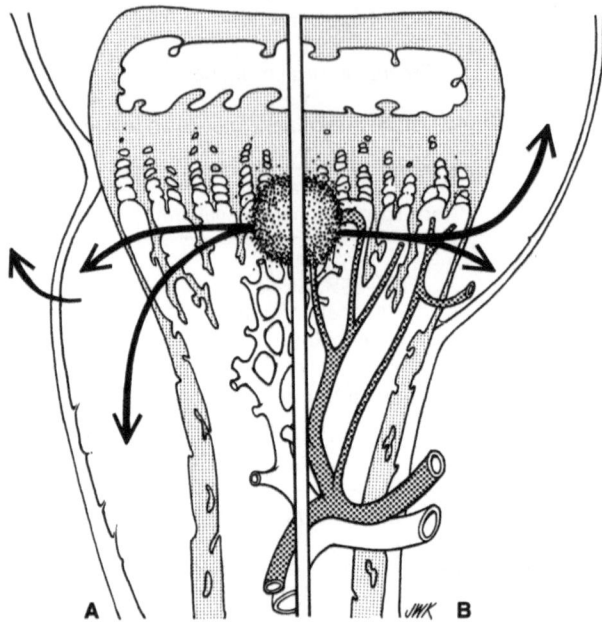

Figure 2.11. Diagram of differing patterns of spread from a nidus of infection located at the metaphysis of a long bone, depending on whether the metaphysis is located within the joint capsule or outside the capsule. The metaphysis is the most common site for acute osteomyelitis, presumably because of capillary looping, as shown. If the metaphysis is outside the joint capsule (**A**), as at the knee, infection can spread subperiosteally down the bone and can ultimately form soft-tissue abscesses by rupturing through the periosteum. However, although a sympathetic joint effusion may be present, joint fluid is sterile. Aspiration of sterile joint fluid from the knee is often misinterpreted as evidence against septic infection, although a sterile knee effusion is a characteristic finding in osteomyelitis of the distal femur or proximal tibia. If the infected metaphysis is within the joint space (**B**), as at the hip, infection commonly spreads laterally, through the cortex into the joint. Joint fluid will be purulent. The finding of purulent fluid in the hip always indicates the possibility of osteomyelitis in the proximal femur. Since the treatment regimen for osteomyelitis is different from that for septic arthritis without bone infection, it is important to exclude bone infection in patients with septic arthritis.

must be made on the basis of the physical examination alone. Inevitably, a few youngsters will be treated initially for osteomyelitis who turn out not to have it; that is the price that must be paid to obtain effective early treatment for those who do.

Radiographic Studies. Conventional radiographs are always negative in early osteomyelitis but are obtained to rule out old disease, associated bone pathology, and fracture. As soon as the diagnosis of osteomyelitis is considered, a technetium-99m bone scan is obtained (Fig. 2.12A-C). Technical aspects of bone scanning are constantly being improved upon and will not be

Table 2.9. Osteomyelitis and Septic Arthritis Laboratory
Studies 1965–1974

	Osteomyelitis (79)	Septic Arthritis (17)
White Blood Count		
Under 10,000/mm^3	38	6
10,000–20,000	34	8
20,000–30,000	3	3
Over 30,000	1	
Not recorded	3	
ESR		
Under 10 mm/h (West)	3	
10–20	13	1
21–40	13	5
41–60	16	5
61–80	15	3
81–100	7	
Over 100	8	2
Not recorded	4	1

Table 2.10. Sources of Diagnosis in
Osteomyelitis

Source of Positive Cultures*	Number
Blood culture only	12
Blood plus bone/joint	8
Bone/joint only	39

Source: Jacobs, ref. 34.
* In 59 of 79 patients.

discussed here. However, combined blood pool and bone imaging with technetium-labeled phosphate compounds often confirms the clinical diagnosis of osteomyelitis, and diagnostic accuracy can be further enhanced by combined gallium-67-citrate and technetium scanning.[39,40]

While bone scans are the first radiologic or laboratory procedure that provides support for the early diagnosis of osteomyelitis, they are not a substitute for skillful interpretive history taking and physical examination. They are often not immediately available and are also not infrequently negative during the first 24 h after the illness begins. False-negative scans may be obtained even after that time for unknown reasons or as a result of misinterpretation. A bone scan is often of help in establishing a diagnosis, but a negative bone scan cannot be taken as a guarantee that a patient does not

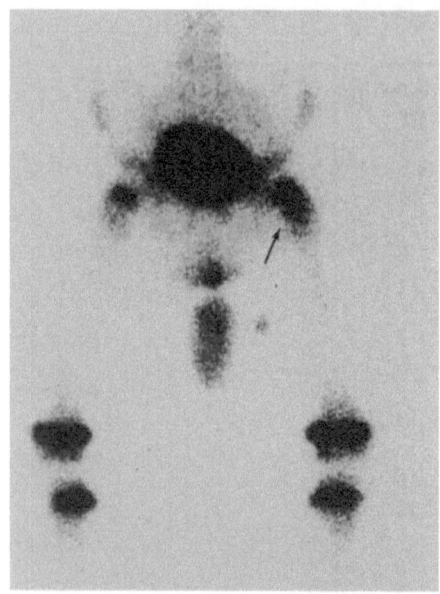

Figure 2.12. Development of radiographic signs of osteomyelitis in the left hip (femur) in a $1\frac{1}{2}$-year-old girl. The technetium bone scan (**A**) was positive at the time of presentation, with mild monarticular synovitis of the left hip. The patient was discharged from the hospital after 2 weeks of intravenous treatment but did not receive the prescribed oral therapy at home. One week later, she was readmitted with a recurrence of subacute hip signs. The radiographs, negative at the time of the initial admission (**B**), showed lytic lesions both at the under-surface of the growth center and breaking through from the femoral metaphysis into the growth plate and joint (**C**).

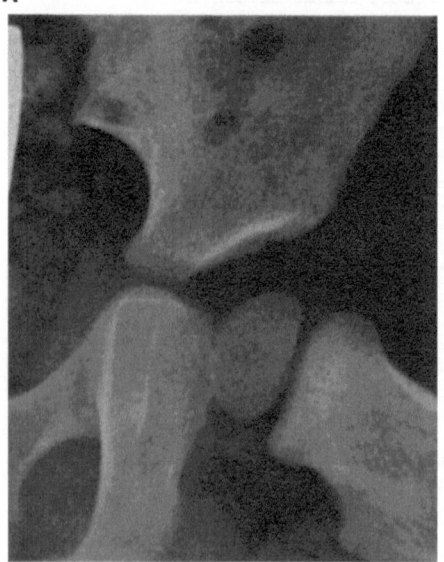

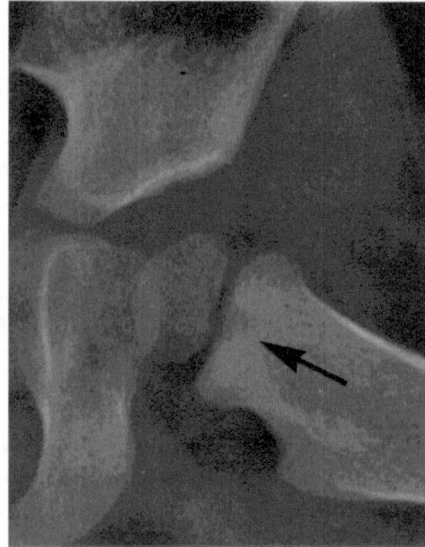

have osteomyelitis,[41–43] and treatment must not be withheld in patients thought to have osteomyelitis (Fig. 2.13).

Treatment. All patients are begun on intravenous medications initially. The choice of drug(s) is based on statistical probability as to the etiologic agent

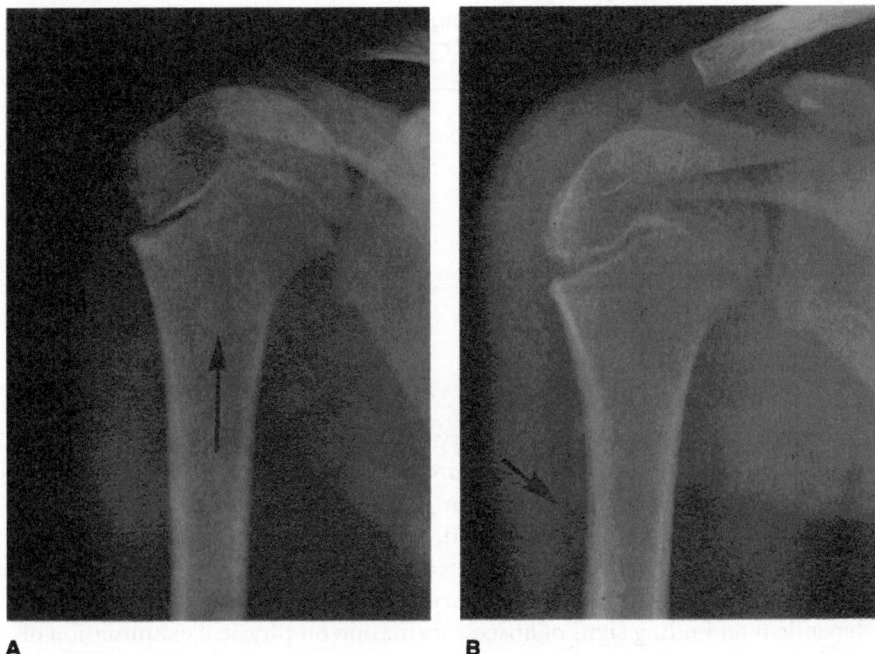

A **B**

Figure 2.13. Admission films of the shoulder of an 11-year-old girl with clinical signs of osteomyelitis of the right humerus were interpreted as normal, although a central metaphyseal lucency has been brought out by the photographer's reproduction (**A**, *arrow*) but is not appreciated, even retrospectively, on the plain film. A bone scan at the time of admission was also interpreted as normal. The patient was promptly treated, and the presumptive diagnosis was confirmed by obtaining *Staphylococcus aureus* from a blood culture. Periosteal new-bone formation, suggestive of evolving osteomyelitis, was first apparent in a film obtained 3 weeks later (**B**).

(Table 2.11). Except in the infant or compromised host or after puncture wounds of the foot, most osteomyelitis is caused by penicillin-resistant staphylococci, so unless the smear suggests gram-negative infection, treatment for this organism alone is administered.[44] A large variety of antistaphylococcal drugs have been shown to be effective; in our own hospital, oxacillin is used in most cases, in a dose of 200 mg/kg/day divided into six 4-hourly doses (maximum 6–12 grams daily).

An etiologic agent has been demonstrated in 75% of cases; in 20–30% of these, the organism was obtained only from the blood culture[34,37] (Table 2.10). This percentage may be expected to increase as fewer patients require surgical drainage. If an organism other than penicillinase-producing *Staphylococcus* is demonstrated, the regimen is appropriately modified.

In our experience, surgical drainage is not necessary when appropriate medical treatment is instituted within 48 h of onset of symptoms. When effective treatment is begun promptly, abscess formation and significant bone

Table 2.11. Organisms Causing Childhood Osteomyelitis

	Number of Case (79) *
Staphylococcus	51
Streptococcus	7
Diplococcus pneumoniae	1
Pseudomonas	1
Hemophilus influenzae B	1
Not proved	20

Source: Jacobs, ref. 34.
*Two multiple organisms.

necrosis do not take place, and surgery would serve no purpose.[37] Not all patients who are diagnosed later require surgery. However, when it is evident that abscess formation has taken place and that there is pus under pressure, surgical drainage is warranted. Since fever may continue for 5 days even in promptly and adequately treated osteomyelitis, fever alone is not a reliable indication of the need for surgery. The decision for surgical drainage is dependent on finding signs of abscess formation on physical examination of the involved bone; the patient should be reexamined frequently. Where there are signs that the infection is spreading down through the marrow cavity or rupturing through the thin cortex to the subperiosteal space, drainage should be promptly performed.

Naturally, all physicians would like to change to oral treatment as soon as possible.[45] However, in all of the reported studies of oral treatment, a large number of patients have had surgical drainage as part of their initial treatment, and the results may not necessarily be applicable to nonoperated patients.[44,46–47] It is also hard to draw firm conclusions from the small series so far reported, and the real advantage of oral treatment would be if it could be successfully accomplished as an outpatient rather than if continued hospitalization is required, as has usually been reported. Our present general policy is to continue parenteral therapy for 21 days and to then change to oral treatment provided the ESR is normal and the patient is asymptomatic. Once the patient is stabilized intravenous therapy can be administered at home. We continue oral treatment for an additional 2 months. There is no question that this constitutes excessive treatment for most patients, but our experience suggests that lesser regimens may be associated with an unacceptable rate of treatment failures,[47] as illustrated by this recent patient.

Case Report

A 21-month-old girl presented with fever and a limp. Physical examination revealed only 5–10° of limitation of full abduction of the left hip without point tenderness in any adjacent bone. The child appeared happy and was running about. However, a bone scan was obtained immediately and demonstrated a focus of infection in the left femoral metaphysis (Fig. 2.12). The ESR was 43, and the white blood count (WBC) was 11,000 with 69% polys. A blood culture taken at this time subsequently was positive for *Staphylococcus aureus*.

Treatment was begun with intravenous oxacillin, and within 48 h fever and the minimal local signs had disappeared. After 2 weeks, the ESR was normal, intravenous medication was discontinued, and the child was discharged to continue oral cloxacillin at home. Unfortunately, she did not receive the oral medicine. Within a week, the limp recurred, but no localizing signs were apparent on examination. The white blood count, which had previously returned to normal, again showed a shift to the left with 22% bands; the ESR was 20 mm/h. X-ray, normal at 2 weeks, now showed a lesion suggestive of a Brodie's abscess (cystic osteomyelitis) at the proximal left femoral epiphyseal growth plate (Fig. 2.12C). Re-treatment with intravenous oxacillin for 3 weeks followed by 3 months of oral cloxacillin was successful in eradicating the infection.

Osteomyelitis in the Sacroiliac Area

Osteomyelitis in the bones articulating at the sacro-iliac joint constituted 15% of all patients with osteomyelitis in our pediatric series (Table 2.6).[34] Prior to 1940, the average delay in diagnosis was 7.3 weeks; horrors are still being reported[48] and in some series, diagnosis is still unusually delayed when compared with osteomyelitis at any site other than the vertebra (3.3 weeks).[48,49] However, in our experience and in retrospective reviews, this delay is unnecessary, as the initial physical findings are so characteristic that it is possible for experienced observers to suspect the diagnosis at the time of initial examination.[48,49]

The distinctive presentation is limp and pain in the buttock, often with radicular sciatic pain. The techniques for diagnosis and management of patients with presumed osteomyelitis in this area are identical to those in any other location; treatment is instituted as soon as the patient with these symptoms is first seen even if the bone scan is negative (45% of initial scans are negative.)[50] Increased awareness of the clinical presentation, improved diagnostic techniques (technetium, gallium, and CT), and prompt, effective treatment have greatly reduced the morbidity previously associated with this infection. Prompt response to treatment confirms the diagnosis; lack of prompt response is an indication for further evaluation.[51]

Subacute Osteomyelitis

A few children with acute osteomyelitis, even without treatment, will spontaneously partially control the infection and enter the less acute phase of bone infection called subacute osteomyelitis. However, the more common situation in subacute osteomyelitis is that at the time of a prior acute illness, skeletal pain was ignored, some other diagnosis was made to explain the fever, antibiotics were given, and the bone infection was partially contained, only to continue to smolder after the antibiotics were discontinued. The signs of infection in subacute osteomyelitis are usually limited to minimal tenderness and local heat. When these bone infections are in or near the knee or ankle joints, they are frequently associated with knee or ankle effusion and may easily be mistaken for monarticular JRA (Fig. 2.14). To help avoid this error, it is our current policy to perform a bone scan on any patient with

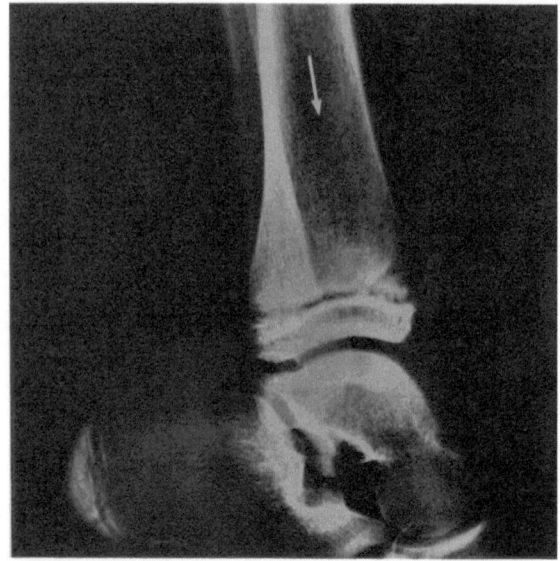

A

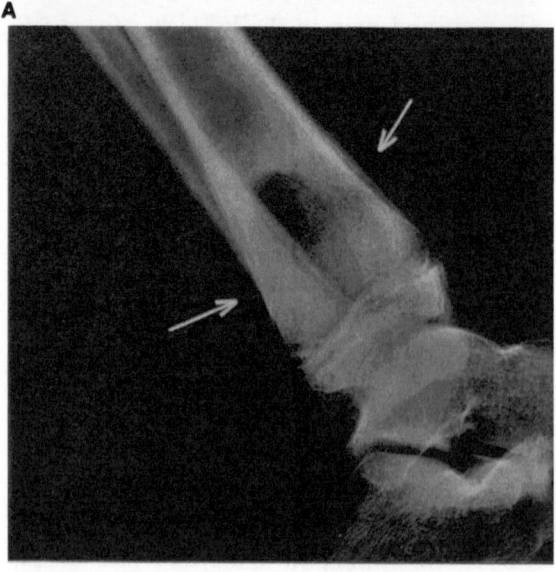

B

Figure 2.14. Staphylococcal osteomyelitis of the right distal tibia, presenting as monarticular arthritis of the ankle several weeks after antibiotic therapy for pneumonia. The patient was followed at two large hospitals in Boston and New York for 4 months (**A**; July 23) before a lytic lesion and periosteal new bone first became radiologically visible (**B**; November 3). The original film is now interpreted as showing a loss of trabecular pattern (**A**, *arrow*). This case precedes the availability of bone scanning. (**B**, Courtesy of Dr. W. Berenberg.)

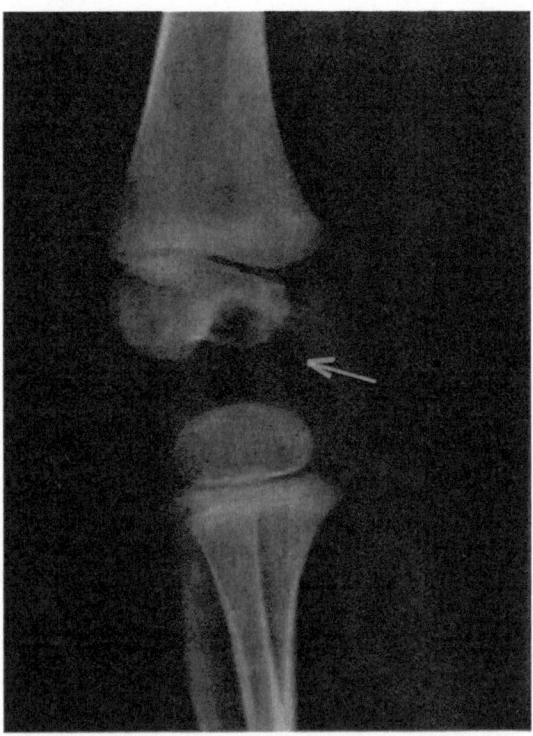

Figure 2.15. Cystic osteomyelitis (Brodie's abscess) of the distal femoral epiphysis, which presented with a monarticular knee effusion. These lesions are sometimes mistaken for tumors.

monarticular arthritis who has had antibiotic treatment just prior to the onset of the arthritis. The bone scan may suggest osteomyelitis, although months may elapse before conventional radiographs demonstrate a well-defined radiolucent lesion in the metaphysis or epiphysis, with surrounding reactive bone, typical of a *Brodie's abscess* (Fig. 2.15). Occasionally, these abscesses are mistaken for bone tumors.[52]

We treat subacute osteomyelitis and Brodie's abscess with 3 months of oral cloxacillin (50–100 mg/kg/day; maximum 2 grams). It is not worth operating to try to establish the bacteriologic or pathologic diagnosis so long as the patient responds satisfactorily to therapy. Clinical improvement is generally apparent within a few days. If the course is not satisfactory, surgery can then always be performed.

Puncture Wounds of the Feet. A special form of osteomyelitis is seen following puncture wounds, primarily in the feet.[53,54] The usual history is that the pain suffered immediately after the puncture disappeared, only to return and get worse after a variable period of time, ranging from 1 day to several weeks. Sometimes the injury was an insect bite or went unnoticed. In patients with this characteristic history, early diagnosis depends on a bone scan; later, conventional radiographs demonstrate destructive changes in one

Table 2.12. Infections In and Around the
Knee

Osteomyelitis of the femur or tibia
Suppurative arthritis of the knee
Prepatella bursitis
Osteomyelitis/osteochondritis of the patella
Cellulitis

of the foot bones. Most, but not all, of these puncturewound infections of foot
bones are caused by *Pseudomonas*—a resident of worn sneaker soles.[53] A variety of other organisms, including rapidly growing mycobacteria, may also be
introduced at the time of penetrating injury.[55,56] Therefore, in this form of
osteomyelitis, debridement should be performed prior to the institution of
antibiotic therapy so that the organism can be identified and an appropriate
antibiotic regimen can be instituted.[56]

Subacute Osteomyelitis of the Patella. Infections of the patella and prepatellar bursa must be distinguished from infections in the knee joint (Table
2.12). Most cases of osteomyelitis of the patella (really mostly suppurative
chondritis in the nonossified portion) occur in children between the ages of 5
and 15 years and are of staphylococcal origin.[57] They are commonly low-
grade infections that are accompanied by sterile knee effusions, and they are
usually confused with pauciarticular JRA. The clinical suspicion of infection
is aroused by patella tenderness to palpation. Abnormalities of technetium
and gallium scan may help in early diagnosis when the radiologist is alerted
to the possibility of patella suppuration. Ultimately, destructive lesions are
visible on radiographs. However, if a lateral film of the opposite (normal)
patella is not obtained for comparison, the radiographic diagnosis of a
destructive lesion in the young child with an incompletely ossified patella
will almost surely be missed (Fig. 2.16). These infections, once diagnosed,
are generally easy to control with oral antistaphylococcal agents by using a
regimen appropriate for subacute osteomyelitis.

Occasionally, subacute osteomyelitis of the patella follows a puncture
wound and, as in the foot bones, is due to *Pseudomonas* infection. The diagnosis is established by obtaining cultures at the time of surgical debridement of
unresponsive patella osteomyelitis.

Suppurative Prepatellar Bursitis

Infection of the patella must be differentiated from suppurative prepatellar
bursitis, a complication of housemaid's or football-player's knee. In suppurative prepatellar bursitis, the bursa generally appears tensely swollen and
obviously infected; this clinical impression can generally be confirmed by

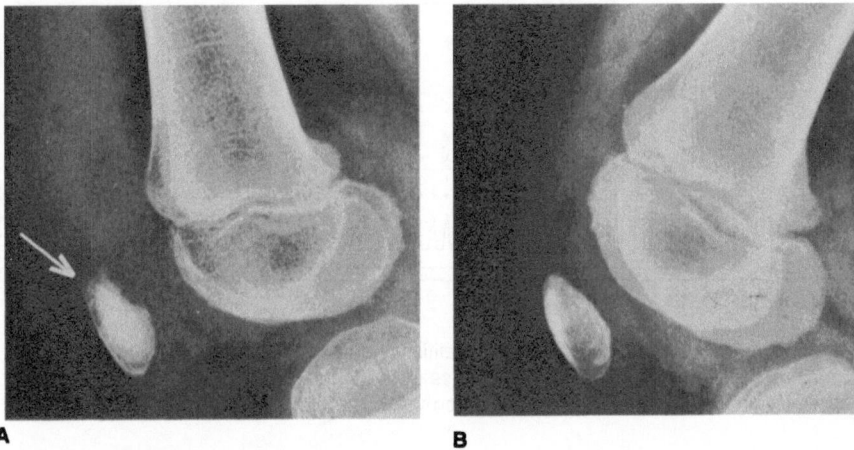

A　　　　　　　　　　　　　　　**B**

Figure 2.16. Osteomyelitis of the left patella presenting as a solitary left knee effusion in a 6-year-old boy. The diagnosis was not apparent for 1 month and was missed until lateral films were obtained of both knees, enabling recognition of the left patellar erosion (**A**, *arrow*), which might pass for normal except when compared with the opposite side (**B**).

aspirating pus from the bursa. A similar lesion, "student's elbow," is occasionally seen at the olecranon bursa (Fig. 2.17). Septic bursitis responds well to oral antistaphylococcal agents after aspiration and initial intravenous therapy.[58-60]

Chronic Osteomyelitis

This complication of inadequately treated acute or subacute osteomyelitis is now fortunately rare and usually presents no problem in differential diagnosis. The chart, published by Dr. Frank Falkner (Fig. 2.18) detailing 56 years

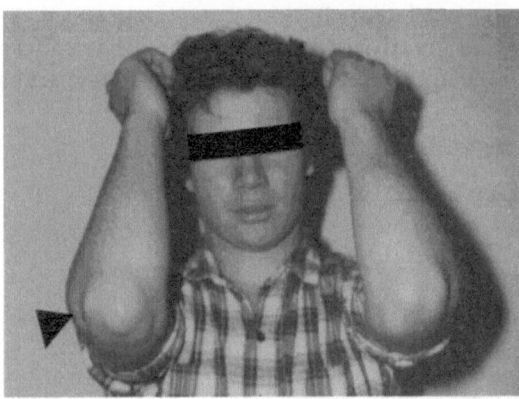

Figure 2.17. Suppurative bursitis of the right elbow (student's elbow) (*arrow*). The olecranon and prepatellar bursae are the most frequently infected in children.

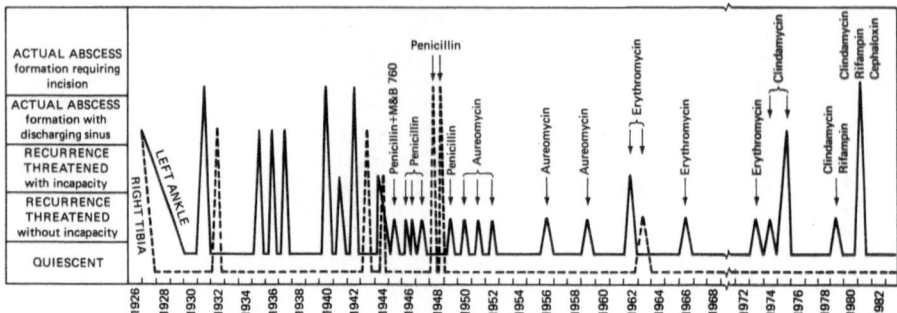

Figure 2.18. The course of chronic osteomyelitis, charted for 56 years, after onset in the right proximal tibia and a "metastatic" abscess in the left ankle at age 8 years. (Modified with permission from Falkner F: Chronic osteomyelitis. Lancet 1:415, 1976.)

of his own disease, provides a multitude of clinical insights and is a reminder of the lifetime disability that can be avoided by prompt, efficient treatment of acute osteomyelitis.

Special Situations—Suppurative Iliac Lymphadenitis and Retroperitoneal (Psoas) Abscess

These two suppurative infections may simulate osteomyelitis of the pelvic bones or septic arthritis of the hip (Table 2.13).[61,62] In general, the clinical picture is less acute, so that the youngster often limps about with hip, back, and abdominal pain and low-grade fever for a week or 2 before he is admitted to a hospital. Examination of the hip in these youngsters (mostly boys) shows little pain with abduction and adduction but great pain on extension of the thigh. The children lie with their hip flexed.[63] In the past, diagnosis was extraordinarily difficult but was generally accomplished by seeing an increased soft-tissue density in the iliac fossa on plain abdominal films or displacement of a ureter on IVP or of the sigmoid colon (in left-sided lesions) on barium enema (Fig. 2.19). We have not had a chance to test the newer technique of gallium scan, which should greatly facilitate the diagnosis of these lesions. However, we have been able to utilize gallium and liver-spleen scans

Table 2.13. Suppurative Causes of Hip Pain

Osteomyelitis of the femur
Suppurative arthritis of the hip
Iliac lymphadenitis
Retroperitoneal abscess
Diskitis
Osteomyelitis of the pelvic bones

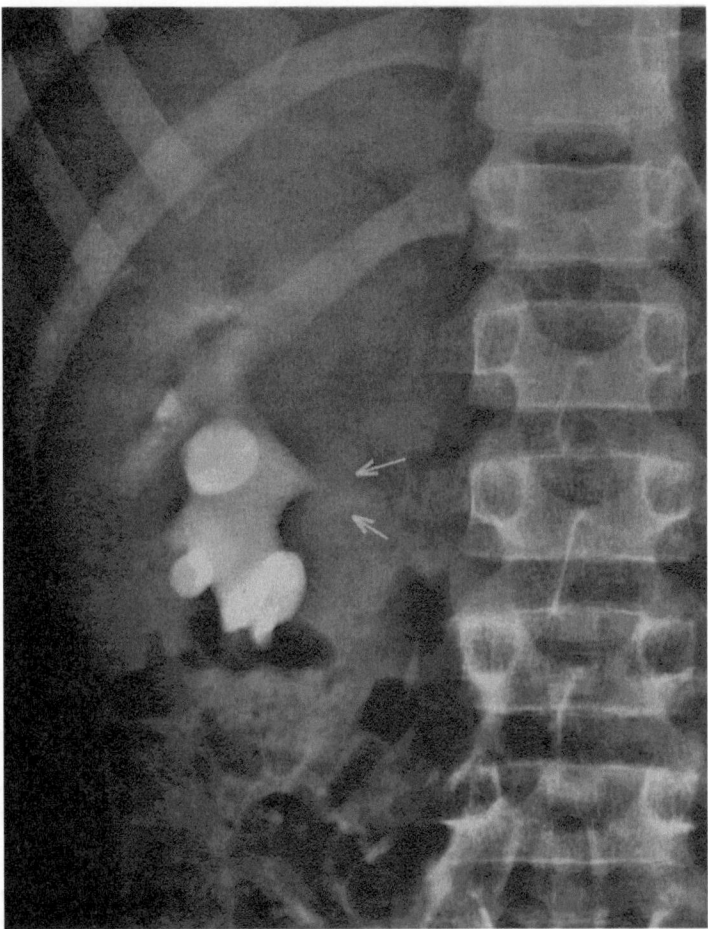

Figure 2.19. Right psoas phlegma in a 10-year-old boy referred as "? JRA" because of unexplained prolonged fever and an elevated ESR. There was a history of antibiotic treatment for "a virus" several weeks earlier. IVP shows swollen medial upper pole of the kidney with partial obstruction of the renal pelvis due to inflammation of the psoas muscle. Abdominal ultrasound is now obtained as a routine part of our workup for unexplained fever.

and ultrasound examinations to show septic abdominal infections[64,65] in other patients referred to us as "possible JRA" because of persistent unexplained fever (Figs. 2.20 and 2.21).

Case Report

An $11\frac{1}{2}$-year-old boy was admitted because of persistent fever and right-hip pain. He had had two hospital admissions for these complaints 4 years previously, with the

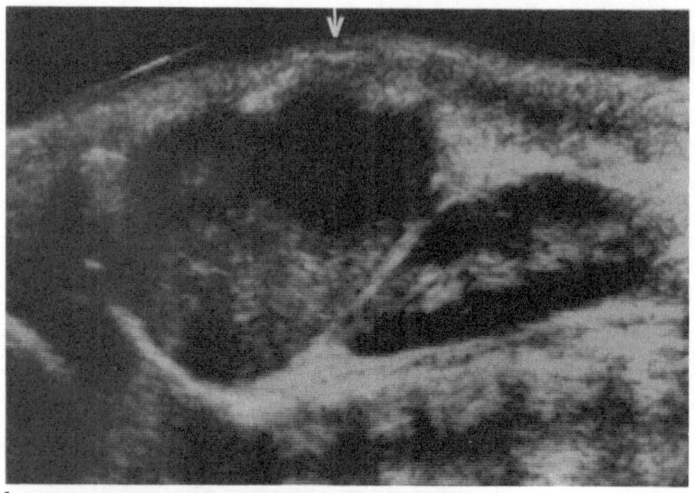

A

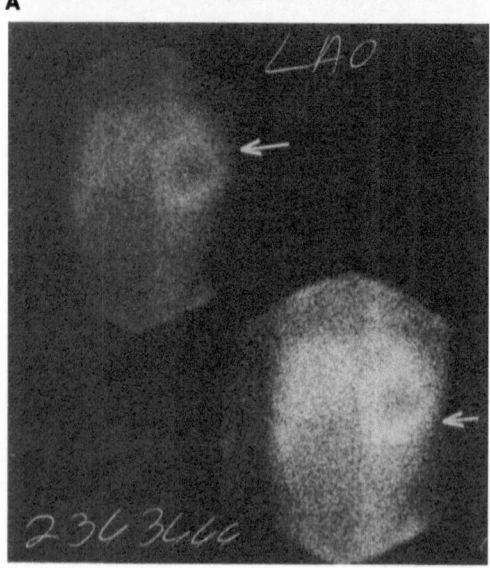

B

Figure 2.20. Ultrasound examination of the spleen (**A**) showing a large abscess cavity in a boy referred for unexplained fever and an elevated ESR. Gallium scan was performed as part of our routine workup for prolonged unexplained fever and showed increased uptake in the splenic area. A liver-spleen scan (**B**) revealed a filling defect caused by the abscess. These newer techniques have dramatically improved our diagnostic ability in patients with unexplained fever.

only abnormality noted being an elevated ESR. Fever disappeared, but intermittently he would limp and complain of hip pain on walking. Physical examination revealed pain on extension of the hip. Laboratory studies showed mild anemia, leukocytosis, and an elevated ESR (102 mm/h). He was treated with prednisone (diagnosis: JRA) and soon developed a mass in the right thigh; a biopsy of the thigh muscle showed perivascular lymphocytic infiltrates. After 1 month of prednisone treatment, the iliac abscess ruptured through the right thigh; *Staphylococcus aureus* was grown from the culture. He was treated with oral erythromycin (allergic to penicillin) and made a complete recovery from the suppurative iliac lymphadenitis.

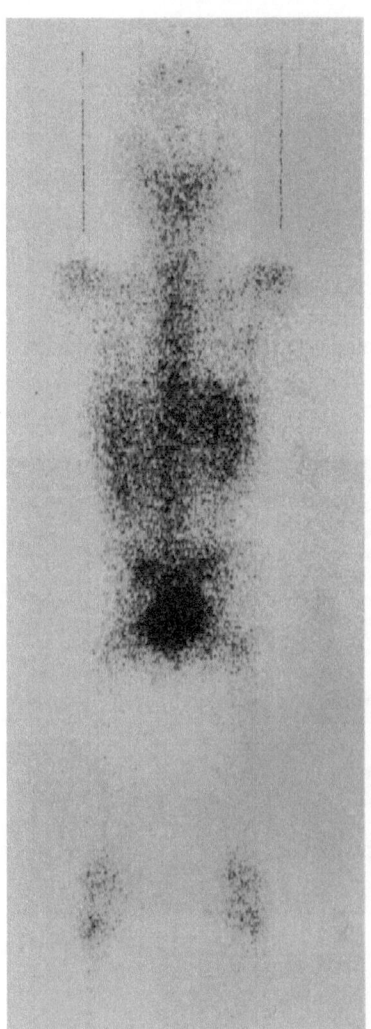

Figure 2.21. Perirectal abscess demonstrated on gallium scan in a 10-year-old boy. The patient was referred for "? JRA" because of unexplained fever and a high ESR.

Pyomyositis

Localized, primarily staphylococcal muscle abscesses, now called pyomyositis, were traditionally thought to occur only in the tropics, where the disorder was termed "tropical pyomyositis." Increasing numbers of cases are now being recognized in the United States.[66,67] The clinical picture is characterized by a child (usually a boy) who appears quite ill and toxic with severe pain and an enlarging area of inflammation in one or both thighs (Fig. 2.22). Although the thighs are extremely tender, there is no bone pain, which differentiates this lesion from osteomyelitis. In some cases, there is a history

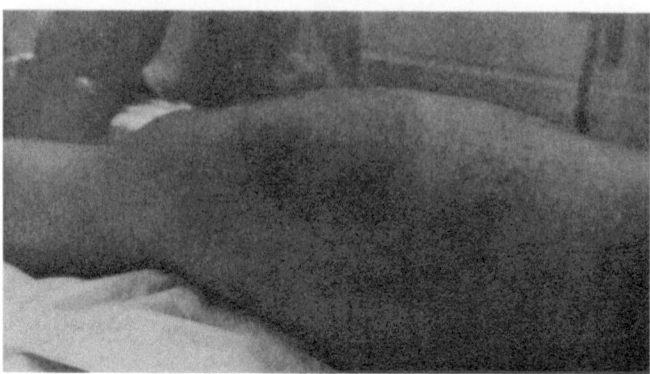

Figure 2.22. Gigantic enlargement of the thigh associated with high fever and prostration required surgical drainage for pyomyositis.

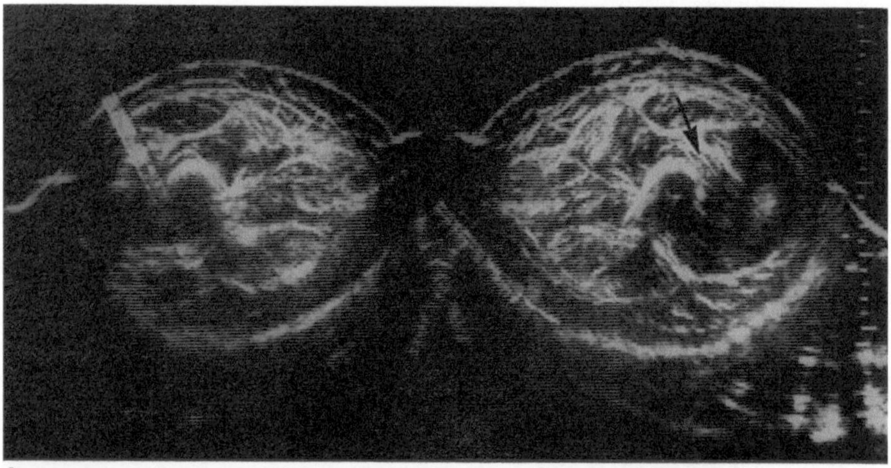

A

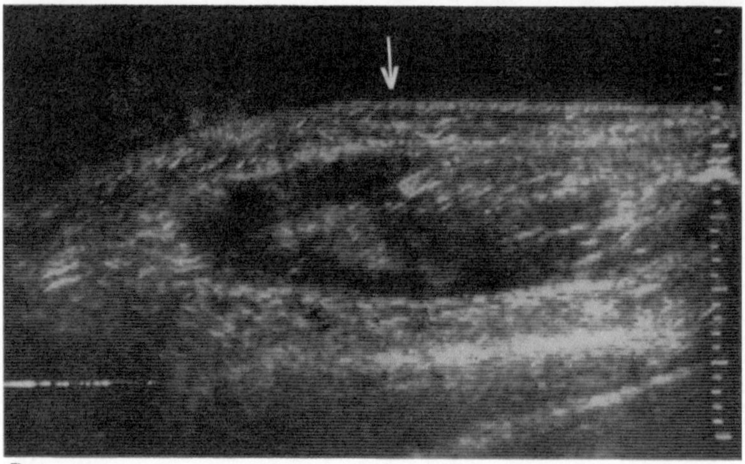

B

Figure 2.23. Pyomyositis, left thigh. Abscess was demonstrated by ultrasound. (**A**) Cross-section of both thighs. (**B**) Supine view of left thigh.

of trauma 1–3 days prior to the onset of the excruciating pain and toxic appearance.

The diagnosis of pyomyositis can usually be confirmed by ultrasound, which shows a mass within the muscle (Fig. 2.23); in some cases, gallium, CT or MRI scans may also be helpful in defining the process.[68,69] Staphylococci can usually be grown from needle aspirants of the muscle abscess but only rarely are found in the blood cultures of these patients.

Pyomyositis requires prompt surgical drainage; treatment with intravenous antibiotics alone has not been satisfactory in our experience or in other reported cases. Rare cases of muscle abscess due to *Gonococcus* have been reported.[70] An increasing incidence of pyomyositis is being reported in AIDS.[70a]

Hemophilus influenzae Cellulitis of the Hand

We have seen two toddlers with septic swelling of the dorsum of the hand, related either to minor trauma or concomitant with respiratory infection (Fig. 2.24). Bone scan showed diffuse inflammation but no evidence for osteomyelitis. Aspiration of the hand grew *Hemophilus influenzae*, type B organisms; in one patient the blood culture was also positive. These youngsters responded to 2 weeks of intravenous therapy. It appears to us that this is another new *Hemophilus* cellulitis syndrome that resembles osteomyelitis or septic arthritis. *Hemophilus* cellulitis syndromes in children may be associated with unrecognized *Hemophilus* meningitis, as is observed in children with *Hemophilus* septic arthritis.[71]

Diskitis

Infection in the intervertebral disk in young children is not rare and constitutes a special syndrome.[72–77] It generally begins with vague leg, hip, or low back pain but may progress over a period of weeks so that the child is unable to walk, then unable to sit, and ultimately lies immobile in bed. Referred abdominal pain, sciatica, and meningeal irritation are less common signs. In the past, diagnosis was extraordinarily difficult; as a result, an extensive literature of untreated children exists. Most got well without specific treatment but were uncomfortable for months, and after narrowing of the disk space finally became apparent on x-rays, they were usually placed in spica plasters. Where an etiology was established, *Staphylococcus aureus* was the most common agent, but less virulent organisms such as *Moraxella kingii* have also been identified.

Previously, diagnosis could not be confirmed for 2–14 weeks until disk-space narrowing was apparent on x-ray or septicemia occurred as the infection spread from the disk into the adjacent vertebral bodies (Figs. 2.25 and 2.26). Earlier (7–14 days) diagnosis is now possible with gallium and technetium scans and MRI. (Fig. 2.27).[39,78] Technetium scans may sometimes be

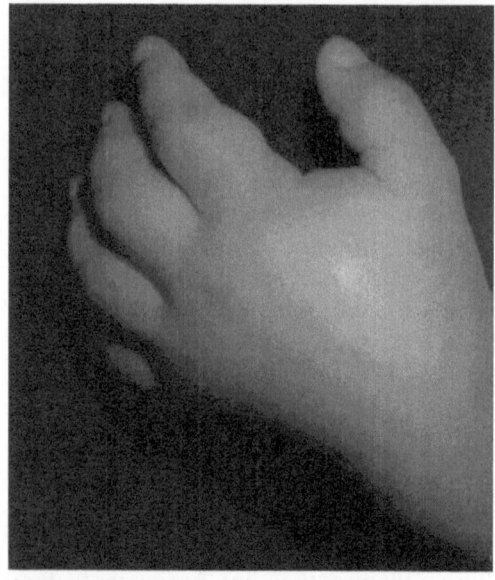

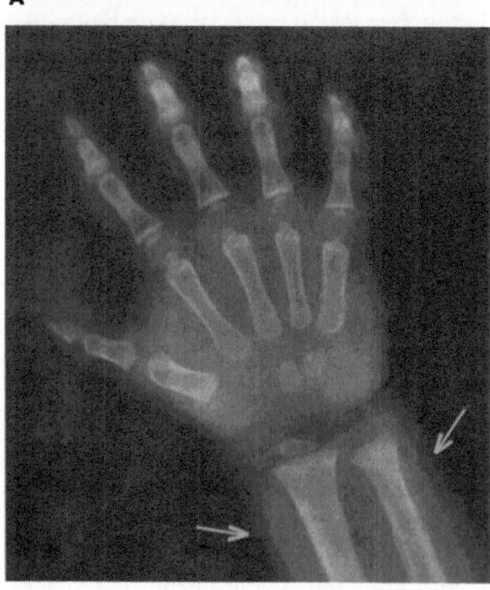

Figure 2.24. (**A**) *Hemophilus influenzae cellulitis* of the hand. (**B**) Dramatic swelling extending up into the arm is shown on film.

negative for many weeks.[39] When the clinical diagnosis is diskitis, after obtaining a blood culture, a needle aspiration of the disk should be performed under fluoroscopy, a specimen should be obtained for culture, and treatment should be begun with an oral antistaphylococcal agent in large doses. It is likely that long periods of disability, hospitalization, and immobilization will be avoided with prompt treatment with oral antistaphylococcal agents. Sev-

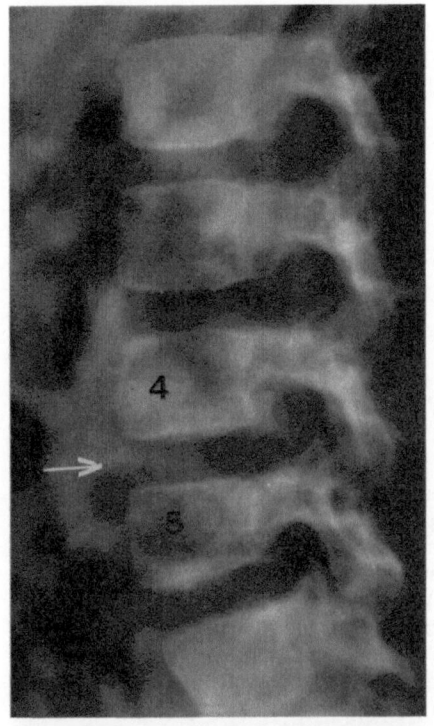

A

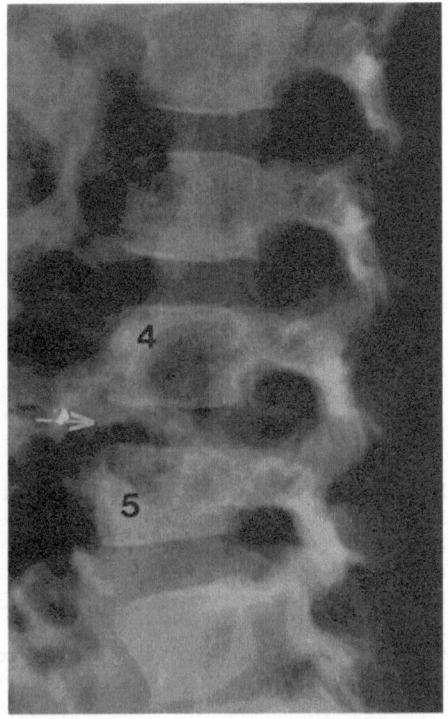

B

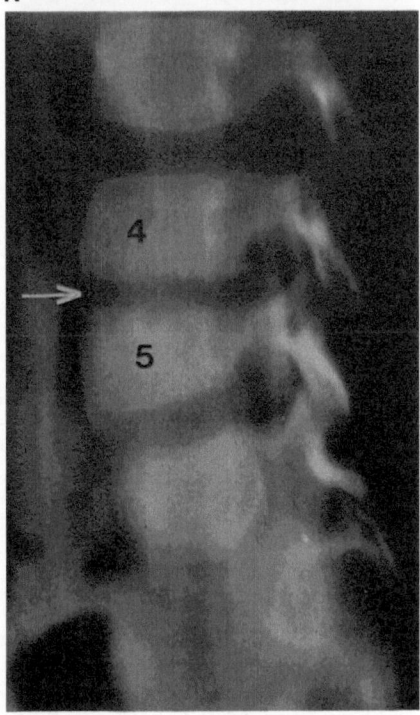

C

Figure 2.25. Radiologic progression of diskitis in a 4-year-old girl. The illness began with a limp in late February and progressed to refusal to walk and then to sit up in bed. Films pictured are from March 5 and 23 and April 20. The initial radiograph (**A**) is normal (A bone scan was also normal at that time.) The intermediate film (**B**) shows beginning of narrowing of the L-4 L-5 disk that was too subtle to be recognized. Film 4 weeks later (**C**) shows obvious narrowing of the disk space with erosions of both adjacent vertebral bodies, a typical radiographic progression of diskitis. Patient was treated with oral antistaphylococcal medication after a few days of intravenous therapy.

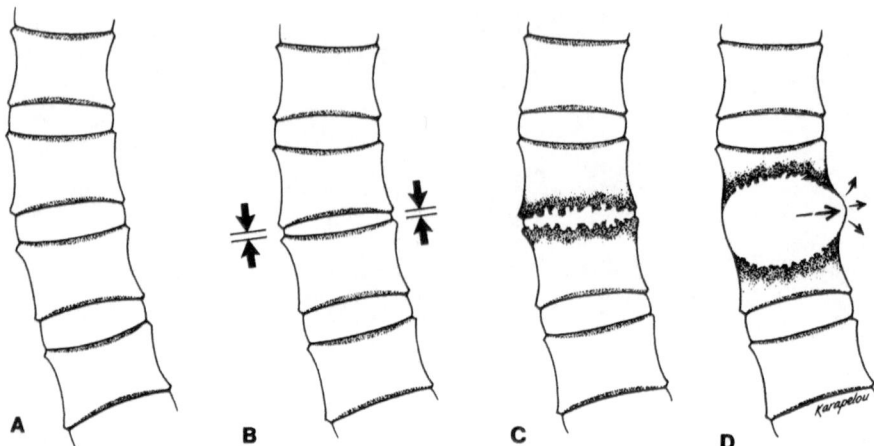

Figure 2.26. Diagram of radiographic progression reflecting pyogenic infection that starts in the intervertebral disk. (**A**) For several weeks, plain films and the technetium bone scan are normal. Gallium scan and MRI are the first studies to become abnormal; the earliest radiologic sign on plain films is narrowing of the affected intervertebral space, but this may be too subtle to appreciate (**B**; and Fig. 2.25B). When the infection causes erosion of the vertebral bone with reactive bone sclerosis (**C**; and Fig. 2.25C), the diagnosis is apparent. In the 16-year-old patient described in the text, there was further ballooning of the infection into the vertebral bodies (osteomyelitis) (**D**), and a myelogram showed posterior extension of the inflammatory granulations. (Modified from Kemp et al.: *J Bone Joint Surg* 55B:698, 1973. Reproduced with permission.)

erely ill patients, however, require intravenous treatment for the vertebral osteomyelitis and sepsis that have ensued.

Many authors have emphasized the benign nature of diskitis in early childhood, and in some institutions it is the policy not to treat this disorder unless suppuration is documented. Even more than in other types of bone and joint infection, proof of diagnosis by culture may be difficult or impossible until very late in the course of the disease. We prefer to treat all these patients and, by doing so, totally avoid the long morbidity associated with the minority (perhaps 35%) of young children who will not recover spontaneously. While in the view of some this constitutes "overtreatment," we find the course of all patients is shortened, and the investment in outpatient oral antistaphylococcal treatment seems, at least to us, to be small compared with the alternative.

Case Report

A healthy 16-year-old basketball star noted a pain in his left foot the day after a game. That night he developed fever that persisted. Two days later, he developed pain in his left hip, followed the next day by pain in his back and right buttock. Many blood cultures were sterile. Extensive evaluation during 3 weeks in his community hospital failed to define the problem. During this time, he became immobile, lying supine in bed, and developed a large decubitus ulcer at his coccyx. After 5 weeks, x-rays

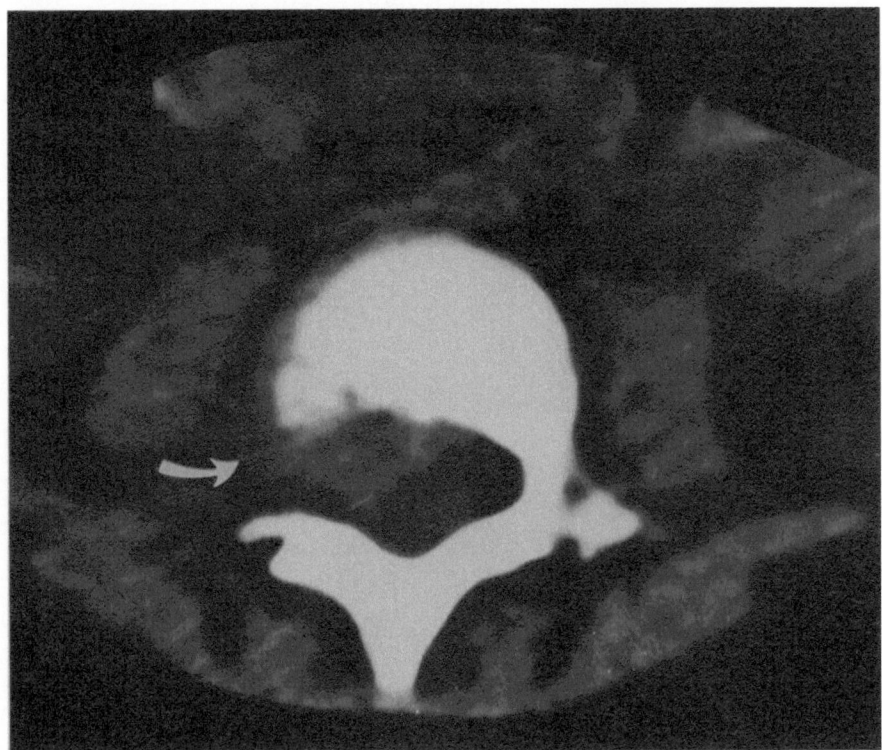

Figure 2.27. MRI in a 2-year-old child with diskkitis; mass (*arrow*) suggested tumor but was inflammatory.

showed narrowing of the T-11-T-12 interspace with associated kyphosis at that level. The end-plates of T-11 and T-12 were eroded. *Staphylococcus aureus* was isolated from multiple blood cultures. Treatment was begun with intravenous oxacillin, which was continued for 4 weeks and followed with oral cloxacillin for 2 months. He was able to walk within 10 days, although back pain persisted for more than a month after treatment was begun. (He was not immobilized in any way as part of his therapy.) He received great acclaim as the "stellar forward" of his team during the next season.

Chronic Recurrent Multifocal Osteomyelitis (CRMO)

Increasing numbers of children are being reported with recurrent attacks of bone pain which generally last from 1 to 12 weeks, associated with radiographic evidence of multifocal, osteolytic lesions, apparently not of infectious origin (Fig. 2.28).[28,29,79-82] These lesions are most frequent in the clavicles and in the distal metaphyses of the long bones but may also occur in the spine causing vertebra plana.[82] In some cases, they have been associated with sterile pustular lesions of the palms and soles—palmoplantar pustulo-

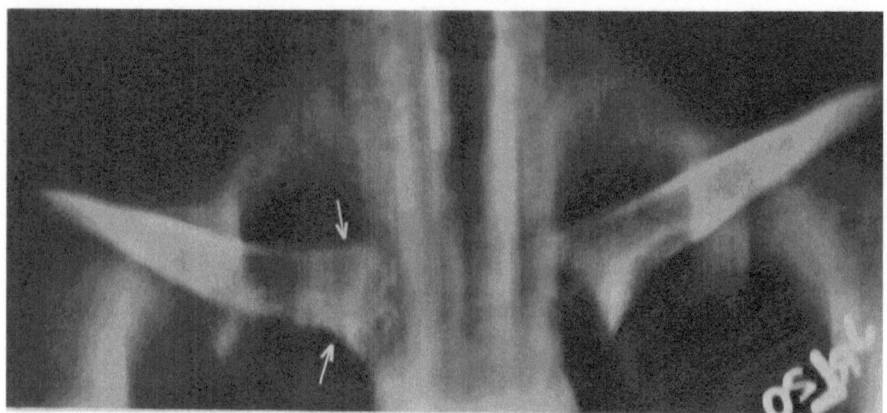

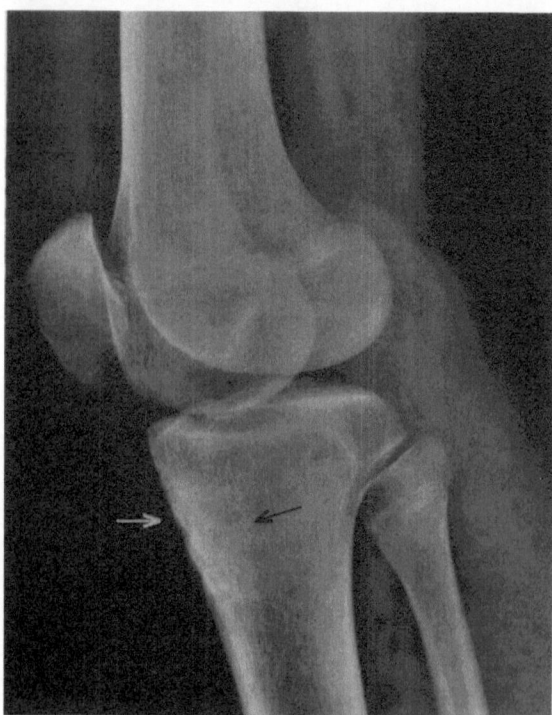

Figure 2.28. Chronic recurrent multifocal osteomyelitis (CRMO) showing sclerosis in the medial right clavicle (**A**) and tibia (**B**) of a 16-year-old girl who complained of pain at these and several other sites. Biopsy of several sites showed only fibrosis. Bone scan showed increased uptake in all symptomatic areas.

sis. There may be local and systemic signs of inflammation, but there is no response to antibiotics. The clinical course may be prolonged and characterized by relapse and remissions for years. Most patients have been reported to respond well to nonsteroidal anti-inflammatory drugs (NSAIDs). Occasionally the lesions are "tumerous" and locally troublesome.

Tuberculosis

Tuberculosis of the bones and joints[83-85] is occurring in increasing frequency in indigent children and may also be acquired from infected caretakers. Children with AIDS may be infected with atypical organisms. Dissemination from BCG vaccination has also been reported in rare instances. A tuberculin test is performed in every patient at the time of the initial visit and if negative *after six weeks of illness*, in the absence of anergy, is accepted as adequate evidence that the arthritis is not tuberculous. In two recent cases of tuberculosis synovitis of the knee we were able to document the diagnosis with a needle biopsy specimen.[86]

Tuberculous rheumatism, Poncet's disease, "a polyarthritis associated with visceral tuberculosis in which there is no evidence of bacteriologic involvement of the joints themselves" (i.e., a reactive arthritis) has also been reported to occur in children.[87] Spina ventosa, tuberculosis of the small bones of the hands that might resemble JRA, has not been seen in our clinic for many years.

Brucellosis

Children who drink raw milk or eat cheese made from unpasteurized milk may develop arthritis and osteomyelitis as manifestions of septicemia with *Brucella melitensis*. Musculoskeletal complaints were predominant in six of 27 American schoolchildren who developed symptoms after an Easter school trip to Spain.[88] Diagnosis is usually a result of serologic testing but the organism can be grown from joint fluid, bone, and blood.[88] The arthritis is most often monarticular in one hip or knee but two joints are affected in 20% and three or more joints is 8% of cases.[89] Combination therapy with trimethoprin-suflamethoxazole (21 days) and gentanycin (5 days) is recommended.[90]

Salmonellosis

Bone and joint infection with *Salmonella* is rare in all pediatric series despite the acknowledged increased susceptibility of children with sickle-cell disease to *Salmonella* infections.[91] Nevertheless, if osteomyelitis or septic arthritis is documented in a child with sickle-cell disease, the chances of the infection being caused by *Salmonella* has been estimated to be 10 times that of it being from any other organism. Clinically, the arthropathy of sickle-cell crisis may be indistinguishable from other arthropathies. We have found bone scans to be helpful in excluding osteomyelitis and demonstrating bone infarcts without evidence of inflammation. However, since bone infarct alone may be the earliest sign of osteomyelitis, even this assumption will lead to an occasional diagnostic error.

Cat-Scratch Disease

This common illness is usually characterized by regional lymphadenitis occurring 1 or 2 weeks after a cat scratch. Occasional patients may present with joint pain secondary to osteolytic bone lesions.[92,93] One child had pain in the knee as the presenting manifestation. X-rays of the hip were initially negative, but after several weeks, a lytic lesion was demonstrated in the right femoral intertrochanteric area. Diagnosis in this and other patients with a lytic bone lesion was achieved by integrating the history of a cat scratch, purulent but "sterile" lymphadenitis, plus a compatible histologic picture of granuloma with central necrosis surrounded by epithelioid cells and lymphocytes. These lesions ultimately healed spontaneously but patients with abscesses of the liver and spleen, overwhelming pneumonia, or encephalitis may be very ill and resemble patients with systemic vasculitis.[94,94a] Recently delicate pleomorphic gram-negative bacilli (*Afipia felis*) have been demonstrated in lesional capillaries and grown from abscesses in immunocompromised hosts. Treatment with gentamycin has been reported to be effective in a seriously ill patient, and ciprofloxacin may be the agent of choice.[94-96]

Acute Septic Arthritis (Nongonococcal)

About one-third of all cases of septic arthritis occur in children; 40% of these are under age 2, and more than half of those occurring under age 2 are due to *Hemophilus influenzae*; 75% of cases occur in weight-bearing joints (knee, hip, and ankle). Large joints of the upper extremity (elbow, wrist, and shoulder) make up almost all of the other affected joints, with the elbow three times as frequent as the shoulder or wrist.[97,98] Over the age of 2, in practically all cases in which a bacteriologic diagnosis is established, *Staphylococcus aureus* is the agent (In one series hemophilus influenza was most frequent in children under 6.)[99] The infection rarely is a complication of local injury and usually is a consequence of bacteremia. An exception is *Pseudomonas* arthritis in metatarsophalangeal joints following puncture wounds of the foot.[100] There is some suggestion that this entity occurs primarily when such wounds have been treated "prophylactically" with oral antibiotics.

The acutely painful, tender, and warm joint with associated muscle spasm and limitation of motion usually presents no diagnostic difficulty. The joint is aspirated with a syringe containing heparin so that the fluid does not clot, and the fluid is examined for cell count, sugar and protein, and stained for bacteria; a separate nonheparinized specimen is obtained for culture. Surgical decompression is advocated for the hip joint regardless of whether the infection is primary or is secondary to osteomyelitis of the femur. All other joints are treated with repeated aspirations as necessary to keep the pressure low. An unsatisfactory clinical response would require surgical drainage of any joint, but we have not had any such experience except where there is an adjacent focus of osteomyelitis that has been diagnosed 48 h or more after onset of symptoms and pus is under pressure in both bone and joint.

As soon as the diagnosis is made clinically and the blood culture and aspirant are obtained, treatment is begun as if for osteomyelitis. Antibiotics are chosen according to the principles detailed by Nelson and Tetzlaff[45,49,101] depending on the age and Gram stain. Children under age 3 are treated for both *Hemophilus* and *Staphylococcus* unless an organism is demonstrated and the appropriate agent is selected. Infections caused by *Hemophilus*, *Streptococcus*, and *Pneumococcus* are treated parenterally for 10 days, *Staphylococcus* for 3 weeks; oral treatment is then continued until the ESR is normal and there are no clinical findings. Thirty percent of children with *Hemophilus* septic arthritis have been reported to have simultaneous purulent meningitis and 22% osteomyelitis which require additional therapy.[71]

It has been repeatedly demonstrated that blood levels of drugs achieved in the joints are adequate without instillation of local antibiotics.[101] Recent evidence presented by Tetzlaff indicates that oral antibiotics are completely satisfactory treatment for septic arthritis when they are administered in the hospital and adjustments in dosage are made to assure a peak serum bacteriocidal titer of at least 1:8.[44,45] It is reasonable to expect that with conscientious parents and doctors, the same regimen could be adapted to outpatient management of septic arthritis, but that remains to be proved.[102]

In our experience, immobilization is unnecessary but may be used for a day or 2 for prevention of pain with movement. The role of steroids and anti-CD18 antibodies at this stage remains to be determined; animal models suggest they may be useful.[102a] We encourage motion with physical therapy as soon as practicable and find NSAID therapy a helpful adjunct during the recovery period when postinfectious inflammatory synovitis and/or reactive arthritis interferes with motion long after all organisms have been destroyed.[103,104] Reactive arthritis may first present during the recovery period after bacterial meningitis.

Although infectious arthritis is said to be a well-recognized and common complication of rheumatoid arthritis[105] we are not certain we have ever seen this or the more recently described pseudoseptic arthritis in JRA patients.

The Gonococcal Arthritis-Dermatitis-Tenosynovitis Syndrome

Disseminated gonococcal infection is the most common cause of infectious arthritis or tenosynovitis in sexually active women. The usual clinical presentation is migratory polyarthritis with fever and chills, often starting within 1 week after a menstrual period.[106] The arthritis then tends to localize in one or two large joints. Painful crops of skin lesions appear, primarily on the extremities. These lesions characteristically begin as a macule or purpuric spot and progress through papular-vesicular stages to pustules. Twenty-six percent of patients have been reported to have tenosynovitis, which may be seen as painful erythema overlying tendon sheaths.

Table 2.14. The Gonococcal Arthritis-Dematitis-Tenosynovitis Syndrome

Migratory polyarthritis starting soon after menses and then localizing in one or two
 large joints
Fever and chills
Painful crops of characteristic embolic skin lesions primarily on the extremities
Tenosynovitis

Diagnosis is usually made on the basis of the characteristic clinical syndrome (Table 2.14), and is proved in only about 50% of cases by culture of the organism from the blood (5%), synovial fluid (25%), or oral, rectal, and genitourinary specimens (20%). Although all patients are presumed to have septicemia, all of the arthritis does not seem to be septic; most instances seem to have the quality of an immune-complex disorder. The response to appropriate treatment for gonorrhea is usually prompt.[107,108] Fatal gonococcal endocarditis may result from inadequately treated gonococcemia.

The clinical picture of chronic meningococcemia is similar.[109–111] Effusions in most cases of meningococcemia are sterile, and cartilage destruction is insignificant even when the joint is truly infected.

Foreign-Body Synovitis

Wood splinters, especially plant thorns such as palm or blackthorn, may dissect in from the surface and produce a chronic synovitis or tendinitis.[112] Plant-thorn synovitis is not rare in children.[113–115] When the inflammation is severe, periosteal new bone may be noted, and when a thorn is sticking into bone, a lytic lesion stimulating osteomyelitis or tumor may be seen radiographically (Fig. 2.29).[116,117] Often, the history of injury has been forgotten, as months may elapse between entry of the fragment and its dissection into the joint.[118] In our experience, careful history-taking in monarticular arthritis provides the clue.

The diagnosis is easier when the foreign body is glass or metal and is itself apparent on x-ray (Fig 2.30). If the splinter is radiographically inapparent but the entry was recent and a tract is apparent, a sinogram may show the splinter.[116] Thermography ultrasound, CT, and MRI studies may also aid in localization. Occasionally, there is secondary infection, and culture of the effusion or operative specimen may produce a soil or water organism such as is found on plants.[115] Only surgical removal of the splinter is effective therapy. Careful surgical exploration may be necessary to prove the diagnosis.

Case Report

A 4-year-old boy rode his bicycle into the "picker tree" (blackberry bramble) and came in crying with thorns in his scalp, which the mother removed. Two days later, he complained of pain in his left elbow, and his arm was placed in a sling; it was

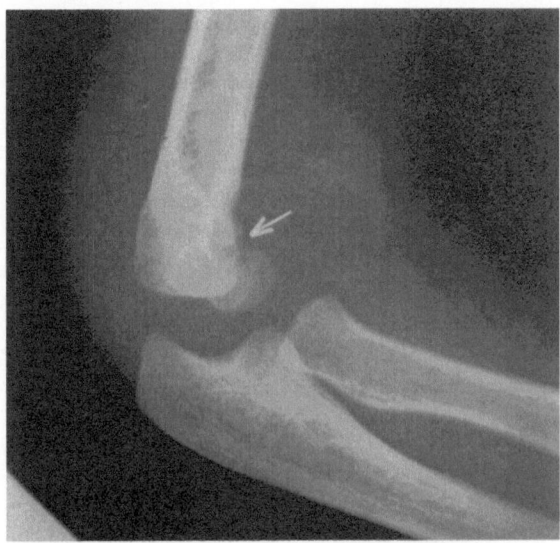

Figure 2.29. Plant-thorn synovitis with erosion of the distal humerus caused by inflammation around the thorn. Monarticular arthritis may mimic septic arthritis or JRA. This condition is not rare in areas where children are exposed to thorny plants and must be considered in cases of unusual monarticular arthritis.

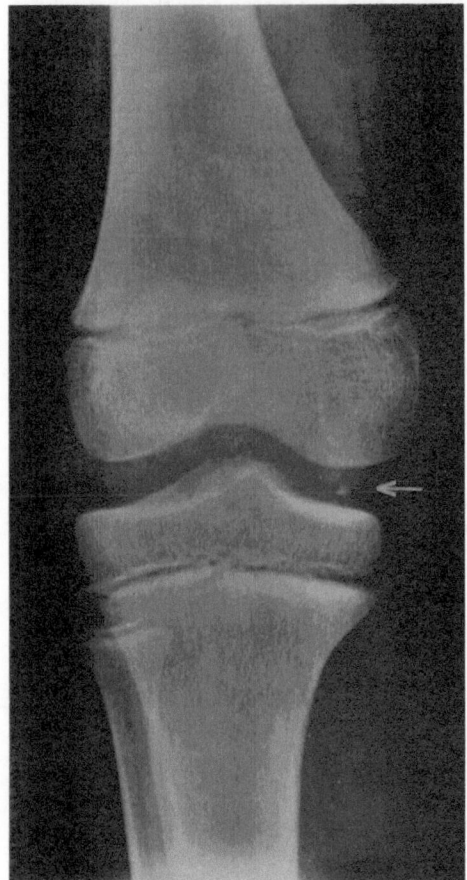

Figure 2.30. Foreign body (glass) causing a right knee effusion in a 8-year-old boy. The glass entered at the time of a fall 6 months earlier. Foreign-body synovitis may take a long time to evolve.

thought he had injured his elbow at the time of the bicycle accident, but the possibility that a thorn was involved not entertained. Two weeks later, the pain became worse, and he developed fever; aspiration of the joint effusion was sterile, and the fluid contained only 1500 WBCs/mm³. Four weeks later, periosteal new-bone formation became apparent along the medial aspect of the humerus, along with a lytic lesion of the humerus (Fig. 2.29). The joint effusion now contained 72,300 WBCs/mm³ (87% polys) and was again sterile. There was no response to intravenous treatment for osteomyelitis. Seven weeks after the accident the elbow was explored surgically, and a thorn was removed from the posterior synovium. Without further therapy, he recovered completely.

Case Report

An 8-year-old boy developed pain and swelling of his knee. Laboratory studies, including a complete blood count (CBC), ESR, and examination of joint fluid, were normal. The pain and effusion continued to get worse, and the ESR rose to 45 mm/h. An x-ray showed a foreign body (Fig. 2.30), and a history of an injury 8 months earlier was then obtained; he had fallen on glass and had a scar over the knee where he had been cut. At surgical exploration, a small piece of glass was removed from the synovium, and he recovered without further therapy.

Fungal Arthritis

Essentially, all fungi may cause arthritis in at least one of four ways: (1) by direct invasion of a joint either from infected adjacent bone or from the skin as in Madura foot; (2) by causing erythema nodosum in which the arthritis is usually associated with the typical skin lesions but may occasionally appear alone; (3) by septicemic spread with formation of granulomas in the joints.[119,120] (this is the most difficult problem diagnostically; the clinical picture may simulate polyarticular rheumatoid arthritis and sometimes may be differentiated only by examination of tissue.) (4) as a complication of intraarticular injection of corticosteroids.[121]

Arthritis and pericarditis were occasional manifestations in a recent urban epidemic of histoplasmosis.[122] Prior to recognition of histoplasmosis as the cause of the illness, many patients were thought to have a rheumatic disease.

Coccidiodomycosis is a common infection in the southwestern United States; it may be acquired there during travel and may disseminate and first become clinically apparent anywhere in the world many years after the initial infection. Of 14 recently reported childhood cases, three presented with musculoskeletal complaints, including knee, thigh, and hand pain and swelling, as manifestations of chronic fungal osteomyelitis.[123] Chest radiographs usually suggest the diagnosis, which can be confirmed with serologic testing and demonstration of the organism in pathologic specimens; skin tests are often negative in disseminated coccidiodomycosis. Treatment with amphotericin B is generally effective.

Neonatal candidiasis with arthritis has been repeatedly reported in sick neonates with predisposing situations. Intra-articular injection of corticosteroids in adults has also resulted in *Candida* arthritis.[121]

Parasitic Arthritis

Immune-complex formation has been demonstrated in many parasitic infections.[124] As a consequence, arthralgia is frequent in malaria and babesiosis;[125,125a] arthritis has occasionally been reported in association with giardiasis, blastocytis hominus, and in overwhelming *Strongyloides* and *Taenia* infections.[124,126,127] We have successfully "cured" arthritis by treatment for giardia and strongyloides, and these infestations may worsen other forms of arthritis.[128] Lymphatic obstruction caused by systemic filariasis may be associated with chylous arthritis of the knee.

Syphilis and Other Diseases Caused by Flexibacteria

Both congenital and acquired syphilis may present with a variety of arthritic manifestations. Although the diagnosis of childhood syphilis was easy for a previous generation of pediatricians, cases seen in our own hospital during the past three decades have been "missed." The importance of the musculoskeletal manifestations is illustrated by our pediatric rheumatologist being called for some recent cases.

In congenital syphilis, a classic presenting manifestation may be pseudoparalysis of an arm or leg, sometimes associated with joint swelling. Syphilitic invasion of bone results in osteochondritis, periostitis, dactylitis, and metaphysitis, which cause the musculoskeletal symptoms and are demonstrable radiographically. These manifestations of syphilitic infection may occur in later childhood if congenital syphilis is not adequately treated in infancy.

Another form of syphilitic arthritis occurs in older children, usually between ages 8 and 16, who had inadequately treated congenital lues. These gummatous infections are called Clutton's joints and most commonly present solely with knee effusions; occasionally, the elbows are also involved.[129] Although Clutton's joints were originally said to be painless, they really are slightly painful and do have minimal inflammatory signs. Diagnosis is made by obtaining serologic tests for syphilis. Both the infantile forms of congenital syphilis and Clutton's joints respond to treatment with penicillin.

Pediatricians may now also expect to see secondary syphilis; recent cases of venereal disease on our service have included two young boys, one an actor in child porno films, the other a young male homosexual prostitute. In a study of 34 adult patients seeking medical care for secondary syphilis, that diagnosis was not entertained by 47% of the physicians who initially examined them.[130]

Polyarthralgias are a common manifestation of secondary lues, and the clinical picture may resemble subacute bacterial endocarditis, acute rheumatic fever, or rheumatoid arthritis.[131] When arthritis occurs, it tends to be symmetrical and nonmigratory, settling most frequently in the knees and resembling Clutton's joints. Sometimes the arthritis is accompanied by tenosynovitis; in general, the tenosynovitis associated with secondary syphilis is "cold" in contradistinction to the heat and redness that is characteristic of the gonorrheal tenosynovitis-arthritis syndrome. Secondary lues is usually accompanied by generalized lymphadenopathy; the postauricular nodes tend to be especially large, tender, and boggy. This characteristic postauricular lymphadenopathy is sometimes accompanied by a maculopapular rash and infectious oral mucous plaques, all good clues to the diagnosis of secondary syphilis. Similar manifestations may occur in yaws.

Migratory arthralgias or arthritis may also occur in other flexibacterial diseases, including rat-bite fever, Haverhill fever, and leptospirosis.[132–135]

Viral Arthritis

Arthritis probably may be associated with or follow practically all viral illnesses and has been reported specifically with mumps,[136] varicella,[137] rubella, Fifth disease (PARVO 19 erythema infectiosum), coxsackie,[138] ECHO, alpha viruses,[139] adenovirus, Herpes simplex,[140] infectious mononucleosis,[141,142] hepatitis, cytomegalovirus disease,[143] vaccinia, and smallpox.[144] Adults are more susceptible than children to at least some of these viral arthritides.

Several different pathogenetic mechanisms may be operative in viral arthritis.[145,146] Rarely, as in vaccinia, the arthritis is a result of virus actually invading the synovial tissue, replicating there, and causing local inflammation and cell necrosis. In other situations such as rubella, arthritis probably results from local host immune response to virus or viral products present in the joint. In most cases, however, the pathogenetic mechanism is probably a systemic serum sickness type of reaction, as in hepatitis, with formation of immune complexes that are demonstrable in both serum and synovial fluid. Nonnecrotizing vasculitis may be seen in synovial membrane biopsy specimens obtained from these patients.

Depending on the mechanism(s) involved, the arthritis may be mild or severe and may be monarticular, pauciarticular, or polyarticular. It may resemble septic infection, be migratory as in acute rheumatic fever, or be mistaken for drug allergy or rheumatoid arthritis. Cases may be seen sporadically or in epidemics. The process is generally brief, although occasional patients may have symptoms intermittently for years, usually with diminishing intensity.[137,147,148]

When the arthritis has the benign quality most typical of viral arthritis, or if the nature of the basic illness is apparent because of an exanthem or other distinctive clinical features or as part of an epidemic of known viral illness, there may be little need to exclude other possibilities. However, as discussed in more detail in the section on Septic Infections of Bones and Joints, 24% of children with osteomyelitis in our series have been misdiagnosed initially as having viral illnesses, and even the most experienced physician will have difficulty sometimes in distinguishing septic from viral arthritis when only a single joint is affected. Synovial fluid examination should be performed whenever there is a possibility of septic infection. The synovial fluid is generally "benign" in viral infection and often contains a preponderance of mononuclear cells (Fig. 2.31).

Three distinctive viral arthritis syndromes deserve special emphasis: rubella and hepatitis and PARVO 19.

Rubella: The "Catcher's Crouch" Syndrome. Brief episodes of polyarthritis are commonly seen in epidemic rubella; adult women are most prone to the arthritis.[139,149] Occasionally, the arthritis precedes the other clinical manifestations, but usually it accompanies the rash or follows it by only a few days. Most patients get well within 2 weeks.

Rubella is now less frequently seen in the United States, and rubella vaccine strains have been developed with little arthritogenic potential, so in infants vaccine arthritis after primary immunization now is also uncommon.

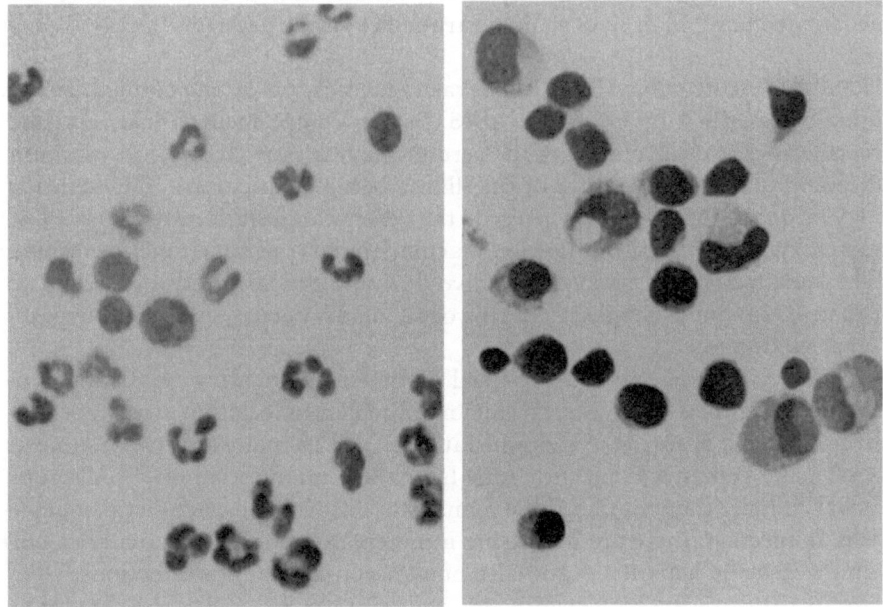

A   **B**

Figure 2.31. Comparison of the cells in the synovial fluid in rheumatoid arthritis (**A**) and in rubella or rubella-vaccine-induced synovitis (**B**). (Reproduced with permission from R.J. Chambers, "Rubella Synovitis," *Annals of the Rheumatic Diseases*, p. 266. 1963.)

Children with rubella vaccine arthritis tend to have a rather distinctive syndrome, awakening in the morning with pain in the knees out of proportion to visible swelling and standing with the knees bent in what has been termed the "catcher's crouch" position.[150] Tenosynovitis may also be seen in the dorsum of the hands. Many children have an associated neuritis, primarily manifested as painful paresthesias of the hands or feet. The history of recent vaccination, characteristic morning stance, and unusual neuritis generally makes the correct diagnosis apparent. Physicians administering rubella vaccine should warn patients of the possibility of this reaction at the time the vaccine is given. Immune individuals may have attacks of arthritis following re-immunization.[151]

The arthritic complaints respond well to aspirin. The child is generally better in the afternoon but for a few days has similar symptoms each morning, with decreasing severity. Most of these reactions are short-lived, but occasionally episodes have recurred over a period of years.[139]

Rubella virus can be demonstrated in the joints in a few of these patients and may persist for months.[152,153] The arthritis would seem to be a manifestation of host immune response to the virus or residual viral products in the joint. There has been no evidence of actual invasion of the synovium by virus. In the few case reports of chronic histologic damage in individuals previously reported to have rubella vaccine arthritis, one cannot be certain that there is any relationship between the current arthritis and the antecedent vaccine arthritis. However, it is possible that a synovial-lining-cell neoantigen may result in chronic postrubella vaccine arthritis.[147]

Hepatitis. Acute polyarthritis and a rash may be a prodrome of hepatitis, as initially described by Graves in 1843. Serum complement is low, and the reaction seems clearly to be of the serum sickness type. It subsides as jaundice appears and the nature of the illness becomes apparent. The arthritis may be quite severe and may precede the other manifestations by weeks. The rash may be urticarial but is often maculopapular and sometimes petechial. The latex fixation test may be positive during the illness and then revert to negative. Immune complex nephritis occasionally occurs, creating a hepatorenal syndrome.

Both circulating and tissue-fixed complement-binding viral antigen-antibody complexes have been demonstrated in association with this syndrome when it is associated with hepatitis B, and as many as 30% of subjects with acute hepatitis B infection may have these manifestations.[154] Although it was initially thought that these manifestations were characteristic of hepatitis B infection, there are increasing numbers of reports of an identical syndrome in acute hepatitis A and also non-A, non-B hepatitis infections.[155,156]

Parvovirus B19.[157,158] This virus causes epidemic erythema infectiosum or Fifth ("slapped cheek") disease, aplastic crises in children with hemolytic anemias, some cases of Henoch-Schonlein purpura, fetal death, and, commonly, arthritis. In adult females anthropathy occurs in 60% of cases; in adult males—30%. Attacks of pain and swelling were usually brief and self-limited (less than 10 days duration) and occurred soon after the onset of rash in the small joints of the hands and feet, or in a knee, but can affect any joint. Some patients have recurrent episodes, each usually less severe and of shorter duration than the prior attack (similar to rubella), and 10% of arthritis-affected adult women have arthritis of sufficient duration to suggest RA. Since up to 30% of the population seroconverts as adults, parvovirus arthritis is a common disorder. Live virus has not been grown from joint aspirants but B19 DNA has been detected in joint fluid of an affected individual.

Joint symptoms are thought to occur in only 5% of children with Fifth disease; the prevalence of B19 infection in children has not been established yet nor has the frequency of parvovirus as a cause of chronic childhood arthritis.[158a]

The spectrum of disease caused by B19 is constantly expanding: hemophagocytic syndromes induced by this or other viruses may resemble systemic JRA,[159] desquamation of the palms and soles following the rash may resemble that seen in Kawasaki disease,[160] and one case of systemic vasculitis seemed to be a manifestation of chronic B19 infection which responded to gamma globulin infusion.[161]

Chronic Active Liver Disease (CALD)

All forms of viral hepatitis may lead to this disorder.[162] Other factors implicated in its etiology include drugs, alcohol, and genetic predisposition, including C4 deficiency.[163] The manifestations of severe CALD are often those of florid autoimmune multisystem disease and may include vasculitis and arthritis.[164] However, the hepatic manifestations are out of proportion to those usually seen in other connective tissue disorders and anti-liver-kidney microsomal antibodies are usually present in significant titer. Women predominate among hepatitis-B-antigen-negative cases, and the frequency of clinical and laboratory manifestations of rheumatic disease is so high in that group that the disorder was formerly called "lupoid hepatitis" (see Chapter 5 under Hepatic Disease). Adequate management of the other features of CALD provides relief of the arthritic manifestations and may be life-saving.[165]

Arthritis Associated with Other Infectious Agents

Migratory polyarthritis has been reported in association with infection with *Mycoplasma pneumoniae*[166,167] and with psittacosis[168] and is commonly seen with *Lymphogranuloma venereum*.

Arthropod-borne Arthritis

Rocky Mountain Spotted Fever. Rocky Mountain spotted fever (RMSF), a rickettsial vasculitis that presents with fever, arthralgias, myalgias, swelling of the hands and feet, and a rash that appears first on the extremities, including the palms and soles, may be mistaken for a rheumatic disease.[125] More than 1100 cases are reported in the United States each year, primarily from outside the Rocky Mountain area. Diagnosis depends on recognition of the clinical pattern of illness and subsequent demonstration of rising serum titers against *Proteus* OX-19 antigen, and specific serologic tests. Treatment with tetracycline should be instituted promptly when this diagnosis is considered. RMSF continues to have a 5–10% fatality rate in the United States! Physicians should consider the diagnosis of RMSF in any patient who, during spring, and summer, has been in a RMSF-endemic area and develops fever.[169]

Lyme Disease. This epidemic multisystem disease initially described in Old Lyme, Connecticut, and termed "Lyme arthritis" is the most common arthropod-borne disease in the United States (Fig. 2.32).[170–176] The tick, usually *Ixodes*, must remain attached for a minimum of 24 hours, and usually 48–72 hours to inject the spirochete.[177] Children are more susceptible than adults; an "epidemic" of JRA reported to health authorities by the mother of one child led to recognition of the disorder as an entity. Infections have been acquired in most states, especially Cape Cod to southern New Jersey and in

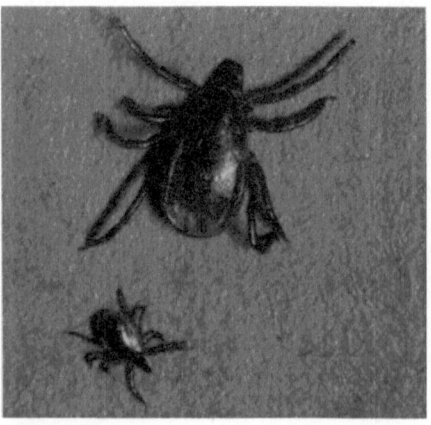 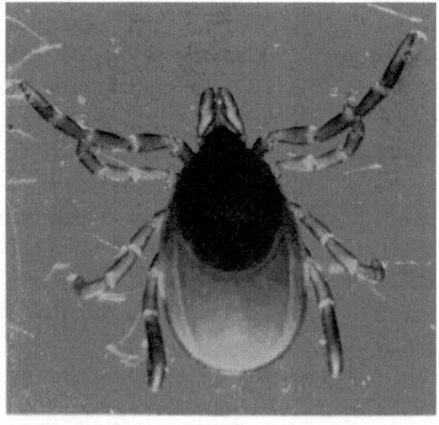

A   **B**

Figure 2.32. (**A**) Appearance of the deer tick *(Ixodes dammini)*, adult and nymph, associated with Lyme disease in eastern United States (note uniformily dark anterior dorsum) as contrasted with the dog tick (**B**) *(Dermacentor andersoni)*, which carries the rickettsia causing Rocky Mountain spotted fever. (**A**, courtesy of Drs. P.A. Rossignol and A. Spielman; **B**, courtesy of Dr. D.D. Despommier.) Other tick vectors occur in other areas.

areas of California, Oregon Minnesota, Wisconsin, Georgia, and Nevada, and in most European countries, Asia, and Australia. As a result of travel, symptoms may first appear thousands of miles from the source of infection.

Erythema Chronicum Migrans (Stage 1). A characteristic skin lesion, erythema chronicum migrans (ECM), occurs at the site(s) of the presumed bite(s) in 40% of patients. The lesion consists of a red spot with a pale center that may grow over a period of days or weeks to a distinctive bright red expanding circle 3–20 inches in diameter (Fig. 2.33). In the few instances in which patients remember having tick bites at the site, 3–32 days elapse from the time of the bite to the onset of the lesion, which, if left untreated, typically lasts about 3 weeks and may be associated with a "flulike" illness. At this stage of organism (*Borrelia burgdorferi*) may be grown from blood culture in 21% of patients tested in a most experienced laboratory.[178]

Arthritis, Neurologic, and Cardiac Manifestations (Stage 2). One to fifty-two weeks after the onset of ECM (median 8 weeks) 10% of untreated ECM patients develop a systemic illness that, in addition to arthritis,[174,179–181] may include Bell's palsy,[174] cranial neuropathy,[182] peripheral neuropathy,[183] aseptic

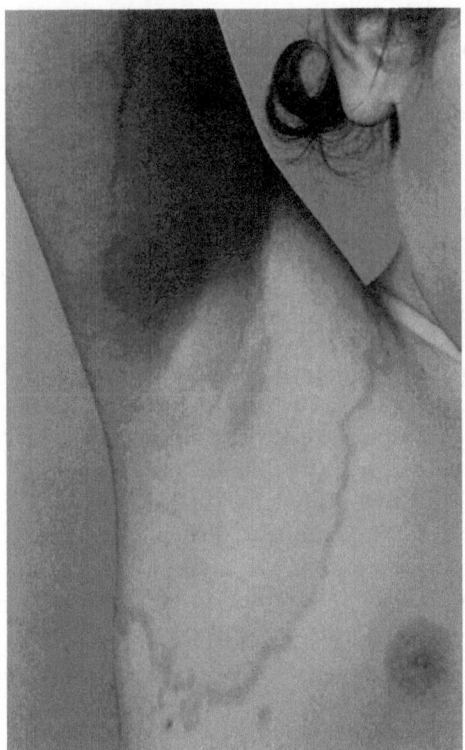

Figure 2.33. Erythema chronicum migrans, the characteristic demal reaction to the tick bite that may later be followed by arthritis, neurologic manifestations, and sometimes cardiac arrhythmia in Lyme disease. Treatment of patients with this skin rash with penicillin reduces the incidence of subsequent arthritis. We question all children with recent onset of arthritis about any prior history of this skin rash, or other unusual rashes. While ECM is a classic finding, other rashes, including urticarial vasculitis, may occur.[22a]

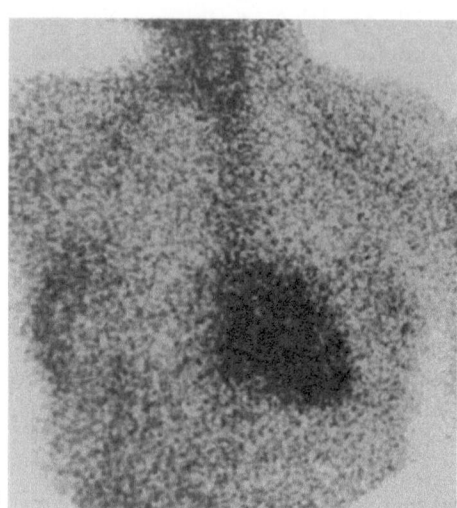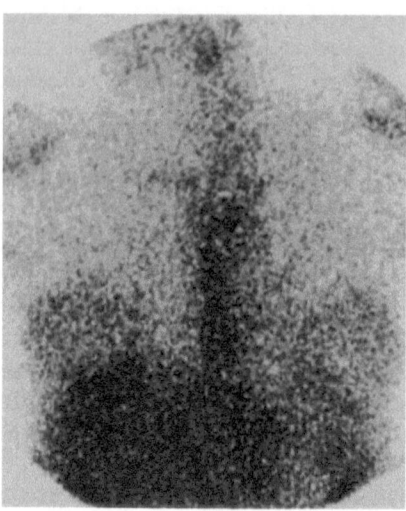

A   B

Figure 2.34. (**A**) Gallium-67 scan showing striking uptake by myocardium (24 h after 3.5 mCi). (**B**) Follow-up scan 8 weeks later, showing normal findings. (Reprinted with permission from Jacobs J.C., ref. 188, with permission of C.V. Mosby Co.)

meningitis, stroke[184] encephalitis,[185-187] hyperesthesia, myocarditis,[188-193] (Fig. 2.34) and/or cardiac arrhythmias.[194-199] Occasional patients develop myositis,[200,201] iritis,[180] or orbital pseudotumor. Organisms may be found in synovium,[179] bone,[180] brain, myocardium,[193] and many other organs (Fig. 2.35).

If Lyme arthritis in children is left untreated most will recover, but 31% will still have occasional episodes of joint pain 10–15 years later. Four percent of these children will also develop keratitis 6 years later.[202] Four percent will also develop a subtle encephalopathy characterized by memory impairment, headache and fatigue, accompanied by intrathecal antibody production typical of Lyme encephalopathy, 11–12 years after the arthritis.[202]

A symptom may subside quickly or last for months. Different manifestations may appear at different times, even months apart. In a group of patients with erythema chronicum migrans who were followed expectantly by rheumatologists, 46% ultimately developed pain on motion of their joints, although only half of these ever had objective evidence of arthritis as characterized by swelling. The knee was the most commonly affected joint; most patients had involvement of only one or a few joints. The attacks were sometimes recurrent, but each episode tended to be milder and to be followed by longer periods of remission. Symptoms in any one joint rarely persist longer than 8 days.

Persistent Lyme Disease (Stage 3). Chronic arthritis, clinically indistinguishable from erosive rheumatoid arthritis; keratitis; and chronic encephalopathic

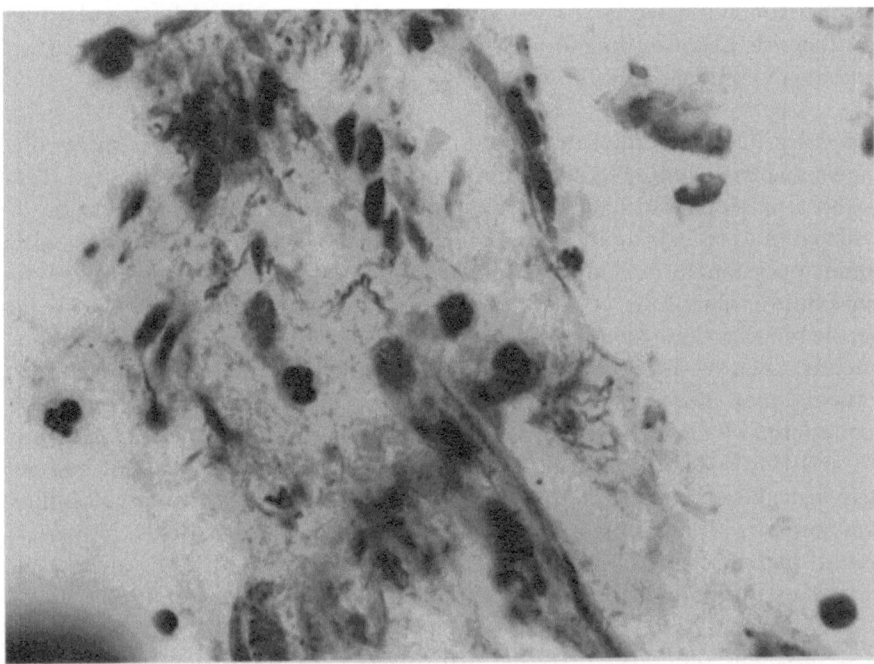

Figure 2.35. Photomicrograph of fibrous connective tissue adjacent to bony tradeculae (needle biopsy of distal femur of a 6-year-old boy with Lyme arthritis); a coiled spirochete (*arrows*) is seen in an area of mild inflammation. (Dieterle stain, ×1250)) (Reprinted with permission from Jacobs J.C., ref. 180. Copyright by the American Medical Association.)

and motor radiculoneuropathies have been reported as late and persistent manifestations of Lyme disease. A late skin rash, violaceous edematous plaque or nodules on the dorsum of the hands and feet called acrodermatitis chronica atrophicans (ACA), has been reported in adults, is histologically identical to lichen sclerosus et atrophicus, and might be confused with localized scleroderma. Morphea, linear scleroderma and Parry-Romberg syndrome have been reported in children (see Chapter 8).

Fatigue and subtle mental disorders and polyneuropathy may be late manifestations of Lyme disease.[202] Two-thirds of patients with unequivocal serological evidence of Lyme disease with chronic neurological symptoms were improved by specific anti-Lyme therapy.[203] However, most patients with these complaints, in our experience, are not helped by treatment for Lyme disease but may be helped by conventional therapy; this has also been found in patients with chronic Lyme arthritis, in whom conventional treatment for their rheumatic complaints is the most effective therapy.[204]

Overdiagnosis of Lyme disease in areas where 20% or more of individuals will test positive for antibodies to *B. burgdorferi* either because of prior exposure or because of polyclonal B-cell activation from other disorders (such as infectious mononucleosis or subacute bacterial endocarditis) has resulted in considerable delay in diagnosis of other conditions and extra morbidity for patients in endemic areas.[205,206]

Laboratory Findings. Laboratory studies in affected patients have generally shown a normal white blood count and hematocrit, with mildly elevated ESR in those patients who have or are about to develop arthritis. Aspiration of synovial fluid reveals an increase in white cells, primarily granulocytes, with counts occasionally reaching as high as 100,000/mm³.[200] In one clinic synovial fluid eosinophilia (34–79%) was typical of Lyme disease.[181] Synovial needle biopsies done on a few patients have revealed a proliferation of mononuclear cells with synovial hypertrophy and vascular proliferation.[179] Patients may have serum cryoprecipitates, in which antibody may be sequestered,[207] elevated serum Clq binding, and diminished levels of serum C3 and C4.[208] Those patients who do have these laboratory abnormalities demonstrable at the time of the ECM, and especially those with cryglobulins containing IgM, are most likely to subsequently develop arthritis. However, not all patients with Lyme disease have had antecedent ECM, and not all children with Lyme arthritis have these immunologic abnormalities.

Diagnosis. The diagnosis of Lyme arthritis is easy when one has seen the characteristic antecedent ECM skin lesion, if the physician can obtain a history of that distinctive rash, or if many of the other features of Lyme disease occur together with arthritis after a known tick bite in an area of the country in which the disorder is endemic.[206] The diagnosis should be considered, however, whenever arthritis and neurologic manifestations or cardiac arrhythmias occur in the same patient or in various family members during the same year or in mini-epidemics within a community (Table 2.15). As in many other diseases, diagnosis often depends upon dependable serologic confirmation.[205a,206]

Serologic Diagnosis. Rising titers of IgM antibodies, which fall as IgG antibodies are produced, provide unequivocal serologic evidence of Lyme dis-

Table 2.15. Clues to the Diagnosis of Lyme Disease

History of tick bite

Erythema chronicum migrans—a distinctive bright red expanding circular skin lesion, 3–20 inches in diameter, 3–32 days after the bite

Arthritis and neurologic manifestations (especially Bell's palsy, peripheral neuropathy, aseptic meningitis, hyperesthesia, pseudotumor of the orbit) and cardiac arrthythmias 1–52 weeks after the skin lesion

Mini-epidemics of some of these manifestations among family members or in the community

ease. (ELISA is the favored technique.) Such conclusive serologic evidence is rarely obtained; the test is poorly standardized with abundant false positives, false negatives, and cross reactions to other spirochetes and disorders such as infectious mononucleosis and SLE with polyclonal B-cell reactions, and a 20% rate of positivity in asymptomatic individuals in certain endemic areas.[209] Western blot tests, now readily available, are more definitive when positive.[205a,210] Cellular immune responses may also help in identifying those ill with Lyme disease.[211] Lyme disease has attracted the public fancy; in endemic areas everyone thinks they have it and many parents demand treatment, and re-treatment of their children with or without serologic evidence of disease, sometimes neglecting proper care of the real problems.[208,211a,212] Only four of 56 patients referred to a neighboring Lyme clinic for possible *late* Lyme disease were thought to have that disorder as an explanation for their symptoms.[213] The presence of positive serologies to *B. burgdorferi* in the presence of other diseases can lead to diagnostic confusion, and misdiagnosis of Lyme disease may lead to delay in recognition and institution of appropriate treatment for a multitude of other conditions.[205,205a]

Treatment. Antibiotic (penicillin) treatment early in the course of ECM has been shown to lessen dramatically the incidence of subsequent arthritis. We have treated ECM in young children with penicillin V just as we treat streptococcal sore throats, and have treated older children with doxycycline, 100mg twice daily; most clinicians in endemic areas now treat for 21 days.[211a] Five daily doses of a new antibiotic, azithromycin, may be preferable.[170] We treat arthritis in children with oral penicillin, 100 mg/kg/day in four divided doses (maximum 4 grams), together with probenecid, 40 mg/kg/day in divided doses (maximum 2 grams) for 21 days; others succeed 96% of the time with less.[175] Treatment regimens are constantly changing;[170,214] Table 2.16 provides the latest guidelines from Dr. Steere.[212] We treat patients who remove *Ixodes* ticks thought to have been attached for 24 hours as if they have ECM.

Treatment of patients with "fibromyalgia" and spondyloarthritic symptoms is apparently universally unsuccessful and should be avoided.[204,206,213] Intravenous ceftriaxone, often insisted upon by parents of children who have not responded to oral treatment (usually because their symptoms are not a result of persistent borrelia infection), results in biliary pseudolithiasis in 50% of cases.[215]

Prognosis. In general, the prognosis for children with Lyme arthritis is excellent, and full recovery without residua should be the expectation.[175,202] However, a few patients with Lyme arthritis, after 4–24 months of recurrent transient attacks of arthritis, have gone on to develop chronic erosive arthritis of the knee pathologically indistinguishable from rheumatoid arthritis.[216,217] Susceptibility to chronic arthritis may be enhanced in patients with HLA-DR4 and DR2.[218] T-cell responses to spirochetal antigens

Table 2.16. Choices of Antibiotic Therapy for Lyme Disease

	Drug	Adult Daily Dosage	Length of Course (Days)
Early disease	Doxycycline	100 mg bid	10–21
	Amoxicillin	500 mg tid	10–21
	Erythromycin	250 mg qid	10–21
Neurologic manifestations			
Facial palsy alone	Doxycycline	100 mg bid	10–21
	Amoxcillin	500 mg tid	10–21
	Erythromycin	250 mg qid	10–21
Other (e.g., meningitis)	Penicillin G	20 million units intravenously	14–21
	Ceftriaxone	2 gm intravenously	14–21
Lyme carditis			
Mild	Doxycycline	100 mg bid	30
Moderate to severe	Penicillin G	20 million units intravenously	14–21
	Ceftriaxone	2 gm intravenously	14–21
Lyme arthritis	Doxycycline	100 mg bid	30
	Amoxicillin* and probenecid	500 mg of each qid	30
	Penicillin G	20 million units intravenously	14–21
	Ceftriaxone	2 gm intravenously	14–21

*We use penicillin V, 100,000 units/kg/day (up to 4 grams daily) in four divided doses in place of amoxicillin and find this regimen excellent. (See also American Academy of Pediatrics, Pediatrics 88:176–179, 1991.) (Modified with permission from: Rahn, D.W., and Malawista, S.E., Clinical Judgment in Lyme Disease, Hospital Practice, 25(3):39–56, 1990.) For use of azithromycin see Ref. 170.

may be excessive in these individuals.[219] This is analogous to the subset of pauciarticular juvenile rheumatoid arthritis of the knees associated with the presence of antinuclear antibodies and uveitis in little girls that is associated with HLA-DR5. These observations in Lyme arthritis seem to confirm the hypothesis that an infectious agent may trigger, in genetically susceptible individuals, a disordered immune response that leads to chronic arthritis and suggest that in this sense Lyme disease may be a model for the DR5 subset of JRA.

Congenital Borellia Infection. When infections takes place during early pregnancy the fetus may be transplacentally infected, resulting in neonatal death or malformation of the fetus. Only a few such cases have been documented so the risk seems small even in highly endemic areas.[220,221]

Special Syndromes Related to Infection

Musculoskeletal Manifestations of Bacterial Infection

Direct invasion of the bones and joints by bacteria results in osteomyelitis and septic arthritis. Dissemination of bacteria to the joints may also occur in less dramatic fashion as part of subacute bacterial endocarditis (SBE) or in the course of brucellosis, chronic meningococcemia, and gonoccemia. However, immune-complex disease seems to be the most frequent pathogenetic mechanism resulting in arthritis as a manifestation of these bacterial infections.

Arthritis as a Manifestation of Subacute Bacterial Endocarditis

The diagnosis of SBE must be entertained in all febrile patients with arthritis; arthritis is the presenting complaint in more than 25% of patients with SBE.[222] In many of these patients, the clinical presentation does not differ significantly from rheumatoid arthritis since the arthritis is a result of immune-complex formation and deposition in joints. Rheumatoid factors (antiglobulins), antinuclear factors, and many other antibodies (including those of Lyme disease) may be demonstrated in many of these patients and lead to diagnostic errors.[205] Multiple blood cultures should be obtained in all febrile patients with arthritis.

Shunt Arthritis

Ventriculoatrial shunts performed to relieve hydrocephalus not infrequently become infected with bacterial organisms. In one instance, intermittent arthralgia, arthritis, and the presence of positive tests for rheumatoid factor in a young child with an infected shunt were interpreted as evidence for JRA for 4 years before blood cultures were demonstrated to be positive, the shunt was removed, and the patient was "cured" of his arthritis.[223] "Shunt nephritis," another complication of immune-complex disease resulting from chronic bacterial infection of ventriculoatrial shunts, has received wider attention in the pediatric literature but may actually be less common than arthritis, and may be associated with arthritis.[224]

Acne Rheumatism

A severe form of acne characterized by the usual findings of acne vulgaris together with double comedones and interconnecting subcutaneous abscesses located primarily on the back and chest, known as acne conglobata or acne fulminans, may be associated with a reactive arthritis similar to that of Reiter's syndrome[225] (see Chapter 4). The musculoskeletal symptoms appear at the time of a clinically obvious flare of the acne, usually in an adolescent male. A similar syndrome may occur in association with hidradenitis suppurativa.[226] Management is the same as for other patients with reactive arthritis.

Arthritis and Rash after Intestinal Bypass Surgery

Many (6–25%) adult patients who have undergone jejunal bypass operations for morbid obesity subsequently developed chronic intermittent polyarthritis involving the knees, ankles, fingers, and wrists, usually with tenosynovitis.[227,228] In HLA-B27-positive patients, the arthritis may have a spondyloarthritic pattern. Vasculitic skin lesions clinically and pathologically identical to acute febrile neutrophilic dermatosis (Sweet's syndrome) often accompany the arthritis. It is thought that this syndrome is a result of bacterial colonization of the blind loop and systemic absorption of intestinal bacterial antigens. Circulating cryoprotein immune complexes containing antibody to these organisms have been demonstrated in affected patients. The arthritis usually responds to appropriate antibiotic therapy for the bowel organisms or to anti-inflammatory drugs. Most episodes are self-limited, although in some cases reanastomosis of the bowel was required to relieve severe disabling arthritis. This syndrome may be a model for some forms of "rheumatoid arthritis," and occurs in inflammatory bowel disease and other bowel infections without bypass surgery.[229]

Whipple's Disease

Another syndrome apparently related to bacterial colonization of the gastrointestinal tract is Whipple's disease,[230–231] a disorder beginning primarily in white middle-age men and characterized by protean manifestations, including diarrhea, abdominal pain, fever, lymphadenopathy, pancarditis, weight loss, anemia, and rheumatic complaints, including arthralgia and arthritis. Diagnosis generally depends on the perioral small-intestinal biopsy demonstration of dense infiltration of the lamina propria with PAS-positive macrophages. In rare cases, similar findings have been demonstrated in a subcutaneous nodule, an inguinal lymph node, bone narrow, pleura, lungs, and myocardium.[232] Childhood cases have not been reported.

Arthritis may precede the other manifestations of Whipple's disease by many years. Attacks may be transient, lasting only a few hours or days, and may be accompanied by the skin over the joint appearing red and hot. All symptoms respond to antibiotic treatment.

The Phalangeal Microgeodic Syndrome

A geode is a hollow stone (Fig. 2.36). Little children with swollen, red, shiny fingers, a high ESR, and multiple punched-out erosions in the phalanges on x-ray have this self-limited syndrome.[233,234] Our experience and review of the literature suggest that this form of "hand-foot" syndrome is a result of bone infarction during a preceding episode of bacterial sepsis, most commonly streptococcal sepsis. Patients recover spontaneously after a few months. Recognition of this syndrome avoids the need for extensive unnecessary studies. No treatment is necessary.

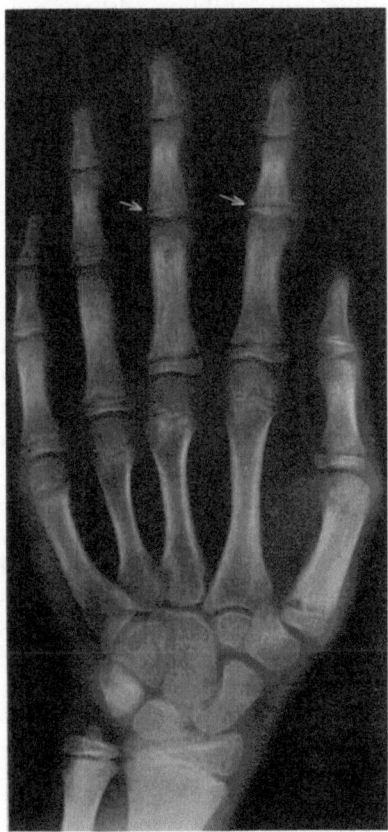 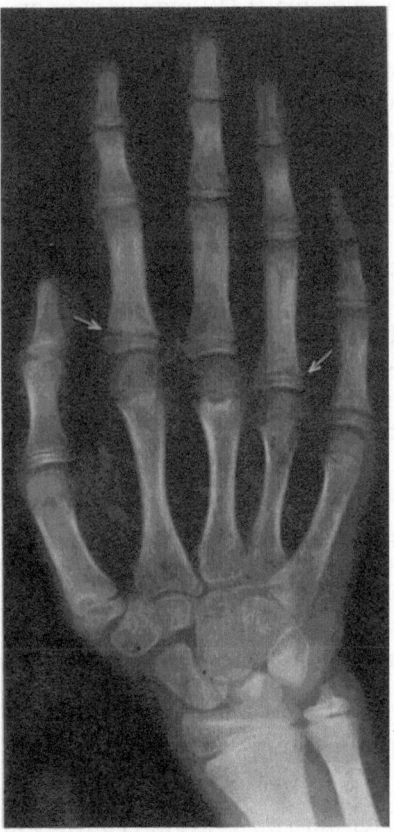

Figure 2.36. The phalangeal microgeodic (holes in stone) syndrome in a 10-year-old girl who developed these multiple lytic lesions at the ends of the phalanges, accompanied by periosteal new-bone formation, and an elevated ESR, several weeks after a streptococcal sore throat. The lesions subsided after several months, leaving no sequelae. The periostitis was better seen in the feet.

AIDS

In New York acquired immune deficiency syndrome must be excluded in every adult seen with rheumatic complaints.[235] So far, no children with AIDS have presented with dermatomyositis but 16 adults and one child with AIDS have been reported to have polymyositis as a feature of that illness.[236,237] In a few cases this may have been associated with toxoplasma infection. Spondyloarthritis in adult AIDS patients may be a result of sexually acquired Reiter's syndrome; at this time AIDS has not been reported to be a cause of arthritis but has been reported in association with lupuslike syndromes in childhood,[238] and is an increasingly frequent cause of bilateral, nontender parotid enlargements.[239,240] Multiple parotid and submandibular gland cysts may be found on ultrasound and characteristic lymphoid interstitial pneumonia (LIP) may be seen on chest x-ray in some children without pulmonary symptoms; these studies should be obtained in all children with symptomatic parotid enlargement. HTLV-I infection may also present with arthritis.[241] Congenital HIV infections may be asymptomatic for many years and patients presenting with Sjögren's syndrome may have only that and recurrent otitis as manifestation for more than 12 years in our experience.

Rheumatic Manifestations of Substance Abuse

Infections of bones, joints, and intervertebral discs are common in IV drug abusers; subacute bacterial endocarditis, hepatitis B, and HIV-associated infections, often associated with rheumatic symptoms, are also frequent in this population. Intramuscular injections, especially of pentazocine, can cause fibrous myopathy with myalgia, stiffness, and weakness, sometimes with a distinctive shoulder abduction or hip flexion contracture. Ipecac ingested to produce vomiting and weight loss may cause generalized myopathy with elevations of serum muscle enzymes. Polyarteritis nodosa and cerebral vasculitis and midline intranasal destruction have been reported as a consequence of amphetamine and cocaine abuse.[242–243a] Cocaine use may also precipitate scleroderma renal crisis.[243b]

Inflammatory Disorders

Transient Synovitis of the Hip

Pediatricians often see a child, typically a 6-year-old boy, who awakens with hip plan and limp which persists for a few days, unaccompanied by significant fever, leucocytosis, or elevation of the erythrocyle sedimentation rate; this is called "transient synovitis of the hip."[244,245] A few days of NSAID therapy enables almost normal activities to be continued, avoiding the old remedies of bed rest, traction, and hospitalization. Septic infection is usually easily distinguished by high fever and more impressive physical findings and laboratory abnormalities. Recurrent or persistent episodes of transient synovitis of the hip in our series are most likely to represent the onset of spondyloarthritis but occasionally represent Legg-Perthes' disease, Lyme disease, Gaucher's disease, or osteoid osteoma.

Inflammatory Bowel Disease (IBD) with Arthritis

Arthritis as a Presenting Manifestation of IBD. Arthritis, with or without erythema nodosum, is frequently the presenting complaint in children with ulcerative colitis or Crohn's disease (regional enteritis or granulomatous colitis).[246–248] The possibility of IBD is considered in every youngster being evaluated for arthritis and special attention is paid to those with a family history of IBD.[249] Boys and girls seem equally affected. The history of diarrhea may be "secret," as schoolchildren often do not volunteer information about chronic diarrhea and parents may be unaware of the child's bowel habits. Careful questioning usually will elicit the hidden history of abdominal cramps, diarrhea, and nighttime bowel movements. Weight loss, recent growth failure, unexplained fever, hypoalbuminemia, and anemia may also be clues to the correct diagnosis (Table 2.17). In children with Crohn's disease, rheumatic complaints so often overshadow the other clinical manifestations at onset that a preliminary diagnosis of "collagen-vascular disease" is first proposed in as many as 35% of cases. Even with a heightened index of suspicion, the diagnosis of IBD is often delayed for about a year; biopsy of normal-appearing proximal colon may suggest IBD.[250]

Arthritis is probably equally common in all forms of IBD but is more likely to cause diagnostic confusion in undiagnosed cases of Crohn's disease that have fewer obvious gastrointestinal symptoms than are usually manifested in ulcerative colitis.

Types of Arthritis in IBD. Although enteropathic and spondylitic forms of arthritis account for most of the arthritis in children with IBD, arthritis may

Table 2.17. Clues to the Diagnosis in Inflammatory Bowel Disease in Children Presenting with Arthritis

Recurrent brief episodes of relatively painless large-joint lower-extremity effusions
Slowing of linear growth and weight loss
Unexplained fever, hypoalbuminemia, and anemia in the presence of pauciarticular arthritis
Erythema nodosum, pustular vasculitis[27]
Abdominal cramps, borborygmi, foul-smelling flatus
Increased frequency of bowel movements
Nocturnal bowel movements

Table 2.18. Types of Arthritis Associated with Inflammatory Bowel Disease

	Incidence in Childhood IBD
Enteropathic	15%
Ankylosing spondylitis	5%
Hypertrophic osteoarthropathy/periostitis	3%
Erythema nodosum	3%
Septic arthritis	
Granulomatous Synovitis ⎫	
Periarteritis with arthritis ⎬	Rare
Aseptic necrosis ⎭	

also be a manifestation of erythema nodosum, hypertrophic osteoarthropathy, granulomatous synovitis, periarteritis, and aseptic necrosis (Table 2.18).[246–252]

Enteropathic Arthritis. This is the most common form of arthritis in IBD and accounts for about 60% of rheumatic complaints associated with IBD. The attacks of arthritis are usually related to the onset or exacerbation of bowel disease and/or reactive to supervening bacterial infections and toxin production in the gut. Large lower-extremity joints are most commonly affected. Elbows and wrists are the most susceptible upper-extremity joints; finger involvement is rare. This pauciarticular pattern is identical to that of childhood spondyloarthritis, but the attacks tend to be briefer (< 6 weeks) and to subside with satisfactory control of the bowel symptoms. Synovial fluid and biopsy findings suggest a reactive process analogous to the arthritis of serum sickness and the short-loop bowel syndrome. No heritable susceptibility marker has so far been demonstrated in these children, but adequate studies have only been reported for HLA-A and HLA-B antigens.

Ankylosing Spondylitis. Ankylosing spondylitis (AS) is much more frequent in patients with IBD (5%) than in control populations; conversely, IBD is much more frequent in patients with AS (17%). HLA-B27 antigen has been identified in 75% of children with IBD and sacroiliitis, and as many as 50% of children with IBD who are HLA-B27-positive will develop AS. Most of these children have peripheral arthritis first, with a spondyloarthritic pattern, and then later go on to a more chronic process involving the sacroiliac joints and sometimes the spine.

Hypertrophic Osteoarthropathy. Asymptomatic clubbing of the fingers is not uncommon in IBD, but periostitis is quite rare. It is possible that some children thought to have enteropathic arthritis have hypertrophic osteoarthropathy.

Erythema Nodosum. In our population, the most common identifiable cause of erythema nodosum is IBD, although the cause of most cases of erythema nodosum is unknown. Children with IBD associated with erythema nodosum almost always have arthritis of the "enteropathic" type. Certainly, IBD must be considered in every child with erythema nodosum (Fig. 2.4).

Septic Arthritis. Complications of IBD include intestinal and psoas abscesses, which may seed or infect joints by direct extention. The hip is most commonly affected. Psoas and iliac abscesses often present with a picture suggesting arthritis of the hip joint.

Granulomatous Synovitis. Three biopsy-proven cases of granulomatous synovitis and one noncaseating granuloma of bone with giant cells causing pain in the femur have been reported in association with Crohn's disease.[251] Monarticular arthritis of the knee was the presenting complaint in an affected 14-year-old boy. The granulomatous synovitis of Crohn's disease must be distinguished from similar lesions caused by infection with atypical mycobacteria or by sarcoidosis or nonmetallic foreign bodies.

Periarteritis. Palpable purpura (cutaneous periarteritis nodosa) has been reported in patients (including one child) with Crohn's disease and may be accompanied by arthritis.[252] We have also seen one child with Crohn's disease, spondyloarthritis, and vasculitis of the gastrocnemius muscle (Fig. 7.34). Recurrent pericarditis resembling that of JRA may also occasionally occur as an immune-complex manifestation of inflammatory bowel disease.[253,254]

Aseptic Necrosis. Children with IBD often require prednisone therapy; a few develop aseptic necrosis, especially of the hips, as a consequence of steroid therapy.

Familial Mediterranean Fever (FMF)

Children with FMF are plagued by recurring attacks of fever, peritonitis, pleuritis, and synovitis.[255-257] Presumably, the recurrent febrile paroxysms are a result of periodic release of a chemical that induces both fever and serous inflammation; the gene causing the disorder in non-Ashkenazi Jews has been mapped to the short arm of Chromosome 16.[258-258b] Periodic disease is not uncommon in people of Mediterranean origin (Greeks, Turks, Armenians, Arabs, Italians, Ashkenazim, and Sephardic Jews) and occurs worldwide. In our series one-quarter were of Irish ancestry and we are now seeing Hispanic patients (Figs. 2.37, 2.38). Most patients do not provide a family history of FMF in prior generations, but in 14% of our cases, a sibling was affected. Inheritance is thought to be autosomal-recessive. FMF is truly

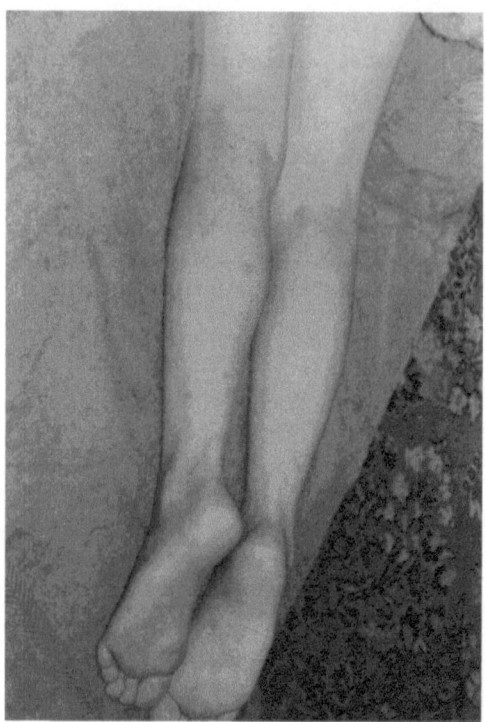

Figure 2.37. Diffuse erythematous erysipeloid rash of the lower extremities associated with painful vasculitic lesions that occur with each febrile episode in a child with Familial Mediterranean Fever.

a pediatric disease; two-thirds of all affected individuals develop symptoms under age 10, and onset in infancy is not rare. The average age of onset in pediatric series is 4.9 years.[259]

Clinical Picture. *Periodic Fever.* The cardinal presenting manifestation is unexplained fever lasting a few days and occurring at regular or irregular intervals but usually every few weeks[260] (Table 2.19). Rarely, the interval between attacks is only a few days. The interval between attacks may vary in the same patient (some attacks may be so mild as to go unnoticed, as in cyclic neutropenia), and remission may occur for a period of years. Fever may rise precipitously over a few hours, may be accompanied by chills, and may result in febrile convulsions in young children.

Serositis. Almost all patients have abdominal pain, which we and others have demonstrated to truly be due to sterile peritonitis. Within a few hours of onset of a severe attack, there may be sufficient generalized abdominal pain, rebound tenderness, and absent bowel sounds to suggest a surgical abdomen. Many children also have pleuritic chest pain, sometimes with transient pleu-

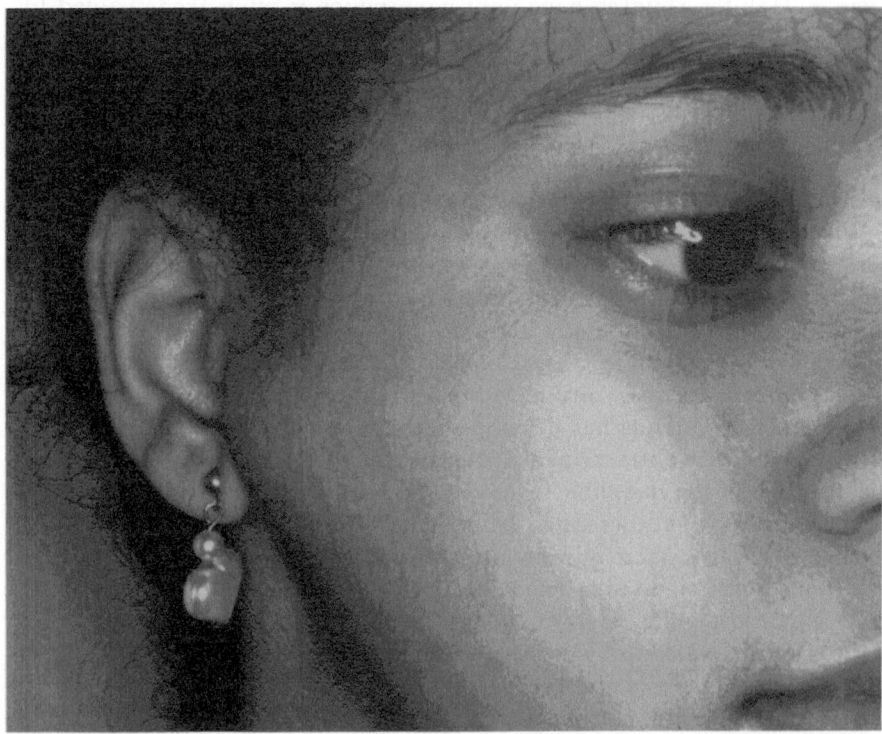

Figure 2.38. Familial Mediterranean Fever presenting with TMJ arthritis; two patients in our series had this manifestation when first seen here.

ral effusion. Some children vomit or have diarrhea with attacks. Paroxysmal pericarditis, meningitis,[261] testicular pain (from inflammation of the tunica vaginalis), and dysuria have also been reported.

Skin Rash. Various skin rashes appear in 31% of patients during the acute attack.[262] The rashes include urticaria, subcutaneous panniculitis nodules, and, in severe cases, extensive, hot, tender, edematous, sharply demarcated red patches (Fig. 2.37). The rashes disappear as the attack subsides.

Table 2.19. Clues to the Diagnosis of Familial Mediterranean Fever

Recurrent episodes of fever (often attributed to other causes) every few weeks

with Arthritis
    Serositis   Only during the febrile episodes
    Skin rash

Arthritis. Half the children have joint pain, which is often accompanied by heat, swelling, and erythema, especially at the knees and ankles.[263] In infants, the arthritis often goes unnoticed; the parents assume the child has abdominal pain because he/she cries and pulls up the legs. Severely affected infants often lie immobile during an acute attack and resist handling. Seeing the child with severe arthritis during such an attack and when he is well a few days later is educational for the physician and helps in making the diagnosis.

When arthritis is the presenting complaint, the diagnosis may be suspected, even in the absence of a family history, because of the repetitive brief attacks of pain. Any joint may be affected. The knees, ankles, hips, and shoulders are most commonly involved, but in some cases arthritis is first evident in a single temporomandibular or sacroiliac joint (Fig. 2.38).[264,265] Most attacks of arthritis subside within a week, but a few persist for months, and one of our patients has developed severe ankylosing spondylitis. Children with recurrent attacks of arthritis as part of FMF may develop growth disturbances of the mandible or at the C-2–C-3 apophyseal joint typical of childhood arthritis at these sites. In patients with recurrent attacks involving the hips and knees, there may be loss of cartilage with joint narrowing, sclerosis, and progressive limitation of motion. Arthrocentesis generally reveals fluid with a low white blood cell count and a predominance of polymorphonuclear cells. Radiographs may show enlargement of the femoral condyles, presumably a result of chronic hyperemia, and double-contour "eggshell" lines on both sides of a radiolucent osteoporotic zone. In our experience, this radiographic finding is not specific for FMF and may also be seen in relapsing polychondritis (Fig. 2.42). It may, therefore, be an indication of recurrent inflammation of chondrocytes.

Growth Retardation. Children who have recurrent severe attacks of FMF often are frail, suffer growth retardation, and have delayed bone age on radiographs.

Renal Amyloidosis. This fatal complication of FMF is very rare in the United States, less rare in untreated cases in Israel, and quite frequent in some poorer areas of the Middle East.[266] It has been suggested that in some populations there may be coincident inheritance of genes favoring both FMF and amyloidosis or that there may be two different forms of FMF, only one of which is associated with amyloidosis.[267,268] In at least some populations, the incidence of amyloidosis is not related to the severity of the disease or the age of onset. In general, patients with FMF who are bound to get amyloidosis do so before they are 30 years old, and children have been diagnosed as early as age 6. Diagnosis is established by finding proteinuria, hypertension, large kidneys, narrow ureters, and a small contracted bladder on intravenous pyelogram and amyloidosis on skin, rectal, buccal, or renal biopsy. Amyloidosis is almost wholly preventable by colchicine treatment.

Making the Diagnosis. FMF is considered a very difficult diagnosis for most Western Hemisphere pediatricians but is considered relatively easy where the disease is commonly seen and the distinctive clinical pattern is readily recognized. In the United States, erroneous diagnoses of recurrent otitis media, "viral" illnesses, or "tonsillitis" have usually been made repetitively by the primary physician although, in retrospect, these are not well documented. To encourage accurate diagnosis, we suggest the following protocol:

1. FMF is considered as a diagnostic possibility in all patients with physician-documented recurrent fevers.
2. A diary of characteristics of the attacks is kept for 6 months and submitted by the patient. We try to document a sudden leukocytosis and elevation of ESR with the onset of attacks.
3. Only aspirin or other NSAIDS are used to treat each attack.
4. A reasonable diagnostic workup is performed, including malarial smears, WBCs at the onset of episodes to exclude cyclic neutropenia, and exclusion of any possibility of hidden urinary tract infection, all of which may also be associated with episodic fevers.

The diagnosis may be confirmed with a therapeutic trial of colchicine, as desired. Failure to respond to colchicine does not exclude a diagnosis of FMF, however, as attacks are prevented by colchicine in only 60% of affected individuals.

Treatment. *Aspirin.* Without proper diagnosis and management, FMF imposes a heavy physical, emotional, and financial burden on afflicted children and their families. Symptoms of the attack may generally be controlled with aspirin, 100 mg/kg/day, begun as the prodrome of the attack appears. Most parents become well aware of subtle premonitory signs of an impending attack and can differentiate these attacks from other illnesses. This has been our traditional approach to the disease, which, together with an optimistic, knowledgeable attitude and avoidance of repetitive hospitalization and "workups," allows a relatively normal life and avoids the emotional handicaps previously considered common in these children and their families. The occasional patient with almost constant symptoms may be maintained on chronic aspirin therapy, just as in JRA. Blood levels are then measured and dosage is adjusted for maximum control (see Chapter 3). Addicting drugs are never prescribed. The patients are seen in the office at yearly intervals, at which time a urinalysis is obtained. No other special care is needed. In these patients, the attack is seen as analogous to a menstrual period. NSAIDs may also be used.

Colchicine. Many drugs and diets had been tried in FMF, all without success, until Goldfinger, in a letter to the editor of the *New England Journal of Medicine* (282:1307, 1972), suggested the efficacy of colchicine. Subsequent double-blind controlled studies and a mass of clinical experience support the efficacy of daily administration of colchicine in preventing attacks in about 60% of patients and reducing the frequency and severity in another 30%.[256,260,268] The drug is of no use in the treatment of an attack as contrasted with its prophylactic value in preventing the episodes. In adults and large children, two tablets (1.2 mg) of colchicine are required daily in some patients and 1.8 mg in others to prevent attacks. "Cheating" by not taking all of the pills after control has been achieved often results in resumption of attacks. Small children are started on 0.02 mg/kg/day, or one tablet daily if they are 30 kg. This dose is increased if attacks are not controlled and the drug is tolerated. Most children tolerate the drug well, although they may have transient diarrhea at first, which subsides without alteration of the dose.

We have found parents of most children with FMF reluctant to give colchicine every day. There are concerns about the long-term effects that might outweigh the potential benefits. In children with severe attacks, with febrile seizures, or children with significant growth retardation, we highly recommend colchicine. While amyloidosis is rare in this country, it seems reasonable to identify these children as the most susceptible. We offer colchicine to all patients in whom we make the diagnosis and will administer it to any affected child with the informed approval of the parent.

Concerns about the daily administration of this drug include fear that growth and development will be adversely affected (this does not seem to be a realistic worry), fear of acute poisoning by a child ingesting many tablets (producing shock, disseminated intravascular coagulation, bone marrow aplasia, central nervous system depression, seizures, severe diarrhea, and dehydration),* and azoospermia and teratogenic effects.[269] These latter problems have been reported in adults, and it is not possible to state with certainty what the long-term side effects of administration of colchicine throughout a child's lifetime might be.

Colchicine has also been reported to induce reversible vitamin B_{12} malabsorption by altering the function of ileal mucosa in adults.[270] Vitamin B_{12} metabolism has not been studied in children receiving daily colchicine. Treated children should be studied, and physicians should be aware of the potential for megaloblastic anemia and possibly other B_{12} deficiency manifestations such as neuropathy and myopathy.[270]

The exact mechanism of action of colchicine in gout or FMF is not known. Colchicine is not the best anti-inflammatory agent in many disorders. However, it is effective in inflammatory reactions dependent on polymorphonuclear leukocytes, such as the Arthus reaction.[271] Its action in FMF suggests that pretreatment with colchicine may prevent the polymorphs from responding to the inducing agent that sets off the attacks of FMF.

---

*Acute poisoning should be treated with immediate induced vomiting and gastric lavage.

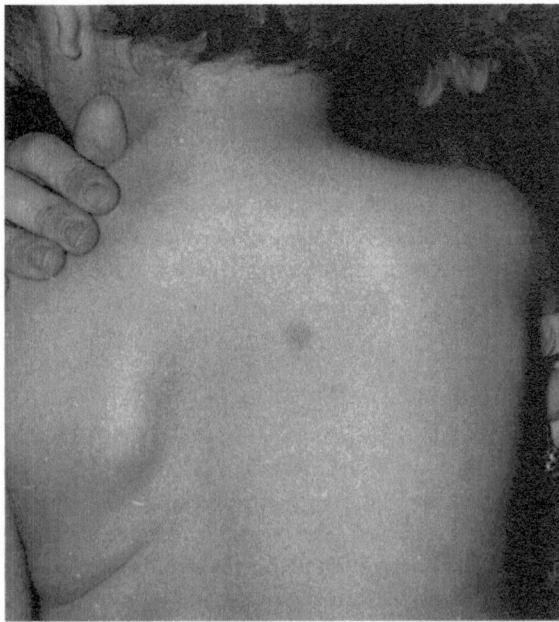

Figure 2.39. Solitary mastocytoma may, if irritated, secrete histamine, causing a sudden spike of high fever and occasionally a febrile convulsion.

Prognosis. The prognosis for American children with this disease has been good. With earlier diagnosis, avoidance of iatrogenic problems, and the availability of colchicine prophylaxis to prevent attacks, the chance for a normal life-style and life-span with minimal disability should be even better.

Solitary Mastocytoma with Flushing

Solitary mastocytomas are relatively common in children.[272,273] These tumors arc generally noted in small infants and have a characteristic pink-brown appearance (Fig. 2.39). The lesions grow during the first few months of life, become more elevated, and usually develop a *peau d'orange* appearance and a rubbery feel to palpation. Rubbing of the lesions often produces some turgescence and may be followed by slight vesiculation. The lesions generally regress spontaneously during childhood. Many are thought to be "moles" by the parent or the physician unfamiliar with this syndrome.

Some infants with these lesions have episodes of generalized flushing accompanied by spontaneous swelling of the mastocytoma. The episodes generally last for a few minutes to $\frac{1}{2}$ h and may be accompanied by diarrhea, high fever, and even by convulsions. These episodes disappear during early childhood as the lesions regress, and we have not found it necessary to remove the tumors. Presumably, the secreted chemical is histamine.

Solitary mastocytomas have not been associated with systemic mastocytosis, a syndrome in which many organs have mast cell infiltrates, which may also be accompanied by episodes of flushing.[274] We have seen a few children who had characteristic flushing episodes with fever in whom we could not find a cutaneous mastocytoma; we do not know if this syndrome could exist with single lesions in viscera, which can also disappear as the infant grows. Carcinoid syndrome may also be associated with episodes of flushing, but I am unaware of this syndrome in youngsters. A few children have been reported to have mast-cell-associated gastritis and arthritis which responded best to antihistamine treatment.[275,276]

Relapsing Polychondritis

Definition and Diagnosis. Relapsing polychondritis (RP) is a relatively rare, episodic, but generally progressive disorder characterized by destructive inflammation of cartilage.[277,278] Ear cartilage is most commonly affected, and the children generally present with recurrent inflammation of the cartilaginous portion of the ear pinnae that ultimately leads to almost total loss of ear cartilage (Table 2.20, Fig. 2.40). In most cases, the diagnosis is obvious and need not be confirmed by biopsy. Other common manifestations of RP include nasal chondritis that may cause a saddle-nose deformity, respiratory obstruction from laryngotracheobronchial chondritis that can be life-threatening, ocular inflammation (conjunctivitis, scleritis, iritis, keratitis), and auditory and vestibular impairment that may result from meatal narrowing and from inflammation about vestibular and auditory nerves. Arthri-

Table 2.20. Diagnostic Criteria for Relapsing Polychondritis

	Incidence (%)
1. Recurrent chondritis of both auricles	89
2. Nonerosive inflammatory polyarthritis	81
3. Chondritis of nasal cartilage	72
4. Ocular inflammation	65
5. Respiratory-tract chondritis	56
6. Cochlear or vestibular damage	46
Associated Diseases	
Cardiovascular (6% aortic insufficiency)	24
Cutaneous vasculitis or other chronic rash	16
Rheumatic diseases (SLE, Sjögren's, scleroderma, RA, spondylitis	15
Autoimmune disease (thyroid, diabetes, colitis, nephritis, pernicious anemia)	10
Malignancy	3

(Modified with permission from McAdam et al., ref. 277.)

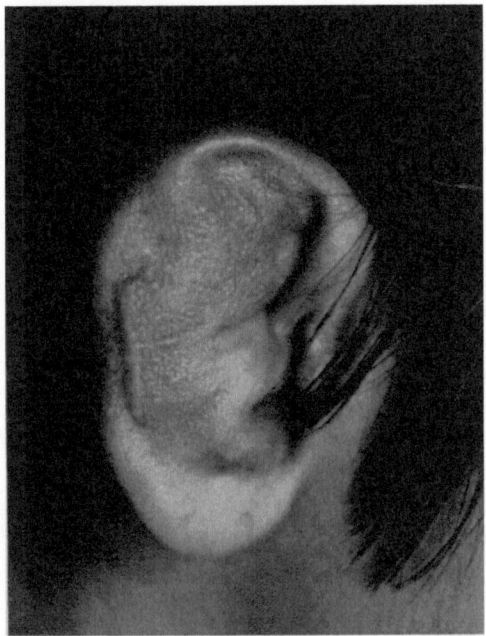

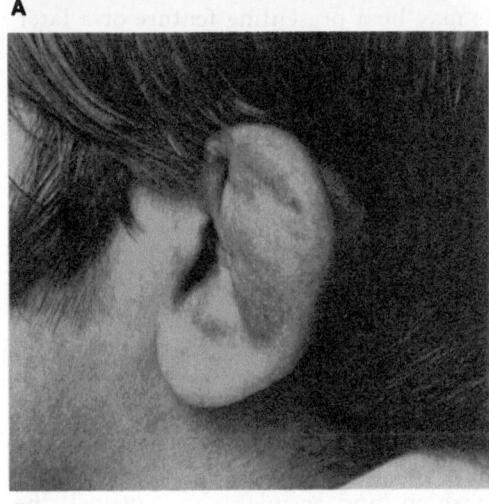

Figure 2.40. Ear in a 15-year-old boy with relapsing polychondritis during an acute episode (**A**) and now, during remission, showing permanent loss of cartilage (**B**).

tis has been reported in 58–81% of patients.[277,279] McAdam[277] has proposed that the diagnosis be established in those with involvement of any three of these six areas, but in childhood we find that recurring inflammation of two or more cartilaginous sites is sufficient for diagnosis provided the ear and/or nasal cartilages are involved and the polychondritis is not part of a systemic vasculitis such as Wegener's granulomatosis or systemic lupus erythematosus (SLE).

Etiology. The triggering mechanism for the dramatic cartilage destruction in RP is unknown. Histopathologically, the inflammation is seen to start at the cartilage margins only and is followed by the appearance of deposits of an undefined diffuse electron-dense material predominantly on the cartilage surface.[280] This may be a result of an immunologically mediated direct insult to cartilage; both cellular and humoral immune processes are active in perpetuating the inflammation in patients with RP, but it is not certain that they cause the initial insult. There is also evidence of an enzymatic attack on proteoglycan, a principal extracellular component of cartilage. It is possible that the immunologic features of the disease are secondary to the release of antigens normally sequestered in cartilage as a result of nonimmunologically mediated enzymatic destruction, but again the trigger for such a process remains unknown. At any rate, when the disease is active, all of these processes can be demonstrated.

Whatever sets off the process can apparently be transferred through the placenta.[281] An infant born to a mother with RP had RP during the first 2 years of her life but subsequently recovered. During the course of the illness, she sustained a permanent saddle-nose deformity and required systemic steroid therapy.

Coexistent Disease. Polychondritis may be a presenting feature or a later manifestation of any systemic vasculitis, especially Wegener's granulomatosis, and in such patients the course and management are what would be expected and appropriate for the primary disorder. About 15% of adults who develop RP have previously fulfilled the diagnostic criteria for some other rheumatic disease, and another 10% subsequently develop persistent arthritis with deformity or radiographic changes characteristic of rheumatoid arthritis. However, at least 75% of patients with RP have no associated disease.

The Arthritis of RP. Arthritis occurs in most patients with RP. In those who do not have any associated rheumatic disease, it tends to have a distinctive quality. The arthritis tends to be intermittent and migratory with attacks that last from several days to weeks and then resolve spontaneously only to recur again months later. Large and small joints of all extremities may be involved, usually in asymmetrical fashion, and as might be expected, the parasternal joints (costochondral cartilages) are involved in 30–60% of the attacks. In adults, this arthritis is nonerosive and nondeforming and responds well to nonsteroidal agents. In young children, metaphyseal inflammation during growth may result in deformity (Fig. 2.41) with a unique radiographic appearance characterized by severe cartilaginous destruction with little or no involvement of adjacent bone or joint, as would be expected in rheumatoid arthritis (Fig. 2.42).[282] The joint fluid is noninflammatory, and in one case in which synovial biopsy was performed in a patient with this "pure" form of RP arthritis, the unusual finding was unique, clear spaces

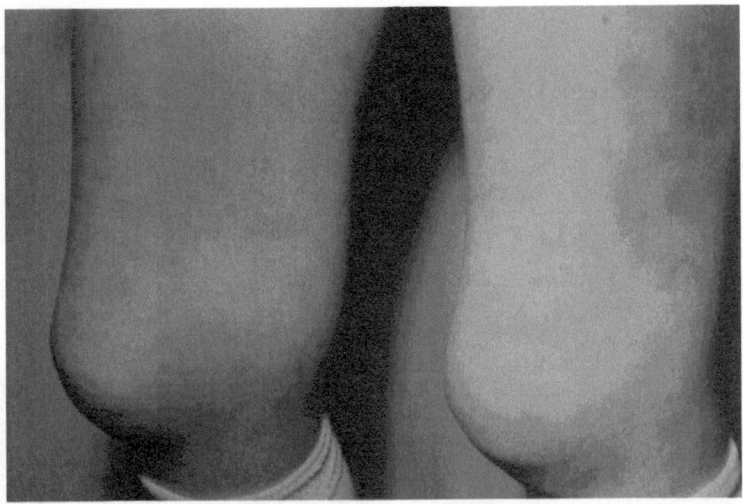

Figure 2.41. Unusual hypertrophic appearance of the knees in a young girl with recurrent episodes of arthritis of the knees, vasculitic rash, keratitis, and nerve deafness since early infancy. The illness has features of relapsing polychondritis, Cogan's syndrome, and Muckle-Wells syndrome, but the arthritis is characteristic of recurrent inflammation of cartilage (see Fig. 2.42). Her sib has congenital nerve deafness. Muckle-Wells patients have a similar rash, limb pains, and progressive nerve deafness, complicated in adult life by amyloidosis (AA).[283]

with multivesicular bodies surrounding the chondrocytes. Laboratory studies arc not helpful in RP; the only consistent abnormality is an elevated ESR. However, laboratory studies are obtained to help exclude other disorders that may be associated with RP.

Course and Treatment of RP. Most patients have a low-grade and smoldering course with exacerbations that can be treated with nonsteroidal anti-inflammatory agents, with alternate-day prednisone, or with combinations of these agents. Attacks of uveitis may require daily steroids, and in those few patients with a fulminant course or with any threat to the airway, daily prednisone is required. Respiratory support and tracheostomy are occasionally necessary in patients with life-threatening airway collapse. Several adult patients were successfully treated with dapsone, an antileprosy drug that has been shown to inhibit hyper-vitamin-A-induced lysosomal enzyme destruction of rabbit cartilage.[284] However, dapsone may be associated with the development of aplastic anemia and is carcinogenic in some animals. Its role in treating RP remains to be determined.

Aortic insufficiency has been reported to develop in some patients with RP; it is not possible to be certain how frequently this was associated with ankylosing spondylitis or Reiter's syndrome as the associated rheumatic disease. However, aortitis coronary arteritis, and heart block do seem to be

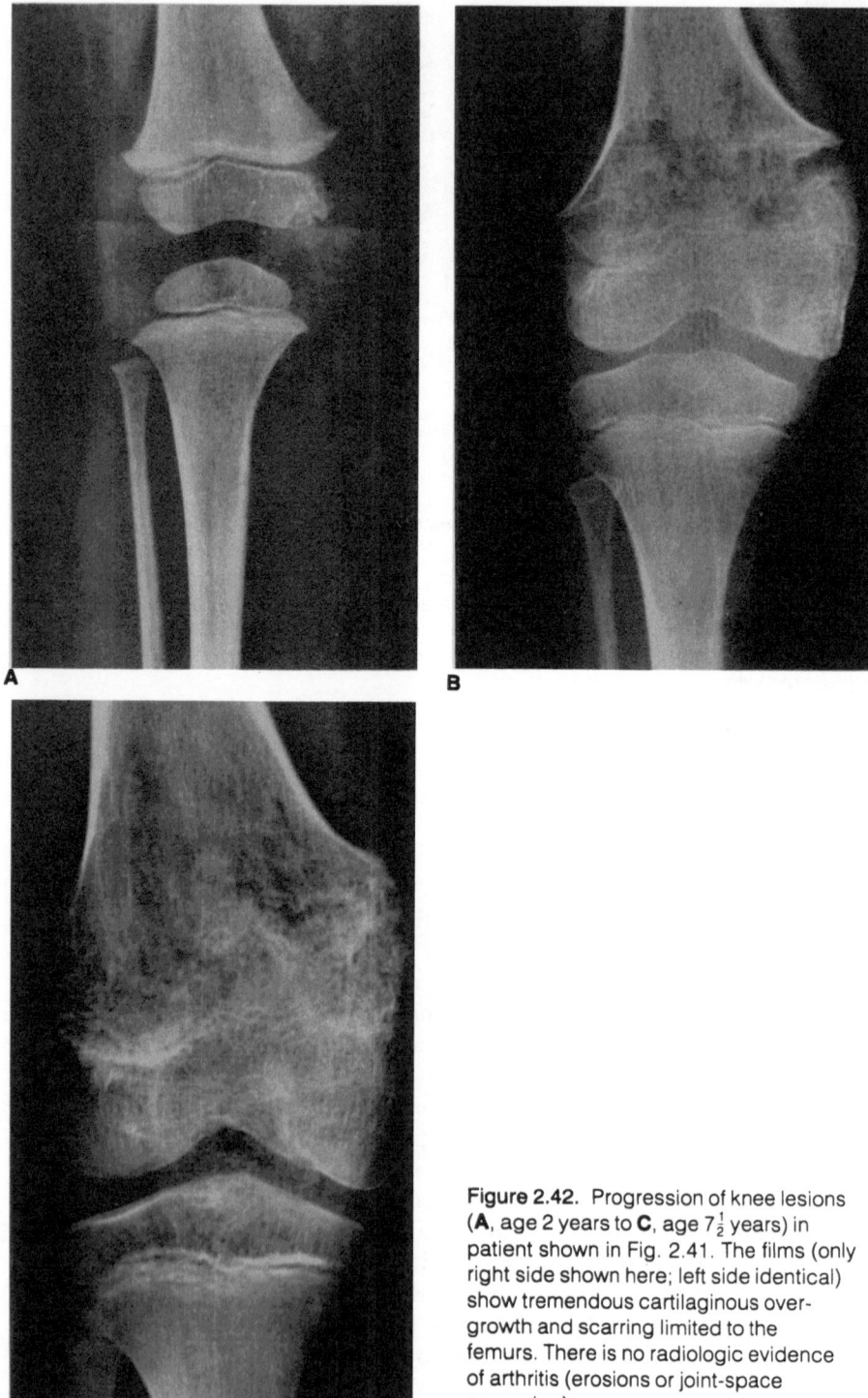

Figure 2.42. Progression of knee lesions (**A**, age 2 years to **C**, age $7\frac{1}{2}$ years) in patient shown in Fig. 2.41. The films (only right side shown here; left side identical) show tremendous cartilaginous overgrowth and scarring limited to the femurs. There is no radiologic evidence of arthritis (erosions or joint-space narrowing).

features of some patients with RP even in the absence of other evidences of systemic vasculitis.[277,278,282,285] In these patients, valve replacement and resection of aortic aneurysms may be lifesaving.

Despite the potential for associated disease, severe manifestations, and cosmetic handicap, most cases of RP are mild, and complete recovery may occur.

Case Report

A 13-year-old Indian boy developed acute unilateral anterior uveitis in October 1976. Customary laboratory studies, including an audiogram, were normal; he was HLA-B27-positive. The uveitis subsided with local corticosteroid eyedrop therapy, but several months later the pinnae of both ears became swollen, red, and painful. Despite treatment with prednisone, dapsone, indomethacin, and penicillamine, continuing inflammation resulted in gradual loss of almost all ear cartilage over the ensuing 2 years (Fig. 2.40). There have been no other manifestations of relapsing polychondritis, and the patient is currently in remission.

Muckle-Wells Syndrome

Muckle-Wells syndrome, characterized by periodic attacks of fever, limb pains, and urticarial rash accompanied by progressive nerve deafness and ultimately amyloid nephropathy in families was first described in 1962.[283]

Idiopathic Periosteal Hyperostosis (Goldbloom's Syndrome)

We have seen three boys with this syndrome of a several-month illness characterized by fever, weight loss, and severe pain in the extremities with very high ESRs and serum gamma globulins.[286] X-rays ultimately show extensive periostitis in long bones (Fig. 2.43). There is limited motion in joints adjacent to the periostitis, and the patients often refuse to walk. Symptoms are relieved with high doses of aspirin or other NSAID, and recovery takes place spontaneously over several months. So far, there have been no clues to the etiology. Bone biopsies (unnecessary) show nonspecific osteitis.[287–289] Our experience suggests that this entity is not as rare as the few case reports would suggest.[287–289] A similar syndrome may result from infusions of prostaglandin.[290]

Case Report

In 1974, this 12-year-old boy developed typical varicella, as did his sibling. Although the chickenpox lesions disappeared, he continued to have daily temperature spikes, fatigue, and musculoskeletal pain for 6 weeks. During this time, he was anorectic and lost more than 10% of his body weight. On admission, the physical examination was

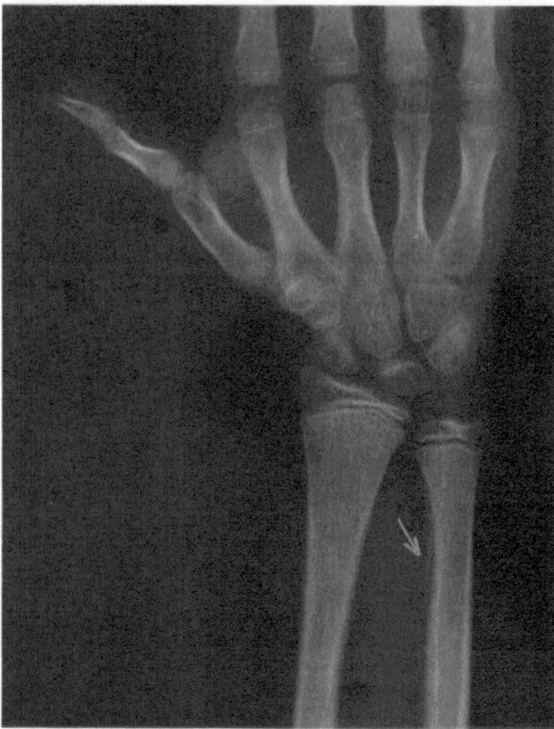

Figure 2.43. Idiopathic periosteal hyperostosis with hypergammaglobulinemia (Goldbloom's syndrome) in an 11-year-old boy referred because of joint pains and effusions. The patient made a full recovery in a few months. Periosteal new bone was formed along the radius, ulna, humerus, and first metatarsal.

remarkable because of generalized bone pain over all the extremities, with only minimal effusions at the ankles but with resistance to motion of all the large joints. X-rays of the extremities had been negative 3 weeks after onset but now showed extensive periosteal new-bone formation along the radius, ulna, and humerus and first metatarsal on one side (Fig. 2.43).

An extensive laboratory workup was unrevealing except for elevation of the ESR and gamma globulin. The pain and systemic symptoms were well controlled with large doses of aspirin that were continued for 6 weeks, following which he made a full recovery and has remained well.

Weber-Christian Disease

Relapsing arthralgia, myalgia, fever, and fatigue together with fluctuant sub-dermal nodules of lobular panniculitis constitute this mysterious syndrome. Systemic manifestations may include pneumonia, sterile visceral abscesses, membranous glomerulonephritis, and mesenteric panniculitis;[291-295] without treatment some children will die.[292,295] Treatment with prednisone is usually effective and patients may then fully recover;[293] the following case report illustrates the reduction in morbidity achieved by diagnosis and steroid therapy:

Case Report

$2\frac{1}{2}$ months following immunization with live measles vaccine at age 16 months,[295] this previously healthy child developed an illness characterized by fever; recurrent sub-cutaneous nodules; and multiple splenic, hepatic, and mesenteric sterile abscesses which were drained at three abdominal surgeries over a 3-month period. (The spleen was removed.) All cultures were sterile, there was no response to antibiotics, and extensive testing of immunologic functions was normal. When the pathology in the skin lesions was recognized as suppurative panniculitis, all antibiotics were replaced with prednisone, 2 mg/kg/day. The patient, who was terribly ill and required hyper-alimentation, recovered fully and in 9 days the medication was changed to qod. Be-cause of the splenectomy, she was given amoxicillin 125 mg tid to prevent infection. The prednisone was gradually weaned away over a 2-year period; the patient has grown and developed normally and is well 8 years after admission to this hospital.

Cyclosporine is said to have been effective in a steroid-resistant case.[296]

Acute Pancreatitis with Arthritis

An acute polyarthritis syndrome has been described in children who are re-covering from traumatic pancreatitis.[297] Symptoms of pancreatitis may be minimal or absent. Some cases are a result of child abuse. Joint pain and effusion first develop 2–3 weeks after the injury and may be accompanied by clinical signs of periostitis. Multiple areas of severe periosteal new-bone formation and punched-out lytic changes in the diaphyses may not be radiographically apparent until 2 months after the precipitating accident or injury when they may be seen in long bones (Fig. 2.44) and especially in the metacarpal and metatarsal bones. Subcutaneous fat necrosis (erythema-nodosum-like skin lesions) may also occur.

Diagnosis is made by demonstrating elevated serum amylase and lipase levels. The excessive lipase causes fat necrosis in the synovium and periar-ticular tissues, producing the arthritis. Bone scan may be a more sensitive diagnostic tool than conventional x-rays, sometimes demonstrating many asymptomatic lesions.

All sorts of pancreatic diseases in adults have been associated with this syndrome, but most childhood cases result from child abuse. The bone changes regress spontaneously over a period of months without specific ther-apy. Recognition of this syndrome is important so as to avoid unnecessary extensive workups for infection and malignancy and to identify abuse, if present, before further harm is done to the child.

Pseudotumor of the Orbit

Pseudotumor of the orbit is characterized by the sudden onset of unexplained eye pain and proptosis accompanied by inflammation and redness of the tissues in and around the eye.[298] Twenty-five percent of affected children also have iritis. This dramatic syndrome is uncommon but not rare in childhood.

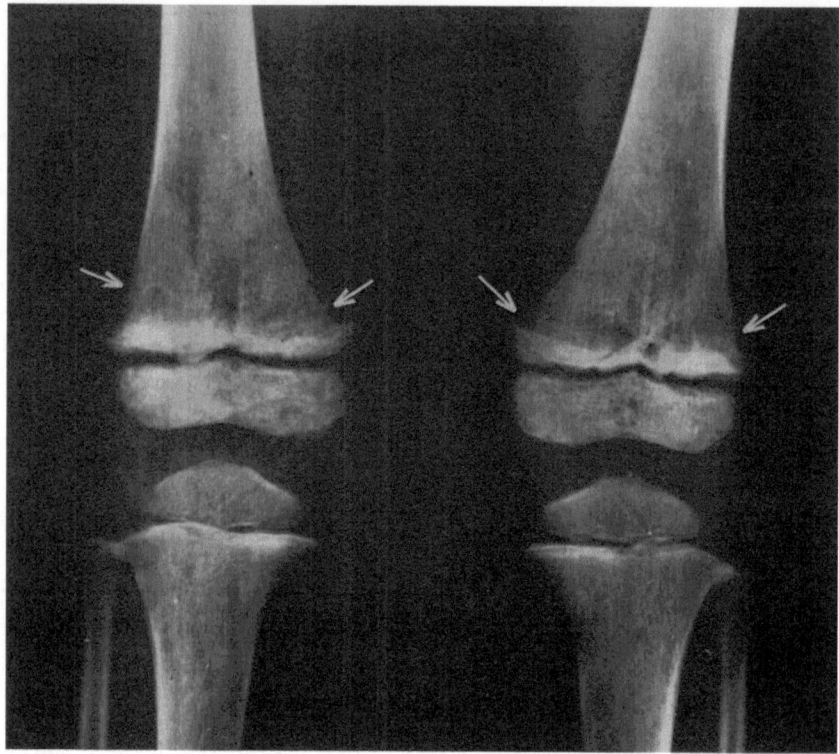

Figure 2.44. Skeletal manifestations of hemorrhagic pancreatitis is a $2\frac{1}{2}$-year-old battered child. Several weeks after injury, the patient began to limp. Radiographs show sclerosis, lucencies, and fragmentation in the distal femoral metaphysis due to bone infarcts.

Mild constitutional symptoms accompany most attacks and include headache, nausea, vomiting, abdominal pain, sore throat, lethargy, and weight loss. Many of these children have recurrent episodes over a period of years, and this is the rule in those with bilateral disease.

A diagnosis of orbital pseudotumor requires exclusion of orbital tumors and metastases. This is usually readily accomplished with radiographs, ultrasound, and computed tomography. The presumptive diagnosis is then confirmed by a prompt, dramatic response (within 48 h) to prednisone. Biopsy is contraindicated, as some cases apparently are a result of orbital trauma, and while the prognosis for vision is generally good, it is much poorer in patients who have been subjected to the surgical trauma of biopsy.

The etiology of this disorder in childhood has been entirely unknown. Biopsy specimens, obtained prior to recognition of the hazards of biopsy, have frequently shown evidence of vasculitis such as perivascular cuffing with lymphocytes and eosinophils but without fibrin, leukocytoclasis, or vascular necrosis. One our of patients, however, was known to have Lyme disease 6 months prior to the onset of orbital pseudotumor and had Lyme arthritis 3 months prior to the pseudotumor. This observation and the pathology observed in prior children in our series suggests that orbital pseudotumor in children is a hypersensitivity vasculitis. In adults, orbital pseudotumor has been reported as a manifestation of systemic vasculitis, especially Wegener's granulomatosis. However, long-term follow-up of 29 children seen at our hospital has not revealed the subsequent appearance of any systemic vasculitis syndrome or generalized disorder. While orbital pseudotumor has not yet been reported as a feature of Lyme disease in other series, we suspect that our one case may actually serve as a natural model for the pathogenesis of orbital pseudotumor in general, albeit with the vasculitis probably incited by many different agents.

Because of the frequency of recurrent attacks, we advise that patients be promptly changed from daily prednisone to an alternate-day steroid regimen, which also controls the manifestations. The prednisone can then usually be withdrawn gradually over a 6-week period. A few patients will require long-term treatment, and exacerbations may be expected in most children.

Cortical Hyperostoses

Caffey's Disease (Infantile Cortical Hyperostosis). Fever and irritability and a greatly elevated ESR in a young infant may be manifestations of this peculiar condition, which is sometimes familial.[299] Diagnosis is generally made by recognizing swelling about the mandible, the most frequently affected bone. Radiographically, cortical thickening may also be seen in long bones, ribs, clavicles, and other bones. Although the disorder is almost always self-limited, treatment with prednisone in small, gradually decreasing doses is generally given because of the severity of the systemic symptoms and their easy control with corticosteroids. NSAIDs have recently been shown to be effective and are the preferable mode of therapy.[300] A similar syndrome occurs in infants following treatment with prostaglandin for ductus-dependent congenital heart disease.[301]

Melorheostosis. This rare, localized (one bone) hyperostosis of childhood appears first as endosteal sclerosis-streakiness of the long bones or as mottled and patchy hyperostosis of the pelvis or small bones of the hands and feet. Only years later does the classic radiologic picture of "melted wax dripping down the side of a candle" appear.[302,303] Most patients are asymptomatic, but occasionally joint swelling and vague joint pain may be the presenting manifestation. Linear sclerodermatous skin changes may overlie affected bones, etiology is unknown, and no treatment is necessary.

Intramedullary Osteosclerosis

We have seen a number of youngsters who presented with mild to moderate lower-extremity pain, worsened by activity, whose x-rays showed intra-

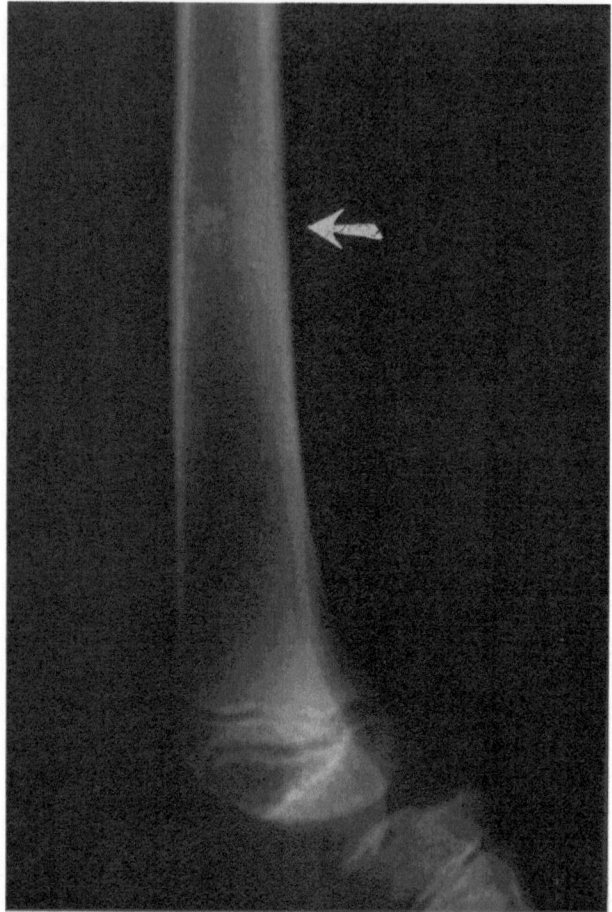

Figure 2.45. Intramedullary osteosclerosis in a 7-year-old boy; (*arrow*). Bone scan showed increased uptake; CT suggested bone infarct. Biopsy showed a reactive lesion characterized by hypervascularity and perivascular lymphocytosis. Pain responded to NSAIDs and subsided after 2 years.

medullary osteosclerois in the tibia or fibula (Fig. 2.45); bone scans showed increased uptake. The erythrocyte sedimentation rate may be slightly elevated. Nonsteroidal anti-inflammatory drugs are effective during the year when the youngster is symptomatic.[304]

Diaphyseal Osteosclerosis

Duffuse diaphyseal cortical thickening may also cause localized intermittent aching pain and discomfort, usually in the lower extremities. Heritable varieties have been described in children (Camurati-Engelmann's disease) and young adults (Ribbing's disease) but there is considerable overlap. In our small experience management is identical to intramedullary osteosclerosis and the major reasons for recognizing these disorders is to provide reassurance and avoidance of biopsy.[305]

Sarcoid Arthritis

The first report of sarcoid arthritis appeared in 1936; the patient was an 8-year-old child. In recent years, many children with sarcoid arthritis have been noted in the literature.[306–308a] The case reports are repetitive, and it is clear that sarcoid arthritis constitutes a special syndrome in infants and young children. The onset of skin rash has been as early as age 4 months and arthritis as early as 9 months. The disease in these young children has been characterized by typical sarcoid cutaneous lesions; severe uveitis; a huge, boggy tendon sheath; and synovial thickening with relatively painless effusions. In contrast to older children and adults fewer have had constitutional symptoms, x-ray changes, hypergammaglobulinemia, or hypercalcemia, and none had hilar adenopathy (Table 2.21), but vasculopathy with large-vessel stenoses has recently been reported.[309] In familial form such patients may be indistinguishable from those with "familial granulomatous arthritis"[310–313] (see Chapter 7; Fig. 2.46). Diagnosis of sarcoidosis in most of these children was established by skin biopsy. The arthritis can be differentiated from JRA by tendon sheath or synovial biopsy showing typical sarcoid granulomas (Fig. 2.47). However, the syndrome of relatively painless, huge, boggy tendon synovial thickening in multiple joints (wrists, ankles, knees, and elbows) in a child with cutaneous lesions proved to be noncaseating sarcoid granuloma is distinctive and, except when familial, may be presumed to be sarcoid arthritis. Systemic steroids may be used to control the uveitis and arthritis.

Table 2.21. Cinical Features in Recorded Cases of Sarcoid Arthritis in Children

	%
Huge boggy synovial thickening and effusion	100
Tendon sheath involvement	100
Onset prior to age 4	100
Uveitis	83
Persistent skin lesions	83
Constitutional symptoms	83
Pain	Minimal
Limited motion	Minimal

(Modified with permission from North et al., Am J Med 48:449–455, 1970.)

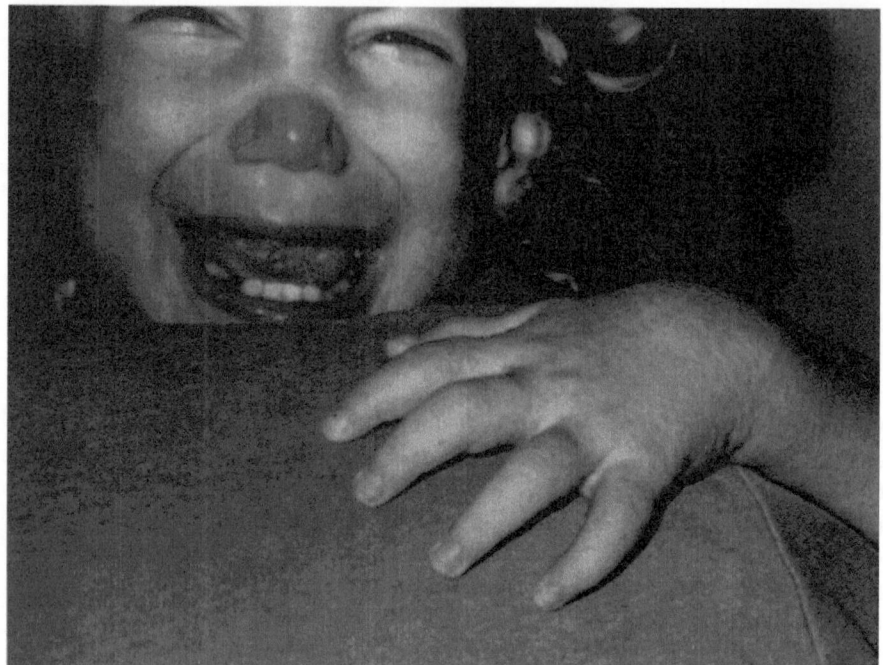

Figure 2.46. Familial granulomatous arthritis; three siblings, mother, and grandmother had similar sarcoidlike rash and arthritis. One child had systemic symptoms; grandmother and an aunt have uveitis. (Courtesy of Dr. C. Balakrishnan.)

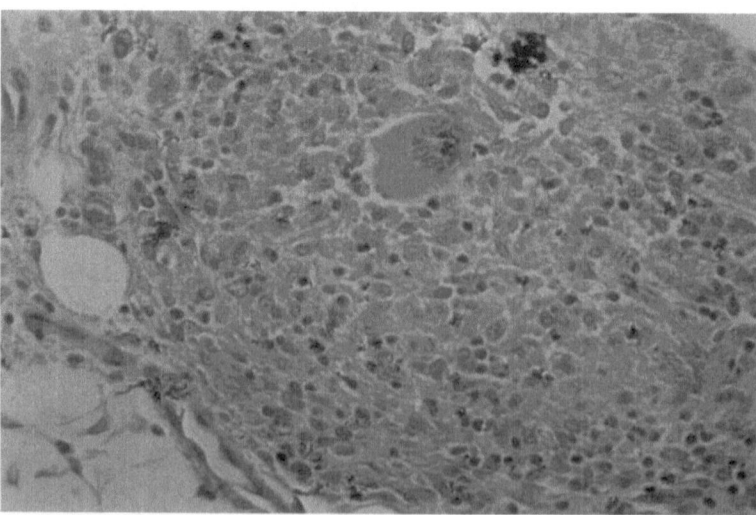

Figure 2.47. Typical sarcoid granuloma found on biopsy of huge boggy tendon sheaths in a young child with sarcoid skin lesions, uveitis, and joint effusions. (Courtesy of Dr. C. Fink.)

Brief attacks of polyarthritis with erythema nodosum are common at the onset of the adult form of sarcoidosis, which may also occur in childhood. Osseous lesions may occur.[313a]

Pseudorheumatoid Nodules

Healthy children occasionally develop asymptomatic subcutaneous nodules, especially on the scalp, eyelids, ankles, and pretibial surfaces of the legs (Fig. 2.48).[314,315] Pseudorheumatoid nodules account for 3% of all superficial lumps in children.[316] The lumps may be only a few millimeters in diameter or may grow to quite a large size (5 cm). The overlying skin is usually normal but rarely may have typical granuloma annulare lesions. These nodules are often multiple, and individual lesions tend to appear and disappear spontaneously over a period of years. The etiology of this syndrome is unknown. Similar nodules have been seen in surfboard users, in whom they are traumatically induced.

Despite a multitude of articles describing over 200 affected children, only rarely does the primary physician or operating surgeon consider this diagnosis preoperatively. Considerable harm is done when, as a result of the unanticipated pathologic resemblance of these nodules to the true rheumatoid nodules seen in rheumatic disease, the children are considered ill and subjected to unnecessary study and treatment. The literature contains case reports of long hospitalization, dangerous medication, mutilating operative excisions, and even biopsy of the heart that have resulted when physicians have tried unsuccessfully to prove these children had systemic illness. Long follow-up studies in our clinic and by others have documented that these nodules are not forerunners of rheumatic or any other disease. Of the thousands of healthy children who have had these nodules only two have been reported to have subsequently developed arthritis.[317]

If one receives an unexpected pathologic report of a "rheumatoid nodule" in a healthy child, it is best to assume the child has pseudorheumatoid nodules. Once aware of these lesions, a presumptive diagnosis may be made and a small biopsy can be taken to confirm the clinical impression. No further studies need then be obtained, and the physician and family may be reassured. Pseudorheumatoid nodules also occur in adults.[318]

Transient Hyperphosphatasemia of Infancy

We have reported two instances in which, at the time we first evaluated new cases of polyarticular juvenile arthritis, we accidentally discovered spectacular elevations of serum alkaline phosphatase (AP) to ten times the upper reference limits for age. The abnormality subsided within 4 to 6 weeks and was not related to drug therapy or liver abnormality or to abnormalities in 25-OH Vitamin D.[319] Serum AP has been measured repetitively on every

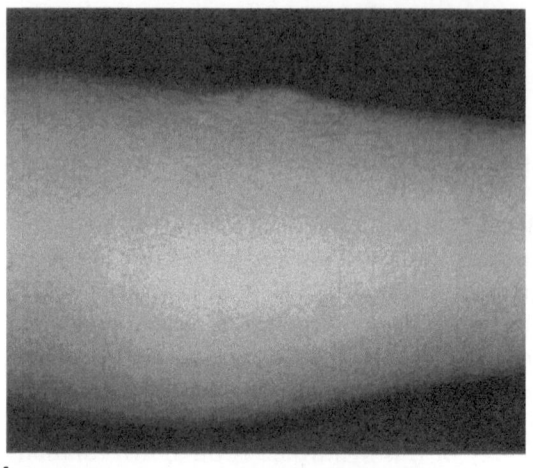

A

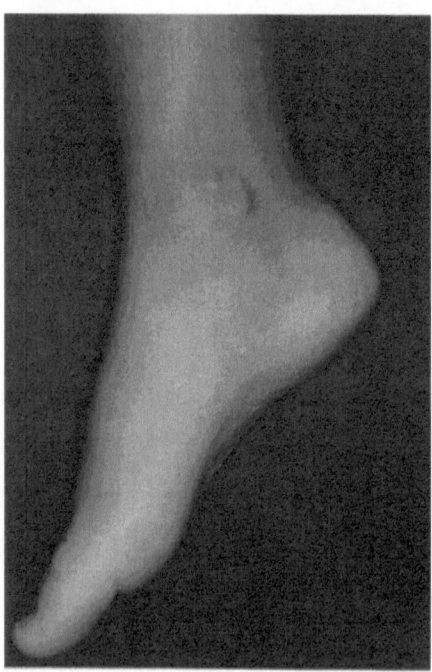

B

Figure 2.48. Typical pseudorheumatoid nodules on the pretibial surface (**A**) and at the ankle (**B**).

visit of about 1000 of our patients with JA as part of an automated chemistry profile and 3 similar pauciarticular cases have been observed. We presume this is an association of two processes which are "reactive" to an antecedent illness. Isoenzyme studies show that elevations of an "atypical" AP derived from liver and bone may follow a variety of childhood illnesses, especially gastrointestinal illness, shown in one recent case to be due to rotavirus. The virus may induce low isoenzyme clearance from the serum.[320]

Erythromelalgia[321]

Recurrent episodes of pain, redness, and heat in extremities exposed to *warmth* (relieved by ice) has been termed erythromelalgia; in children this is an extremely rare disorder but we have seen one 14-year-old male who suffered these symptoms, unrelated to any primary hematologic, vascular, neurologic, or rheumatic disease and are presently caring for a 14-year-old girl with erythromelalgia and periodic fever.

Hypertrophic Osteoarthropathy

Secondary Hypertrophic Osteoarthropathy

Most pediatricians associate hypertrophic osteoarthropathy (HO) with clubbed fingers and cardiopulmonary disease. The full syndrome actually includes periostitis with new-bone formation, especially at the distal ends of the long bones, arthritis in large joints, and, occasionally, autonomic dysfunction (flushing, blanching, sweating). The arthritis is frequently present without clubbing, especially in children with malignancy. Secondary HO is by no means rare in children and constitutes an important and underemphasized form of childhood arthritis.[322–325] Table 2.22 lists the many childhood disorders that may cause this form of arthritis.

The pathogenesis of HO is poorly understood. None of the proposed explanations satisfactorily explains the productive periostitis that proceeds through the usual inflammatory cycle from edema to lymphocytic and plasma-cell inflammation to subperiosteal new-bone formation and the formation of a pseudocortex that ultimately fuses with and expands the original cortex. The inflammation of synovial tissue is indistinguishable from that of rheumatoid arthritis and progresses in a few uncontrolled cases to pannus formation and crippling. The radiographic demonstration of periosteal new bone along the shaft of long and tubular bones is diagnostic but depends on the x-rays being taken at the stage where new-bone formation has taken place. Our experience with periostitis is that x-rays are frequently negative during the acute painful stage of inflammation and that radiographically visible new bone represents healing, sometimes of a lesion that was painful a year earlier. Technetium bone scans have also not been helpful in the acute stage. Acute periostitis is, however, very painful, and patients often complain of the slightest touch, requiring elevation even of the bed sheets. The pain may not be continuous in one area, and the migrating quality and the severe complaints in the absence of visible arthritis or radiographic evidence of periostitis may seem puzzling and suggest hysteria. In

Table 2.22. Hypertrophic Ostoarthropathy (HO) in Childhood

Secondary HO	
Pulmonary	*Endocrine*
Cystic fibrosis	Thyroid acropachy (hyperthyroidism)
Infections	Myxedema (hypothyroidism)
Fibrosis	Hyperparathyroidism
Cardiovascular	*Neoplasma*
SBE	Leukemia
Cyanotic congenital heart disease	Hodgkin's disease
Patent ductus arteriosus	Neuroblastoma
	Medulloblastoma
Gastrointestinal	Osteogenic sarcoma
Inflammatory bowel disease	Others
Cirrhosis of the liver	
Becterial or parasitic colitis	
Subphrenic abscess	

Primary HO (Familial)	
With pachyderma	*Without pachyderma*

our experience, nothing induces "hysterical" behavior quite as much as periosteal inflammation, and nothing helps more in diagnosis than recognition of the characteristic pain pattern in an appropriate clinical setting.

HO is generally treated with aspirin or other nonsteroidal anti-inflammatory drugs and is often responsive to these agents. Several patients have been successfully treated with atropine or Pro-Banthine, based on the theory that pulmonary HO results from a neuroreflexogenic afferent stimulus conducted by the vagus nerve.[326]

Cystic Fibrosis (CF). Two types of arthritis are commonly associated with CF in older children: (1) hypertrophic osteroarthritis, sometimes with clubbing and/or radiographic evidence of periostitis and (2) "recurrent, short lived, episodic attacks of a debilitating, asymmetric, non-nodular, effusive, and non-erosive synovitis involving large and small joints above and below the waist in a classic *palindromic* pattern."[322] The attacks last from hours to weeks and can be controlled with nonsteroidal anti-inflammatory agents. One girl was followed for palindromic rheumatism for 14 years (from the age of 7) before the diagnosis of CF was made[322] (i.e., cystic fibrosis presenting as palindromic rheumatism)!

Ultimately many of these CF patients with arthritis do develop joint space narrowing, permanent damage, and erosions. A few children with CF develop seropositive RA with nodules (Fig. 3.21).[322,327] Some others have arthritis associated with erythema nodosum or rashes suggestive of intestinal bypass syndrome.[328,329]

Hypertrophic osteoarthropathy in CF sometimes responds to more vigilant control of pulmonary infection. CF patients with extensive periostitis have a significantly increased mortality rate (36%/4 years).[330]

Celiac Disease. Rheumatic symptoms may accompany any sort of bowel inflammation. Celiac disease may coexist with JRA but enteropathic arthralgia/arthritis may be a manifestation of unrecognized celiac disease and disappear following institution of a gluten-free diet.[331]

Arthritis Associated with Absence of the Bile Ducts: Alagille's Syndrome. Arthritis has not been described as a feature of Alagille's syndrome (infantile cholestasis with paucity of intralobular bile ducts, peripheral pulmonary artery stenosis, butterfly vertebrae, coloboma or posterior embryotoxon of the eye, and striking "birdlike" facies) but we follow one patient (Fig. 2.49) and have been privileged to see another followed at Yale.[332] The arthritis in these two children is extremely destructive (Fig. 2.50) and crippling but without effusions; at the time of foot surgery we obtained a synovial biopsy which was not distinctive in any way. So far as we can determine, this arthri-

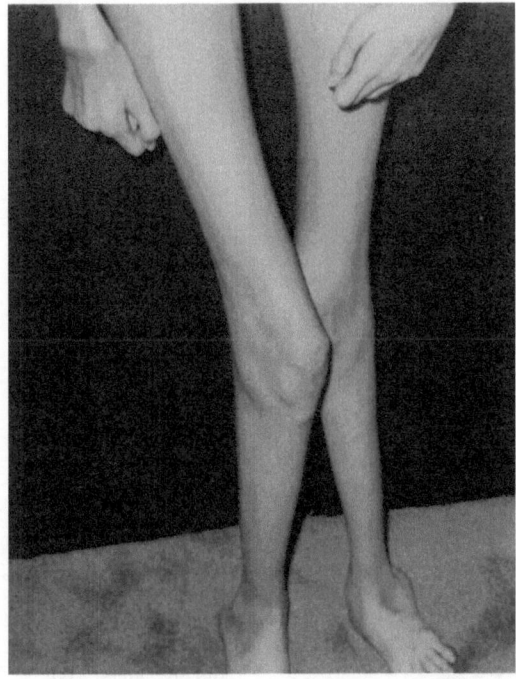

Figure 2.49. Alagille's syndrome with arthritis.

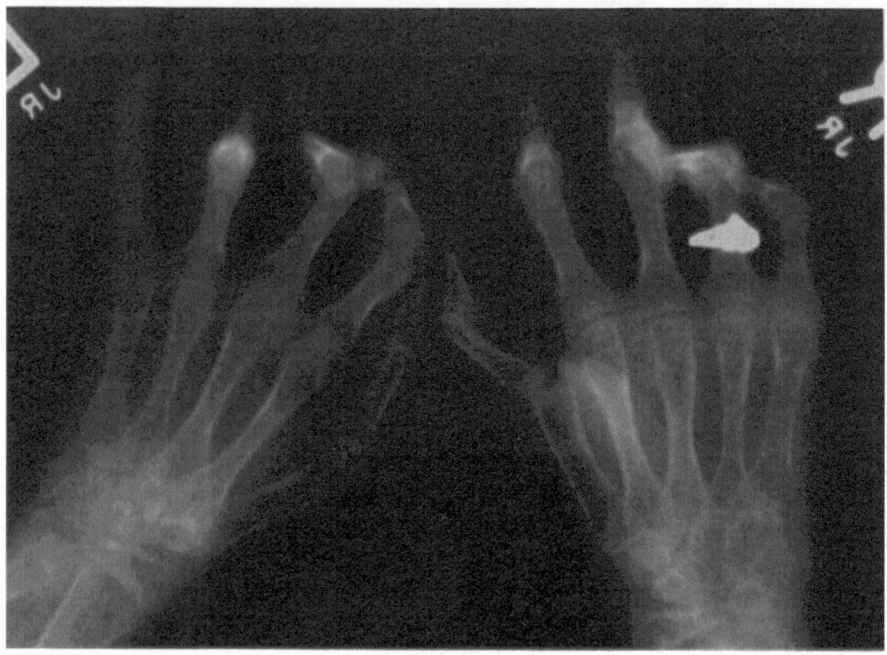

A

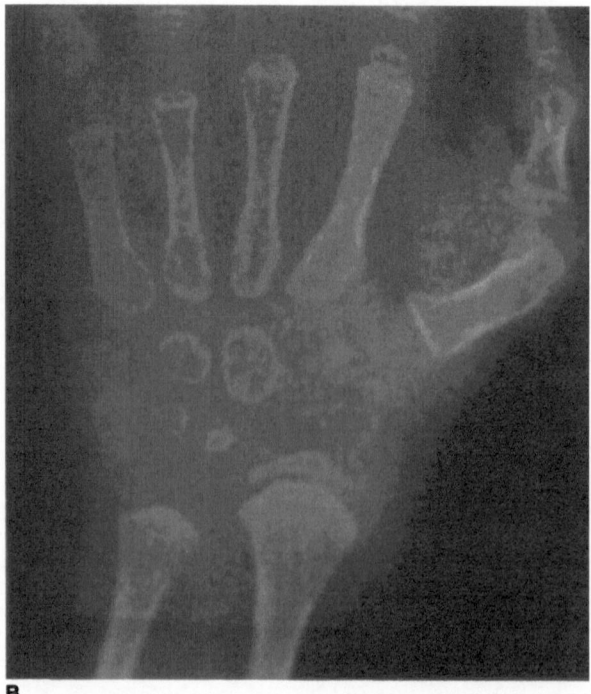

B

Figure 2.50. Destructive arthritis in Alagille's syndrome, age 15 (**A**); other joints are similar. (**B**) second patient, age 5.

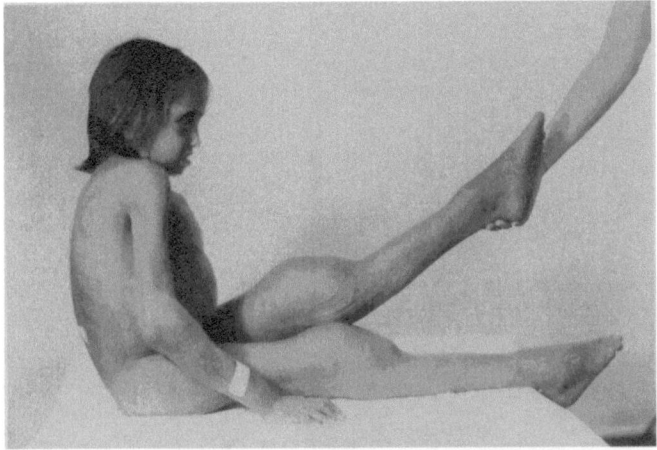

Figure 2.51. Pseudoarthritis associated with congenital absence of the intrahepatic bile ducts.

tis is unresponsive to drugs. We have inquired and similar cases have not been seen by Dr. Alagille.

Pseudoarthritis Associated with Congenital Absence of the Intrahepatic Bile Ducts. Patients with preductal bile stasis as a result of congenital absence or progressive loss of the intrahepatic bile ducts develop a striking pseudoarthritis late in the first decade of life (Fig. 2.51).[333] Joint deformity and limitation of motion simulating hypertrophic osteoarthropathy results from the formation of multiple bursal lipomas analogous to the cutaneous xanthomas seen in these patients with severe hyperlipidemia.

Malignant Disease in Childhood Presenting with Musculoskeletal Pain. The first diagnosis to consider in a child with evanescent bone pain, especially with episodic refusal to walk or to use an arm, is malignancy (Fig. 2.52).[323–325,334–339] There are a variety of pathogenic mechanisms for bone pain in children with cancer (Table 2.23). Joint effusions may result from leukemic infiltrates of the synovial membrane.[340] Bone pain may result from direct invasion of the cortex or marrow by tumor, especially in Hodgkin's disease and neuroblastoma. Leukemia and lymphoma may present with a very high serum uric acid from white-cell destruction, resulting in acute gouty arthritis;[340a] and bone pain and arthritis may be a manifestation of hypertrophic osteoarthropathy, caused either by the primary tumor or by pulmonary metastases, especially from osteogenic sarcomas. Bone-marrow examination, abdominal ultrasound, and appropriate skeletal x-rays and scans must be performed and generally enable prompt diagnosis. We have recently discovered a reversal of the usual marrow MRI characteristics

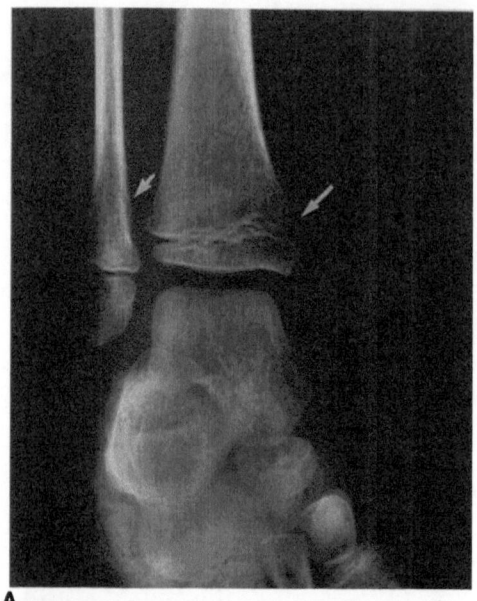

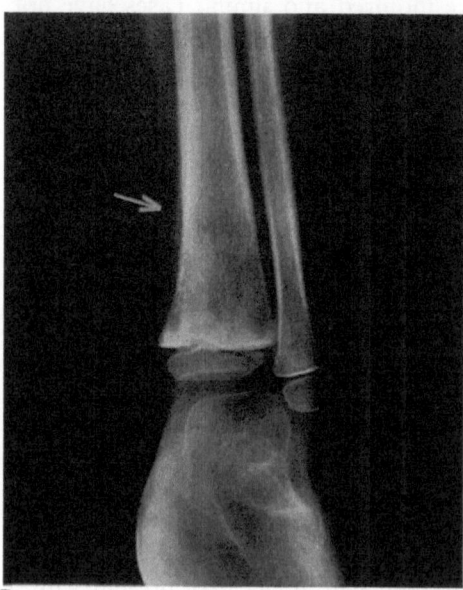

Figure 2.52. (A) Acute leukemia presenting as monarticular arthritis of the ankle in a 4-year-old boy referred as "JRA." The moth-eaten appearance, metaphyseal lucencies, and periostitis at the distal tibia and fibula were not recognized at the referring hospital. **(B)** Metastatic neuroblastoma mistaken for JRA in a 3-year-old boy. The moth-easten appearance of the metaphyses of the long bones (ankle) and periostitis (less apparent on the original radiograph than on this photograph) were unrecognized even at a large pediatric rheumatology center.

on T1/T2-weighted images in children with cancer.[339] This may be the sole clue to diagnosis in some patients but many radiologists are not yet aware of this sign.

Of all of the disorders discussed in this chapter, the most common to be confused with JRA is cancer, especially leukemia, neuroblastoma, and lymphoma. Malignancy must be well sought after in every child with mysterious

Table 2.23. Causes of Musculoskeletal Pain in Malignancy

Bone infarction from marrow or cortical invasion
Periostitis
Invasion of synovium and soft tissues by leukemic cells[341]
Secondary gout in leukemia
Hypertrophic osteoarthropathy
Immune complexes in synovium
Referred pain from spinal-cord tumors
Dermatomyositis*, erythema nodosum*, polymyalgia rheumatica*, Sjögren's
  syndrome*

* Not reported in childhood malignancy.

musculoskeletal pain before a diagnosis of JRA is presumed (Figs. 2.52–2.54). Bone pain out of proportion to visible signs of arthritis, and/or fever or anemia or leucopenia, thrombocytopenia, or lymphocytosis, always suggest the possibility of cancer.[337] But monarticular or polyarticular arthritis indistinguishable from JRA may also be a presenting manifestation of malignancy.[335-337] Intermittent sciatic root pain caused by malignancies in or invading the spinal cord (Figs. 2.53, 2.54) may be referred to the lower extremity and present as hip, thigh, or knee pain with or without objective joint findings.

Primary Hypertrophic Osteoarthropathy

There are two rare, primary heritable forms of HO, both presumably autosomal-dominants with much greater severity in males.[338,341]

Pachydermoperiostosis. In addition to clubbed fingers and then periostitis appearing in late childhood (adolescence), these patients (89% males) have a progressive thickening of the skin of their face and head producing an angry, grotesque bulldog (cutis verticis gyrata), aged lepromatous (leonine), or acromegalic facies. Increased sweat-gland activity causes dilated sebum-plugged facial pores. The hands and feet become enlarged as a result of increased soft tissue and bone. Effusions, primarily in the knees and ankles, and usually the presenting complaint, are "sympathetic" noninflammatory reactions to periostitis.[341a]

Although patients are grossly disfigured, the disease tends to slow in its progression. In some cases, however, ossification at the entheses ultimately results in ankylosis of the spine and peripheral joints.

Familial HO without Pachyderma. This type of HO is less common than that associated with pachyderma and is characterized by clubbing from infancy, onset of other features under age 5, and anomalous ossification of the skull with delayed suture closure and Wormian bones.

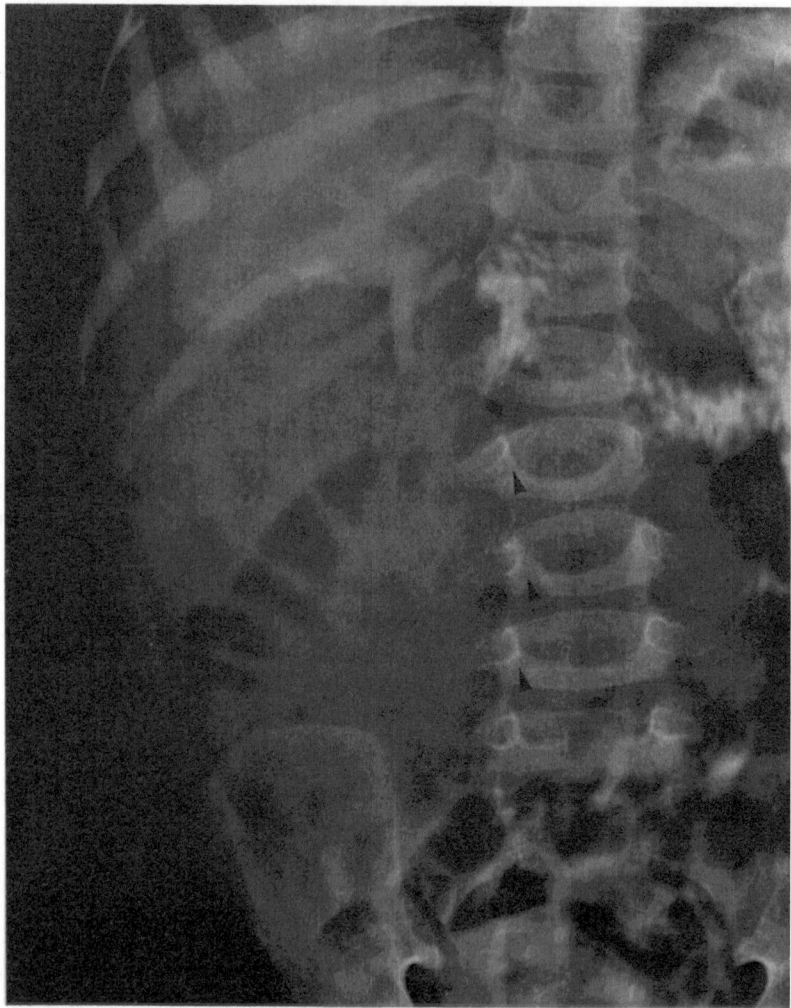

Figure 2.53. IVP in a 6-year-old boy referred for recurrent episodes of leg pain (sciatica), showing the right kidney elevated by a soft-tissue mass that is pushing the duodenum toward the midline. A dumbbell tumor is evidenced by pedicle changes at L-1, -2, -3 (*arrows*). A ganglioneuroblastoma invading the extradual space was found at surgery.

Unusual Traumas and Unusual Responses to Trauma (Table 2.24)

Stress Fractures

Stress fractures occur in normal bone subjected to repeated episodes of minor stress associated with the normal daily activities of a child or athletic

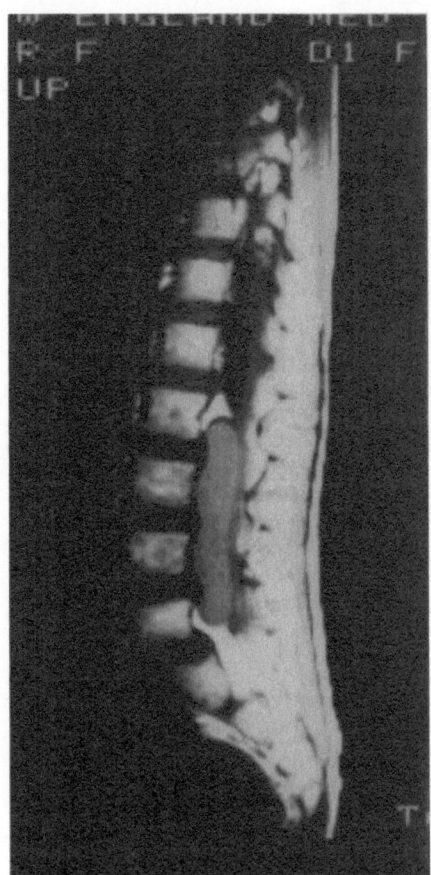

Figure 2.54. MRI revealing Ewing's sarcoma invading spinal cord in a child who presented with polyarthralgias and intermittent leg pain thought to be JRA. (Courtesy of Dr. Marisa Klein-Gitelman.)

adolescent.[342–345] They are most common in the tibia of young children. In the usual case, the youngster complains of pain below the knee and limps. Radiographs are normal for many weeks but ultimately show radiolucency along the posteromedial or posterolateral aspect of the proximal tibia fol-

Table 2.24. Unusual Forms of Traumatic Bone and Joint Pain in Children

Stress fractures
Child abuse
Frostbite
Congenital indifference to pain
Foreign-body synovitis
Acute chondrolysis of the hip
Transient demineralization of the hip

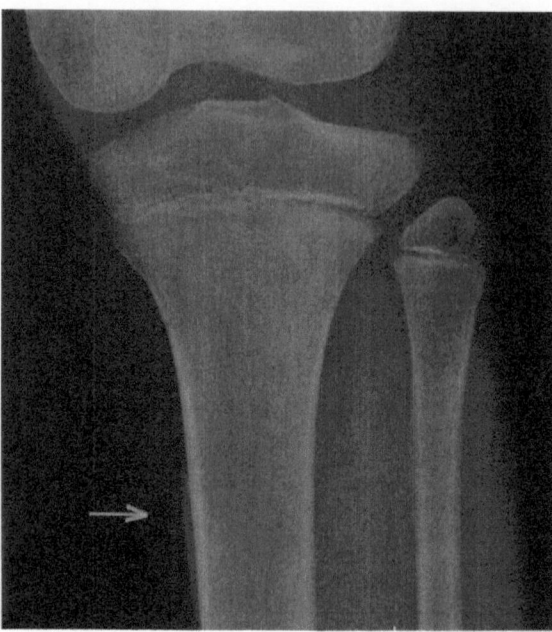

Figure 2.55. Periosteal new-bone formation at typical site of a stress fracture along the tibia of an 8-year-old boy. Biopsy (performed because of unwarranted fear of malignancy) showed the corrent diagnosis. Symptoms may be confused with subacute osteomyelitis.

lowed later by abundant periosteal new-bone formation (Fig. 2.55). The importance of making the diagnosis is avoidance of unnecessary biopsy (and possibly further mischief from mistaking the pathologic findings for a tumor) or long, inappropriate antibiotic therapy for osteomyelitis.

Case Report

An 8-year-old orthopedic physician's son complained of intermittent aching in the anteromedial aspect of the left tibia, just below the knee. The pain occurred primarily at night and tended to subside with rest. One month later, he began to limp; x-rays were thought to be normal. The discomfort increased, and a tender area became apparent on examination. X-rays now showed periosteal new-bone formation (Fig. 2.55). Biopsy was performed, the findings were misinterpreted as osteomyelitis, and treatment was given with antibiotics for 2 months. Cultures of the tissue were negative, as were all usual laboratory studies. He was in a long leg cast for 6 weeks before gradually resuming normal activities. Review of the biopsy specimen showed a healing fracture.

Acute Chondrolysis of the Hip (Juvenile Lamellar Coxitis)

It has long been recognized that occasional patients with a slipped capital femoral epiphysis will develop acute necrosis of the hip cartilage.[346-348] This is visualized radiographically as the joint space rapidly becomes narrow and

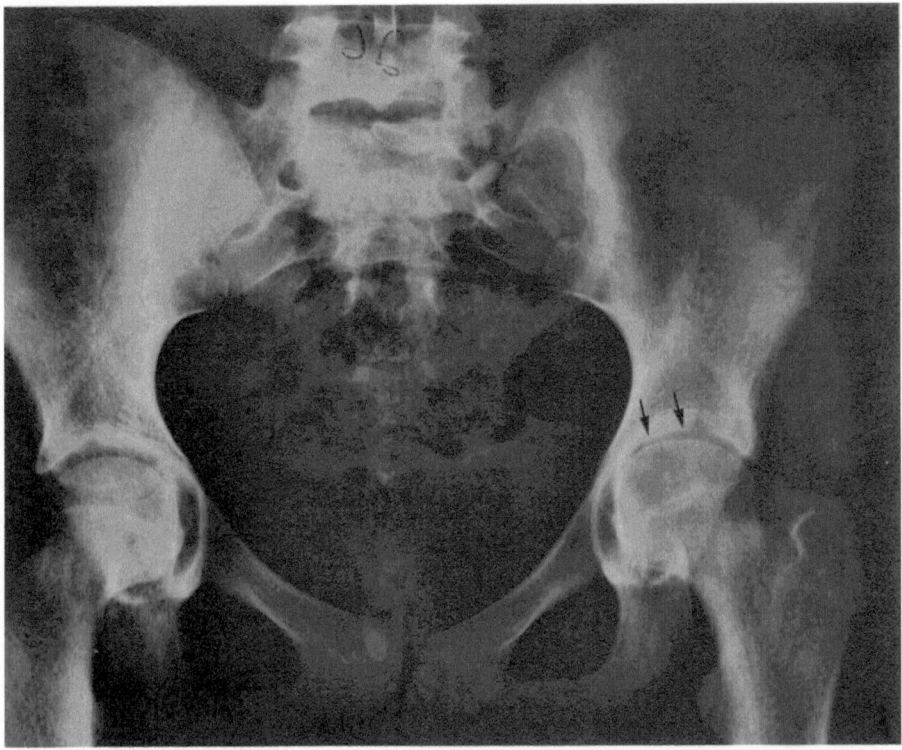

Figure 2.56. Lamellar coxitis (sudden narrowing of the hip joint) in a 15-year-old girl who had pain while doing a split. Follow-up films 9 months later were normal, and she was asymptomatic (see also Fig. 3.36).

irregular. Pathologic examination in these youngsters has shown that the cartilage destruction is not necessarily avascular and that the cartilage is replaced by fibrous vascular granulation tissues (pannus). Taillard and Grasset first recognized that acute chondrolysis alone may also result from trauma and be seen independently of apparent slipped capital femoral epiphysis.[348]

Our experience suggests that following sudden extreme motion, as in jumping into the swimming pool or doing a "split" in ballet, there may be immediate pain and limitation of all hip motions, followed by rapid radiographic evidence of cartilage dissolution (Fig. 2.56). Symptoms respond to aspirin or other nonsteroidal anti-inflammatory agents. Unlike reports of this complication in association with a slipped epiphysis, these patients may recover completely, both functionally and radiographically, over a 6-month period. Our management has been predicated on reports of improved cartilage regeneration in children and animals allowed weight bearing and given anti-inflammatory drug therapy.[349] Experimental evidence suggests that immobilization following cartilage injury prevents rather than enhances recovery. We have seen several young girls who had rapid chondrolysis of both hips, without trauma, which was permanent.[347,350]

Case Report

A 15-year-old female cheerleader developed a sudden pain in her left hip while doing a split. She was able to continue cheerleading during the game, but by the next day was limping severely and had increased pain. Radiographs were said to be normal. When seen by us 3 months later, there was considerable limitation of motion of the left hip and severe narrowing of the hip-joint space radiographically (Fig. 2.56). She was treated with aspirin and gradually improved. Nine months after the incident, examination of the hip was normal, and she no longer required medication. Radiographs now were normal.

Transitory Demineralization of the Hips

We have seen transitory demineralization of the hip (Fig. 2.57) in children, although affected youngsters have not previously been reported.[351,352] As in acute chondrolysis, there is onset of pain and limitation of motion of the hip joint following sudden extreme motion such as doing splits in gym or dance class. The pain progresses, and demineralization becomes evident radiographically. By definition, cases included in this category have not progressed to avascular necrosis, which may initially be suspected, have not had neurovascular changes or other features suggestive of reflex sympathetic dystrophy, and do not have evidence of stress fractures. We treat these children with aspirin and maximum tolerated weight bearing. Symptoms disappear, and the radiographs return to normal in a few months.

Case Report

A 9-year-old female gymnast felt pain in the left thigh while doing a split. The pain subsided with bed rest but recurred with ambulation. Radiographs were said to be normal. Pain continued, and when first seen by us several months later, the examination revealed pain on full range of motion of the hip and demineralization of the femoral head on radiographs (Fig. 2.57A). She was treated with aspirin with relief of symptoms. Radiographs 5 months later were normal, and the femoral head had remineralized (Fig. 2.57B).

Special Forms of Trauma

Child Abuse. Although abused children frequently have skeletal trauma, arthritis has not been a reported feature of child abuse. However, we have

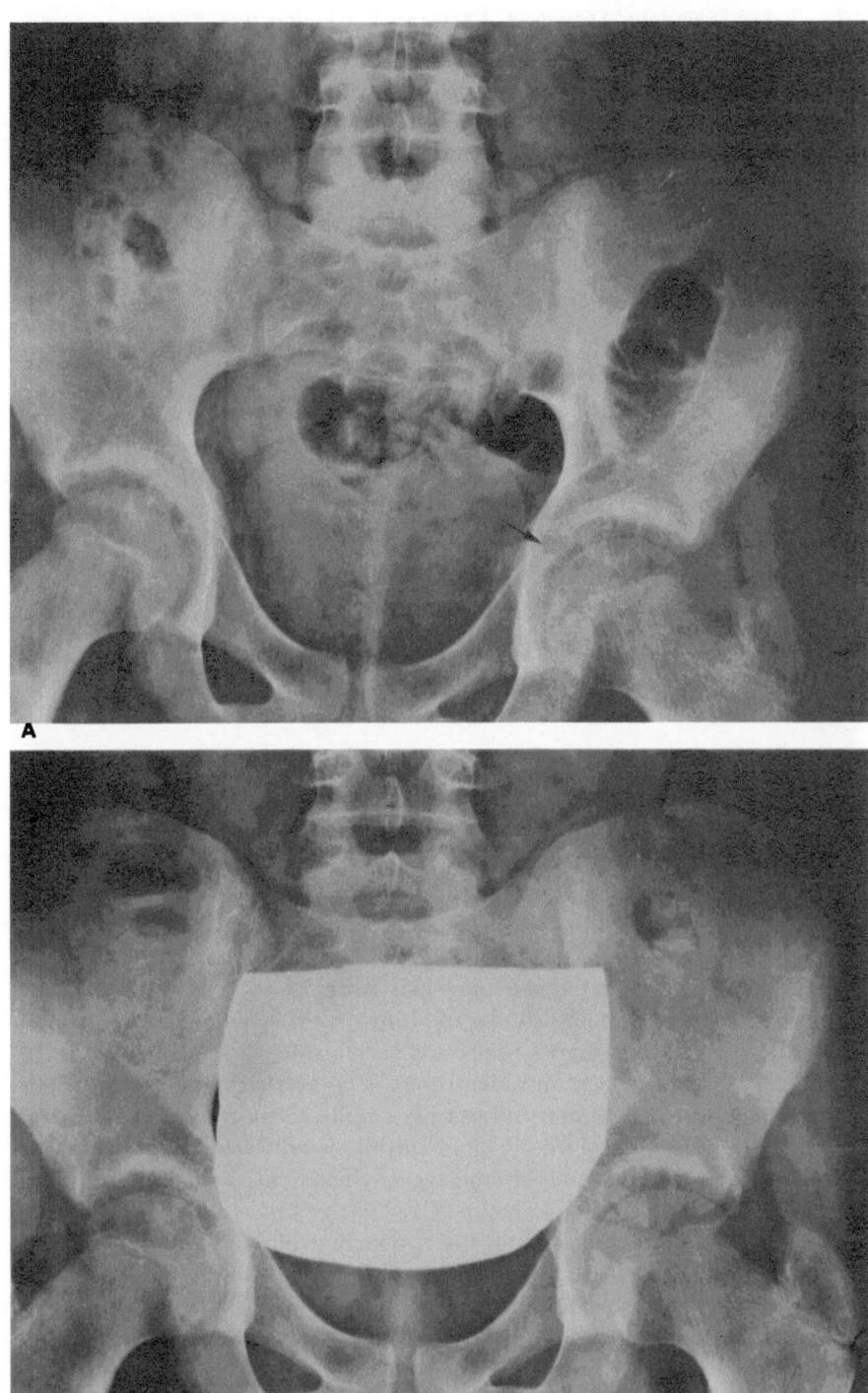

Figure 2.57. (**A**) Transient demineralization of the hip with pain following performance of a split by a 10-year-old girl. (**B**) The hip films are normal 4 months later.

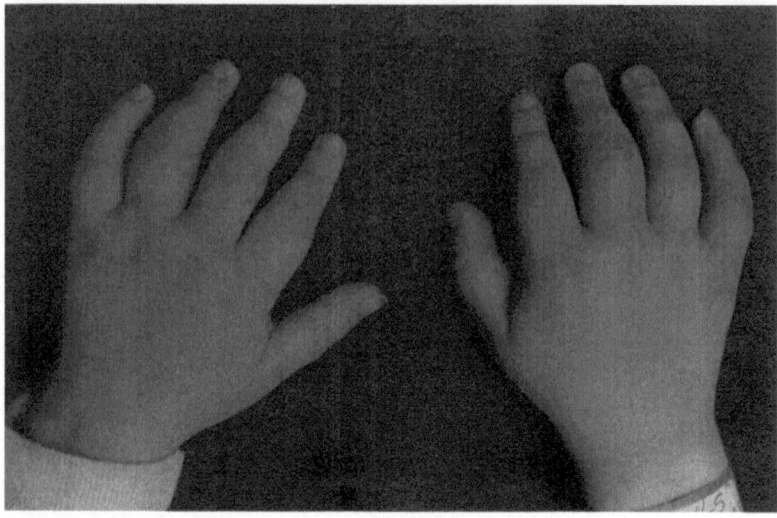

Figure 2.58. Thick brawny induration over and just proximal to the second through fifth proximal interphalangeal joints is a clue to child abuse (beating the child across the fingers with a ruler).

recognized three cases of child abuse characterized by thick, brawny induration over and just proximal to the second through fifth proximal interphalangeal joints (Fig. 2.58). Radiographs show thick, dense phalangeal bones, suggesting chronic hyperemia (Fig. 2.59). In our first two cases, bone chips and periosteal new-bone formation were characteristic features; while periosteal new-bone formation is usually associated with trauma, it had been interpreted in these patients as suggestive of JRA.

Dr. John Caffey suggested the diagnosis to us in 1956 in the first case, stating immediately on being shown the film with the bone shards, "Somebody is beating the child across the hands with a ruler," a punishment technique more commonly used in olden times. The abusive individuals in our cases were found to be regular babysitters employed daily in two cases and the foster mother in the third. Prompt improvement was seen when these children were removed from the abusive environment, and ultimately the fingers returned to normal.

One of our patients had a history of a poorly explained femoral fracture prior to the onset of the traumatic arthropathy, and one child had associated recurrent mouth ulcers. While these were attributed to his chewing on his own gums, we found no evidence of this habit during hospital observation, and the mouth lesions disappeared within a few days of admission, confirming our impression that they were either thermal or chemical burns. Thus, other signs of trauma may provide some clue to this diagnosis, as in other forms of child abuse.

While this syndrome of child abuse is rare (we have recognized only one

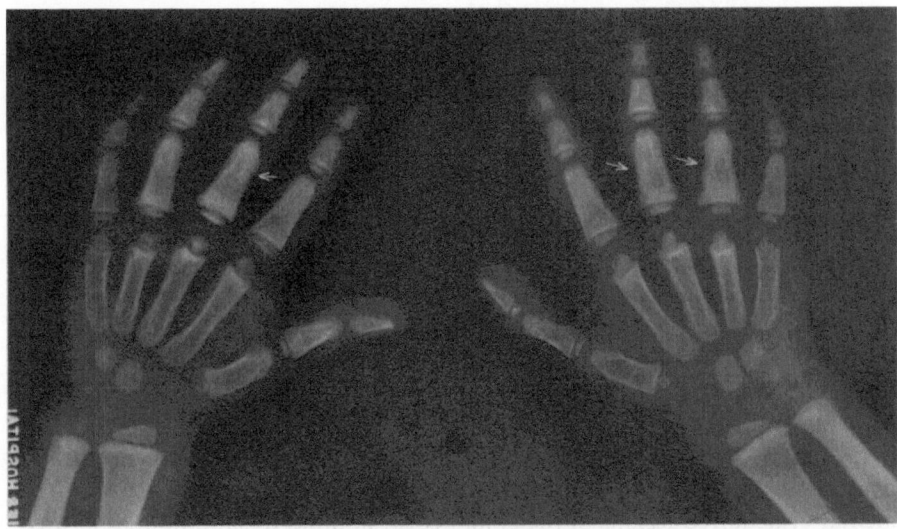

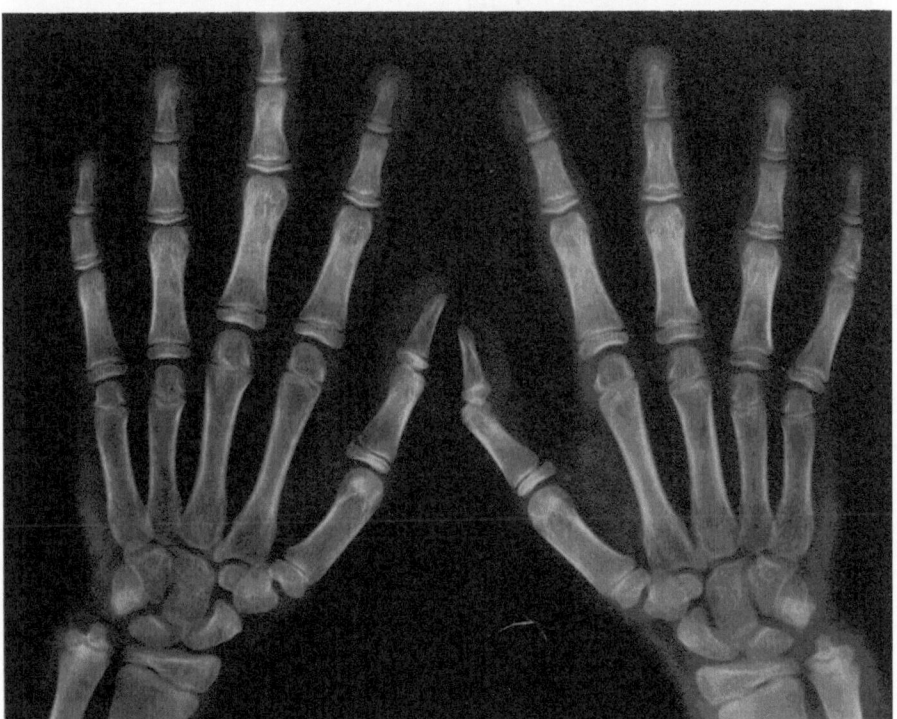

Figure 2.59. (A) Increased density and thickening of the proximal phalanges together with periosteal reaction and sometimes bone shards enables radiographic recognition of this form of child absure (see Fig. 2.58), which in our experience is always confused with JRA. **(B)** Follow-up films 9 years later show remodeling to normal.

case per 7 years), we suspect that such cases are not as rare as this sole report would imply and that they are generally not recognized. One case of self-mutilation produced the same findings.[352a]

Congenital Indifference to Pain (Charcot's Joints in Childhood)

Swollen but painless joints with distal necrosis of the toes and fingers together with bizarre destructive and sclerotic radiographic changes seen in the fingers and toes are characteristic of this rare inborn incapacity to feel superficial or profound pain (Fig. 2.60).[353] These youngsters or their affected sibs often perform "daring feats" or have scars from unrecognized burns or injuries to fingertips or tongue, all clues to the correct diagnosis. Surprisingly, the family may not recognize that their pain sensations are different from normal. Neurogenic arthropathy in childhood may also be seen in developmental or acquired lesions of the spinal cord, familial dysautonomia, or any other condition where there is impairment of deep sensation to a joint. When impaired sensation is not recognized, diagnosis is suggested by the character-

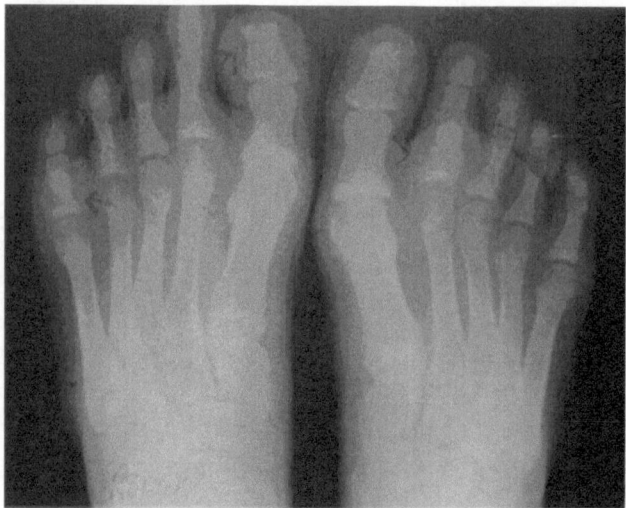

Figure 2.60 Wearing away of the end of the distal first toe phalanx with bizarre fractures and periosteal new-bone formation indicative of unusual trauma in a young girl with congenital indifference to pain. Foot lesions were presumably from overly vigorous bowling. Hand lesions were also a result of unrecognized trauma. Her affected brother had put his hand in a fire as a demonstration of bravado. The father has no lesions but had learned to "take care of my hands." The condition was unrecognized by all family members, and the patient was referred because the appearance of the damaged fingers and toes raised a question of JRA.

istic x-ray findings of (1) erosion of articular cartilage, (2) subchondral sclerosis, (3) periosteal new-bone formation, and (4) loose bodies (bone shards) and marginal fractures.

Frostbite

Occasionally, a small child presents with swollen red fingers and color changes that have suggested a diagnosis of Raynaud's syndrome to the primary physician. History reveals the onset after cold exposure; the parents were not aware of the particular sensitivity of the baby's hands to cold injury. Cold injury to immature digital blood vessels may result in Raynaudlike hypersensitivity for months or years thereafter. Radiographs sometimes show narrowed "pointing" of the terminal phalanges (Fig. 2.61).

Less commonly seen sequelae of frostbite are shortened fingers due to epiphyseal cold injury that resulted in premature closure of the damaged epiphysis and growth deformity.[354] These damaged distal interphalangeal joints may also develop deformities, and the children may have arthritic symptoms in these damaged joints.[355] The arthritic manifestations may appear many years after the initial insult and represent an inflammatory response in an "osteoarthritic" joint rather than JRA, as might be suspected, especially if the history of cold injury was not obtained.

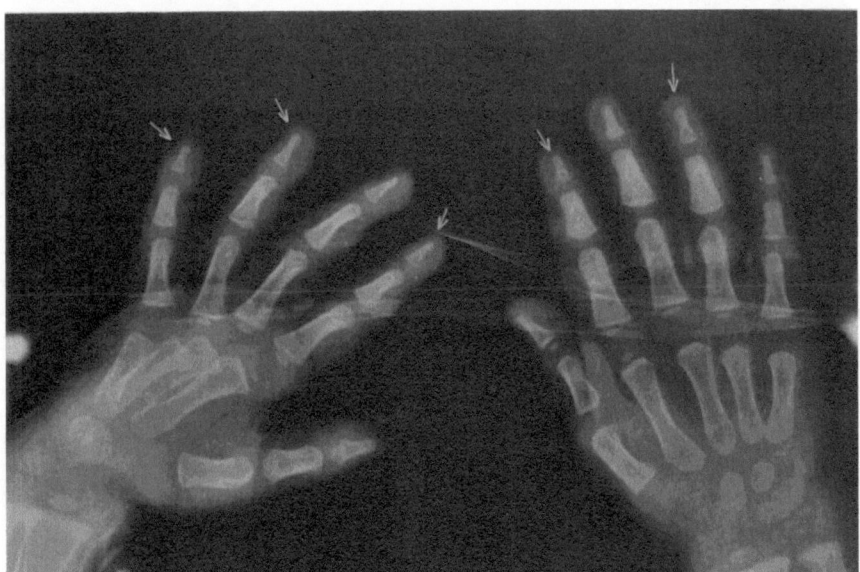

Figure 2.61. Penciling of distal phalanges in a toddler following unrecognized frostbite. This boy was referred for Raynaud's phenomenon because of vascular instability in the fingers.

Eosinophilic Synovitis

Recurrent episodes of acute monarticular arthritis occur as a manifestation of familial Mediterranean fever, Lyme disease, cystic fibrosis, Whipple's disease, sitosterolemia, and gout. Synovial fluid eosinophilia may be seen in parasitic infection, Lyme disease, in atopic allergy, or in patients with hypereosinophilia of any etiology including malignancy. A few patients have been reported with synovial fluid hypereosinophilia as a response to trauma. Episodes are recurrent and tend to subside spontaneously in 1–2 weeks without therapy.[356]

Erythrocyte and DNA Autosensitivity

At least some cases of this disorder, characterized by recurrent painful ecchymoses of the extremities with intermediate-type skin reactions to lysed autologous erthrocytes,[357] or leukocytes and heterologous DNA, are due to self-inflicted injury or injury by a caretaker.[358] However, some cases are apparently not factitious and these may respond to treatment with hydroxychloroquine.[359]

Degenerative Disorders

Avascular ("Aseptic") Necrosis of Bone (AVN)

These lesions occur in a number of clinical settings in children and may be divided into five subgroups (Table 2.25). In each instance, damage is thought to be secondary to circulatory compromise and inadequate nutrition of cancellous bone, most frequently of the femoral head and neck.[360] It is easy to understand the hypothesized pathogenesis in cases of direct trauma, vasculitic diseases, diseases with storage or sluggish infarcts, or air or fat emboli, all of which could be expected to obstruct circulation. The pathogenic mechanisms in the idiopathic or steroid-induced forms are harder to comprehend. In AVN of bone, pain is initially present only on standing or walking and is absent at rest and at night, characteristics that help to differentiate the pain of AVN from that of JRA or other rheumatic diseases. Diagnosis de-

Table 2.25. Types of Avascular Necrosis of bone Seen in Children

"Idiopathic"
Heritable
Vasculitic
Drug-induced
Posttrauma, infection

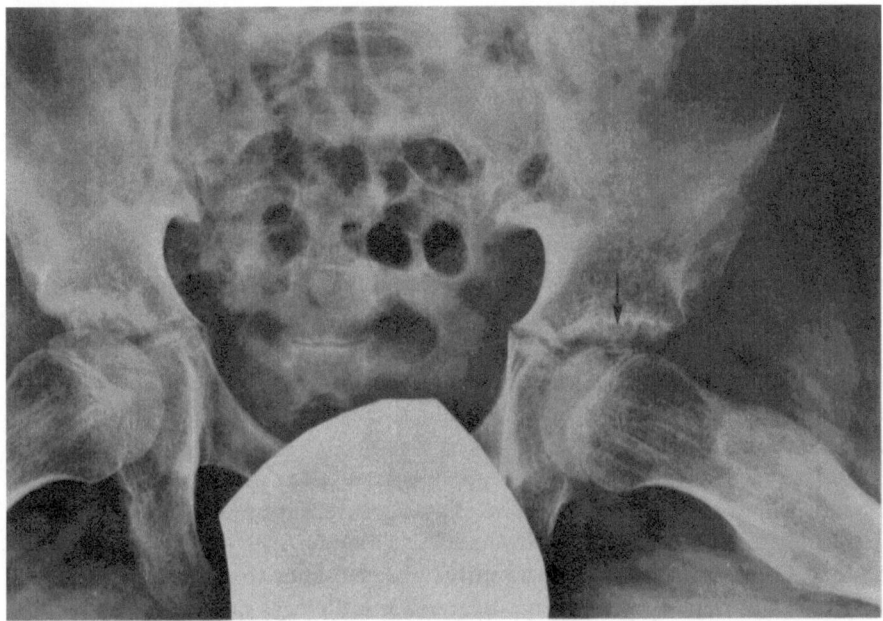

Figure 2.62. Avascular necrosis in left hip of a 15-year-old boy following corticosteroid therapy for a brain tumor; he was referred as "JRA." Films showed flattening of the femoral head with a subchondral curved lucency (*arrow*).

pends on radiographs, which should be obtained in any painful bone or joint (Fig. 2.62). Bone scans and MRI may be helpful before x-ray changes are apparent.

Idiopathic. Although many bones may be affected, each with its own eponym, Legg-Calvé-Perthes disease is the most frequent. Aseptic necrosis of the femoral head is predominantly a disease of young boys (average age 7) and is unfortunately bilateral in 10% of patients. In bilateral disease, hypothyroidism and skeletal dysplasia must be excluded.[361] Painless limp alone is the clinical presentation in 25% of these boys, but hip, knee, or groin pain plus limp is the more frequent presentation. X-rays may be negative when initially obtained, and scans and repeat films are sometimes necessary to establish the diagnosis. This disorder is so common that every pediatrician is taught to take an x-ray of the hip in every case of unexplained limp or knee pain. Optimal treatment has been a subject of controversy.[362]

What was previously called osteochonditis of the tibial tubercle (Osgood-Schlatter disease) is not aseptic necrosis at all and is now recognized as an avulsion of bone from the tibial tiberosity growing into the patellar ligament. Complaints of pain and swelling at the tibial tuberosity are very common in pediatric practice; the diagnosis is generally made clinically and the patient is reassured. No treatment is necessary.

A derangement of endochondral ossification in multiple vertebrae has been called juvenile (adolescent) kyphosis (Scheuermann's disease, Schmorl's nodes). Schmorl's nodes are often limited to the thoracic area and usually go unnoticed unless there is pain or an incidental x-ray is obtained for another reason. X-rays show dorsal kyphosis, narrowed anterior vertebral bodies and disk spaces, and herniation of intervertebral disk tissue into the vertebral bodies. Some cases are familial.[363]

Heritable Disorders. Patients with hemoglobinopathies may have sludging of cells in small vessels, causing aseptic necrosis of the precariously vascularized femoral head. SS, SC, SD, and SA diseases have all been associated with avascular necrosis. Storage diseases such as Gaucher's and Fabry's disease may first present with musculoskeletal complaints and aseptic necrosis of the femoral head.

Another cause of mysterious aseptic necrosis is the group of skeletal dysplasias, which may be familial. The clinical presentation may resemble JRA with multiple joint pains. Family history, short stature, stubby hands with blunted fingers, and elbow contractures may be clues to the correct diagnosis. In the spondyloepiphyseal type, lateral spine x-rays may show characteristic vertebral changes (humping of bone in the central plate and lack of bone in the apophyses).

Vasculitic Diseases. What appears to be local bone death apparently may occur in all of the vasculitic diseases. We have seen it at the knees elbows, shoulders, ankles, and hips of children with SLE (Figs. 5.25 and 5.26), Goodpasture's syndrome, and various forms of systemic vasculitis. All of our patients have had corticosteroid treatment, but it is well documented that AVN may also occur in these disorders even without steroid treatment.[364] The diagnosis suggests itself in youngsters who, as they are generally improving from the primary disease, suddenly develop rather severe pain in a hip or knee out of proportion to any evidence of arthritis elsewhere as a part of their basic disease. X-rays most commonly show a crescentic area of rarefaction in subchondral bone, but there may be patchy sclerosis of the femoral head or irregularity and flattening of the epiphysis (Fig. 2.62). Earlier diagnosis is possible with bone scan or MRI.

We treat this pain with aspirin or other nonsteroidal anti-inflammatory agents and allow full weight bearing and normal activities. Most of the children recover with this judicious neglect, but an occasional youngster goes on to complete hip-joint destruction and may require joint replacement.

Corticosteroids. Patients treated with corticosteroids for asthma and other disorders may develop aseptic necrosis, especially of the hips.[365] The mechanism is unknown, but the condition is also seen in naturally occurring Cushing's syndrome. When a patient with a vasculitis has been treated with steroids, the risk of aseptic necrosis seems to be increased, although in an individual instance it is impossible to know whether the cause is related to the basic disease or the steroid therapy or both.

In children, remineralization without sequelae is possible; in our experience, this is the most frequent end result. In the absence of proof that any of the proposed treatments—medical or surgical—affects the outcome, we have chosen to relieve pain and secondary synovitis with aspirin or other nonsteroidal antiinflammatory drugs and not to restrict the children in any way. It is possible that adequately controlled studies will, in the future, indicate a better approach (see also Chapter 5, section on AVN).

Cracking Joints

Crepitus (creaking joints) may signify loss of cartilage and apposition of underlying bone or synovial hypertrophy with alteration of joint mechanics.[366] It is sometimes demonstrable in spondyloarthritic children in joints without other objective signs of disease. Some children voluntarily "crack" their knuckles (metacarpophalangeal joints), a feat that is accomplished by traction in the joint, causing the formation of a gas bubble within the joint. Release of the tension collapses the bubble, producing the "crack." Transient symptomless cracking occurs occasionally in adults and more frequently in children, whose joints are more mobile. Occasionally, it elicits concern; in the absence of other evidence of disease, the child and parents may be reassured. Obsessive knuckle cracking may be the cause of joint damage and should be discouraged.

Chondromalacia Patellae

Vague complaints of diffuse aching knee pain, sometimes with sensations of buckling or instability, are not uncommon in teenage girls. These complaints have been related to softening of some of the patellar cartilage, which can be seen in various stages on arthroscopy.[367] However, we have no knowledge of whether these same findings might be found as frequently if one arthroscoped teenage girls who had no complaints. Operative treatment has been generally unsatisfactory (over 150 different operative procedures have been described) and leaves an unattractive scar unless performed arthroscopically.

We will entertain a diagnosis of chondromalacia in youngsters with patellar pain without objective or radiographic findings but recommend no further diagnostic or therapeutic procedures. Any procedure, even arthroscopy, sometimes makes the situation worse. Activities are not limited, and we offer NSAID treatment only if desired. We assume that these youngsters are likely to improve with "judicious neglect," and they generally do. The patients and their families seem more amenable to this approach when told the problem is "chondromalacia," as contrasted with "an unexplained pain in the patella."[368]

Osteochondritis Dissecans

Loose bodies, especially in the knees or ankles, may occur without a history of trauma, but more frequently the patient with osteochondritis dissecans presents with persistent pain following a known injury.[369] Initial x-rays may be negative, and repeat films are required in patients with persistent unexplained symptoms. Orthopedic opinion differs, but most youngsters are said to respond to conservative therapy; a few who do not improve benefit from operative procedures. The disease is sometimes familial and multifocal. One family with a mother and two affected children whose disease was mistaken for JRA has been reported.[370]

Slipped Capital Femoral Epiphysis

Adolescent boys, and occasionally girls, just prior to the time when the femoral head is scheduled to unite with the shaft, sometimes insidiously develop a medial/posterior displacement of the head of the femur (a slipped capital femoral epiphysis) (Fig. 2.63). Pain and limitation of motion of the hip may be accompanied by knee pain; or limp, groin, thigh or knee pains may be the only complaints.[370a] In 25% of cases, the condition is bilateral. Diagnosis is made by x-ray, and prompt surgical treatment is required in an effort to avoid the three major complications of a slip: acute cartilage necro-

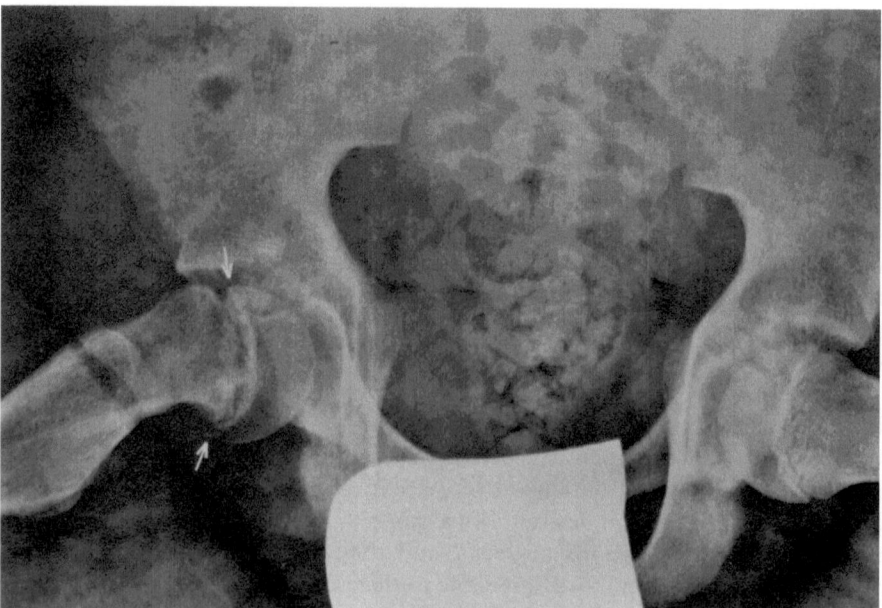

Figure 2.63. Slipped capital femoral epiphysis, a common cause of hip pain in adolescent boys.

sis, osseous necrosis of the femoral head, and late osteoarthritis. There is some evidence that low androgens may be a factor contributing to the development of a slipped capital femoral epiphysis.

Osteoarthritis in Childhood

Primary osteoarthritis is a disorder of aging not seen in children except as a rare feature of progeria or its adolescent equivalent, Werner's syndrome. However, once the joint cartilage is damaged as a result of any primary process, secondary degenerative changes may take place, especially in weight-bearing joints. Secondary osteoarthritis (OA) is seen in children following septic hips, Legg-Calvé-Perthes disease, congenital dislocation of the hip, slipped capital femoral epiphysis, JRA, and all of the metabolic and other disorders discussed in this chapter.

There are many theories but so far no final understanding about the pathogenesis of this common form of progressive joint destruction.[371] Various studies show alterations in collagen and proteoglycan chemistry, release of harmful enzymes, altered biomechanics, and acceleration of damage with occupational trauma. Each probably plays a role in the pathogenesis of OA.

Children with damaged hips sometimes have episodes of "traumatic synovitis" associated with sudden increase in pain and limitation of motion. If the inflammation is sufficiently severe, it may be accompanied by systemic signs such as fever and an elevated ESR. The possibility of reactivation of old infection or onset of new infection must always be considered. We have seen a number of these youngsters who were referred for evaluation for rheumatoid arthritis. The history of prior joint damage and lack of evidence of arthritis elsewhere make it easy to exclude JRA as a cause of the symptoms. Relief of these acute synovitis episodes in damaged joints may be effectively achieved with aspirin or nonsteroidal anti-inflammatory drugs.

Attacks are usually brief, and the medication, if promptly administered in effective quantities, allows the child to continue normal activities. Chronic administration of anti-inflammatory drugs is rarely necessary for these children.

Metabolic Diseases

Ordinarily, a pediatrician doesn't think about metabolism and the joints at the same time. But the joints contain connective tissues, cartilage, and bone, all potentially altered by abnormalities in structure, biosynthesis, and metabolism. There must be thousands of potential abnormalities. We have divided the recognized metabolic abnormalities into those discussed in this section, those grouped together because of characteristic joint laxity or joint stiffness, and those resulting from the presence of abnormal red blood cells or plasma proteins (Table 2.26).

Table 2.26. Metabolic Abnormalities with Musculoskeletal Manifestations

Abnormality of	*Manifestation*
Carbohydrate	Diabetic cheiroarthropathy
Amino acid	Alcaptonuria
	Homocystinuria
	Sulfite oxidase deficiency
Organic acid	Lowe's syndrome
Lipid	Familial hyperlipoproteinemia
	Fabry's disease
	Gaucher's disease
	Farber's disease
Endocrinopathies	Cushing's syndrome
	Addison's disease
	Thyroid acropachy
	Myxedema
Purine/Pyrimidine	Gout
Heavy metal	Hemachromatosis
Blood cells	Hemoglobinopathies
	White-blood-cell bacterial-killing defects
Plasma proteins	Hemophilia
	Complement and gamma globulin deficiencies
	Streaking leukocyte factor
Bone and calcium and phosphorus	Hypophosphatemic D-resistant rickets
	Bone and cartilage dysplasias
	Hyperparathyroidism
	Vitamin A and D poisoning
	Fluorosis
	Calcific periarthritis
	Juvenile osteoporosis
	Tumor- and drug-induced rickets
Connective tissue	Ehlers-Danlos syndrome
	Marfan's syndrome
	Mucopolysaccharidoses
	Mucolipidoses
	Leri's plenocytosis
	Familial hypertrophic synovitis
	Weill-Marchesani syndrome
	Vanishing bone diseases
	Stickler arthro-ophthalmic syndrome
	Myositis ossificans (FOP)

Diabetic Cheiroarthropathy (Diabetic Hand Syndrome)

Thickening and tightening of the soft tissues of the fingers with progressive stiffness and flexion contractures, first of the distal interphalangeal joints and then of the proximal interphalangeal joints, has been called juvenile diabetic

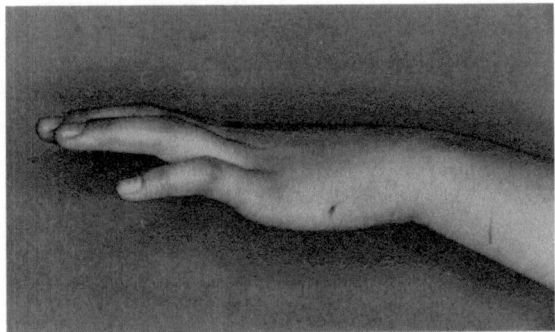

Figure 2.64. Diabetic cheiroarthropathy, early stage. (Courtesy of Dr. A. Benedetti.)

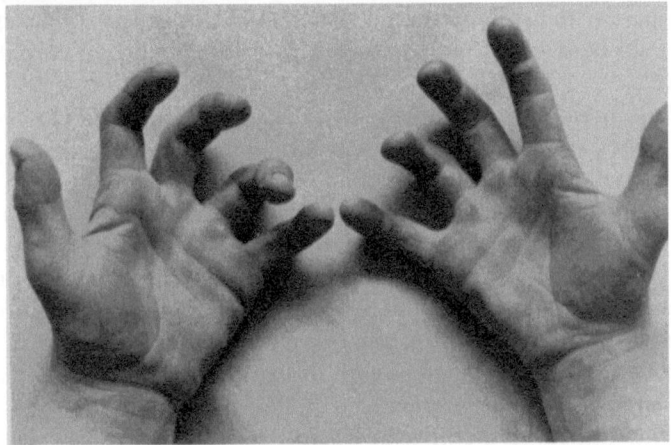

Figure 2.65. Diabetic cheiroarthropathy, late stage, with inability to flatten the hand. In older series of patients with JRA prior to description of this entity, we found that these patients were thought to have both diabetes and JRA. (Courtesy of Dr. A. Benedetti.)

cheiroarthropathy (Figs. 2.64 and 2.65).[372] The manifestations seem to be a result of increased deposition of collagen in the lower dermis and may precede other signs of diabetes.[373,374] Although this syndrome is rare in diabetic adults, surveys of diabetic children suggest that cheiroarthropathy is a common feature in adolescents who had the onset of diabetes in infancy and early childhood (67% after 8 years of disease),[375] especially if control of hyperglycemia has been difficult and inadequate. As a result, patients with this manifestation of diabetes also have an increased incidence of retinopathy and nephropathy.[376]

There is generally no pain, although occasional patients may have paresthesias and hyperesthesias, probably from associated diabetic neuropathy. Review of our old clinic records reveals that most children previously thought to have diabetes and JRA actually had this nonrheumatic syndrome, although occasionally both disorders do coexist.[377] The differentiation is important since antiarthritic drugs are not useful in diabetic cheiroarthropathy.

As the syndrome progresses, other joints may also develop limited motion, resulting in asymptomatic mild flexion contractures of the wrists, knees, neck, elbows, and hips. Restrictive pulmonary lung disease can be demonstrated with special pulmonary function studies, analogous to that seen in scleroderma.[373]

When it became apparent that carpal tunnel syndrome might also complicate diabetes, electrical studies were performed on both children and adults with diabetic hand syndrome. Delayed transmission of nerve impulses has been frequently demonstrated in both the median and ulnar nerves of these patients. Recent studies suggest that packing, cross-linking, and turnover of collagen is abnormal in these patients, perhaps as a result of nonenzymatic glucosylation. Since the ulnar nerve does not travel through the carpal tunnel, it is apparent that carpal tunnel release will not relieve this syndrome. Surgery should be avoided unless there is certain evidence of carpal tunnel entrapment.

The pathogenesis of this syndrome has not been defined. However, the thickened tissues and abnormal nerve conduction studies suggest to us that the nerves may indeed be entrapped, not in the carpal tunnel but as a result of being bound down in abnormal connective tissue. The joint limitations also seem likely to be a result of periarticular deposition of an undefined abnormal ground substance, but animal models suggest that it may be a result of saturation of the sorbitol dehydrogenase pathway enzymes resulting in increased production of sorbitol and other polyols and depletion of various intracellular mediators. Treatment with the aldose reductase agent sorbinil, an experimental agent, has been reported to provide dramatic reversal of this syndrome with improved mobility and grip strength.[373]

Disorders of Bone Metabolism

"Weak bones" (osteopenia) may result in limp with pain in the knees and ankles, presumably as a result of subclinical impaction fractures in weight-bearing metaphyses.[378] Fractures of long bones after minimal trauma and collapse of vertebral bodies may also occur. This group of conditions has been divided into those seen primarily as defects in the rate of synthesis or breakdown of bone matrix (osteoporosis), as contrasted with those that are a result of defective mineralization of bone (osteomalacia), such as rickets. The differentiation is often difficult or impossible but may sometimes be accomplished with x-rays, chemical and metabolic studies, and bone biopsy.

Idiopathic Juvenile Osteoporosis. Children with this rare disorder usually present as preadolescents with back, knee, and ankle pains.[379-382] All have stopped growing or are actually losing height; this may have escaped notice, and review of the growth chart may provide an important clue to the diagnosis. Definitive diagnosis depends on the radiographic demonstration of demineralization of the spine and documentation that the child has adequate intake of calcium and vitamin D and is not on corticosteroids or anticonvul-

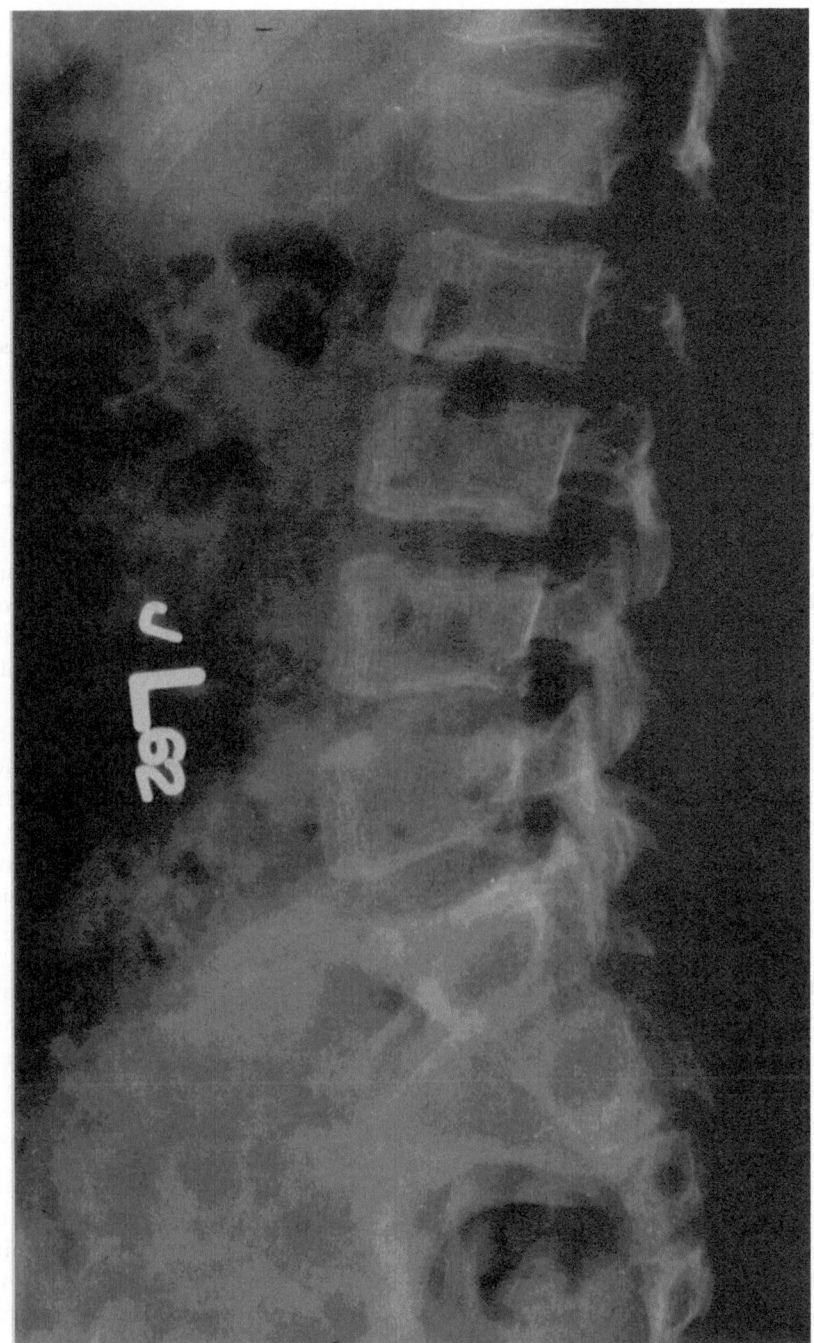

Figure 2.66. Juvenile osteoporosis of the spine in an 11-year-old boy with back pain. The patient made a spontaneous recovery without treatment. We have seen similar cases in a child placed on a milk-free diet, and in a child taking corticosteroids for asthma, and in leukemia.

sant drugs (Fig. 2.66). In later stages, there may be multiple compression fractures and fractures of the long bones, especially around the joints. All other disorders that may cause demineralization or these other findings must be excluded, especially leukemia, which may mimic this disorder.

Children with idiopathic juvenile osteoporosis always recover during adolescence, usually without residua. A few severe cases are left with deformities. Although the etiology of this disorder is unknown, bone resorption at the metaphyseal ends of long bones seems to be especially accelerated, presumably due to some hormonal imbalance triggered by the prepubertal growth spurt that is spontaneously relieved by the onset of puberty. In two patients treatment with biphosphonate or calcitriol has been efficacious.[382,383]

Hyperparathyroidism. Primary hyperparathyroidism is an exceedingly rare condition in childhood, but hyperparathyroidism secondary to renal disease is not uncommon. In addition to bone pain, symptoms include those due to hypercalcemia (weakness, hypotonic muscles, hyperextensible joints, anorexia, nausea, mental changes); those due to increased excretion of calcium in the urine (polyuria, polydipsia, nocturia, frequency, calculi, and renal colic); and those due to soft-tissue ("metastatic") calcium deposits in the eyes (band keratopathy), and in the ligaments, cartilage, and periarticular tissues, which are occasionally associated with joint effusions.

Bone pain is often the complaint that first brings the patient to the doctor. Radiographs show demineralization with thinning of the cortex of the bones. Cystlike areas of rarefaction with a moth-eaten appearance of the skull and osteoblastic (brown) tumors appear later (osteitis fibrosa). Diagnosis may be apparent radiographically but is documented by appropriate chemical studies. The differential diagnosis of hypercalcemia with bone pain in childhood is shown in Table 2.27.

Dialysis Arthritis. Articular and periarticular beta-2 microglobulin amyloidosis manifested by carpal tunnel syndrome, arthralgias, bone cysts, and destructive arthritis occurs in 14% of adults on long-term hemo- or peritoneal dialysis.[384] Similar lesions were described in adults with hyperparathyroidism many years ago.[385]

Late-Onset Rickets. Osteoporosis and bone pain may be seen in late-onset vitamin-D-resistant rickets (phosphate diabetes). Bony overgrowth of the wrists and knees in hypophosphatemic rickets may cause significant limitation of motion and, together with painful subperiosteal erosions in the fingers, may be mistaken for JRA. One such patient was referred to us after a 1-year trial of gold injections.

There are two curable forms of late-onset rickets seen in childhood. Anticonvulsant therapy may result in osteomalacia and rickets through a number of metabolic interactions,[386,387] and a number of children have been reported

Table 2.27. Differential Diagnosis of Hypercalcemic Disorders

Hyperparathyroidism, primary or secondary (renal)
Vitamin D intoxication
Leukemia, neuroblastoma, hepatoblastoma, and other malignancies
Immobilization with fractures
Sarcoidosis
Hypothyroidism and Addison's disease
Hypophosphatasia

with bone pain, rickets, and myopathy of late onset that was cured by removal of a nonossifying fibroma or other benign tumor of bone.[388–390] We have seen one such patient;[390] the incidence of this disorder (oncogenous rickets) may be more common than has been recognized. A thorough search for skeletal or mesenchymal tumors is essential in all patients with unexplained acquired rickets. Medical reversal of acquired hypophosphatemic osteomalacia has been reported where the tumor could not be found or was in extensive sebaceous nevi.[391,392]

Case Report[390]

A 13-year-old girl was seen because of intermittent pain in the knees for 1 year and pain in the heels for 2 months. The ankles were occasionally noted to swell. Pain was worse when walking and especially on climbing stairs. Physical examination was normal except for slight swelling about the right ankle. A mass of laboratory data was normal except for phosphorus, 1.7 mg/dl, and alkaline phosphatase, 1725 units/liter. X-rays showed florid rickets (Fig. 2.67) and benign cortical defects in the left femur, thought to represent a nonossifying fibroma. The tumor was removed, blood chemistries returned to normal within 1 month, and the rickets completely healed over a 2-month period.

Endocrinopathies with Arthritis. There is evidence of endocrine control of the synthesis and degradation of connective-tissue molecules, so it is not surprising that rheumatic syndromes may be associated with hypo- and hyperthyroidism and with Addison's disease and Cushing's syndrome.

Hypothyroidism. Joint effusions were reported as part of myxedema 100 years ago and have been noted in the knees and metacarpo- and metatarsophalangeal joints in many hypothyroid patients.[393] Despite synovial thickening and stiffness, patients have little pain. Thyroid replacement therapy completely relieves the arthritis. Episodic arthralgia[394] and inflammatory polyarthritis[395] have been reported in Hashimoto's thyroiditis in the absence of hypothyroidism and do not respond to thyroid replacement therapy.

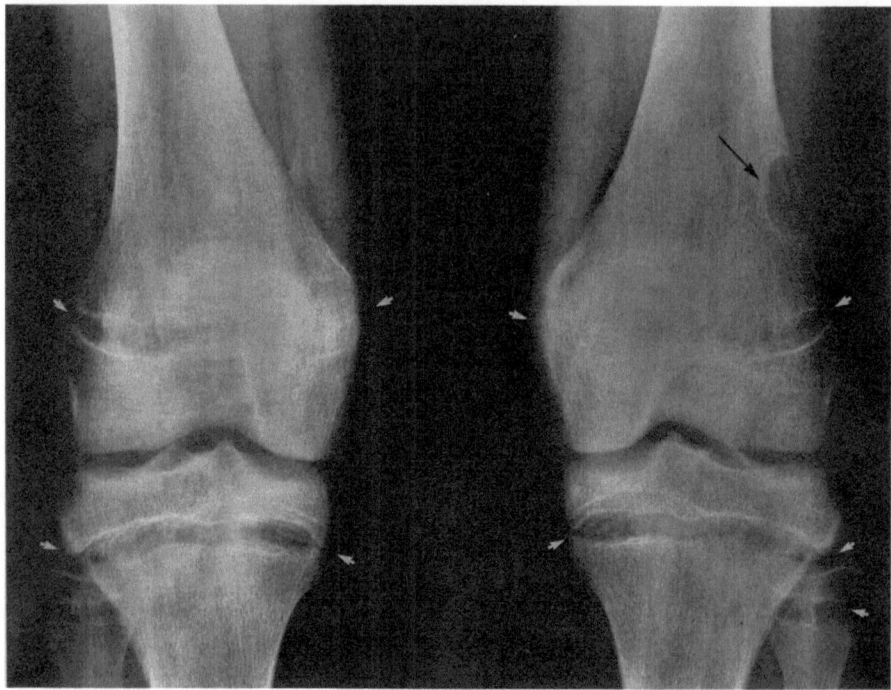

Figure 2.67. Tumor-induced rickets in a 12-year-old girl with nonossifying fibroma (*black arrow*) of the distal left humerus. The patient presented with muscloskeletal pain suggestive of arthritis, but was found to have florid rickets on the radiograph (widened osteoid accumulation) (*white arrows*). Removal of the benign tumor was followed by prompt relief of symptoms and disappearance of radiographic evidence of rickets. (Courtesy of Dr. R. Asnes. Reprinted with permission from Asnes, RS, ref. 390)

Arthritis is a common side effect of treatment of hyperthyroidism with propylthiouracil and represents drug allergy rather than hypothyroidism.[396]

Hyperthyroidism. Hyperthyroidism in adults has been associated with a distinctive form of arthritis, thyroid acropachy. The main features are swelling of the subcutaneous tissues, fluffy subperiosteal new-bone formation in the hands, and clubbing of the fingers and toes. Unlike other forms of hypertrophic osteoarthropathy, no heat or pain is manifested in these patients. Hyperthyroidism is usually present for many years before acropachy develops, which makes this an extraordinarily rare form of arthritis in childhood.[397]

Cushing's Syndrome and Addison's Disease. Patients with Cushing's syndrome often have bone pain as a result of osteoporosis and avascular necrosis at multiple sites.[398] Addison's disease is usually accompanied by myalgias, but occasionally joint stiffness may simulate rheumatic disease[399] Addison's disease may be a presenting manifestation or feature of SLE and anticardiolipin syndrome; some cases are due to thromboembolism of adrenal blood vessels.[400]

Vitamin and Fluoride Poisoning

Most vitamin poisoning is iatrogenic, induced by the physician using vitamins to treat acne or other conditions or by the mother (who thinks vitamins can only be beneficial) giving excess vitamins to the child. However, we have also seen one case in which a teenage boy secretly took large amounts of vitamins purchased in a health-food store.

Vitamin A Poisoning. Chronic excess ingestion of vitamin A alters bone metabolism and results in cortical thicking of bone. Synthetic retinoids prescribed for ichthyosis, psoriasis, or other skin diseases, may also cause hyperostosis and spinal and extraspinal tendon and ligament calcifications.[401–403] Pain in the bones and joints is often the most troublesome symptom in hypervitaminosis A and the symptom that brings the patient to the doctor.[404] Other symptoms include painful muscular stiffness, fatigue after exercise, anorexia, alopecia, generalized pruritus, and dry, scaling, eczematous skin with yellow palms (Fig. 2.68). If ingestion continues, increased intracranial

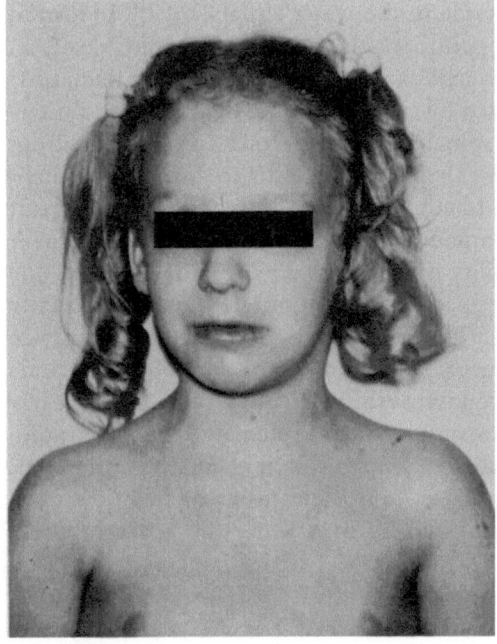

Figure 2.68. Arthralgia and bone pain were the presenting manifestations in this child, who was noted to have frontal bossing, alopecia, and excoriated rash, and papilledema typical of vitamin A poisoning. The sicker she got, the more vitamin A the mother gave her!

pressure (pseudotumor cerebri) may develop. The entire clinical picture may simulate connective-tissue disease.[402]

Diagnosis is usually established by careful history taking in cases with the characteristic clinical picture and may be confirmed with determination of high serum levels of vitamin A and, particularly in early cases, retinal esters.[401] During the early stages of intoxication, vitamin A is deposited in the liver, and serum levels are not as high as they become after the liver is saturated. Occasionally, hypercalcemia is also a consequence of vitamin A poisoning and may be a clue to diagnosis.[402]

All of the symptoms disappear over a period of months after withdrawal of vitamin A. Repeated lumbar punctures may be necessary to lower intracranial pressure and protect vision. Accurate diagnosis helps avoid unnecessary neurosurgical procedures.

Vitamin D Poisoning. Excess vitamin D administered by the parent or taken by the teenager produces bone pain from demineralization, just as in hyperparathyroidism. However, the major presenting manifestations are usually the result of soft-tissue deposits of calcium, especially in the kidney, resulting in obstructive uropathy from stones; in the eyes, resulting in band keratopathy; or in the periarticular structures, resulting in limitation of motion of the joints.

Fluorosis. Endemic fluorosis as a cause of chronic rheumatic symptoms is common in certain areas of the world, especially in parts of India, and has been reported in the United States and in many other countries in areas with especially high natural levels of fluoride in the water supply.[405–409] Industrial and environmental poisoning by pollution also occurs and may result in either chronic symptoms or in the accidental creation of epidemic fluorosis.

Crippling fluorosis is characterized by calcified spinal ligaments and intervertebral disks with a narrowed spinal canal and cord compression from bony overgrowth and generalized calcification of all the entheses (attachments of ligaments and tendons to bone). These severe manifestations result from continuous ingestion of large amounts of fluoride (20–80 mg daily) over a period of many years. Joint mobility is progressively limited. The first clue to diagnosis is often mottling of the enamel of the permanent teeth, especially the premolars and second molars. The most frequent early complaints in children are vague pains in the knees, spine, and small joints of the hands and feet that simulate JRA or spondyloarthritis. Radiographs at an early stage may be normal or may show only increased density of bone. Radiographic abnormalities are usually first noted in the spinal column and pelvis. Later, all the bones may become dense, and metastatic calcifications may also be seen. The diagnosis is confirmed by measuring the serum fluoride level.

There is no evidence that controlled fluoridation of low-fluoride public water supplies can cause adverse effects. However, levels only twice those that effectively prevent dental caries cause dental mottling, so proper care must be exercised in the use of fluoride-containing dental preparations, vitamins, and supplements.[410] Accidental increases in the fluoride content of fluoridated water supplies have caused epidemics of rheumatic symptoms.

Familial Hyperlipoproteinemia

Type IIa Hyperlipoproteinemia. Achilles tendinitis and migratory tenosynovitis are the most common presenting manifestations of heterozygous type II hyperlipoproteinemia.[411] The episodes are generally gradual in onset, last 2 or 3 days, and subside spontaneously. Diagnosis is by demonstrating significant elevations in plasma cholesterol, phospholipids, and low-density lipoproteins with normal levels of triglycerides. These "rheumatic" symptoms may antedate the development of cutaneous xanthomas and may lead to recognition of hypercholesterolemia in other family members.

Homozygous type II hyperlipoproteinemia is characterized by the youthful development of xanthomas on the skin and in the Achilles tendons. Homozygous individuals often have episodes of migratory polyarthritis simulating acute rheumatic fever; persistent arthritis for periods as long as a month occurs in a few patients.

Type IV Hyperlipoproteinemia. Type IV hyperlipoproteinemia, characterized by high levels of triglycerides with normal cholesterol, has been associated with the development of bilateral asymmetrical oligoarthritis of the lower extremities during the fifth decade of life.[412] This syndrome has not yet been reported in children.

Sitosterolemia

Recurrent brief attacks of arthritis are usually part of this rare familial (recessive) storage disease in which children accumulate plant sterols as well as cholesterol, presumably due to deficiency of the enzyme hydroxymethylglutaryl—Co A reductase.[413] The arthritis responds to treatment with cholestyramine and a low-sterol diet;[414] diagnosis depends on recognition of tuberous and tendinous xanthomata.

Gout

Primary gout is a storage disease resulting either from overproduction of uric acid due to defined or unknown defects in purine biosynthesis, or from defects in renal excretion of uric acid including familial defects in tubular reabsorption of uric acid distal to secretory sites.[415]

Hippocrates is said to have stated that "the young man does not take Gout until he engages in coition"; this is presumably a result of the relatively ele-

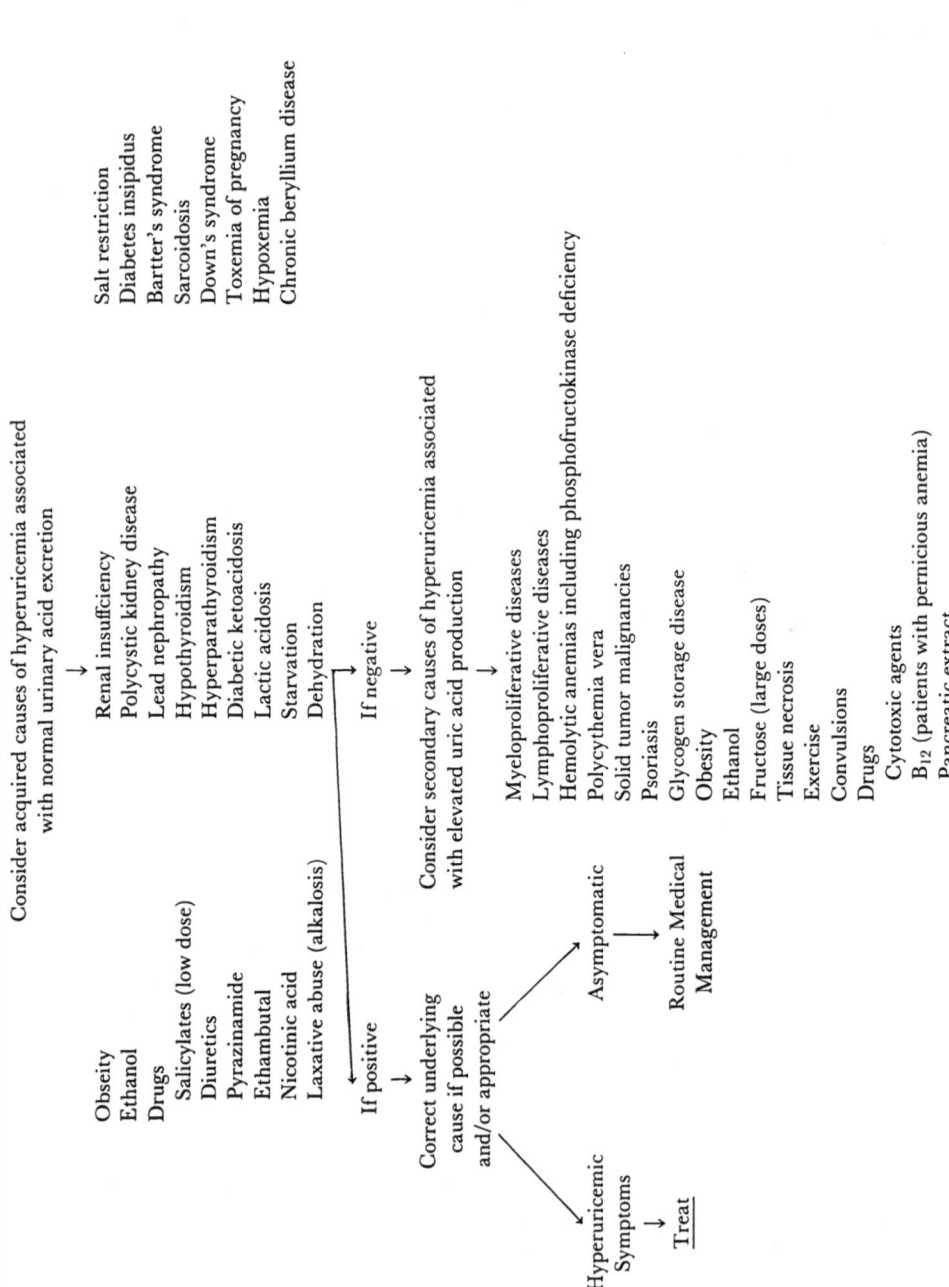

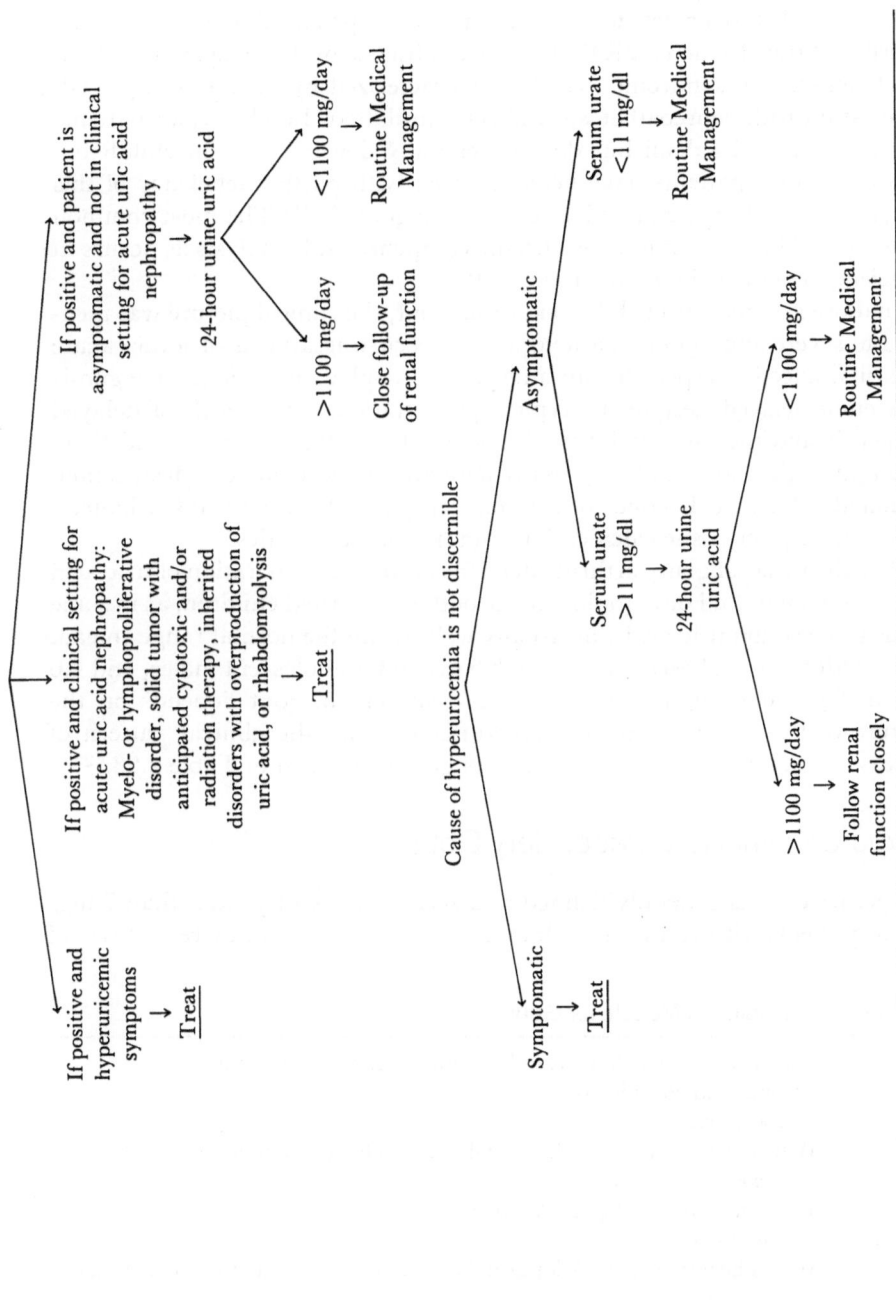

Figure 2.69. Evaluation of the patient with hyperuricemia. (Modified with permission from Kelly WN, ref. 422, p. 575.)

vated renal uric acid clearance characteristic of childhood. The exceptions are a result of hyperuricemia caused by other diseases (Fig. 2.69) or as a consequence of congenital superactivity of phosphoribosylpyrophosphate (PRPP) synthetase or deficiency of the enzyme hypoxanthine-guanine phosphoribosyl transferase (HPRT). Complete absence of this enzyme results in the Lesch-Nyhan syndrome, which is characterized by mental and growth retardation with choreoathetosis and self-mutilation. Lesch-Nyhan patients develop uric acid calculi but do not generally develop gout in childhood. However, some patients have been reported with partial deficiency of this enzyme who did present in adolescence with gout.[416,417] The most common cause of childhood gout may be chronic compensated hemolysis as occurs in deficiencies of phosphofructokinase.[418,419]

In those rare reports of childhood-onset gout, the clinical picture was identical to severe adult gout, characterized by recurring attacks of severe acute arthritis, affecting especially the first metatarsophalangeal joint. Diagnosis was often delayed despite the typical presentation. As a result of delayed diagnosis and the unavailability of modern drugs, tophi formed, and there was radiologic evidence of progressive joint and subcortical bone destruction, terminal phalangeal bone resorption, epiphyseal growth disturbances, osteoporosis, soft-tissue calcification, and flexion deformities.

The diagnosis of gouty arthritis depends on the demonstration of uric acid crystals in joint fluid or in tophi. In one of these reported children, as in some adults, the serum uric acid was usually well within the normal range (mean, 3.6 mg/dl for prepubescent children, 5.5 mg/dl for adolescent males, and 4.0 mg/dl for adolescent females).[420] The treatment of gout depends on the nature of the defect producing hyperuricemia and the clinical pattern of disease.[421] A scheme for the treatment of gout is detailed in Table 2.28.[422]

Hyperuricemia and Secondary Gout

Hyperuricemia is generally defined as a serum uric acid greater than 7 mg/ dl, as patients with consistent values above this level are at increased risk of

Table 2.28. Treatment Module for Gout

   I. Acute gouty arthritis: Colchicine, indomethacin, or naproxen only
  II. Hyperuicemia and chronic gout:
     A. Overproducers:
       1. With a history of gout: Allopurinol plus colchicine, indomethacin, or naproxen
       2. Without a history of gout: Allopurinol
     B. Underexcretors:
       1. With a history of gout: Allopurinol plus a uricosuric agent (probenemid or sulfinpyrazone)
       2. Without a history of gout: observe without therapy

eventually developing gouty arthritis or renal stones.[422] In some population studies, 2–17% of all individuals studied had levels over 7 mg/dl. In most cases, the hyperuricemia cannot be explained, and most such individuals never develop gout or renal stones.

A scheme for the investigation and management of hyperuricemia is summarized in Figure 2.69. The finding of hyperuricemia requires a search for a disorder known to produce secondary hyperuricemia; elevated serum uric acid is occasionally an initial clue to the diagnosis of myeloproliferative or lymphoproliferative disorders.

When hyperuricemia reflects the presence of a condition associated with normal uric acid excretion, no further studies are generally necessary. In disorders associated with increased urine excretion of uric acid, treatment may be urgently required to prevent uric acid nephropathy.[422]

Lowe's (Oculocerebrorenal) Syndrome

Patients with this syndrome of organic acidemia, decreased renal ammonia production, hydrophthalmos, and severe mental retardation may develop erosive arthritis and tenosynovitis in the second decade of life.[423] The arthritis is noninflammatory and presumably a result of the undefined metabolic abnormality.[424]

Williams (Elfin Facies) Syndrome

Stiff gait and flexion contractures of proximal and digital interphalangeal joints, wrists, elbows, knees, and ankles occur in 50% of children with Williams syndrome. In addition to the characteristic facies this syndrome includes transient hypercalcemia in infancy, intellectual dysfunction, and supravalvular aortic and peripheral vascular stenosis.[425]

Alcaptonuria

Teenagers with this rare (autosomal-recessive) deficiency of the enzyme homogentisic acid oxidase may excrete urine that turns black on standing and may begin to deposit visible black pigment in the sclerae and in ear and nasal cartilages (ochronosis). However, the degenerative arthritis that results from deposition of this material in articular cartilage does not occur until middle age. As in all other forms of degenerative arthritis, there may be periods of acute inflammation that resemble rheumatoid arthritis.

Hemochromatosis

Primary hemachromatosis is not a pediatric disorder, generally having its onset between 20 and 30 years of age with arthritis alone or in association with amenorrhea, cardiac abnormalities, or a triad of skin pigmentation, diabetes, and cirrhosis.[426,427] The disease seems to represent a genetically controlled error in iron metabolism resulting in increased movement of iron from plasma into storage.[428] Genetic linkage studies of families with hemachromatosis show a susceptibility locus on chromosome 6. Although the susceptibility allele at this locus cannot be reliably detected, it is marked within an individual family by a particular HLA haplotype; different HLA antigens are involved in different families. Once an affected individual has been identified and his particular HLA haplotype has been determined, susceptibility can be predicted within this family; homozygotes develop severe disease; heterozygotes have a wide spectrum of clinical or subclinical disorder. It is possible that the disorder may ultimately be preventable with environmental or genetic manipulation for susceptible individuals.

The arthritis of hemachromatosis is usually progressive, starting in the small joints of the hands and progressing to involve the wrists, elbows, hips, knees, and ankles. The arthritis seems to be a manifestation of articular chondrocalcinosis, which has also been reported to be a finding in patients with hemolytic anemia. Some patients have acute arthritis typical of pseudogout with demonstration of calcium pyrophosphate crystals in joint aspirants. Serum transferrin saturation values are elevated.

Some cases of Kashin-Beck disease (see below) have been attributed to excess amounts of iron in water and foodstuffs. Patients with transfusion hemosiderosis also may have similar arthritis with iron deposition in the synovium.

Kashin-Beck Disease (Urov Disease)

Children living in remote, mountainous, impoverished areas of southeastern Siberia, northeastern China, and Korea develop a chondrodysplasia without inflammation, which is thought to be a result either of ingestion of unknown toxic products associated with bread grain fungi soil, or water, or a deficiency of trace elements in soil or water.[429–431] A similar disease has been induced in experimental animals (rats and puppies) fed the fungus *Fusarium sporotrichiella*. The disease, which is endemic in the area where grain is infected, is reported not to occur in children fed uninfected imported bread and not to progress in children moved to a new home in unaffected areas.

Interphalangeal, wrist, knee, and ankle joints are symmetrically progressively thickened with progressive limitation of motion. There are no effusions or signs of inflammation until late in the disease when they are presumably secondary to osteoarthritis Patients ultimately develop a dwarfed appearance suggestive of a storage disease or a bone dysplasia with short, stubby fingers. The arthritis resembles that seen in hemochromatosis and has also been attributed to ingestion of excess amounts of iron in water and foodstuffs.

Mselini Joint Disease

A similar disease occurs in remote parts of Zuzuland.[432]

Calcific Periarthritis

Pseudogout, an acute inflammatory syndrome in elderly patients with chondrocalcinosis, is caused by precipitation of calcium pyrophosphate dihydrate crystals in the synovial space (crystal synovitis). No exactly analogous situation has been seen in children. However, a familial ankylosing form of chondrocalcinosis starting in the second decade has been reported in Chiloe Islanders (Chile),[433] and one of our patients with familial hypertrophic synovitis has developed chondrocalcinosis in adult life (see Familial Hypertrophic Synovitis later in this chapter.)

Patients with chronic renal failure being treated with dialysis may develop recurrent attacks of periarticular pain and tenosynovitis caused by precipitation of calcium pyrophosphate crystals in tendons and periarticular tissues. There are no detectable microcrystals in the joint fluid.[434] The syndrome is related to the hyperphosphatemia of chronic renal failure and may be prevented by more frequent dialysis, limiting phosphate intake, and the administration of aluminum hydroxide gel to bind phosphates in the gastrointestinal tract and prevent their absorption.

Abnormal Blood Proteins

Hemoglobinopathies—Sickle-Cell Disease

Musculoskeletal pain is common in sickle-cell (SS) disease (Table 2.29).[435] Stagnant blood flow and oxygen desaturation in terminal blood vessels cause thrombosis and infarction of bone. Reactive periostitis is frequent. Joint capsules, tendons, and synovial membranes may all be similarly affected.

Because patients with SS disease are especially prone to infection, these bone infarcts commonly become infected. Over 50% of these instances of osteomyelitis in SS patients are due to infection with *Salmonella*, a rare cause of osteomyelitis in normal individuals. Although osteomyelitis in SS disease may be staphylococcal or pneumococcal, it is most frequently due to gram-negative organization. It may be difficult to distinguish between uncomplicated bone infarcts and osteomyelitis. Technetium, gallium and MRI scans may be helpful in this differentiation.

Migratory polyarthritis is a typical feature of sickle-cell crisis. When the child is anemic and has fever and a heart murmur, it may be difficult to distinguish these episodes from acute rheumatic fever. Joint effusions tend to subside in a few days.

Table 2.29. Causes of Skeletal Pain in
the Hemoglobinopathies

Bone infarction due to oxygen
    desaturation
Synovial, joint capsule, and tendon
    infarction
Bone-marrow infarction
Periostitis
Aseptic necrosis
Septic infection
Coincident connective-tissue disease

During the second half of the first year of life, as the percentage of protective fetal hemoglobin declines, sickling may be accentuated in the most distal
bones of the body, resulting in sickle-cell diactylitis—the hand-foot syndrome of sickle-cell anemia (Fig. 2.70). Swelling of the hands and feet with
exquisite pain is followed in several weeks by characteristic radiographic
changes, including periosteal elevation, subperiosteal new-bone formation,
and a moth-eaten appearance of bone. This syndrome is rarely seen after the
toddler age, presumably because the red marrow of these distal bones has
been replaced by fibrous tissue that has lower oxygen requirements and
fewer blood vessels susceptible to infarction.

Synovitis of the hip secondary to avascular necrosis of the head of the
femur is another manifestation of sickle-cell disease. Although bone necrosis
is most common in SS disease, sludging may occur in all hemoglobinopathies, depending on oxygen saturation and the concentration of less soluble hemoglobin.

Hemophilias and Thrombasthenias

The most common causes of hemorrhage into the joints are trauma and
bleeding disorders. The history of trauma is usually easily established except

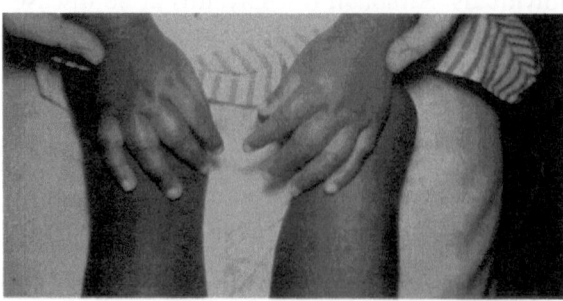

Figure 2.70. Fever and painful
swelling of the proximal digits
with radiographic evidence of
periostitis led to recognition
of sickle-cell anemia in this
toddler.

in cases of child abuse. Severe classic hemophilia, while a cause of severe crippling arthropathy, is usually diagnosed prior to the first episode of hemarthrosis, which generally occurs without known trauma in the second year of life. However, mild hemophilia and more subtle bleeding disorders due to deficient activity of other clotting factors may have traumatic hemarthrosis as their initial manifestation.[436] Patients often present with a single knee effusion, usually with a clear history of trauma. Except in child abuse, bleeding into joints is generally intracapsular and unaccompanied by visible bruising or superficial swelling. Arthrocentesis reveals bloody fluid. Detailed coagulation studies are necessary to establish the diagnosis.

More than 80% of the episodes of hemorrhage in severe hemophiliacs are bleeds into joints or muscle. The mechanism of joint destruction in hemophilia is unknown, but clearly an inflammatory reaction results from blood in the joint, and chronic arthropathy is related to repetitive episodes of articular hemorrhage. Modern management of hemophilia is aimed at the prevention of hemarthrosis by prompt home infusion of clotting factors at the first premonitory sign of bleeding into the joint. Chronic hemophilic arthritis may respond to penicillamine.[437]

Bleeding associated with platelet disorders is usually in the superficial microcirculation, resulting in recurrent bruises, epistaxis, menorrhagia, and bleeding after dental extraction. The few patients reported to have bled into joints have usually had single episodes in the knee. In one case, recurrent subclinical bleeding led to destructive arthritis similar to that seen in hemophilia. Diagnosis is suggested by a prolonged bleeding time and confirmed with special platelet studies.[438]

Other rare causes of bloody joint fluid include synovial hemangioma (see Figs. 2.92 and 2.93) and congenital and acquired disorders of connective tissue. Scurvy is an example of an acquired metabolic disorder in which hemarthrosis may be a major manifestation. Ehlers-Danlos syndrome is an example of a congenital disorder with abnormal structural integrity of the connective tissue which is sometimes also accompanied by platelet dysfunction and other coagulation defects; in these situations, normal activities or minor trauma may result in synovial hemorrhage (see Fig. 2.77).

More children are on chronic anticoagulant therapy now, following heart-value replacement or for other reasons. Administration of many drugs may enhance the anticoagulant effect and cause bleeding into joints. We have seen this situation present in an eight-year-old boy as polyarthritis of the hips and elbow. He had been given trimethaprin-sulfa for an earache!

Immunologic Deficiency Disorders with Arthritis

Many forms of arthritis may occur as features of immunologic deficiency disorders. In agammaglobulinemia, osteomyelitis and septic arthritis result from increased susceptibility to bacterial infection. Hypertrophic osteoarthropathy occurs secondary to chronic suppurative lung disease. Arthritis may be the first manifestation of chronic echovirus meningitis in agamma-globulinemic children.[439] When agammaglobulinemic patients have a rheumatoid-arthritis-like syndrome, however, they generally have transient episodes of oligoarthritis rather than severe or erosive disease, and they rarely have any functional disability. The arthritis frequently disappears after increases in frequency or dose of gamma globulin injections.[440] Synovial biopsy specimens in such individuals are characterized by synovial-cell hyperplasia and vascular endothelial proliferation without leukocyte or plasma cell infiltrates. One case of erosive arthritis with persistent adenovirus infection in synovial tissue has been well documented in an agammaglobulinemic man.[441]

All forms of immunologic deficiency have also been associated with an increased susceptibility to autoimmune disorders such as rheumatoid arthritis, and lupus, which may be the presenting manifestation.[440,442] About 4% of children with JRA have been reported to have selective deficiency of IgA.[443] In some of these patients, the deficiency was transient, and the arthritis disappeared coincident with the appearance of normal levels of IgA in the serum.[444] In most children with IgA deficiency and arthritis, the arthritic symptoms are mild. Occasionally, severe erosive polyarticular arthritis is seen in IgA-deficient individuals, but the incidence of IgA deficiency and of arthritis in the population is such that it is not possible to be certain that the association between severe arthritis and IgA deficiency is anything more than coincidence.

There have been several reports of improvement in symptoms associated with IgA deficiency, including arthritis, following plasma transfusions.[445] However, some IgA-deficient patients have high titers of anti-IgA antibodies, and in these individuals transfusions or injections of blood products such as gamma globulin may induce fatal anaphylactic reactions. Children with IgA deficiency should be tested for such antibodies prior to transfusion or injection of gamma globulin.

Complement deficiencies, especially C2 deficiency, may also be associated with increased susceptibility to arthritis and lupus. Job's syndrome, a phagocytic immunodeficiency disorder, has also been associated with SLE.[446]

Familial Lipochrome Histiocytosis

Three girls in one family have been reported with this syndrome, characterized by recurrent pulmonary infection and arthritis.[447] The immunologic defect is reported to be identical to that of chronic granulomatous disease (CGD) with deficient ability of white blood cells to kill ingested staphylococci. Generalized lipochrome pigmentation of histiocytic cells is common to both this syndrome and CGD. However, the patients did not form granulomas (boys with CDG do); these girls all developed symmetrical polyarthritis. Two also had positive latex fixation tests, and one had rheumatoid nodules, none of which has been reported in boys with CGD. The two most severely affected girls died of pulmonary infection at 19 and 34 years of age. The exact relationship of this disorder to CGD remains to be determined.

Schaller initially described a syndrome of discoid lupus, arthritis, and stomatitis in female carriers of the CGD defect;[448] many cases have now been reported.[449] These women were not reported to have lipochrome histiocytosis, however. One child with CGD has developed convincing clinical, serologic, and pathologic evidence of SLE, and a few others have had features of discoid lupus.[449]

Arthritis, Pyoderma Gangrenosum, and Streaking Leukocyte Factor

In this syndrome first reported by us in 1975,[450] a 2-year-old boy developed massive monarticular joint effusions and later pyoderma gangrenosum following minor trauma (Figs. 2.71 and 2.72). Repeated episodes of sterile pyarthrosis in a joint resulted in progressive bony overgrowth with mild limitation of motion (Fig. 2.73). The major early handicap was repetitive, erroneous diagnosis of spetic arthritis with unnecessary long hospitalizations, surgery, and antibiotic therapy. The arthritic episodes were ultimately self-limited or could be controlled by the administration of prednisone.

Pyoderma gangrenosum initially occurred at the site of intramuscular alum injections (DPT), later with minor trauma, and more recently as a complication of teenage acne. It remains a major problem. The patient is now 32 years old. As he grew older, arthritis disappeared, perhaps because he has required almost continuous administration of alternate-day prednisone to control the scarring pyoderma lesions on his face and the leg ulcers. When these lesions are most threatening, prednisone must be administered every 2 h around the clock to achieve healing. The disorder could not be controlled with plasmapheresis but in 1991 was completely controlled, we are told, by administration of FK 506.[451]

The etiology of this syndrome was related to the finding of a leukocyte-migrating-enhancing factor in the patient's serum. This heavy-molecular-weight factor reversibly enhances in vitro random migration of both polymorphonuclear and mononuclear leukocytes. Chemotaxis is secondarily (but not primarily) increased. The exact mechanism of action and identity of the enhancing factor are unknown. It is hypothesized that increased leukocyte random migration and other activity at the site of inflammatory exudation after minor trauma prevent repair and healing, resulting in arthritis and pyoderma gangrenosum.

We have recently seen a second case presenting with pyoderma gangrenosa at the site of DPT injection and subsequently at sites of minor trauma. At age 2 the boy developed cardiac failure secondary to aortitis and inflammation of the large arteries taking off from the aorta. The picture on ultrasound and MRI resembled Takayasu's arteritis but the pathology in the

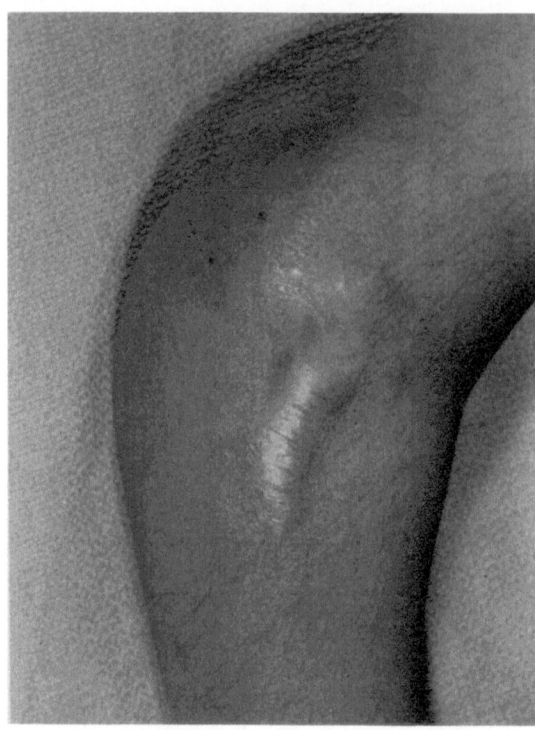

A

Figure 2.71. Clinical appearance of effused right elbow in a boy with "streaking leukocyte factor." Aspiration yielded purulent (WBC > 100,000/mm³) but sterile fluid. (Reprinted with permission from Jacobs, ref. 450. Copyright by the American Academy of Pediatrics.)

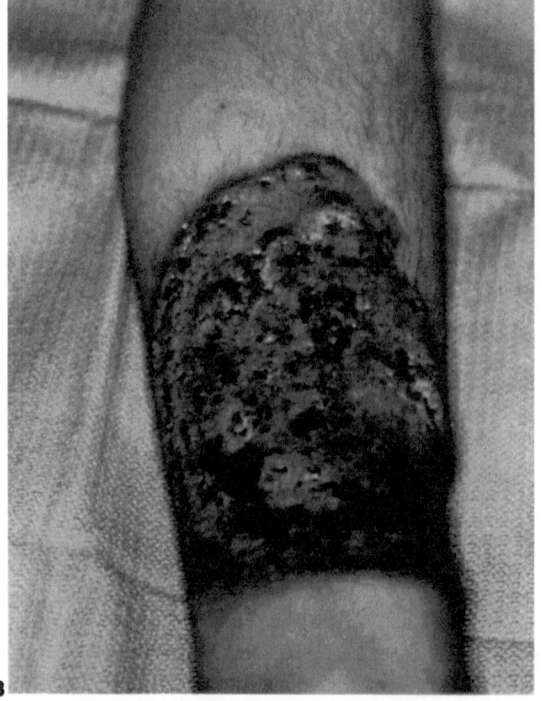

B

Figure 2.72. Giant leg ulcer typical of those that patient continues to suffer. Local treatment and grafting were unsuccessful, but the ulcers healed promptly when large doses of prednisone were administered. These lesions have caused considerable facial scarring and continue to be a major problem in this patient, now age 32. (Reprinted with permission from Jacobs, ref. 450. Copyright by the American Academy of Pediatrics.)

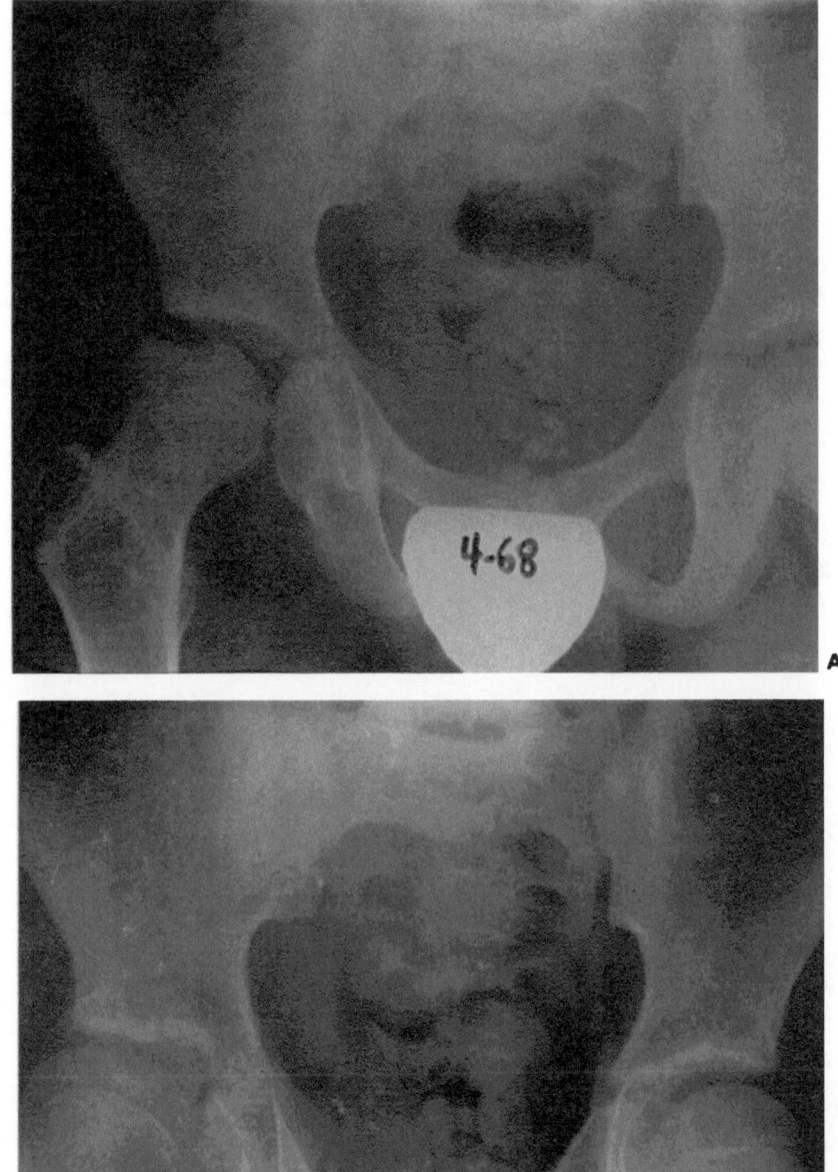

Figure 2.73. X-rays of the hips showing progressive overgrowth and flattening of the head of the right femur (**A**, at age 8 years; **B**, at age 11 years). (Reprinted with permission from Jacobs, ref. 450. Copyright by the American Academy of Pediatrics.)

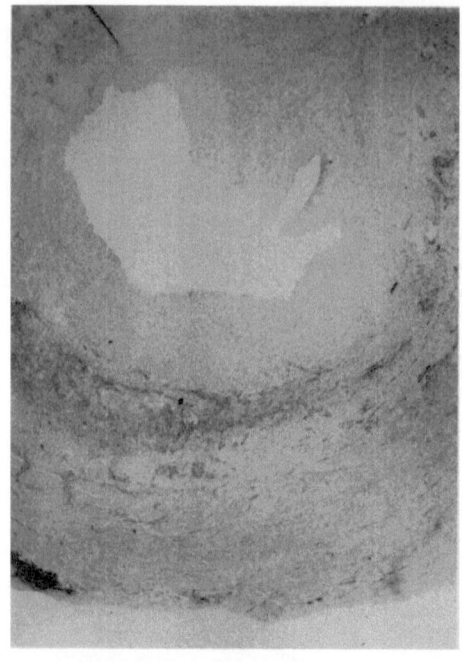

A

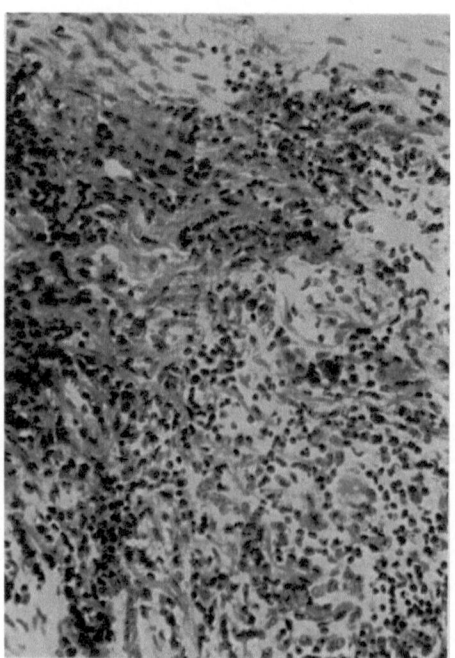

B

Figure 2.74. Streaking leucocyte factor, case 2. Innominate artery infiltrate similar to infiltrates in synovium and pyoderma lesions of case 1 (see pictures in ref. 450). **A** × 20; **B** × 200).

innominate artery (Fig. 2.74) was identical to the pyoderma gangrenosa lesions. The child died following grafting of the aneurysms, unfortunately just prior to our learning that the lesions in our prior patient had been completely controlled by FK 506[451] and that some patients with refractory pyoderma gangrenosum respond to cyclosporine.[451a]

Waldenström's Hypergammaglobulinemic Purpura

A few children, primarily of Greek origin, have been reported to have relapsing purpura of the lower extremities which, if one is not familiar with the entity, may be confused with arthritis because of diffuse leg swelling, a very high ESR, and a positive test for rheumatoid factor (Fig. 2.75).[452] The hypergammaglobulinemia consists of large amounts of intermediate sedimenting complexes consisting of IgG-anti-IgG antibodies. These IgG anti–gamma globulins are characteristic of this disorder, but their etiology is obscure. The symptom complex may be temporarily relieved by recurrent plasmapheresis. The few reported children, including our patient, have had unusual suscepti-

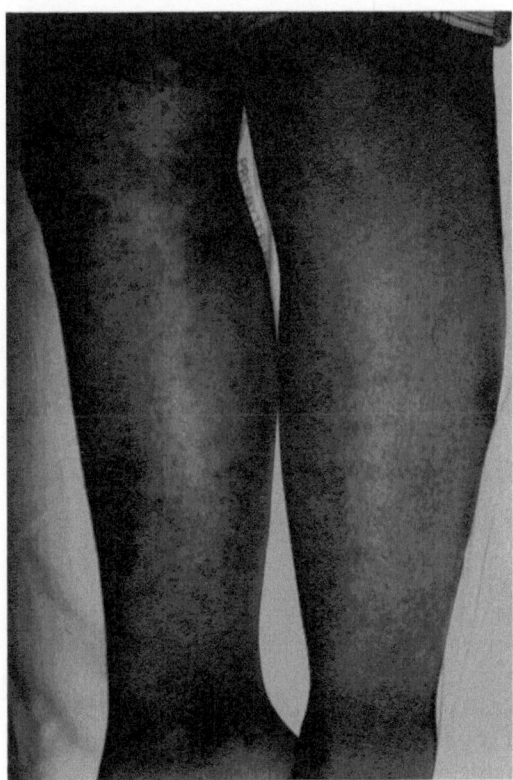

Figure 2.75. Purpura of the legs typical of Waldenström's (hypergammaglobulinemic) purpura.

bility to *Salmonella* infections. In adults, this disorder may be a manifestation of other connective-tissue disease or lymphoreticular malignancy.[453]

Hereditary Angioedema (HAE)

This disorder is manifested by attacks of body swellings and colicky abdominal pain that last for a few days and disappear without sequelae.[454,455] When the swellings compromise the airway, death may be instantaneous. The disorder is heritable (autosomal-dominant) and has been shown to be a result of deficient C1 esterase-inhibitor ($C1_{1H}$) activity. Diagnosis may be suspected in patients with the clinical syndrome who have low serum C2 and C4 and confirmed by showing either low levels of $C1_{1H}$ or functional impotence of the $C1_{1H}$ that is present; both forms of the disease exist. Recent studies show that almost all attacks can be prevented by daily administration of an androgenic agent, danazol. This disease often becomes apparent in childhood and worsens during adolescence. Patients with HAE are at increased risk for autoimmune disease, especially SLE, and also for non-SLE glomerulonephritis.[456,457] An acquired form, rare, and usually associated with lymphoproliferative disease, also occurs.[458,459] A few cases due to acquired inhibitors of $C1_{1H}$ have also been reported.[459]

Cold Fibrinogenemia

Minor trauma may be the triggering event for inflammation in human skin called dematographia,[460] demonstrable in 5% of normal children, and in a much higher percentage of those with rheumatic disease (? 100% in systemic JRA). Cold challenge may produce similar lesions characterized by erythema, pruritis, and edema, and termed cold urticaria.[461] Mediators may include histamine, chemotactic factors for eosinophils and neutrophilis, platelet factor 4, and platelet-activating factor.[462] Cryofibrinogenemia, associated with malignancy or thromboembolic disease in adults, may be a transient response to infection in children. Children may present with lesions resembling H-S purpura associated with erythema and swelling of the toes.[462]

In searching for cryoproteins it is mandatory that samples be kept at 37°C until processed by centrifugation.

Arthritis as a Manifestation of Food Allergy

It is extremely difficult to get patients to diligently follow elimination diets, even in those rare instances in which a single item such as milk has been well documented as the sole cause of severe chronic juvenile arthritis.[463] As a result, there has been a paucity of scientific studies which adequately address this important issue.[464,465] If patients want to try a dietary approach, on the

Table 2.30. Heritable Disorders
Associated with Joint Laxity

Marfan's syndrome
Ehlers-Danlos syndrome
Benign hypermobility
Larsen's syndrome

basis of what is known, they might be encouraged to eliminate dairy products for a month as the initial approach. Next they might try corn products; corn and dairy products may be used as filler for medications and in arranging elimination diets this problem must be addressed.[466]

Heritable Disorders Associated with Joint Laxity

A number of heritable disorders may be associated with joint laxity, which results in increased risk of joint injury, bleeding, and effusion (Table 2.30).

Marfan's Syndrome

Long, thin extremities (dolichostenomelia) with proportionately more lengthening of the distal extremities (arachnodactyly) result in a tall individual with arm span greater than total height and this constitutes the Marfan habitus (Fig. 2.76). Associated skeletal features include thoracic asymmetry, scoliosis, high arched palate, long great toes, and pronounced flat feet ("rocker bottoms"). Occasional patients have considerable myopathy. Cardiac manifestations include prolapse of the mitral valve with mitral insufficiency. Ocular manifestations are characterized by high myopia and upward dislocation of the lens (as contrasted to the downward ectopia lentis of homocystinuria). The inborn weakness of the tunica media of the aorta results in dilatation of the aortic ring with aortic insufficiency followed by ascending thoracic and sometimes descending abdominal aortic aneurysm, ultimately with rupture and death.[467] Certain diagnosis depends on typical features plus upward ectopia lentis or a certain family history. Marfan's syndrome is an autosomal-dominant defect of collagen organization, probably due to a deficiency in chemically stable collagen cross-links.[468]

The arthritic manifestations of Marfan's syndrome (a result of loose-jointedness) are really the least of the patient's problems and present no diagnostic difficulty. The heritable disorders of connective tissue are magnificently reviewed in McKusick's textbook and cannot be adequately reviewed here.[471] However, it is important to recognize Marfan's syndrome despite the lack of any final understanding of its chemical pathogenesis as a model of connective-tissue disease. For it is in this syndrome that one can

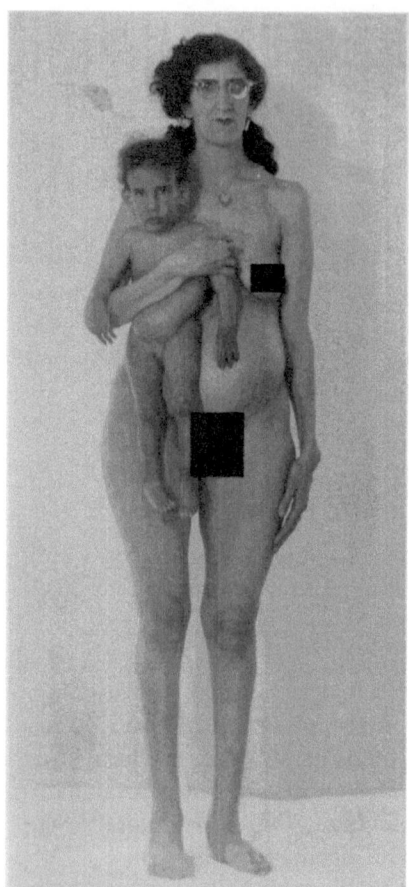

Figure 2.76. Arachnodactyly, dolichostenomelia, and cardiac and eye findings typical of Marfan's syndrome in a mother and child. The mother died a few years later of a ruptured aortic aneurysm; most such deaths are now preventable with elective repair.[469] However, diagnosis continues to be missed even in athletes in public view.[470]

most clearly see the effects of what surely must be a chemical abnormality in determining structure, function, and deterioration of organs. These syndromes result in congenital abnormalities, in disturbances of growth and development, and in *abiotrophy*, hereditary (but not congenital) defects that result from progressive degeneration of specific tissues.

Ehlers-Danlos Syndrome (EDS)

This term is applied to a heterogeneous group of genetic disorders of collagen structure and biosynthesis characterized by hyperextensible skin, hypermobile joints, and in some forms, fragile tissues and a bleeding disorder (Fig. 2.77).[472,473] The most elastic (type III) are the professional circus contortionists ("rubber men"). In some patients, the skin splits apart in minor trauma, and many have typical "cigarette paper" scars from minor injury to

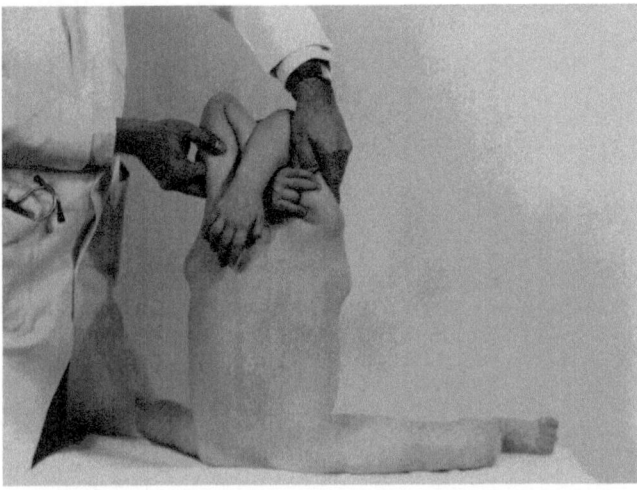

Figure 2.77. This patient with Ehlers-Danlos syndrome was recognized following recurrent dislocation of the hips. He had typical papyruslike skin lesions of his forehead from recurrent falls; the mother kept these scars hidden with bangs. She and her mother had all the same features as the child, but the disorder had not been recognized.

the forehead and shins. Joint effusions are common in those with recurrent dislocations or instability, especially in the ankles and knees. Bleeding may be due to abnormal blood vessels and supporting tissues or to platelet dysfunction and other coagulation abnormalities.

In Table 2.31 are charted the nine currently proposed subgroups of EDS with the biochemical features of abnormalities so far defined and the inheritance patterns. New forms are described each year, and not all patients fit this schema;[473a] complicated as it seems, this subdivision of EDS is surely an oversimplification.[471,472,474,475]

EDS must be differentiated from cutis laxa, a disorder characterized by lax rather than hyperelastic skin (Fig. 2.78).[476]

Benign Hypermobility

Children with those hereditary disorders of connective tissues associated with hyperextensible joints, Marfan's or Ehlers-Danlos syndromes, or forme frustes of these syndromes[477,478] may have damage to their joints as a result of recurrent subclinical dislocations. Temporomandibular joint dysfunction may be presenting manifestation.[479] Youngsters with significant isolated hypermobility and joint laxity may also have recurrent joint pain and effusion following strenuous exercise.[480] However, mild, generalized, and often familial ligamentous laxity is relatively-common in the general population

Table 2.31. Subgroups of the Ehlers-Danlos Syndrome

Type	Inheritance	Elastic Skin	Joint Hypermobility	Bruising, Skin Splits, Cigarette-Paper Scars	Mitral Valve Prolapse	Death from Bowel, Uterine, Vessel Rupture	Eye Globe Rupture	Hip Recurrent Dislocation	Biosynthetic Error
I	AD	++++	++++	++++	+++				?
II	AD	++	++	++	++				?
III	AD	±	++++		++				?
IV	AD	±	±	++++	++	+++			*1
V	X-R	++	++	++	++				?
VI	AR	++	++	++	++	+*	++++		I-(2)
VII	AR	++	++					+++	E*2
VIII	AD	++	++	++	++				?
IX	X-R	+	+	+	+				*3

Key: AD = autosomal-dominant; AR = autosomal-recessive; X-R = sex-linked recessive; I-(2) = intracellular processing error (decreased lysyl hydroxylase); E = extracellular processing error (increased aminopropeptide in procollagen alpha-2 chains). *Vessel only.
*1 = point mutations (deletions) and splicing errors in Type III procollagen.
*2 = splicing mutations that delete amino-terminal propeptide cleavage sites.
*3 = defective copper metabolism.

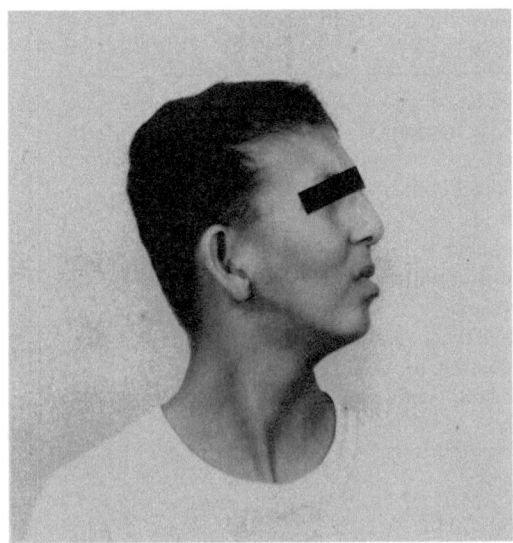

Figure 2.78. Although cutis laxa is sometimes confused with Ehlers-Danlos syndrome, these patients do not have lax joints, and their skin is lax rather than hyperelastic. The typical "bloodhound" facies, illustrated here, is characterized by drooping and ectropion of the eyelids, sagging facial skin (jowls), and accentuation of the nasolabial and other facial folds. The child appears older than his stated age, and the skin of the body appears too large for his frame.

and can be demonstrated in 9% of adults and 34% of children.[475,481–484] Recurrent bland effusions, especially in the knees of athletic teenagers, are frequent complaints.[485] Increased susceptibility to injury is not usually significant and rarely, if ever, requires restriction from sports.[485a,b]

Down's Syndrome (Trisomy 21)

Bland effusions may be seen in association with Down's syndrome as a result of the characteristic hypermobility of the joints and gout may also occur as trisomy 21 patients have an undefined tendency to hyperuricemia.[486] However, approximately 1% of children with Down's syndrome seem to develop inflammatory arthopathy, most of which is polyarticular; this increased susceptibility is most likely related, to the known immunologic dysfunctions associated with Down's syndrome.[487,488] Arthritis has also been reported in children with chromosome 18 deletions[489] and Turner's (45X0) syndrome.[490]

Larsen's Syndrome

Extraordinary laxity of the joints with recurrent dislocations, widely spaced eyes with a depressed nasal bridge ("dish face"), and malformed fingers with a spatulate thumb characterize this unusual group of syndromes.[491] Radiographic demonstration of an extra ossification center in the calcaneus is an important diagnostic feature. Desbuquois syndrome and spondyloepiphyseal dysplasia are other skeletal dysplasias with prominent joint laxity.[475,492]

Table 2.32. Syndromes Associated with Joint
Contractures Present at Birth

Nail-patella syndrome
Arthrogryposis multiplex congenita
Fetal alcohol syndrome
Congenital contractual arachnodactyly
Chromosome abnormalities
Punctate epiphyseal dysplasia
Congenital joint contractures with facial abnormalities
   Marden-Walker syndrome
   Schwartz-Jampel (mask face) syndrome
   Freeman-Sheldon (whistling mouth) syndrome
   Cerebro-oculofacioskeletal syndrome (COFS)
The stiff-skin syndromes

Joint Contractures at Birth (Table 2.32)

Nail-Patella Syndrome (Onycho-osteo-arthro Dysplasia)

This congenital syndrome with restricted elbow extension due to posterior dislocation of the radial heads is associated with:

1. Symmetrical vertical ridges of the thumbnails.
2. Vertical moons of all other fingernails.
3. Small, laterally placed or absent patellae. The knee dysplasia is often the chief complaint that brings the patient to the physician's attention.
4. Posterior iliac horns.
5. Inability to fully flex the distal interphalangeal joints.

The nail-patella syndrome is an autosomal-dominant, relatively common anomaly.[493,494] Up to 40% of affected children have nephritis; 25% of them die of renal insufficiency. The renal pathology is unique, with collagen fibers within the lamina densa of the basement membranes, presumably a result of trapping of abnormal collagen fibers but possibly due to an abnormality of the membrane itself.

Arthrogryposis Multiplex Congenita

This term is applied to a variety of undefined disorders of unknown origin, usually not heritable, characterized by restricted articular mobility at birth.[491] Although nonprogressive, there may be considerable disability. Long bones may be fractured during delivery. Muscular hypotonia, congenital dislocation of the hips, and talipes equinovarus clubfoot are frequently present. A few families with an autosomal-dominant form of distal (hands and feet) arthrogryposis have been reported.

A similar disorder (Koskokwim disease) has been reported in Alaskan eskimos who are accomplished knee walkers.[495]

Fetal Alcohol Syndrome

Alcohol ingestion during pregnancy may result (if the offspring survives at all) in mental retardation, impaired linear growth, cardiac septal defects, and abnormalities of joint mobility. These include camptodactyly, clinodactyly, inability to completely flex the metacarpophalangeal joints, and inability to completely extend the elbows.[496]

Congenital Contractual Arachnodactyly

This autosomal-dominant syndrome is characterized by (1) congenital flexion contractures of the fingers, elbows, and knees that improve with age; (2) kyphoscoliosis that is progressive; and (3) abnormal ear crura and "Abe Lincoln" habitus without the specific features of Marfan's syndrome.[497]

Chromosomal Abnormalities

Hypertonia with congenital flexion deformities of various joints may be seen in 18 trisomy, the 13q-deletion syndrome, and other syndromes associated with chromosomal abnormalities (Fig. 2.79).

Punctate Epiphyseal Dysplasia

Twenty-seven percent of patients with the autosomal-dominant Conradi-Hunermann phenotype stippled epiphysis syndrome have large joint contractures at birth.[491]

Congenital Joint Contractures with Facial Abnormalities

Limited joint mobility is a frequent finding in the Weaver overgrowth syndrome identified by characteristic facies, dysharmonic osseous maturation, and unusual metaphyseal splaying of the long bones.[498] Significant congenital hip, knee, and elbow contractures are one characteristic feature, together with blepharophimosis (small palpebral fissures) and low-set, oddly formed ears, of the Marden-Walker syndrome, and of two syndromes characterized by these features plus myotonia: the Schwartz-Jampel (mask face) and Freeman-Sheldon (whistling mouth) syndromes.[499] Various other anomalies may be present in each of these syndromes.

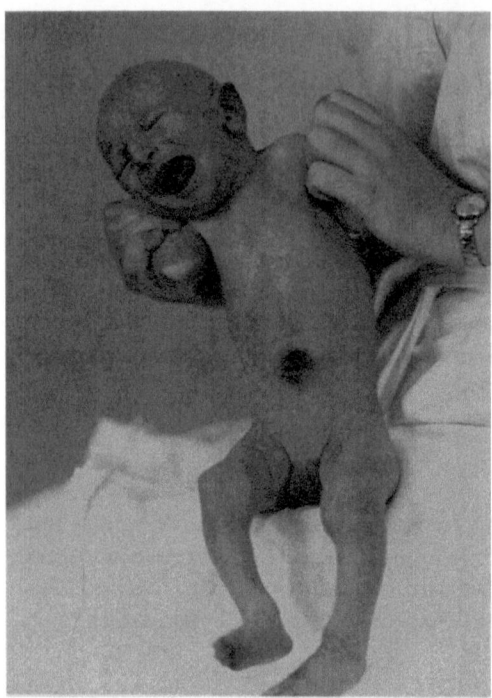

Figure 2.79. Joint contractures may be present at birth in many syndromes. This patient had a chromosomal abnormality (the 13q-deletion syndrome). (Reprinted with permission from *Am J Hum Genet*, 21:499–512, 1969).

The cerebro-occulofacioskeletal syndrome (COFS) is a more severe and generalized rare dysplasia leading to early death.

The Stiff-Skin Syndromes

Limited extension of joints together with stony-hard (marble!) skin have been reported in one family (autosomal-dominant) by Esterly and McKusick.[500] Some of the patients were affected at birth. A similar but more severe recessive syndrome has been reported in several families in Parana, Brazil. The enzymatic defects in these syndromes have not been defined but in acquired adult stiff-man syndrome impaired neuronal pathways that operate through gamma-aminobutyric acid appear to be a result of autoimmune disease.[501] We are aware of a child with juvenile arthritis misdiagnosed as having stiff-man syndrome.

Hypomobile (Stiff-Joint) Syndromes Appearing after Birth

These stiff-joint syndromes represent a relatively large number of phenotypes for a relatively small number of affected individuals (Table 2.33). In general, the defects may be explained in the following schematic form:

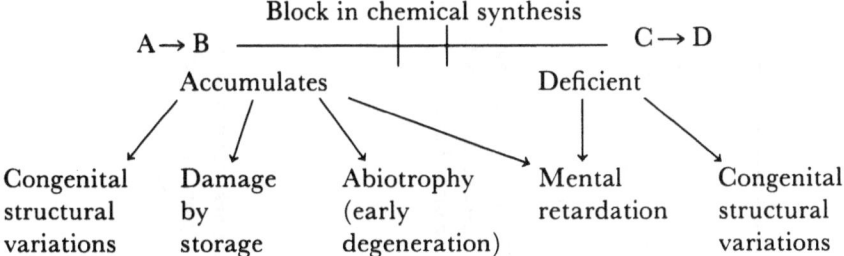

Table 2.33. Syndromes Associated with the Appearance of
Joint Contractures after Birth

Mucopolysaccharidoses and mucolipidoses
Weill-Marchesani disease
Leri's plenocytosis
Myositis ossificans
Stickler syndrome
Multicentric reticulohistiocytosis
The lipidoses
   Gaucher's disease
   Fabry's disease
Ceramidosis (Farber's disease)
Bone and cartilage dysplasias
The vanishing-bone diseases
Familial hypertrophic synovitis
Congenital arthropathy with rash appearing in the newborn
Williams syndrome

Damage begins early in intrauterine life and continues after birth. Most of these conditions are autosomal-recessive, suggesting enzymatic defects, as contrasted with the dominantly inherited loose-joint syndromes in which there is no progressive damage by storage and the defects are most likely due to structural abnormalities in nonenzymatic proteins.

Where the enzyme defect is known, the diagnosis is confirmed by the demonstration of decreased activity of the appropriate lysosomal hydrolase in cultured fibroblasts (Table 2.34).

The Mucopolysaccharidoses and Mucolipidoses

Limitation of motion with flexion contractures of the fingers is seen in Hurler's, Hunter's, Morquio's, Maroteaux-Lamy, and Sly's type of mucopolysaccharidoses and in type III mucolipidosis (pseudo-Hurler polydystrophy).[471] Differential features are detailed in Table 2.34.

Table 2.34. Inherited Disorders of the Lysosome with Arthritic Manifestations

Disease	Defective Enzyme(s)	Major Accumulated Substrates or Lysosomal Defects	Major Phenotypic Manifestations	Major Arthritic Manifestations
Defects of Specific Lysosomal Hydrolases				
I. Lipidoses				
A. Glycosidase deficiencies				
A. 1. Ceramide trihexosidosis (Fabry)	α-Galactosidase A	Galactosyl-galactosyl-glucosylceramide; digalactosylceramide	Juvenile onset; angiokeratoma; corneal opacity; acroparesthesias; renal and cardiovascular insufficiency; death usually in fourth decade; X-linked inheritance	Polyarthritis in adolescent boys; aseptic necrosis of bone
2. Glucocerebrosidoses a. Type 1 (adult Gaucher)	Acid β-Glucosidase	Glucosylceramide; glucosylsphingosine;	Juvenile or adult onset; hepatosplenomegaly; pancytopenia; Gaucher cells in bone marrow	Attacks of hip and knee pain; aseptic necrosis of bone

B. Esterase and deacylase deficiencies				
1. Ceramidosis (Farber)	Ceramidase	Ceramide	Infantile onset; psychomotor retardation; death by 2 years from granuloma of larynx and epiglottis with pneumonia	Arthropathy a major manifestation with large nodular masses on tendon sheaths and over pressure points beginning at age 1 month
II. Mucopolysaccharidoses				
1. MPS I-H (Hurler)	α-L-Iduronidase	Dermatan sulfate; heparan sulfate	Infantile onset; characteristic craniofacial dysmorphism; mental retardation; dysostosis multiplex; growth retardation; corneal opacities; hepatosplenomegaly; coronary death by 20 years	Short hands, limited motion with flexion contractures of fingers, elbows, shoulders, knees, wrists, costovertebral joints
2. MPS I-S (Scheie)	α-L-Iduronidase	Same as I-H	Milder than MPS I-H, normal intelligence; moderate short stature; normal life-span, aortic insufficiency	Severe DIP joint contractures, carpal tunnel syndrome with claw hand

continued

Table 2.34. (*Continued*)

Disease	Defective Enzyme(s)	Major Accumulated Substrates or Lysosomal Defects	Major Phenotypic Manifestations	Major Arthritic Manifestations
3. MPS II (Hunter) a. Type A	Sulfoiduronate sulfatase	Dermatan sulfate; heparan sulfate	Similar to but milder than B; normal-to-mild retardation; survival up to 60 years; X-linked inheritance	Same as in II, 2
b. Type B	Sulfoiduronate sulfatase	Same as type IIA	Infantile onset; deafness, mental retardation, hepatosplenomegaly; dysostosis multiplex; no corneal opacities; death by 20 years; X-linked inheritance	Same as in II, 1
4. MPS III (Sanfilippo) a. Type A	Heparan-N-sulfate sulfatase	Heparan sulfate	Onset noted around age 4 years; progressive intellectual deterioration; dysostosis multiplex; hepatosplenomegaly; clear corneas; death by 20 years	Same as II, 2
b. Type B	α-N-acetylglucosaminidase	Same as type IIIA		

5. MPS IV (Morquio)	Chondroitin-6-sulfate sulfatase	Keratan sulfate	Normal at birth, severely dwarfed by 2 years; severe skeletal abnormalities; corneal opacities; normal intelligence	Unstable hyperextensible deformed joints
6. MPS VI (Maroteaux-Lamy)				
a. Type A	Chondroitin-4-sulfate sulfatase	Dermatan sulfate	Mild form of type B	Mild stiffness of the fingers, carpal tunnel syndrome
b. Type B	Chondroitin-4-sulfate sulfatase	Same as type VI A	Infantile onset, type I-H-like phenotype; severe dysostosis multiplex; severe growth retardation; normal intelligence	Same as in II, 1, carpal tunnel syndrome, Dupuytren's contracture; aseptic necrosis
7. MPH VII (Sly)	β-Glucuronidase	Chondroitin-4-sulfate Chondroitin-6-sulfate	Onset noted by age 2 years; moderate psychomotor retardation; dysostosis multiplex; short stature; hepatosplenomegaly	Puffy hands and feet
III. Cystinosis	Unknown	Cystine	Infantile onset; renal failure; rickets; growth retardation by 1 year; corneal cystine deposits; death before puberty	Rachitic changes

continued

Table 2.34. (Continued)

Disease	Defective Enzyme(s)	Major Accumulated Substrates or Lysosomal Defects	Major Phenotypic Manifestations	Major Arthritic Manifestations
Defects of Lysosomal Apparatus				
I. Mucolipidoses				
A. Type II (I cell; Leroy disease)	UDP-N-Acetylglusosamine-1-Phosphotransferase	Inclusion bodies; most lysosomal hydrolases decreased in cultured skin fibroblasts with concomitantly increased lysosomal hydrolases in culture media; elevated plasma levels of most lysosomal hydrolases	Infantile onset; dysostosis multiplex; short stature (<80 cm); mild-to-severe psychomotor retardation; gingival hypertrophy; death usually in childhood from pneumonia and heart failure	Limitation of shoulder motion and tight, thick skin in neonates; severe periostitis in infancy; progressive limitation of motion-flexion contractures
B. Type III (pseudo-Hurler polydystrophy)	Same as Type II	Similar to mucolipidosis II	Juvenile onset; mild mental retardation; dysostosis multiplex; ± corneal opacities	Same as in II, 2

Adapted with permission from Grabowski GA, Ludman MD, Desnick RJ: The kidney in metabolic disorders. In Edelmann CM, et al. (eds) *Pediatric Kidney Disease.* Little, Brown, Boston, 1992, pp. 1600–1605.

The Weill-Marchesani Syndrome

Short stature with particularly short hands and feet (brachymorphia, the antithesis of Marfan's syndrome), *downward* ectopia lentis, and immobile, flexed, thick fingers are found in these children. This very rare autosomal-recessive syndrome is compatible with long life.[471]

Leri's Pleonosteosis

Youngsters with this autosomal-dominant condition develop progressive generalized limitation of joint movement with flexion contractures as a result of fibrous hyperplasia of joint capsules, tendons, and ligaments.[491] The affected individuals are short and have broad, deformed thumbs and great toes. The hands are short, square, and thick. Fibrous hyperplasia causes carpal tunnel syndrome in the hands and Morton's metatarsalgia from compression of the digital nerves of the feet.

Myositis Ossificans (Fibrodysplasia Ossificans Progressiva)

These children have recurrent episodes of spontaneous localized tendon, fascial, and fibrous-tissue inflammation that calcifies, causing progressive disability with limitation of joint motion.[471] The disorder is autosomal-dominant with irregular penetrance. Susceptibles may be recognized at birth by the presence of a small great toe, sometimes also present in a parent. Radiographs show synostosis of the phalanges of the great toe.

Symptoms may begin at any age, but in infancy a common presentation resembles torticollis. When fibrodysplasia ossificans progressiva begins at a later age, it may be confused with dermatomyositis, with calcinosis universalis, and with Weber-Christian disease.

Stickler Syndrome

This is the most common autosomal-dominant connective tissue dysplasia in the American midwest.[502] Enlargement of the knee, ankle, and wrist joints may be present at birth, and incapacitating degenerative arthropathy, sometimes mistaken for JRA, occurs in childhood. The arthropathy is frequently associated with congenital joint hyperextensibility and Marfanoid slender-body habitus. Associated anomalies may include the Pierre Robin syndrome, deafness, and an ocular symptom complex including myopia, cataract, retinal degeneration or detachment, and blindness. The familial occurrence of arthropathy and ocular disease suggests the diagnosis. No biochemical abnormalities have been discovered, and the variable pleiotropic manifestations make diagnosis difficult. Stickler syndrome, like the Marfan and Ehlers-

Danlos syndromes, is genetically heterogeneous and probably may result from a variety of biochemical defects.

Multicentric Reticulohistiocytosis

Complaints of pruritis followed by the appearance of brownish histiocytic wartlike nodules on the face, ears, and dorsum of the hands heralds this syndrome of nodules, arthritis of the hands, wrists, elbows, and knees, and mutilating degeneration of the distal interphalangeal joints.[503,504] One family with an autosomal-dominant variant of this syndrome has been reported; in addition to the dermatoarthritis, these children had severe ocular disease, including uveitis, cataracts, and glaucoma.[505] The pathology of the tumors of both types includes histiocytic granulomas. However, giant cells laden with PAS-positive material seen in all of the sporadic cases have not been seen in the familial form. So far, only the familial form has been reported in children.

The Lipidoses

Gaucher's Disease. Musculoskeletal pain, especially hip, knee, and thigh pain, which is sometimes accompanied by fever and simulates osteomyelitis ("bone crisis"), is often the earliest sign of Gaucher's disease.[506] Mis-sense mutations of the enzyme β-glucosidase result in bone and bone-marrow deposition of glucosyl-ceramide, causing "blood sludge," bone infarction, and avascular necrosis (Fig. 2.80).

Gaucher's disease is a relatively common lysosomal storage disorder inherited as an autosomal-recessive trait. Diagnosis may be suspected because of unexplained splenomegaly or because of the Erlenmeyer flask x-ray appearance produced by widening of the distal femur. Serum acid phosphatase is usually elevated. Bone-marrow examination reveals large kerasin-filled Gaucher cells. The diagnosis may be confirmed by enzymatic analysis of skin fibroblasts grown in tissue culture. Alglucerase is now available as the specific treatment for Gaucher's disease,[507] replacing anti-inflammatory drug treatment of the bone pain and secondary synovitis of the hips, and replacing splenectomy which has been reported to worsen the musculoskeletal symptoms.[507a]

Fabry's Disease. This X-linked deficiency of alpha-galactosidase A (measurable in leukocytes, serum, or tears) may present with episodes of polyarthritis, fever, and elevated ESR in hemizygous adolescent boys.[508]

Excruciating burning pain in the fingers and toes may be intolerable. The recurrent episodes tend to last a few days. Limitation of motion becomes apparent in the fingers and sometimes the elbows, shoulders, and spine. Confusion with JRA is not unusual.

Musculoskeletal symptoms are produced by both storage of the glyco-

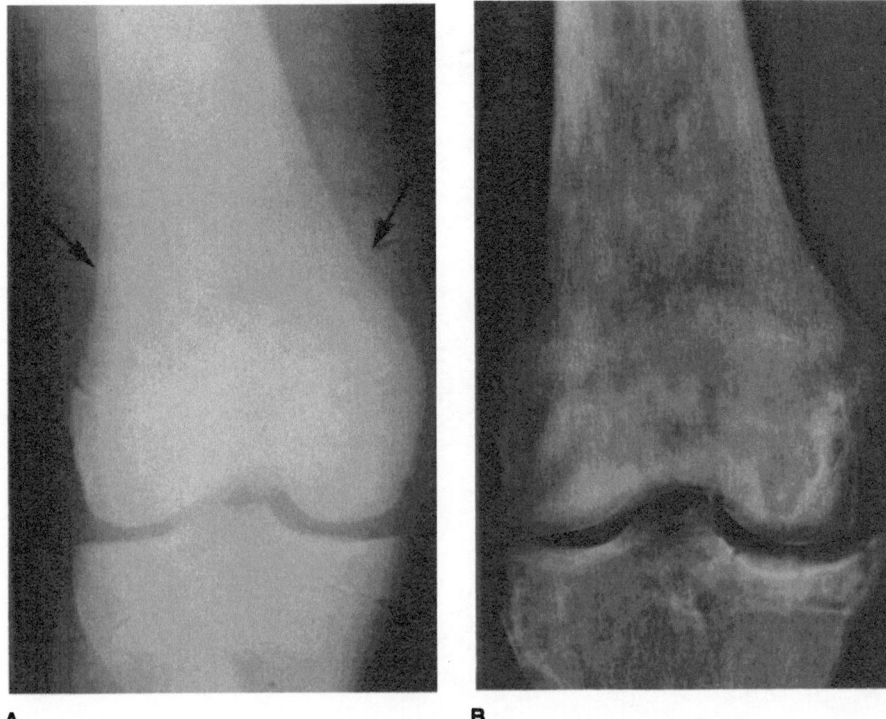

A

B

Figure 2.80. Radiographs in a 12-year-old girl with hip and knee pain (**A**) showed Erlenmeyer-flask widening of the distal femur, typical of Gaucher's disease. Musculoskeletal pain continues to be the major symptom. Repeat films at age 23 (**B**) show extensive infarction but no longer any evidence of Erlenmeyer-flask appearance. It is easy to understand the bone and joint pain in a patient with this radiographic appearance.

sphingolipid trihexosyl ceramide in synovium and by aseptic necrosis of bone and neuroischemia caused by occlusion of blood vessels. The best clue to diagnosis is recognition of the skin manifestation: angiokeratoma—hundreds of tiny red or blue-black flat spots (angiectasias) or papules concentrated between the umbilicus and the knees with a predilection for the lower back, buttocks, and scrotum, which usually appear during childhood. Cornea verticillata, thin opaque lines ("fingerprints") radiating from a central area of the cornea, may be seen in both affected males and carrier females. The corneal lesion is similar to that seen with chloroquine toxicity. Cardiac, neurologic, and renal manifestations result in shortened life-span.

Isolation and sequencing of the gene has led to recognition of variant forms of Fabry's disease.[509]

Ceramidosis (Farber's Disease). Arthritis is a major manifestation of this syndrome.[510] Deficiency of the enzyme ceramidase results in an accumulation of ceramide, causing proliferation of histiocytes, lymphocytes, and

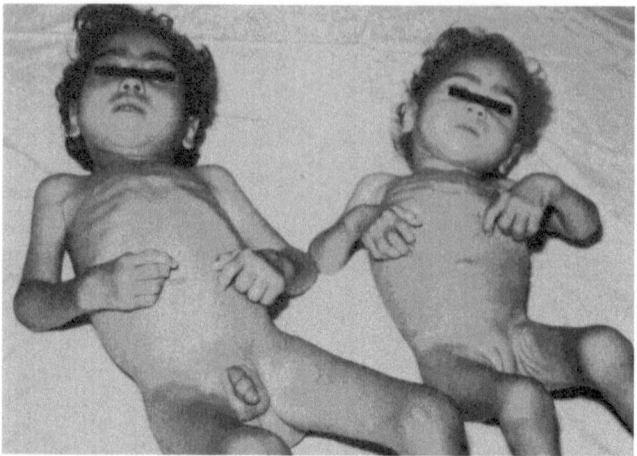

A

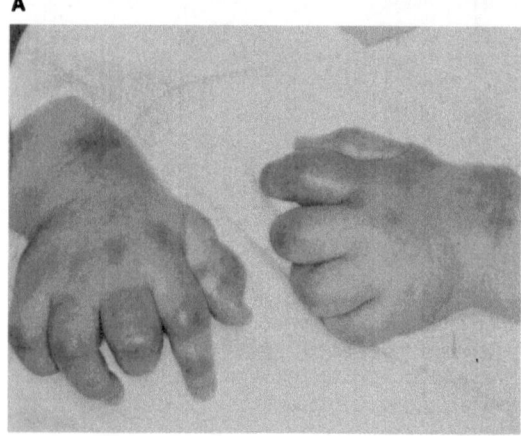

B

Figure 2.81. **(A)** Severe arthritis with atrophy and flexion contractures in 1- and 3-year-old siblings with Farber's disease; the clinical appearance of the children resembles that of severe JRA. (Both children died shortly after this photo.) **(B)** Close-up view of hands in another patient, showing nodular swelling and erythema about the wrists and phalangeal joints. Note the accentuation of the process over the medial aspects of the wrists about the biopsy scars. (**A**, courtesy of Dr. H. Zazif, Damascus University, Syria; **B**, courtesy of Dr. S. K. Abul-Haj; reprinted with permission from ref. 510.)

fibroblasts in skin, subcutaneous tissues, tendons, synovium, viscera, and the nervous system.[511] As a result, affected infants present with a hoarse voice and noisy respirations; subcutaneous nodules; joint swellings and restrictions; general malaise with irritability, poor growth, and development; and sometimes fever (Fig. 2.81). The large nodular masses on the tendon sheaths and in the periarticular tissues, especially over pressure areas, are distinctive

(Fig. 2.81B). Granulomas of the epiglottis and larynx cause recurrent pneumonia and death, most commonly during the second year of life. However, a few milder cases have survived.[511] Diagnosis may be confirmed by demonstrating deficiency of ceramidase in plasma or leukocytes.[512]

Bone and Cartilage Dysplasias

Heritable disorders causing abnormal epiphyseal ossification frequently lead to early progressive degenerative arthritis, especially in the hips and knees, which may mimic and be mistaken for JRA.[513–516] When the epiphyseal dysplasia is part of a generalized syndrome with obvious dwarfism such as in Morquio's disease, Ellis-van Creveld syndrome, diatrophic dwarfism, gargoylism, achondroplasia, pseudoachondroplasia, or cretinism, the diagnosis is usually apparent. However, diagnosis may be very difficult in less severely affected individuals.

Suspicion should be aroused whenever there is a family history of many individuals with early symmetrical joint destruction, especially of weight-bearing joints.[517] Short stature is characteristic of these disorders and may be accompanied by stiff joints, small hands, and a waddling gait. Lateral-spine radiographs obtained when this diagnosis is considered may show flattened vertebral bodies with irregular end-plates, particularly in the thoracic spine, before other radiographic signs are apparent. Other abnormal roentgenographic findings may include short metacarpals; flattened humeral heads; oblique acetabuli; flat, large, deformed femoral heads; and slanting ankle mortices.

More than 100 chondrodystrophy syndromes have been described, including Kniest syndrome (Swiss cheese cartilage), Stickler arthro-ophthalmopathy, multiple epiphyseal dysplasia, spondyloepiphyseal dysplasia, and dysplasia epiphysealis hemimelia. Erroneous diagnoses of JRA are avoided by obtaining appropriate radiographs of patients with unusual family histories, short stature, and small hands.

Trichorhinophalangeal Dysplasia (TRPS)

This usually heritable dominant disorder, which causes enlargement of the interphalangeal joints, has been mistaken for JRA. The syndrome is recognized by the strikingly large pear-shaped nose, thin upper lip, sparse brittle hair, and short stature.[518] Suspicion is aroused by the family history and appearance of the affected parent. Radiographs show cone-shaped middle-finger epiphyses and small capital femoral epiphyses. As in the epiphyseal dysplasias, aseptic necrosis of the hips often occurs. Some authors have suggested obtaining hand films in all children with bilateral Perthes' disease to exclude TRPS; children may present with unilateral hip disease.[519]

Multiple Cartilaginous Exostoses

This common autosomal-dominant failure of bone modeling results in bony protuberances, usually at the ends of long bones (Fig. 2.82).[520] The lesions grow during childhood, and symptoms may begin around the age of 10. Where tendons are irritated by the pointed lesions, the pain patterns may simulate arthritis, most frequently in boys. Radiographs frequently reveal more exostoses than are clinically apparent.

Metachondromatosis

Enchondromatosis (Ollier disease) and Maffucci syndrome (enchondromatosis with multiple cavernous hemangiomata) affect bones all over the skeleton; metachondromatosis (Fig. 2.83) is a combination of enchondromatosis and exostosis in which the lesions are primarily in the hands and feet. Lesions disappear as new ones grow.[521]

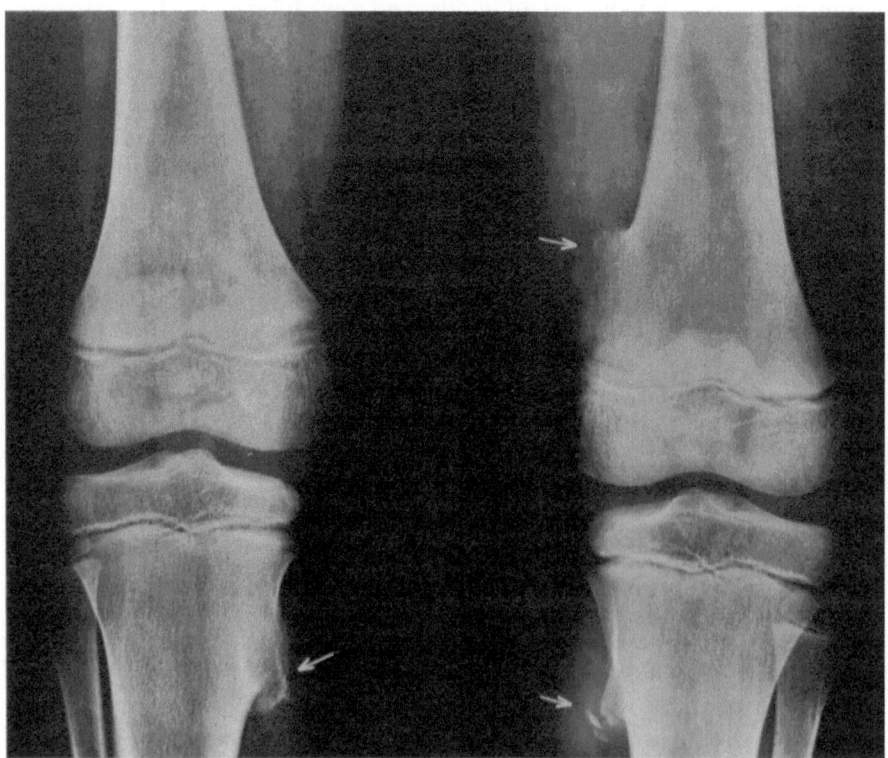

Figure 2.82. Multiple cartilaginous exostoses (*arrows*) causing knee pain in a 9-year-old boy.

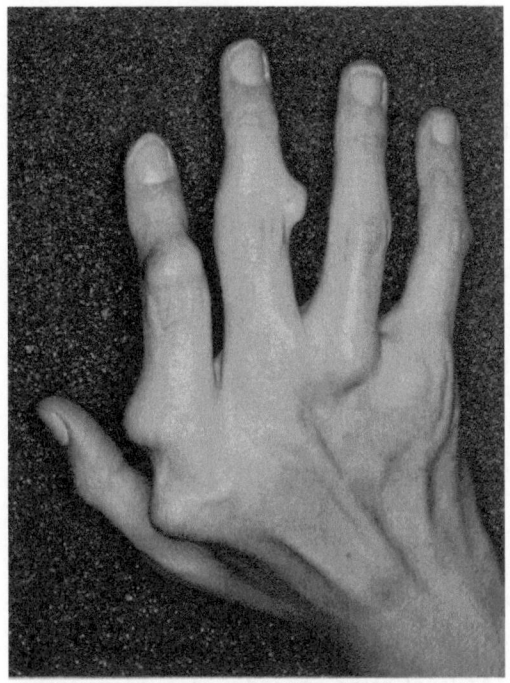

A

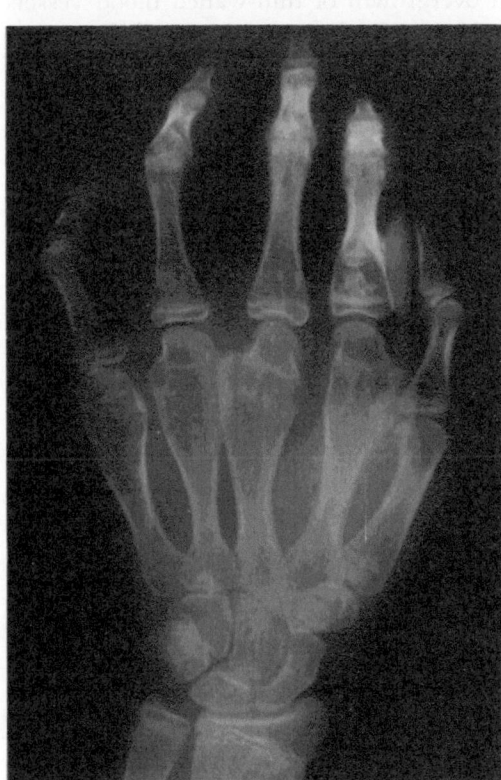

B

Figure 2.83. Metachondromatosis; clinical appearance (**A**); (**B**) radiograph showing a combination of exostosis and enchondromatosis primarily in the hands and feet.

Table 2.35. Differential Diagnosis of the Vanishing Bone Diseases (Acro-osteolysis)

Gorham's disease
Idiopathic multicentric osteolysis
Carpotarsal osteolysis
Farber's disease
Multicentric reticulohistiocytosis
Pseudo-Hurler dystrophy
Winchester syndrome
Hajdu-Cheney syndrome (phalangeal osteolysis)[524]

The Vanishing Bone Diseases

There are a variety of disorders in childhood that may be associated with disappearing bones (Table 2.35). At least some sporadic cases seem to be related to the development of an overgrowth of thin-walled blood vessels (angiomatosis), as originally described by Gorham and Stout.[522] The forms that are of most concern to the rheumatologist are characterized by carpal-tarsal osteolysis.

Carpotarsal Osteolysis. *Clinical Features.* There are many different, poorly understood syndromes that start in childhood with crippling progressive osteolysis of the wrists and ankles.[523] Initially, the preschool child is seen for what seems to be JRA with heat, tenderness, swelling, and flexion contractures. At about age 6, generalized demineralization of the carpal and tarsal bones begins to be apparent radiographically. This is followed by localized destruction of carpal and tarsal bones and then complete resorption and disappearance of these bones, along with partial destruction of the metacarpals and metatarsals and of the epiphyses of the radius and ulna. In some forms of these diseases, elbows and knees ultimately may also be affected. The early childhood symptomatic phase of the carpotarsal osteolytic syndromes is generally followed by a relatively pain-free period in adolescence, during which time the bones are disappearing. In middle-age adults, deformity may again accentuate with extrusion of involved bones in some cases.

Some of these syndromes are associated with hypertension and renal disease in childhood.[525] Although the renal disease may be severe and ultimately fatal, it has not been well characterized. What evidence is available suggests arterial and arteriolar sclerosis.

Pathology. Although the synovium in these disorders contains greatly thickened arterioles, there is a total absence of inflammation. A degenerative proliferative reaction is seen on the periosteal surface. The periosteum forms a thick fibrous structure invading the cortical bone, which is demineralized and replaced with fibrous tissue.

The presence of metachromatic staining mucopolysaccharides and hyperplastic fibroblasts suggests that these various disorders are primarily enzymatic defects resulting in storage or biochemical abnormalities involving fibroblasts. These hypotheses are supported by finding osteolysis as one feature of Farber's disease (ceramide deficiency) and pseudo-Hurler mucolipidoses, a defect of the lysosomal apparatus. Other syndromes, which include osteolysis as a primary feature, are listed in Table 2.35.

Winchester Syndrome

Arthritis is characteristically the first manifestation of this heritable (? autosomal-recessive) disorder.[526] Symmetrical swelling in the fingers, hands, wrists, and ankles may be accompanied by pain and limited motion in the hips and elbows and generalized osteoporosis (Fig. 2.84). Osteolysis of carpal-tarsal bones results in arthritis mutalans (the opera-glass hand). Associated features include short stature, corneal opacities, coarse facial features, and generalized osteoporosis. The basic abnormality is thought to be ultrastructurally abnormal fibroblasts.

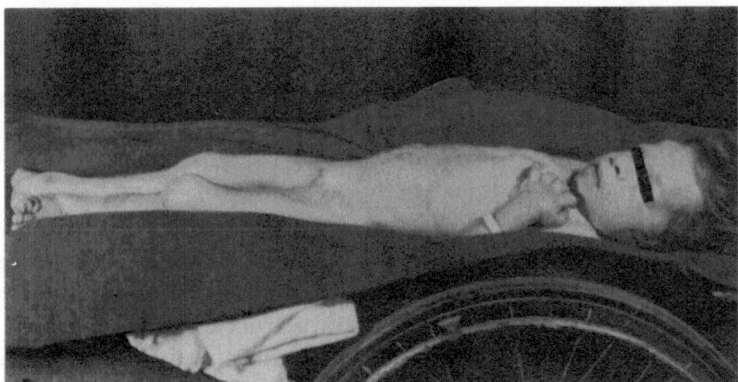

Figure 2.84. Arthritis is usually the first manifestation of Winchester's syndrome, which progresses to total crippling. Carpal-tarsal osteolysis is a prominent finding. Although this was though to be a mucopolysaccharidosis at first, the nature of this familial disorder remains uncertain. There is some clinical resemblance to Farber's disease. (Courtesy of Dr. P. Winchester. Reprinted with permission from Winchester et al. *Am J Roentgenol* 106:121–128, 1969.)

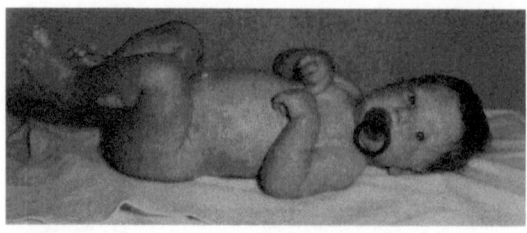

A

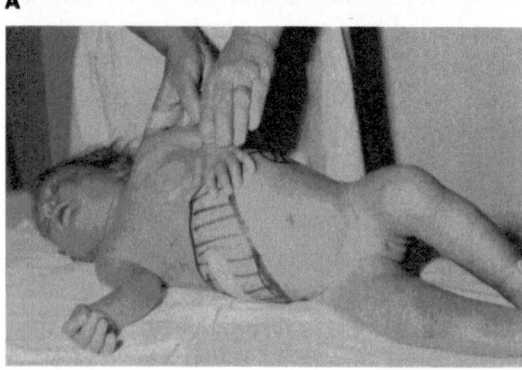

B

Figure 2.85. Congenital arthropathy with rash. (NOMID or CINCA syndrome). The rash was noted in the newborn nursery; within a few months this baby began having episodes of high fever and was noted to have lymphadenopathy and hepatosplenomegaly. Radiographs revealed extensive periosteal new-bone formation in all long bones and the phalanges. Photographs were taken at ages 8 months (**A**) and 20 months (**B**). The child died at age 23 months, after months of chronic pneumonia. The joints contained cellular infiltrates identical to those seen in all of the viscera and throughout the musculoskeletal system.

Congenital Arthropathy with Rash Appearing at Birth; Infantile Multisystem Inflammatory Disease (CINCA, NOMID Syndrome)

More than 30 cases of an unusual chronic arthropathy recognizable by the appearance of a severe persistent rash at or a few days after birth have been reported.[527] Two children in one family were affected. We have seen a similar patient (Fig. 2.85). In addition to the rash and progressive erosive arthritis and periostitis, most of the affected children have had recurrent fever, lymphadenopathy, hepatosplenomegaly, and mental retardation; some had uveitis, deafness, and chronic meningitis.[528] Pathologic examination in reported cases revealed infiltration of the skin, lymph nodes, and meninges by polymorphonuclear cells. In our patient, at autopsy, all organs except the brain showed a granulomatous inflammatory process characterized by lymphocytes, histiocytes, and plasma cells, with fibrinoid necrosis, principally around blood vessels. There was intensive calcification in some of the blood vessels in the brain.

Infantile Systemic Hyalinosis

Neonatal onset of painful joint contractures with papules on the face and trunk, gingival hypertrophy, persistent diarrhea, failure to thrive and periostitis in long bones also occurs in a newly described syndrome, infantile systemic hyalinosis. There is some overlap with Winchester syndrome, infantile multisystem inflammatory disease, and another new syndrome, juvenile hyaline fibrosis.[529]

Familial Hypertrophic Synovitis

Clinical Description. In 1965, we first reported a family of nine children, five of whom had a unique arthropathy characterized by flexion contractures of the fingers ("trigger fingers") apparent during the first few months of life and noninflammatory joint effusions (Fig. 2.86).[530] We later reported a second family with three of five affected children,[531] and a third family with three of five affected children was recognized by Athreya[532] in 1978. Large symmetrical effusions in knees, ankles, and wrists are characteristic. There is little or

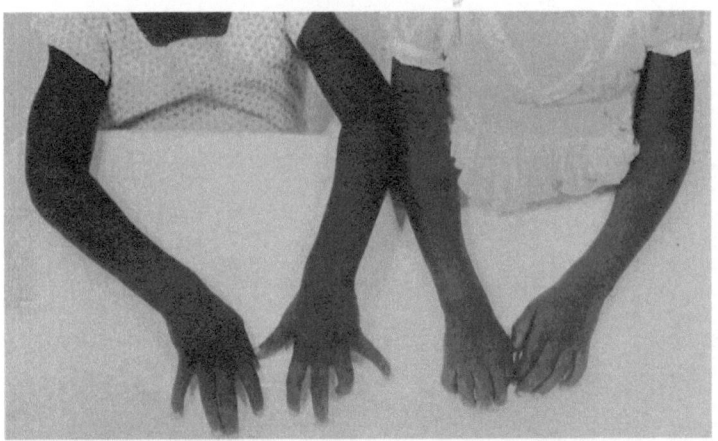

A

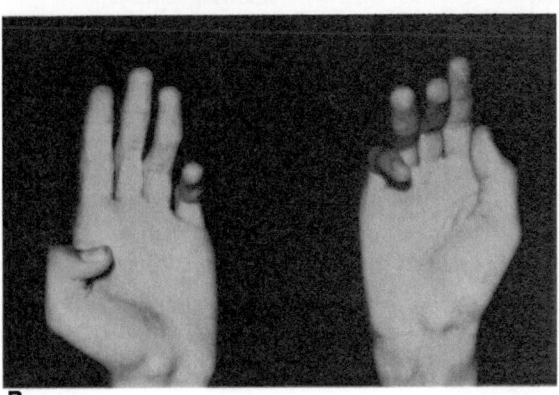

B

Figure 2.86. Trigger fingers and large-joint effusions in two of six sibs with familial hypertrophic synovitis (**A**) and in one of three affected sibs in another family (**B**). The bent thumb appears soon after birth and is the first clue to the diagnosis. (**A**, Reprinted with permission from Jacobs, ref. 530.)

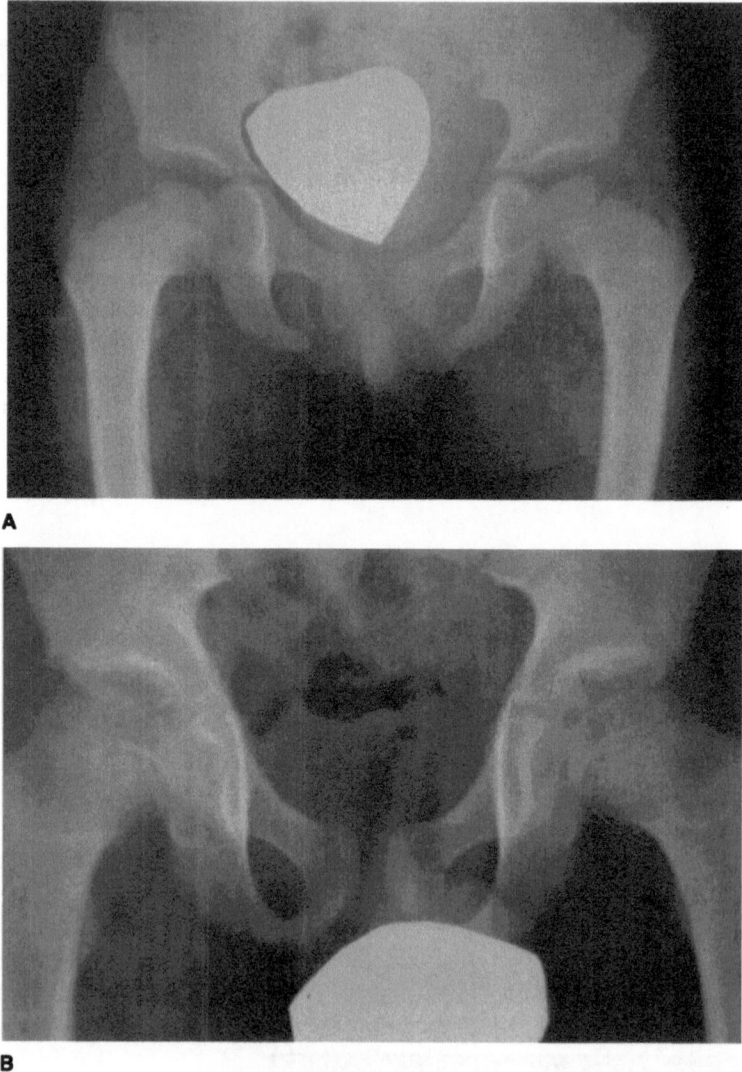

Figure 2.87. (**A** and **B**) Curious proximal flattening of the femoral ossification centers, suggesting tendon contractures analogous to trigger fingers in two children with familial hypertrophic synovitis.

no pain, and there are no systemic manifestations or laboratory abnormalities. As the children grow older, there is some limitation of motion in large joints, especially in the hips, where radiographs show a curious proximal flattening of the femoral ossification centers, suggesting tendon contractures analogous to the trigger fingers (Fig. 2.87). One patient has developed chondrocalcinosis during the third decade of life.

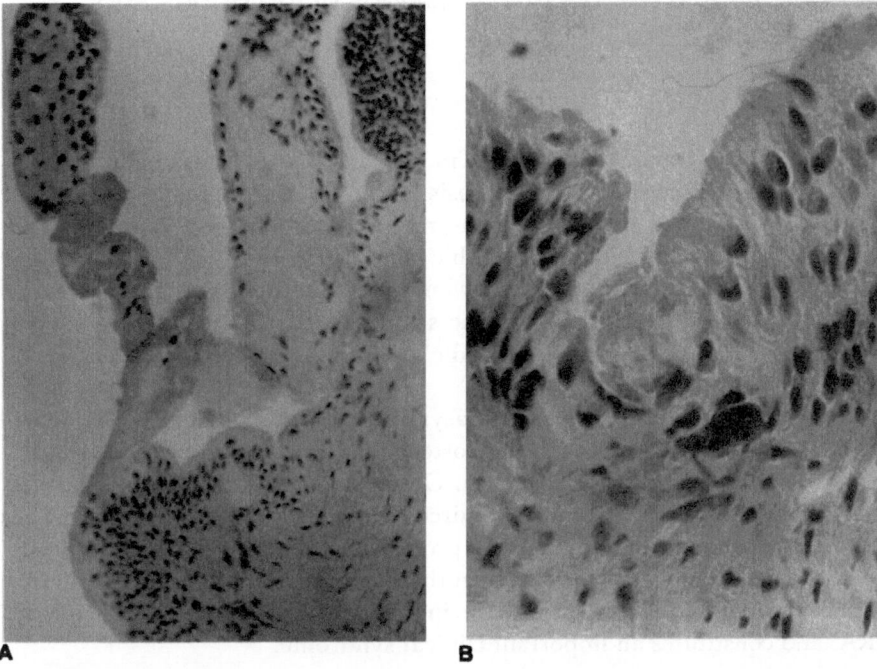

A   B

Figure 2.88. Unique synovial pathology seen in familial hypertrophic synovitis consists of large hypertrophic avascular villi and giant cells but no underlying inflammation (**A**). The hypertrophy is due solely to extraordinary hyperplasia of the lining cells **B**). There was no change when two of these patients were rebiopsied 10 years later. (Reprinted with permission from Jacobs et al., ref. 531. Copyright by the American Academy of Pediatrics 1978.)

Pathology. The synovial pathology is unique, characterized by large hypertrophic avascular villi with giant cells but no inflammation.[531,532] The hypertrophy is due solely to extraordinary hyperplasia of synovial lining cells (Fig. 2.88). There was no change in patients rebiopsied after a 10-year interval. The inborn stimulus for the synovial lining cell hyperplasia has not been identified.

Genetic Study. Genetic studies in one family showed an autosomal-dominant mode of inheritance, but surprisingly, none of the parents of these children have been affected. The three families have been of Irish, Pakistani, and American black origins, suggesting that this condition occurs worldwide. While the presence of trigger fingers in infancy should alert the physician to this condition, we suspect most cases have not been distinguished clinically from JRA and that this disorder is more common than might be presumed from the few reported cases.

Neoplasms and Neoplasmlike Lesions of the Bones and Joints (Table 2.36)

Tumors of Bone

Malignant bone tumors are not rare in childhood and occasionally present with joint pain or swelling.[533] Diagnosis is usually immediately apparent on x-ray, with accurate prediction of the tumor type based on the age of the child and the location and radiographic characteristics of the tumor. Malignant tumors adjacent to the sacroiliac joint may not show on plain x-rays but may show up as "hot spots" on bone scan. CT scan is helpful in showing these lesions.[51] Occasionally, a Brodie's abscess has been mistaken for a malignant tumor.[52]

Benign tumors of bone are usually asymptomatic and coincidentally noted on x-rays obtained for other reasons (osteochondroma, enchondroma, simple bone cyst, and nonossifying fibroma). Occasionally, a nonossifying fibroma may be secretory and produce acquired vitamin-D–resistant rickets. The secreted substance and method of production of the syndrome has not been proved. Removal of the tumor in these cases has resulted in cure of the rickets. Osteoid osteoma is not rare in childhood, may be confused with JRA, and constitutes an important clinical syndrome.

Osteoid Osteoma

This relatively common benign tumor of bone produces characteristic localized aching or boring bone pain, worse at night and at rest or with elevation, and exquisitely responsive to aspirin and naproxen. Boys are affected twice as often as girls. Half of the reported cases occurred between the ages of 11 and 20; 75% were in the femur or tibia.[536]

Histologically, this tumor consists of a tiny nidus of osteoid and new bone within highly vascularized osteogenic connective tissue. Radiographically, a reactive layer of sclerotic bone is seen around the lucent or calcified nidus. The pain may result from nerve fibers within the nidus but in our experience is more typical of periostitis; periosteal new-bone formation and cortical thickening are characteristically associated with osteoid osteoma. Saville hypothesized that the pain was a result of metabolites of arachidonic acid produced by the tumor and at highest concentration at rest.[537]

Pain from these tumors may be referred to adjacent joints. Synovitis, sympathetic effusions, demineralization, and muscle atrophy occur and may be apparent long before the lesion itself is radiographically demonstrable[536-539] (Fig. 2.89). When the tumor is in the vertebrae, painful scoliosis or radicular pain down the arm or leg may be the major complaint, sometimes with muscle atrophy. It was not unusual for these children to be subjected to many procedures and therapies or to be often misdiagnosed as malingerers during the long period (sometimes 2 years) it could take for the

Table 2.36. Tumors in and Around the Joints

Benign
Ganglions
Pigmented villonodular synovitis
Hemangioma
Osteochondromatosis, chondroblastoma[534]
Xanthoma
Lipoma
Neuroma, neurofibroma,[535] myxoma,
 myoma, glomus

Malignant
Synovial sarcoma
Epithelioid sarcoma
Clear-cell sarcoma
Malignant giant-cell tumor
Synovial chondrosarcoma
Leukemic (or metastatic) infiltrates

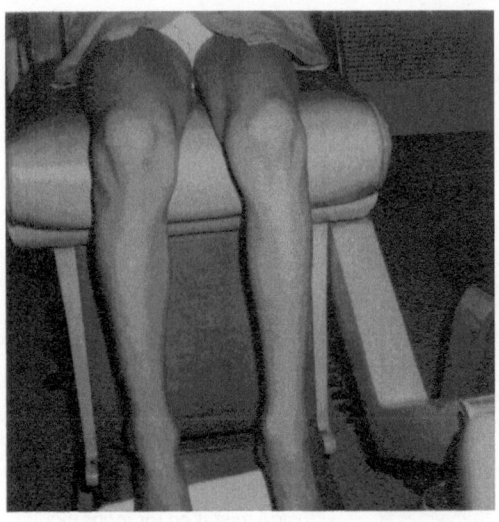

Figure 2.89. Atrophy of entire leg caused by an unrecognized osteoid osteoma in the foot.

lesion to become radiographically apparent (Fig. 2.90). Technetium bone scanning and CT are more sensitive diagnostic tools for these lesions, enabling, prompt diagnosis. We do not yet know the incidence of false-negative bone scans.

Osteoid osteomas in childhood are generally surgically removed with complete relief of symptoms.[540] Recently, symptoms have been relieved by re-

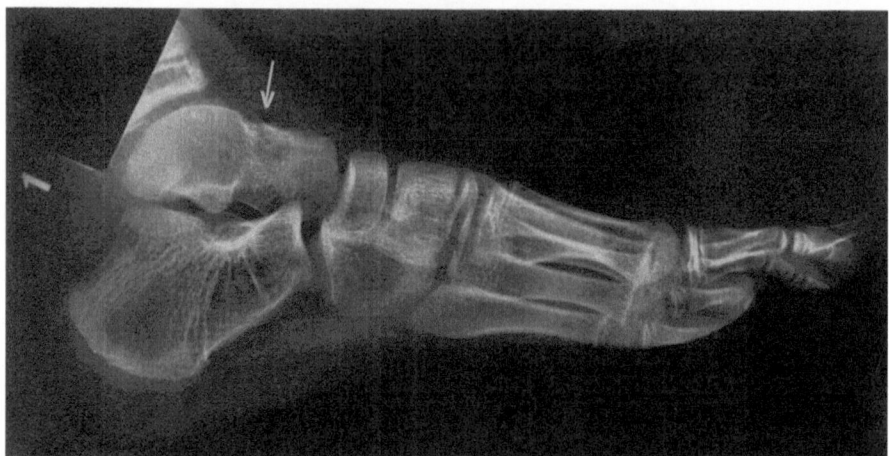

A

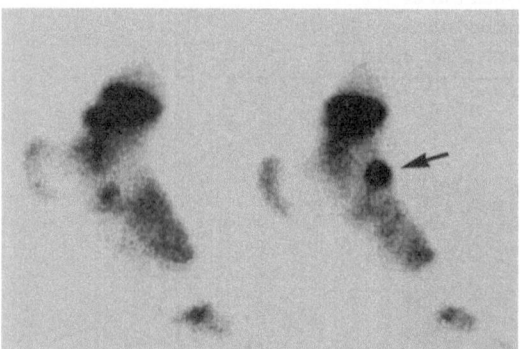

B

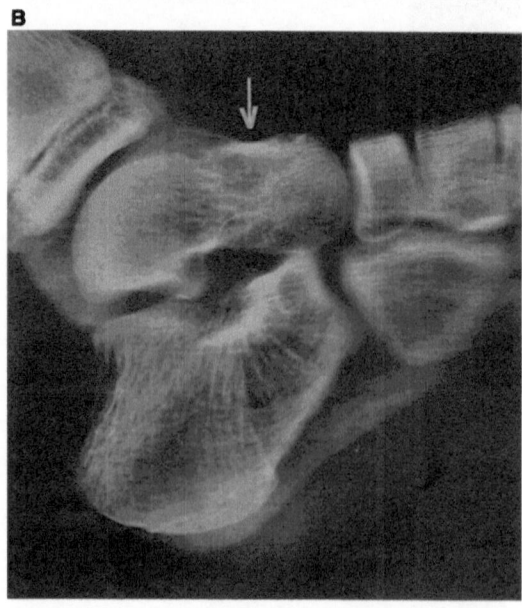

C

Figure 2.90. Unrecognized osteoid osteoma, left talus, with effusion mistaken for monarticular JRA of the ankle. After $1\frac{1}{2}$ years, a bone scan was obtained (**B**) and was positive, but the lesion was still not recognized on plain films (**A**). The lesion was clearly visible on tomograms (**C**) and, in retrospect, can be seen on the plain films. Over a period of years the lesion healed completely and was no longer visible radiographically.

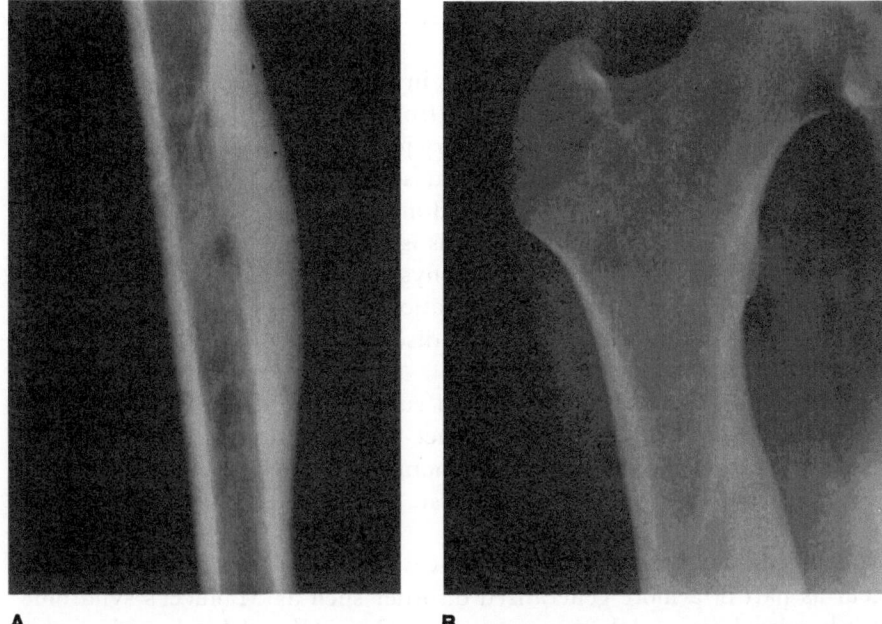

A   **B**

Figure 2.91. (A) Osteoid osteoma (femur) in a 15-year-old boy. Pain disappeared after 1 year of aspirin therapy. **(B)** The lesion, now asymptomatic, is radiologically visible 11 years later.

moval of the nidus alone with a Craig needle guided by CT.[541] Some parents elect not to have surgical removal and choose NSAID therapy as the alternative.[537] Relatively small doses of aspirin or naproxen are required for relief. Over a period of years, the pain disappears, and a sclerotic "scar" may be all that remains visible radiographically. In many patients, this medical regimen is an excellent alternative to surgery (Fig. 2.91).

Benign Neoplasms of the Joints

Tumors in or about the joints may arise from nonspecialized soft tissues such as fat and blood vessels or from the synovial cells themselves (Table 2.36). Ganglions are frequent; the others are all rare.

Ganglions. These cystlike outpouchings of tendon sheaths or joint capsules are common in children; are called Baker's cysts when located in the posterior medial aspect of the knee; usually disappear spontaneously if you wait long enough; tend to recur if surgically removed; and are said to account for over 4000 unnecessary operations per year in the United States. They are thought to be a response to local irritation,[542,543] resulting in increased production of joint fluid and causing the narrow neck between joint and bursa to act as a ball valve, preventing the fluid from reentering the joint. No treatment is necessary.

Outpouchings of the wrists and knees in rheumatoid arthritis are usually soft, multiple, and easily distinguishable from ordinary ganglions. Such cysts contain turbid low-viscosity inflammatory joint fluid, unlike the clear jelly of the simple ganglion. Occasionally, what seems like a ganglion (or simple Baker's cyst) is the first sign of JRA and may be noted when the balance of the physical examination is normal. This is so infrequent that children with ganglions afforded a thorough normal physical examination of their musculoskeletal system and slit-lamp examination of their eyes require no additional studies and no "exclusion" of disease; moreover, no aggravating advice to their parents is necessary.

Popliteal cysts sometimes dissect and rupture into the calf and simulate thrombophlebitis, or, rarely, may dissect into the anterior leg or into the thigh.[544] Ultrasonography is a safe and noninvasive technique for confirming the suspicion of a dissecting popliteal cyst.

Synovial Hemangiomas. These blood-vessel tumors (malformations) may occur as part of a more generalized disorder such as Maffucci's syndrome (dyschondroplasia and hemangiomata) or Von Hippel-Lindau syndrome (visceral angiomatosis) or may be limited to the joints and periarticular tissues. One joint or multiple joints may be affected.

Symptoms generally begin in childhood, but the correct diagnosis is rarely made until young adulthood.[545-547] The patients characteristically have episodic attacks of excruciating pain after mild trauma, sometimes with only minimal swelling and discoloration of overlying skin. Aspiration yields grossly bloody joint fluid. The knee is most frequently involved, but elbow and ankle tumors have also been reported. A mass may be palpated adjacent to the joint, or there may be signs of internal derangement, leading to operative treatment and diagnosis at the time of surgery.

Recurrent brief attacks of excruciating pain with effusion should suggest this diagnosis; aspiration of bloody joint fluid on repeated occasions in the absence of a bleeding disorder confirms that suspicion. In the past, preoperative diagnosis was dependent on the radiographic appearance of a phlebolith in muscle adjacent to the joint (Fig. 2.92). Recently, preoperative diagnosis has been achieved by computerized tomographic joint scan (Fig. 2.93), arteriography, phlebography, and thermography.[547,548] Improvement follows surgical removal, but it may be impossible to completely remove diffuse lesions, and recurrences are common.

Case Report

The patient was first seen at age $4\frac{1}{2}$ years with a history of having screamed with pain in the left knee 6 days earlier. One day later, the area appeared slightly ecchymotic. Over the next few days, she again screamed, because of intermittent pain in the

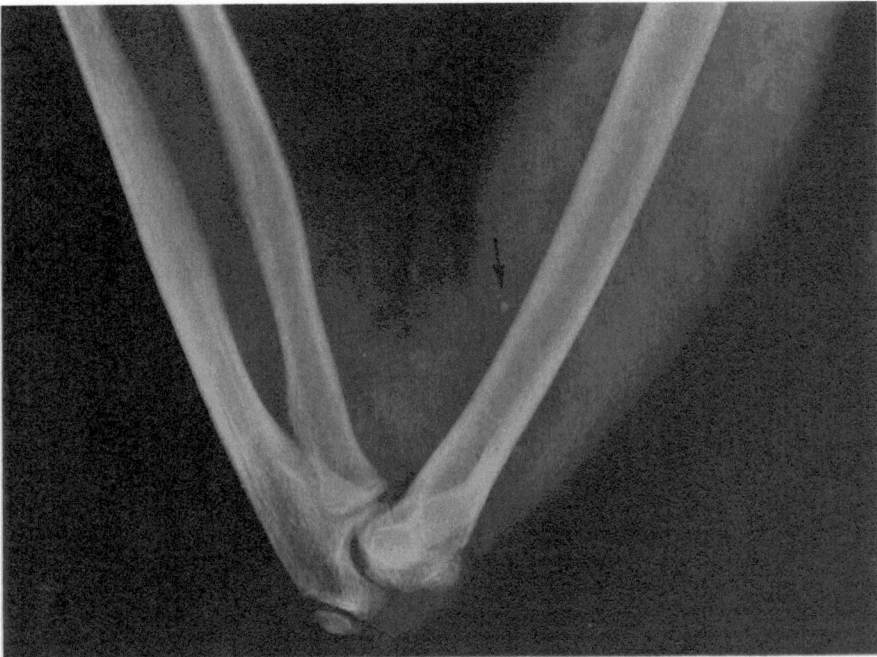

Figure 2.92. Hemangioma near elbow causing recurrent elbow effusion with transient diffuse ecchymotic swellings. Onset occurred at age 5 years. Diagnosis was not made until after a phlebolith became apparent *(arrow)* at age 10 years. Earlier diagnosis might now be possible with the use of CT scans (see Fig. 2.93).

opposite knee or wrists, although no color changes were noted. Physical examination and laboratory studies were normal. One year later, she had a similar episode in the right elbow and was seen by an orthopedist who made a diagnosis of JRA. When examined here 18 days later, there was subsiding ecchymosis about the elbow but no other signs. ESR was 36 mm/h. Beginning at age 7, the episodes in the elbow became more frequent, each brief but each exquisitely painful and associated with visible ecchymotic change; she related the episodes to having been hit by her brother. In 1977, an x-ray showed calcification in the muscle above the elbow (Fig. 2.92). The area was explored, and a cavernous hemangioma was removed from the muscle. However, the hemangioma dissected down into the bone and could not be totally excised. Symptoms were improved following surgery, but the tumor is now palpable in the triceps muscle. A sibling had similar complaints at age 6 for a brief time but has been well for the past 6 years.

Pigmented Villonodular Synovitis. Teenagers and adults may develop pigmented villonodular synovitis (PVNS), a unique diffuse chronic synovitis almost always limited to a single knee, which is clinically suggested by the finding of chocolate-brown synovial fluid at arthrocentesis. The disease is not

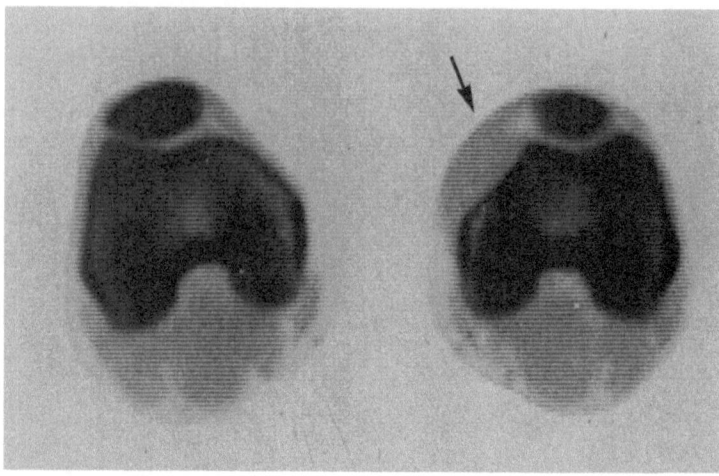

Figure 2.93. Synovial hemangioma of the knee demonstrated by CT scan showing loss of normal contour of the medial femoral condyle and a soft-tissue mass in the bony defect (*arrow*). Recurrent brief episodes of nontraumatic bloody knee effusions began at age 2 years. Roentgenograms were normal. (Courtesy of Drs. M.A. Linson and I.P. Posner. Reprinted with permission from Linson M.A. Synovial Hemangioma as a Cause of Recurrent Knee Effusions. *JAMA* 242:2214–2215, 1979. Copyright by the American Medical Association.)

seen in young children.[549,550] The diagnosis is best established by arthroscopy where the synovium is seen to be thrown into multiple coarse and fine villi ("a scraggly beard") colored deep brown to light yellow. A biopsy obtained at the time of arthroscopy will show a dense cellular infiltrate of the synovium without lining-cell hyperplasia but with numerous microscopic villi. The cellular infiltrate consists of multinucleated giant cells, lipoid-loaded foam cells, and hemosiderin-pigment-loaded stromal cells; definitive diagnosis depends on the demonstration of this characteristic pathology.

The etiology of this uncommon disease is unknown; most authors consider it an unusual benign inflammatory response to a local stimulus, which in some cases is probably blood. Others consider PVNS a histiocytic tumor. A localized form also occurs in adults, generally presenting as a solitary mass on a finger. PVNS may extend into surrounding tissues—tendons, ligaments, muscle, bone, and skin. Invasion of bone is reflected by the radiographic appearance of cystic lesions on both sides of the joint space.

The course of PVNS is uncertain; many patients can be adequately managed with aspirin and nonsteroidal anti-inflammatory drugs, and the disease may remit without surgery. While some authorities advocate surgical excision, many patients have recurrences and an unsatisfactory course after surgery. In some series, only 17% of cases were cured with surgery. It would, therefore, seem reasonable to reserve surgery for cases that cannot be adequately managed with anti-inflammatory drugs.

Synovial Chondromatosis. These patients develop intrasynovial cartilaginous nodules that ultimately project above the surface and may calcify.[551] Some shed into the joint space as loose bodies, producing pain, swelling, and mechanical limitations. The male knee is most commonly affected, occasionally bilaterally. The youngest reported patient was age 14. Unless the lesions calcify and are apparent on x-ray, the diagnosis cannot be made clinically but might be made by arthroscopy. Therapy has usually consisted of removal of the loose bodies and affected synovium, but occasional patients have been reported to have spontaneous regression of the tumor. The disorder is apparently self-limited since even partial removal has resulted in relief of symptoms without evident regrowth of tumor.

Langerhans'-cell Histiocytosis. Previously called eosinophilic granuloma, this nonmalignant tumor may present with neck pain and torticollis suggestive of JRA.[552] Patients referred to us as having JRA because of torticollis have had histiocytosis, chromophobe adenoma, and unrecognized cervical spine fractures, all of which could be identified with CT films of the spine with contrast if not apparent on routine spine films.

Malignant Synovial Tumors

Synovial, epithelioid, and clear-cell sarcomas have all been reported in children. However, these malignant synovial tumors are extremely rare in children and are usually located in soft tissues *outside* the joints.[553–554a] It is for this reason that joint biopsies are generally not necessary to exclude this diagnosis.

Synovial Sarcoma. This is the most common of these tumors, and although most cases occur between 15 and 30 years of age, the youngest reported patient was only 20 months old at the time of diagnosis, and 9.5% of patients are under 16 years of age. Of all soft-tissue sarcomas in childhood, 7% are synovial. Although males have been most commonly affected as adults, two-thirds of the children are girls.

The most common clinical presentation is a firm or elastic soft-tissue lump that is usually painless. Anatomic continuity with a joint or surrounding tissues is very rare, and even when the lesions are contiguous with a joint capsule, the joint itself is rarely invaded, although these may be a reactive joint effusion if the tumor is near a joint. Although pain in the knee without a visible lump has been mistaken for arthritis in a few adults with synovial sarcoma, diagnosis has not usually been difficult in pediatric patients, as all reported cases have presented with obvious extra-articular soft-tissue masses that demanded biopsy. Our most recent case (Fig. 2.94) is an unfortunate exception.

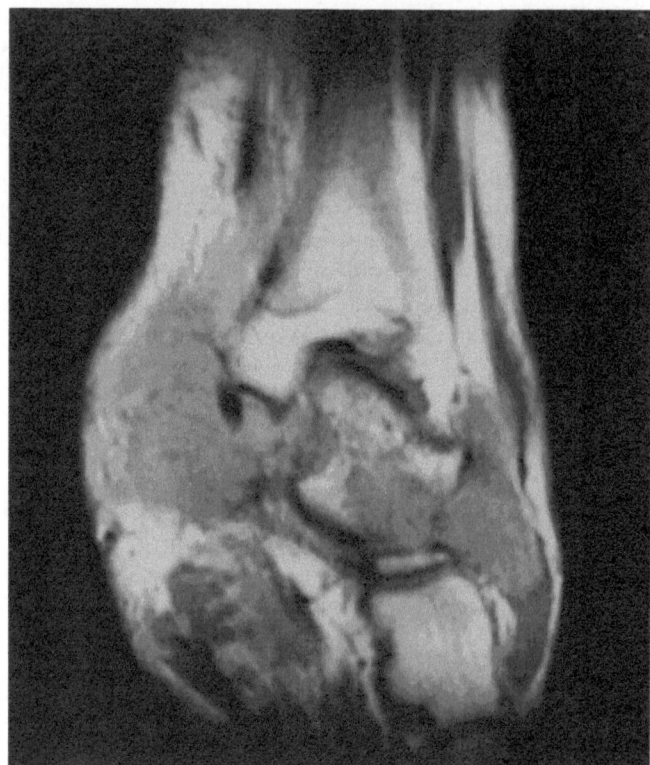

Figure 2.94. MRI demonstrated a large synovial sarcoma in the ankle of a 15-year-old boy previously treated for $1\frac{1}{2}$ years for ligamentous injury, Lyme disease, and JRA, Although the tumor originated outside the joint, it was not palpable or apparent on radiographs. Bone scan was negative and the tumor was not seen at a previously performed arthroscopy.

Epithelioid Sarcoma. These tumors arise from fascia, tendon sheath, and periosteum. Although related to synovial sarcomas, they are morphologically distinctive, with a characteristic nodular pattern that, with low-power microscopy, can be confused with an inflammatory granuloma. This is the most common soft-tissue sarcoma of the hand and generally presents as a painless mass on the fingers, hand, or wrist; it is rare elsewhere. A similar tumor on the ankle, heel, or plantar region of the foot, said to most resemble an epithelial neoplasm, has been termed a *clear-cell sarcoma.*

Epithelioid Hemangioendothelioma. This tumor, in some cases related to exposure to vinyl chloride, which in some children may be result of living near a toxic-waste dump, may present with joint pain; x-rays show an osteolytic lesion in nearby bone.[554]

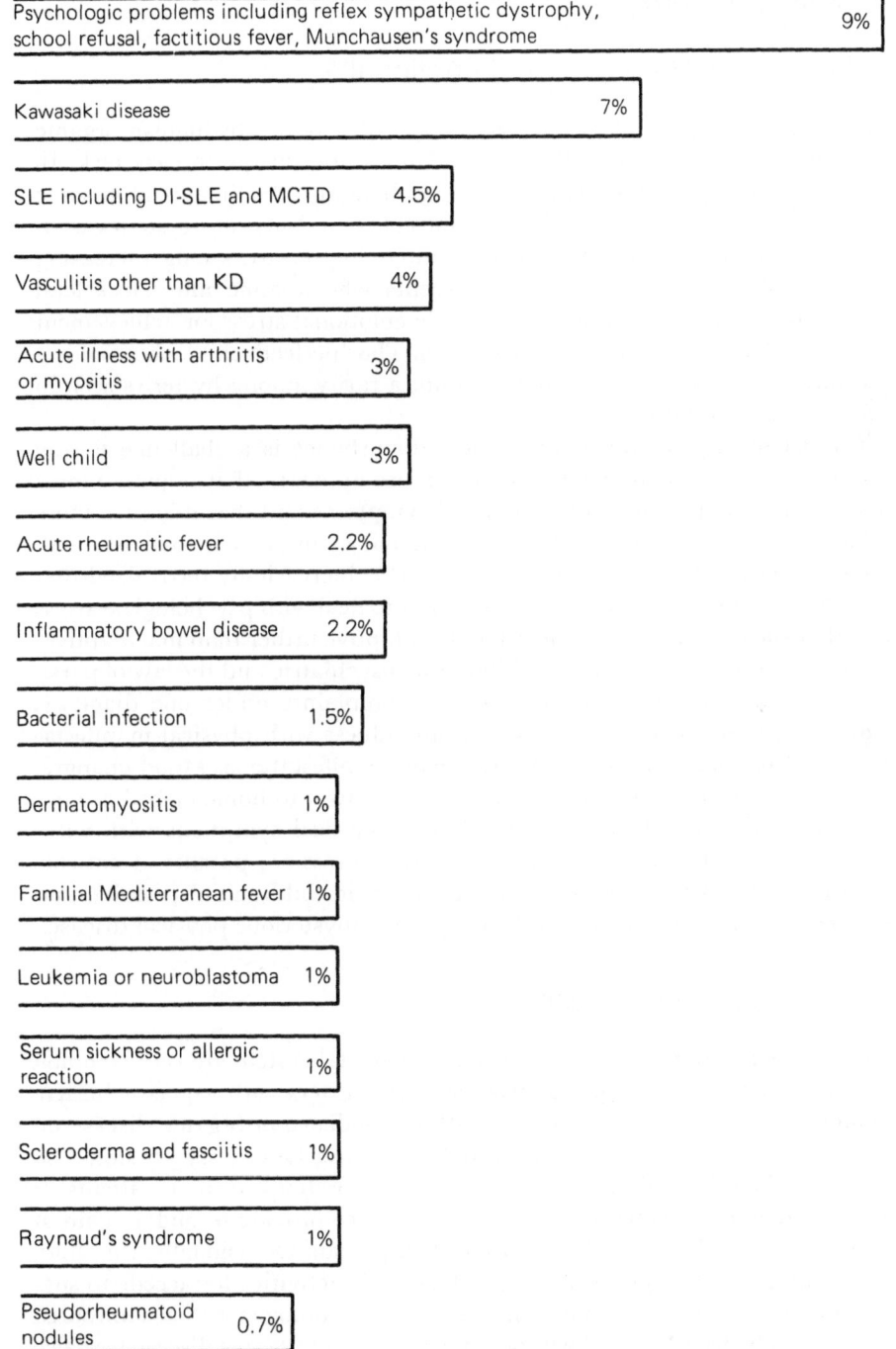

Figure 2.95. Most common diagnoses (other than arthritis) in children referred for rheumatologic consultation. Of those referred, 42% had childhood arthritis and 15% had other less frequent diagnoses than those shown here. (See also Ref. 555).

Psychiatric Disorders

Is the Disease "Organic" or "Functional"?

The pediatric rheumatologist is frequently called on to distinguish organic from functional symptoms (Fig. 2.95). This is not always an easy task. In SLE, behavioral manifestations previously thought to be functional in some cases now seem clearly to be manifestations of central-nervous-system vasculitis. On the other hand, pediatric rheumatologists are seeing increasing numbers of adolescents and preadolescents who assume musculoskeletal symptoms as a defense against unbearable emotional stress for achievement either in schoolwork or on the athletic field. The "perfect" child who couldn't possibly have an emotional problem is not a rarity among hysterics seen in rheumatology practice.

Coexistent organic and psychological disturbance is a challenge to any physician. Yet it has become more and more apparent that organic illness does not protect patients from emotional symptoms and that it is even more difficult to evaluate and deal with emotional symptoms in patients with known physical illness. At the same time, it is increasingly recognized that the sick may use the sickness they know best to deal with psychological stress and that such use may even sometimes be adaptive rather than maladaptive.

Fear of misdiagnosis of physical illness as psychiatric and the law of parsimony that subsumes all of the patient's complaints under one diagnosis cause diagnostic error in both psychogenic illness with physical manifestations and physical illness with psychogenic manifestations. Mood changes, loss of interest in normal activities, and withdrawal to home or bed are not symptoms of physical illness. Unexplained physical symptoms with withdrawal and mood change are diagnostic of depression; parents of patients with these manifestations do not recognize their children's depression and routinely ascribe these behavioral changes to a mysterious physical disease.

Psychogenic Rheumatism

Conversion reactions involving the musculoskeletal system are very common in children.[556–559] Every pediatrician sees youngsters with vague or bizarre complaints of musculoskeletal pain without evidence of organic disease on physical examination and with normal x-ray and laboratory studies. "La belle indifference" and absent gag are common findings in these patients. If the pain does not succeed in excusing disability or provide secondary gain, it usually is easily dealt with by the primary physician. Occasionally, the child, the family, and their physicians limit the child's activities (or accede to suggestion or demand for limitations), and the rheumatologist is then confronted with a totally disabled child without any evidence of organic disease (see also Chapter 1, Evaluation of the Functional State of the Child).

When disability exceeds visible evidence of organic disease, the child must be directed back to full activities. When resistance is met from the child or family, psychiatric help is needed. Repeated studies have demonstrated that long school absence for any reason forebodes a poor prognosis for later achievement in life.[560]

When one keeps constantly in mind the regular school attendance of our most severely crippled children with rheumatoid arthritis, dermatomyositis, and scleroderma, children who are using musculoskeletal pain for school or life avoidance are easily recognized. We find it best to identify two separate problems in our discussions with these families: (1) the problem of the child's complaints: we acknowledge the possibility that some organic process may exist despite our inability to document such a process at this time. Of course, we hope that no bad disease does exist; and (2) the emotional problem, which is self-evident: the withdrawal from normal activities appropriate for the child. It is crucial to emphasize that the complaints do not warrant or excuse the withdrawal since children with much greater objective evidence of disease have not withdrawn from the same activities. Thus, the child must be directed back to the normal activities immediately, and if the child does not resume normal activities, it is for psychiatric rather than medical reasons. The physician must be sympathetic but must assume a confident and firm stance.

These severe disabilities do not occur in a vacuum. Most parents today are committed to as normal a life-style as possible even for their crippled children and understand the benefits of such a philosophy for the child. Therefore, when disability greatly exceeds objective evidence of disease, the parents have played a role in its creation, and one can anticipate resistance from them in the physician's attempts at rehabilitation.[561] Mothers obsessed with obtaining medical care for nonexistent illness in their children have been termed "doctor addicts."

It is easier to prevent these situations than to treat them. Prevention requires that the physician have an orientation to full function without restrictions. There is no place for limiting activities of children with chronic musculoskeletal complaints. The physician's role is to promote, not restrict, function; to enable crippled children to have as full a life as possible; and to not contribute to the crippling, either physical or emotional.

Fibrositis/Fibromyalgia/Tension Myalgia

Some physicians have labeled patients who complain of diffuse musculosketel aches, pains, and stiffness with point tenderness in a number of areas but without any other signs, symptoms, or laboratory evidence of any disease as having what they term tension myalgia, fibrositis, or fibromyalgia.[562–564] All published series emphasize disturbed (nonrestorative) sleep, fatigue, headaches, irritable bowels, paresthesias, and numbness as frequent associated complaints. Reduction in stress and antidepressive medications are said to provide modest relief in adults. The long-term prognosis is for continued symptoms although remissions may occur. This disorder is not a prodroma of rheumatic disease, and while adults with well-defined rheumatic diseases may have similar complaints, my experience with thousands of arthritic children suggests that these symptoms are not noted in children with arthritis.

We do not make the diagnosis of fibrositis/fibromyalgia tension myalgia syndrome; Hadler[565,566] defines our approach: (1) "explain to patients that we do not understand the pathophysiology of their complaints," (2) "reassurance," and (3) "redress psychologic stresses," which to us means identifying the factors which are involved and teaching the family/child to deal with them in a way which avoids the need for conversion into musculoskeletal and other physical symptoms and minimizes the importance of symptoms in the absence of evidence of organic disease.

Reflex Sympathetic Dystrophy

Hysterical edema (reflex sympathetic [neurovascular] dystrophy) is not rare in childhood but is almost never recognized by the pediatrician.[567,568] The important diagnostic clue is that the child suddenly assumes a bizarre immobile posture of a hand or foot that is soon accompanied by diffuse juxta-articular swelling and continuous burning pain (causalgia) that is greatly intensified by light touch. The swelling is often accompanied by color and temperature (trophic) changes either from spasm of vessels or from dilatation (Table 2.37). Uniquely, the child refuses to move the hand or foot, although, obviously, muscular effort is required to maintain the bizarre posture (Fig. 2.96). Anyone can reproduce the syndrome by partially flexing all the joints of the hand and then forcing the muscles into spasm as in a fixed claw. I recommend that the reader try this right now and notice how quickly numbness and tingling and color changes appear. Imagine the pain associated with maintaining such a posture for a long period of time!

There has been considerable argument over the etiology and pathogenesis of this syndrome. While in rare instances reflex sympathetic dystrophy may be an unusual response to a minor injury (a "contused nerve"), most affected children have no history of trauma. Occasionally, however, trauma or even localized abnormalities accompanied by pain such as arthritis may have hysterical edema superimposed as a result of the child holding the hand or foot immobile.

Table 2.37. Early Signs of Reflex Sympathetic Dystrophy

Bizarre spastic posture of a hand or foot with refusal to move the extremity
Diffuse, puzzling swelling and vasomotor changes
Continuous burning pain greatly intensified by light touch and associated with numbness and tingling

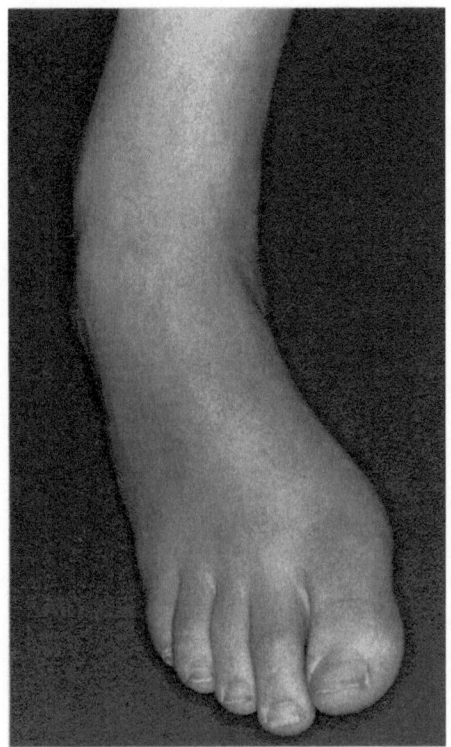

Figure 2.96. Foot held in bizarre spastic posture typical of reflex sympathetic dystrophy. The foot was edematous, cold, and suffused.

Reasonable diagnostic studies are often unavoidable except in very early cases and help to reassure both the physician and the family.

It is important to remember, however, that after a period of time, x-rays will show patchy demineralization (Sudeck's atrophy) and that Doppler studies and technetium and gallium scans may reflect the excessive autonomic activity and increased or decreased blood flow (Fig. 2.97).[569] It is important not to misinterpret these findings as indicative of other disorders. Repeated investigations by inexperienced physicians who are made anxious by the bizarre and incomprehensible symptoms may reinforce the child's disordered function and foster prolonged and intractable illness. Prompt, confident diagnosis fosters easy management and prevents harmful treatments and procedures that may result in permanent disability.

Psychopathogenesis. Sherry and Weisman[570] provide new insights into the psychopathogenesis of this disorder; as in other series, 83% of their patients were girls. Although half had difficulties with school, they were also very frequently involved in a wide variety of extracurricular activities. In our recent experience, this most frequently involves sports, with many patients "female jocks"—members of several competitive teams. "All were extremely

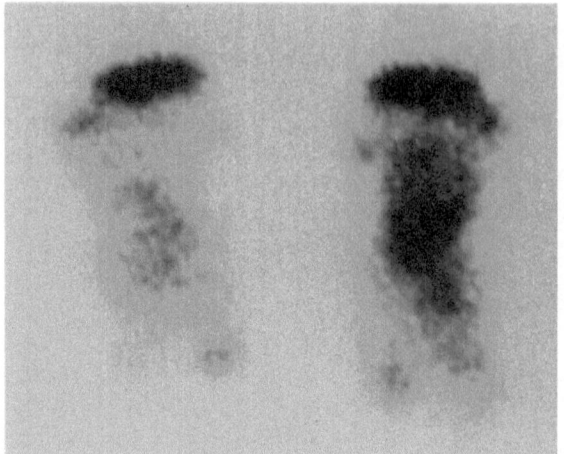

A

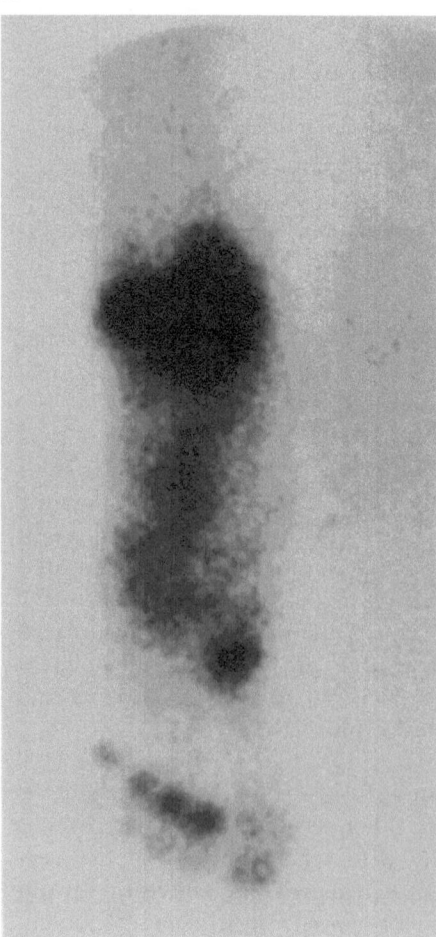

Figure 2.97. Bone scans in two patients with reflex neurovascular dystrophy. Patient 1 (**A**) had decreased uptake in the left foot due to disuse. Patient 2 (**B**) had increased uptake due to neurovascular effects. Either pattern may be seen.

B

compliant and had difficulty expressing their own needs." In every case, there was "inappropriate closeness and involvement of the child" in the parents' affairs and of the parents in the child's decision-making, or what should have been the child's decision-making. This family "enmeshment" usually involved mother and daughter, and this unusual compliance of the child with the achieving mother's sometimes covert (vicarious) goals was put to good use by physiotherapists who observed that the girls performed their exercises with fewer complaints than those with rheumatic disease. This finding is not so surprising, because once the need for the symptom is removed, exercise relieves the pain in this syndrome.

Other important observations in this study include recognition that the symptom is a conscious or unconscious effort to relieve stress by, in our experience, avoiding the activities the child cannot verbalize she simply cannot participate in any longer. These are often cited by both child and parent as the ones she "loves" and cannot live without. The syndrome "offered a way for the children to be less responsible for their families and have attention focused back on themselves." The symptoms provide an opportunity for regression and give the children back "the nurturing and freedom from responsibility that normally accompanies childhood." The children and their parents deal better with physical handicap as an excuse for nonperformance than with recognition and acceptance that one could "just say no." Recurrent attacks occurred when family pressures again mounted and the child perceived the need to be "caretaker, mediator, or super-child," and could be relieved by helping the child find "alternate ways of relieving stress" and providing support for the role of childhood.

Treatment. Familiarity with the disorder and having a dynamic, well-organized treatment plan in mind are essential (Table 2.38). Simple discussion of family psychodynamics and secondary gain often provide prompt insight into the function of the symptom in the family's psychic economy. An ordinary relaxed conversation about what was going on when the symptom appeared and what was supposed to happen that couldn't because of this disability often leads to an understanding of its development and an opportunity to manipulate the environment to at least temporarily remove the necessity for the symptom.

Table 2.38. Treatment of Reflex Sympathetic Dystrophy

Assure child and family that the "mysterious" symptom is understood and is readily amenable to treatment.

Demonstrate the neurovascular disturbance created by holding the hand in a bizarre posture associated with muscle spasm.

Prohibit the acitivity that the symptom guards against.

Provide physical therapy, reassurance, and repetitive exercise.

Psychotherapy is required for patients who are not fully functional within 3 days.

Any form of immobilization is contraindicated. Physiotherapy aimed at encouraging motion is of undisputed benefit and is sometimes enhanced with related modalities. We demonstrate to the patient and parents how immobility with muscle spasm creates the pain and symptoms, having them create the symptom in their own hands. We then gently massage the extremity and begin motion, showing how motion relieves pain and swelling and trophic changes. The great pain created by this posturing is acknowledged, and guilt and embarrassment are avoided. We emphasize that the problem is relatively common (at least in a pediatric rheumatologist's practice) and is the body's way of dealing with an unreasonable demand being made upon it, a demand that we will prohibit so that the symptom can go away.

Although many cases are just this simple and are relieved with 1 h or 2 of experienced evaluation and discussion, once the symptom has become "fixed" for a long period of time, more formal psychotherapy may be required. We had one unusual patient who held his neck to one side for a year despite a multitude of hospitalizations and many psychotherapeutic sessions.[571,572] However, in most cases, hospitalization is not needed; we specify that hospitalization and psychiatric evaluation will be required if the youngster is unable to resume normal activities within 3 days.

In our experience the prognosis is good except for long-standing cases with prolonged school absence. However, mild recurrences at times of stress are not uncommon.

Chronic Fatigue Syndrome

Patients with persistent or recurrent fatigue, sleep disturbances, lymphodenopathy, sore throat, and inability to concentrate or remember or go to school or work, all without objective evidence of disease or with disability far in excess of objective signs, often prefer antiviral treatment for chronic Epstein-Barr (EB) virus or chronic enterovirus infection to having to face up to and deal more satisfactorily with their life situations.[573] Serologic tests for these disorders, briefly popular, have not stood the test of time.[574,575] Magnesium is the latest treatment.[576]

Munchausen's Syndrome and Factitious Fever

Most psychiatrically determined musculoskeletal illness may be classified as malingering (conscious and volitional, sometimes factitious), or hysterical (nonvolitional and unconscious), or a combination of these mechanisms.[560,577,578] Occasionally, illness may be self-inflicted; this rare syndrome was named for Baron von Munchausen, who was famous for telling tall tales.[579] Pediatricians may also be confronted with parentally inflicted bizarre illness, a form of child abuse termed Munchausen's syndrome by proxy.[358,580,581] These cases are more common than has been recognized.[578] The difficulty of diagnosis is illustrated by a report of a teenager who repetitively injected fecal material into her joints.[579] That patient had 23 hospitalizations and 13 major surgical procedures before the diagnosis was confirmed by finding the syringe with a feculent suspension among her possessions. A high index of suspicion is necessary to make this diagnosis, but physicians must overcome their reluctance to consider self-inflicted illness or child abuse in patients with repetitive bizarre manifestations; 4–9% of all prolonged, unexplained fever in childhood is factitious (Table 3.5).

References

1. Schumacher HR Jr, Klippel JH, Robinson DR: Primer on the Rheumatic Diseases, 9th ed. Arthritis Foundation, Atlanta, GA, 1988, pp. 1–355.
2. Markowitz M, Gordis L: Rheumatic Fever, 2nd ed. Saunders, Philadelphia, 1972.
3. Pope RM: Rheumatic fever in the 1980's. Bull Rheum Dis 38:1–8, 1989.
4. Griffiths SP, Gersony WM: Acute rheumatic fever in New York City (1969 to 1988): A comparative study of two decades. J Pediatr 116:882–887, 1990.
5. Zangwill KM, Wald ER, Londino AV Jr.: Acute rheumatic fever in western Pennsylvania: A persistent problem into the 1990's. J Pediatr 118:561–563, 1991.
6. Wallace MR, Garst PD, Papadimos TJ, Oldifeld EC III: The return of acute rheumatic fever in young adults. JAMA 262:2557–2561, 1989.
7. Hicks R, Yim G: Post-Streptococcal Reactive Arthritis (PSRA)—A Manifestation of Acute Rheumatic Fever (ARF). Arthritis Rheum 33:S145, 1990.
8. Kusala GA, Doshi H, Brick JE: Rheumatic fever and post-streptococcal glomerulonephritis: A case report. Arthritis Rheum 32:236–239, 1989.
9. Raz I, Fisher J, Israeli A, et al.: An unusual case of rheumatic pneumonia. Arch Intern Med 145:1130–1131, 1985.
10. De Cunto CL, Giannini EH, Fink CW, et al.: Prognosis of children with post-streptococcal reactive arthritis. Pediatr Infect Dis J 7:683–686, 1988.
11. Wilson MG: Rheumatic Fever. The Commonwealth Fund, New York, 1940.
12. Crea MA, Mortimer EA Jr: The nature of scarlatinal arthritis. Pediatrics 23:879–884, 1959.
13. Austin III HA, Balow JE, Henoch-Schonlein Nephritis: Prognostic features and the challenge of therapy. Am J Kid Dis 2:512–520, 1983.
13a. Olson JC, Kelly KJ, Pan CG, Wortmann DW. Pulmonary disease with hemorrhage in Henoch-Schonlein purpura. Pediatrics 89:1177–1181, 1992.
14. Stewart M, Savage JM, Bell B, McCord B: Long term renal prognosis of Henoch-Schonlein purpura in an unselected childhood population. Eur J Pediatr 147:113–115, 1988.
15. Blomgren SE: Erythema nodosum. Semin Arthritis Rheum 4:1–24, 1974.
16. Spear JB, Kessler HA, Dworin A, Semel J: Erythema Nodosum Associated with Acute Cytomegalovirus Mononucleosis in an adult. Arch Intern Med 148:323–324, 1988.
17. Weston WL, Brice SL, Jester JD, Lane AT, et al.: Herpes Simplex virus in childhood erythema multiforme. Pediatrics 89:32–4, 1992.
18. Kunnamo I, Kallio P, Pelkonen P, Viander M: Serum-sickness-like disease is a

common cause of acute arthritis in children. Acta Paediatr Scand 75:964–967, 1986.

18a. Heckbert SR, Stryker WS, Coltin KL, et al.: Serum sickness in children after antibiotic exposure: Estimates of occurrence and morbidity in a health maintenance organization population. Am J Epidemiol 132:336–342, 1990.

19. Rasmussen JE: Update on the Stevens-Johnson syndrome. Clev Clin J Med 55:412–413, 1988 (see also pp. 467–469).

20. Levy M, Shear NH: *Mycoplasma pneumoniae* infections and Stevens-Johnson syndrome. Report of eight cases and review of the literature. Clin Ped 30:42–49, 1991.

21. Prendiville JS, Herbert AA, Greenwald MJ, Esterly NB: Management of Stevens-Johnson syndrome and toxic epidermal necrolysis in children. J Pediatr 155:881–887, 1989.

22. Gern JE, Yang E, Evrard HM, Sampson HA: Allergic reactions to milk-contaminated "nondairy" products. N Eng J Med 324:976–979, 1991.

22a. Olson JC, Esterly NB: Urticarial vasculitis and Lyme disease. J Am Acad Dermatol 22:1114–1116, 1990.

22b. Massarotti EM, Liu NY, Mier J, Atkins MB. Chronic inflammatory arthritis after treatment with high-dose Interleukin-2 for malignancy. Am J Med 92:693–697, 1992.

23. Braverman IM: Skin Signs of Systemic Disease. Saunders, Philadelphia, 1981, pp. 444–452.

24. Longley J, Demar L, Feinstein RP, et al.: Clinical and histologic features of pityriasis lichenoides et varioliformis acuta in children. Arch Dermatol 123:1335–1339, 1987.

25. Baron F, Sybert VP, Andrews RG: Cutaneous and extracutaneous neutrophilic infiltrates (Sweet Syndrome) in three patients with Fanconi anemia. J Pediatr 115:726–729, 1989.

26. Moreland LW, Brick JE, Kovach RE, et al.: Acute febrile neutrophilic dermatosis (Sweet Syndrome): A review of the literature with emphasis on muscloskeletal manifestations. Semin Arthritis Rheum 17, 3:143–155, 1988.

27. Jorizzo JL, Solomon AR, Zanolli MD, Leshin B: Neutrophilic vascular reactions. J Am Acad Dermatol 19:983–1005, 1988.

28. Majeed HA, Kalaawi M, Mohanty D, et al.: Congenital dyserythropoietic anemia and chronic recurrent multifocal osteomyelitis in three related children. J Pediatr 115:730–734, 1989.

29. Yu L, Kasser JR, O'Rourke E, et al.: Chronic Recurrent Multifocal Osteomyelitis. J Bone Jt Surg 71-A:105–112, 1989.

30. Cho KH, Shin KS, Sohn SJ: Behcet's disease with Sweet's syndrome-like presentation—A report of six cases. Clin Exp Dermatol 14:20–24, 1989.

31. Webb JG, Butany J, Langer G, et al.: Myocarditis and myocardial hemorrhage associated with thrombotic thrombocytopenic purpura. Arch Intern Med 150:1535–1537, 1990.

32. Onundarson PT, Rowe JM, Heal JM, Francis CW. Response to plasma exchange and splenectomy in thrombotic thrombocytopenic purpura. Arch Int Med 152:791–796, 1992.

33. Bell WR, Braine HG, Ness PM, Kickler TS: Improved survival in thrombotic thrombocytopenic purpura-hemolytic uremic syndrome. Clinical Experience in 108 Patients. N Eng J Med 325:398–403, 1991. (See also: Editorial pp. 426–427).

34. Jacobs JC: Acute osteomyelitis; medical management in children NY State J Med 78:910–912, 1978.
35. Shulman, ST, Ayoub EM: Severe staphylococcal sepsis in adolescents. Pediatrics 58:59–66, 1976.
36. Hieber JP, Nelson AJ, McCracken GH: Acute disseminated staphylococcal disease in childhood. Am J Dis Child 131:181–185, 1977.
37. Dich VD, Nelson JD, Haltalin KC: Osteomyelitis in infants and children. Am J Dis Child 129:1273–1278, 1975.
38. Edwards MS, Baker CJ, Granberry WM, Barrent FF: Pelvic osteomyelitis in children Pediatrics 61:63–67, 1978.
39. Nolla-Solé JM, Mateo-Soria L, Rozadilla-Sacanell A, et al.: Role of technetium-99m diphosphonate and gallium-67 citrate bone scanning in the early diagnosis of infectious spondylodiscitis. A comparative study. Ann Rheum Dis 51:665–667, 1992.
40. Lisbona R, Rosenthall L: Observations on the sequential use of ^{99m}Tc-phosphate complex and ^{67}Ga imaging in osteomyelitis, cellulitis, and septic arthritis. Radiology 123:123–129, 1977.
41. Sullivan DC, Rosenfield NS, Ogden J, et al.: Problems in the scintigraphic detection of osteomyelitis in children. Radiology 135:731–736, 1980.
42. Handmaker H: Acute hematogenous osteomyelitis: Has the bone scan betrayed us? Radiology 135:787–789, 1980.
43. Fleisher GR, Paradise JE, Plotkin SA, et al.: Falsely normal radiouclide scans for osteomyelitis. Am J Dis Child 134:499–502, 1980.
44. Tetzlaff TR, McCracken GH, Nelson, JD: Oral antibiotic therapy for skeletal infections of children. II. Therapy of osteomyelitis and suppurative arthritis. J Pediatr 92:485–490, 1978.
45. Nelson JD: A critical review of the role of oral antibiotics in the management of hematogenous osteomyelitis. In: Remington JS, Swartz MN (eds.) Current Clinical Topics in infectious diseases 4. McGraw-Hill, New York, pp. 64–74, 1983.
46. Blockey, NJ, Watson JT: Acute osteomyelitis in children. J Bone Joint Surg 52B:77–87, 1970.
47. Kolyvas E, Ahronheim IG, Marks MI, et al.: Oral antibiotic therapy of skeletal infections in children. Pediatrics 65:867–871, 1980.
48. Dangles CJ: Two unusual presentations of pyogenic sacroiliitis. Orthopaedic Review 16:77–80, 1987.
49. Schaad UB, McCracken GH, Nelson JD: Pyogenic arthritis of the sacroiliac joint in pediatric patients. Pediatrics 66:375–379, 1980.
50. Reilly JP, Gross RH, Emans JB, et al.: Disorders of the sacroiliac joint in children J Bone Joint Surg 70A:31–40, 1988.
51. Milgrom C, Kaplan L, Fields S, et al.: Osteolytic osteogenic sarcoma of ilium in a 46 month old boy. Ortho Rev 16:187–189, 1987.
52. Cabanela ME, Sim FH, Beabour JW, Dahlin DC: Osteomyelitis appearing as neoplasms; a diagnostic problem. Arch Surg 109:68–72, 1974.
53. Fisher MC, Goldsmith JF, Gilligan PH: Sneakers as a source of Pseudomonas aeruginosa in children with osteomyelitis following puncture wounds. J Pediatr 106:607–609, 1985.
54. Congeni BL, Weiner DS, Izsak E: Expanded spectrum of organisms causing osteomyelitis after puncture wounds of the foot. Orthopedics 4:531–533, 1981.
55. Harrison CJ, Kiely L, Fowler SL: Puncture wounds of the foot. Pediatr Res

25S:180A, 1989.

56. Subbarao EK, Tarpay MM, Marks MI: Soft-tissue infections caused by Myco-bacterium fortuitum complex following penetrating injury. Am J Dis Child 141:1018–1020, 1987.

57. Wadlington WB, Hatcher H, Turner DJ: Osteomyelitis of the patella. Clin Pediatr 10:577–580, 1971.

58. Ho G, Tice AD, Kaplan SR: Septic bursitis in the prepatellar and olecranon bursae. Ann Int Med 89:21–27, 1978.

59. Raddatz DA, Hoffman GS, Franck WA: Septic Bursitis: Presentation, treat-ment and prognosis. J Rheumatol 14:1160–1163, 1987.

60. Pien FD, Ching D, Kim E: Septic Bursitis: Experience in a community practice. Orthopedics 14:981–984, 1991.

61. March AW, Riley LH, Robinson RA: Retroperitoneal abscess and septic arthri-tis of the hip in children. J Bone Joint Surg 54A:67–74, 1972.

62. Maull KI, Sachatello CR: Retroperitional iliac fossa abscess; a complication of suppurative iliac lymphadenitis. Am J Surg 127:270–274, 1974.

63. Stefanich RJ, Moskowitz A: Hip flexion deformity secondary to acute pyogenic psoas abscess. Orthopaed Rev 16:25–35, 1987.

64. Korobkin M, Callen PW, Filly RA, et al.: Comparison of computed tomogra-phy, ultrasonography, and gallium-67 scanning in the evaluation of suspected abdominal masses. Radiology 129:89–93, 1978.

65. Taylor KJW, Sullivan DC, Wasson JFM, et al.: Ultrasound and gallium for the diagnosis of abdominal and pelvic abscesses. Gastrointest Radiol 3:281–286, 1978.

66. Sirinavin S, McCracken GH Jr.: Primary suppurative myositis in children. Am J Dis Child 133:263–265, 1979.

67. Beavers BR: Fusobacterium Nucleatum Pyomyositis. Orthopedics 15:208–211, 1992.

68. Minor RL, Baum S, Schulze-Delrieu KS: Pyomyositis in a patient with progres-sive systemic sclerosis: case report and review of the literature. Arch Intern Med 148:1453–1455, 1988.

69. Yuh WTC, Schreiber AE, Montgomery WJ, Ehara S: Magnetic resonance im-aging of pyomyositis. Skeletal Radiol 17:190–193, 1988.

70. Swarts RL, Martinez LA, Robson HG: Gonococcal pyomyositis. JAMA 246:246, 1981.

70a. Fleckenstein JL, Burns DK, Murphy FK, et al. Differential diagnosis of bac-terial myositis in AIDS: evaluation with MR imaging. Radiology 179:653–658, 1992.

71. Rotbart HA, Glode MP: Haemophilus influenzae type b septic arthritis in chil-dren: Report of 23 cases. Pediatrics 75:254–259, 1985.

72. Taylor TKF, Bye WA: Role of antibiotics in inflammatory disc lesions in chil-dren. Lancet 2:881–882, 1977.

73. Fischer GW, Popich GA, Sullivan DE, et al.: Diskitis: A prospective diagnostic analysis. Pediatrics 62:543–548, 1978.

74. Bolivar R, Kohl S, Pickering LK: Vertebral osteomyelitis in children: Report of four cases. Pediatrics 62:549–553, 1978.

75. Wenger DR, Bobechko WP, Gilday DL: The spectrum of intervertebral disc-space infection in children. J Bone Joint Surg 60A:100–108, 1979.

76. Waldvogel FA, Vasey H: Osteomyelitis: The past decade. N Engl J Med 303:360–370, 1980.

77. Boscamp JR, Steigbigel NH: Disk space infection. In: Orthopedic infection, Schlossberg D (ed.) Springer-Verlag, New York, pp. 49–68, 1988.

78. Meyers SP, Wiener SN: Diagnosis of hematogenous pyogenic vertebral osteomyelitis by Magnetic Resonance Imaging. Arch Intern Med 151:683–687, 1991.

79. Bjorksten B, Gustavson KH, Eriksson B, et al.: Chronic recurrent multifocal osteomyelitis and pustular palmoplantaris. J Pediatr 93:227–231, 1978.

80. Van Howe RS, Starshak RJ, Chusid MJ: Chronic, recurrent multifocal osteomyelitis. Case report and review of the literature. Clin Pediatr 28:54–59, 1989.

81. Mortensson W, Edeburn G, Fires M, Nilsson R: Chronic recurrent multifocal osteomyelitis in children. A roentgenologic and scintigraphic investigation. Acta Radiol 29:565–570, 1988.

82. Yu L, Kasser JR, O'Rourke E, et al.: Chronic recurrent multifocal osteomyelitis. J Bone Jt Surg 71-A:105–112, 1989.

83. Berney S, Goldstein M, Bishko F: Clinical and diagnostic features of tuberculous arthritis. Am J Med 53:36–42, 1972.

84. Wallace R, Cohen AS: Tuberculous arthritis. Am J Med 61:277–282, 1976.

85. Sutker WL, Lankford LL, Tompsett R: Granulomatous synovitis: The role of atypical mycobacteria. Rev Infect Dis 1:729–735, 1979.

86. Jacobs, JC, Phillips PE, Johnston AD, Needle biopsy of the synovium of children. Pediatrics 57:696–701, 1976.

87. Southwood RT, Hancock EJ, Petty RE, et. al: Tuberculous rheumatism (Poncet's disease) in a child. Arthritis Rheum 31:1311–1313, 1988.

88. Arnow PM, Smaron M, Ormiste V: Brucellosis in a group of travelers to Spain. JAMA 251:505–508, 1984.

89. Lubani M, Sharda D, Helin I: Brucella arthritis in children. Infection 14:233–236, 1986.

90. Lubani MM, Dudin KI, Sharda DC, et al.: A multicenter therapeutic study of 1100 children with brucellosis. Pediatr Infect Dis J 8:75–78, 1989.

91. Diggs LW: Bone and joint lesions in sickle-cell disease. Clin Orthop 52:119–143, 1967.

92. Collipp PJ, Koch R: Cat scratch fever associated with an osteolytic lesion. N Engl J Med 260:278–280, 1959.

93. Margileth AM, Wear DJ, English CK: Systemic cat scratch disease: Report of 23 patients with prolonged or recurrent severe bacterial infection. J Infect Dis 155:390–402, 1987.

94. Rizkallah MF, Meyer L, Ayour EM: Hepatic and splenic abscesses in cat-scratch disease. Pediatr Infect Dis 7:191–195, 1986.

94a. Case records of the Massachusetts General Hospital. Case 22-1992. NEJM 326:1480–1489, 1992.

95. Bogue CW, Wise JD, Gray GF, Edwards KM: Antibiotic therapy for Cat-scratch disease? JAMA 262:813–816, 1989.

96. Holley HP Jr.: Successful treatment of Cat-scratch disease with ciprofloxacin. JAMA 265:1563–1565, 1991.

97. Nelson JD: The bacterial etiology and antibiotic management of septic arthritis in infants and children. Pediatrics 50:437–440, 1972.

98. Goldenberg DL, Cohen AS: Acute infectious arthritis Am J Med 60:369–377, 1976.

99. Barton LL, Dunkie LM, Habib FH: Septic arthritis in childhood: A 13 year

review, Am J Dis Child 141:898–900, 1987.

100. Chusid MJ, Jacobs WM, Sty JR: Pseudomonas arthritis following puncture wounds of the foot. J Pediatr 94:429–431, 1979.

101. Nelson JD, Howard JB, Shelton S: Oral antibiotic therapy for skeletal infections of children. I. Antibiotic concentrations in suppurative synovial fluid. J Pediatr 92:131–134, 1978.

102. Bryson YJ, Connor JD, LeClere M, et al.: High-dose oral dicloxacillin treatment of acute staphylococcal osteomyelitis in children. J Pediatr 94:673–675, 1979.

102a. Jafari h, Friedland I, Ehrett S et al. Effects of dexamethasone and anti-CD18 antibodies on *H. Influenzae* Type B induced joint destruction. Pediatr Res 31 (#4, Pt.2):165A, 1992.

103. Rush PJ, Shore A, Inman R, et al.: Arthritis associated with Haemophilus influenzae meningitis: Septic or Reactive? J Pediatr 109:412–415, 1986.

104. Likitnukui S, McCracken GH, Nelson JD: Arthritis in children with bacterial meningitis. Am J Dis Child 140:424–427, 1986.

105. Goldenberg DL: Infectious arthritis complicating rheumatoid arthritis and other chronic rheumatic disorders. Arthritis Rheum 32:4596–4502, 1989.

106. Britigan BE, Cohen MS, Sparling PF: Gonococcal infection: A model of molecular pathogenesis. N Eng J Med 312:1683–1694, 1985.

107. Hook EW III, Holmes KK: Gonococcal infections. Ann Intern Med 102:229–243, 1985.

108. Kerr JM, LeBlanc W, Heagarty MC: Genitourinary Gonorrhea Presenting as Mild Arthritis. Clin Pediatr 30:388–389, 1991.

109. Leibel RL, Fangman JJ, Ostrovsky MC: Chronic meningococcemia in childhood. Am J Dis Child 127:94–98, 1974.

110. Rosen MS, Myers AR, Dickey B: Meningococcemia presenting as septic arthritis, pericarditis, and tenosynovitis. Arthritis Rheum 28:576–578, 1985.

111. Schaad UB: Arthritis in disease due to Neisseria meningitidis. Rev Infect Dis 2:880–887, 1980.

112. Reginato AJ, Ferreiro JL, O'Connor CR, et al.: Clinical and pathologic studies of twenty-six patients with penetrating foreign body injury to the joints, bursae, and tendon sheaths. Arthritis Rheum 33:1753–1762, 1990.

113. Kelly JJ: Blackthorn inflammation. J Bone Joint Surg 48B:474–477, 1966.

114. Sugarman M, Stobie DG, Quismorio FP, et al.: Plant thorn synovitis. Arthritis Rheum 20:1125–1128, 1977.

115. Barton LL, Saied KR: Thorn-induced arthritis. J Pediatr 93:322–323, 1978.

116. Kleiman MB, Elfenbein DS, Wolf EL, et al.: Periosteal reaction due to foreign body induced inflammation of soft tissue. Pediatrics 60:638–641, 1978.

117. Swischuk LE, Jorgenson F, Jorgenson A, et al.: Wooden splinter induced "pseudotumors" and "osteomyelitis-like lesions" of bone and soft tissues. Am J Roentgenol Radium Ther Nucl Med 122:176–179, 1974.

118. O'Connor CR, Reginato AJ, Delong WG: Foreign body reactions simulating acute septic arthritis. J Rheumatol 15:1568–1571, 1988.

119. Cuellar ML, Silveira LH, Espinoza LR: Fungal arthritis. Ann Rheum Dis 51:690–697, 1992.

120. Bayer AS, Choi C, Tillman D, et al.: Fungal arthritis I: *Candida*. Semin Arthritis Rheum 8:142–150, 1978 (see also 8:200–211; 9:66–74, 145–151; 10:218–227).

121. Katzenstein D: Isolated Candidia arthritis: report of a case and definition of a distinct clinical syndrome. Arthritis Rheum 28:1421–1424, 1985.

122. Rosenthal J, Brandt KD, Wheat LJ, Slama TG: Rheumatologic manifestations

of histoplasmosis in the recent Indianapolis epidemic. Arthritis Rheum 26:1065–1070, 1983.

123. Kafka JA, Catanzaro A: Disseminated coccidiodomycosis in children. J Pediatr 98:355–361, 1981.

124. Bocanegra T, Espinoza LR, Bridgeford P et al.: Reactive arthritis induced by parasitic infection. Ann Int Med 94:207–209, 1981.

125. Zaki MH: Selected tickborne infections: A review of Lyme disease, Rocky Mountain spotted fever, and babesiosis. NYS J Med 89:320–335 1989.

125a. Krause PJ, Telford SR III, Pollack RJ, et al. Babesiosis: An underdiagnosed disease of children. Pediatrics 89:1045–1948, 1992.

126. Gunasekaran TS, Hassall E: Giardiasis mimicking inflammatory bowel disease. J Pediatr 120:424–426, 1992.

127. Lakhanpal S, Cohen SB, Fleischmann RM: Reactive arthritis from Blastocystis hominis. Arthritis Rheum 34:251–253, 1991.

128. Shaw RA, Stevens MB: The reactive arthritis of giardiasis: A case Report, JAMA 258:2734–2735, 1987.

129. Borella L, Goobar JE, Clark GM: Synovitis of the knee joints in late congenital syphilis. JAMA 180:190–192, 1962.

130. Chapel TA: Physician recognition of the signs and symptoms of secondary syphilis. JAMA 246:250–251, 1981.

131. Reginato AJ, Schumacher HR, Jiminez S, et al.: Synovitis in secondary syphilis. Arthritis Rheum 22:170–176, 1979.

132. Gould K: Clinical recognition of leptospirosis. Intern Med 2:51–58, 1981.

133. Raffin BJ, Freemark M: Streptobacillary rat-bite fever: A pediatric problem. Pediatrics 64:214–217, 1979.

134. Shanson DC, Gazzard BG, Midgley J, et al. Streptobaccilus moniliformis isolated from blood in four cases of Haverhill Fever. Lancet 2:92–94, 1983.

135. Madden, M: Polyarthritis due to rate bite fever. IM:16–19, 1991.

136. Gordon SC, Lauter CB: Mumps arthritis: unusual presentation as adult Still's disease. Ann Intern Med 97:45–47, 1982.

137. Cwajgenbaum M, Azem I, Weisbrod M, et al.: Arthritis in chickenpox. Am J Dis Child 140:502, 1986.

138. Roberts-Thomson PJ, Ahern MJ, Southwood TR, et al.: Adult onset Still's disease or Coxsackie polyarthritis? Aust NZ J Med 16:509–511, 1986.

139. Hawkes RA, Boughton CR, Naim HM, Stallman ND: A major outbreak of epidemic polyarthritis in New South Wales during the summer of 1983/1984. Med J Aust 143:330–333, 1985.

140. Remafedi G, Muldoon RL: Acute monarticular arthritis caused by Herpes Simplex Virus Type 1. Pediatrics 72:882–883, 1983.

141. Sigal LH, Steere AC, Niederman JC: Symmetric polyarthritis associated with heterophile-negative infectious mononucleosis. Arthritis Rheum 26:553–556, 1983.

142. Ray CG, Gall EP, Minnich LL, et al.: Acute polyarthritis associated with active Epstein-Barr virus infection. JAMA 248:2990–2994, 1982.

143. Marshall GS, Starr SE, Witzleben CL, et al.: Protracted mononucleosis-like illness associated with acquired cytomegalovirus infection in a previously healthy child: Transient cellular immune defects and chronic hepatopathy. Pediatrics 87:556–562, 1991.

144. Petty RE, Tingle AJ: Arthritis and viral infection. J Pediatr 113:948–949, 1985.

145. Phillips PE: Evidence implicating infectious agents in rheumatoid arthritis and juvenile rheumatoid arthritis. Clin Exp Rheumatol 6:87–94, 1988.

146. Vaughan JH: Infection and Rheumatic Diseases: A Review. Bulletin on the Rheumatic Diseases 39: #1 & 2, 1990; Arthritis Foundation.
147. Chantler JK, Tingle AJ, Petty RE: Persistant rubella virus infection associated with chronic arthritis in children. N Eng J Med 313:1117–1123, 1985.
148. Niklasson B, Espmark A: Ockelbo disease: Arthralgia 3–4 years after infection with a sindbis virus related agent. Lancet 1:1039–1040, 1986.
149. Fraser JRE, Cunningham AL, Hayes K, et al.: Rubella arthritis in adults. Isolation of virus, cytology and other aspects of the synovial reaction. Clin Exp Rheumatol 1:287–293, 1983.
150. Spruance SL, Metcalf R, Smith CB, et al.: Chronic arthropathy associated with rubella vaccination. Arthritis Rheum 20:741–747, 1977.
151. Jacobs, JC: Childhood arthritis following rubella booster immunizations: Is arthritis more frequent in immune individuals? Pediatr Res. 29(#4.Pt2):175A, 1991.
152. Utsinger PD: Immunopathogenesis of chronic post-rubella vaccination arthritis. Arthritis Rheum 22:667–668, 1979.
153. Grahame R, Armstrong R, Simmons N, et al.: Chronic arthritis associated with the presence of intrasynovial rubella virus. Ann Rheum Dis 42:2–13, 1983.
154. Wands JR, Mann E, Alpert E, et al.: The pathogenesis of arthritis associated with acute hepatitis-B surface antigen-positive hepatitis. Complement activation and characterization of circulating immune complexes. J Clin Invest 55:930–936, 1975.
155. Perrillo RP, Pohl DA, Roodman ST, et al.: Acute non-A, non-B hepatitis with serum-sickness-like syndrome and aplastic anemia. JAMA 245:494–496, 1981.
156. Dan M, Yaniv R: Cholestatic hepatitis, cutaneous vasculitis, and vascular deposits of immunoglobulin M and complement associated with hepatitis A virus infection. Am J Med 89:103–104, 1990.
157. Woolf AD, Campion GV, Chishick A, et al.: Clinical manifestation of human parvovirus B19 in adults. Arch Intern Med 149:1153–1156, 1989.
158. Naides SJ, Scharosch LL, Foto F, Howard EJ: Rheumatologic manifestations of human parvovirus B19 infection in adults. Initial two-year clinical experience. Arthritis Rheum 33:1297–1309, 1990.
158a. Nocton JJ, Miller LC, Tucker LB, Schaller JG. Human parvovirus B19 arthritis in children. Pediatr Res 31(#4,Pt.2):172A, 1992.
159. Bruchoff SE, Woda BA, Pihan GA, et al.: Parvovirus B19-Associated hemophagocytic syndrome. Arch Intern Med 150:897–899, 1990.
160. Dinerman JL, Corman LC: Human parvovirus B19 arthropathy associated with desquamation. Am J Med 89:826–828, 1990.
161. Finkel TH, Gelfand EW, Harbeck R, et al.: Chronic parvovirus infection presenting as juvenile polyarteritis nodosum. Arthritis Rheum 33:S132, 1990.
162. Kaplan MM: The spectrum of chronic active liver disease. Hosp Practice pp. 67–75, October 1983.
163. Vergani D, Larcher VF, Davies ET, et al.: Genetically determined low C4: a predisposing factor to autoimmune chronic active hepatitis. Lancet 2:294–297, 1985.
164. Fitz JG, Petri M, Hellmann D: Chronic active hepatitis presenting with rheumatoid nodules and arthritis. J Rheumatol 14:595–598, 1987.
165. Maggiore G, Porta G, Bernard O, et al.: Autoimmune hepatitis with initial presentation as acute hepatic failure in young children. J Pediatr 116:280–282, 1990.

166. Ponka A: Arthritis associated with *Mycoplasma pneumoniae* infection. Scand J Rheum 8:27–32, 1979.
167. Davis CP, Cochran S, Lisse J, et al.: Isolation of Mycoplasma pneumoniae from synovial fluid samples in a patient with pneumonia and polyarthritis. Arch Intern Med 148:969–970, 1988.
168. Bhopal RS, Thomas GO: Psittacosis presenting with Reiter's syndrome. Br Med J 284:1606, 1982.
169. Helmick CG, Bernard KW, D'Angelo LJ: Rocky Mountain spotted fever: Clinical, laboratory, and epidemiological features of 262 cases. J Infect Dis 150:480–488, 1984.
170. Massarotti EM, Luger SW, Rahn DW et al. Treatment of early Lyme disease. Am J Med 92:396–403, 1992.
171. Steere AC: Lyme disease. N Eng J Med 321:566–596, 1989.
172. White DJ, Chang Hwa-Gan, Benach JL, et al.: The geographic spread and temporal increase of the Lyme disease epidemic. JAMA 266:1230–1236, 1991.
173. Alpert B, Esin J, Sivak SL, Wormser GP: Incidence and prevalence of Lyme Disease in a suburban Westchester County community. NYS J Med 92:5–8, 1992. (See also: Editorial pp 2–4)
174. Williams CL, Strobino B, Lee A, et al.: Lyme disease in childhood: clinical epidemiologic features of ninety cases. Pediatr Infect Dis J 9:10–14, 1990.
175. Eichenfield AH, Goldsmith DP, Benach JL, et al.: Childhood Lyme arthritis in an endemic area. J Pediatr 109:753–758, 1986.
176. Benach JL, Bosler EM: Lyme disease and related disorders. Ann NY Acad Sci 539:1–150, 1988.
177. Piesman J, Mather TN, Sinskey RJ, Spielman A: Duration of tick attachment and Borrelia burgdorferi transmission. J Clin Microbiol 25:557–558, 1987.
178. Nadelman RB, Pavia CS, Magnarelli LA, Wormser GP: Isolation of Borrella burgdorferi from the blood of seven patients with Lyme disease. Am J Med 88:21–26, 1990.
179. Johnston YE, Duray PH, Steere AC, et al.: Lyme arthrtis: Spirochetes found in synovial microangiopathic lesions. Am J Pathol 118:26–34, 1985.
180. Jacobs JC, Stevens M, Duray PH: Lyme disease simulating septic arthritis. JAMA 256:1138–1139, 1986.
181. Kay J, Eichenfield AH, Atheya BH, et al.: Synovial fluid eosinophilia in Lyme disease. Arthritis Rheum 31:1384–1389, 1988.
182. Farris BK, Webb RM: Lyme disease and optic neuritis. J Clin Neuro-ophthalmol 8:73–78, 1988.
183. Meier C, Grahmann F, Englehardt, Dumas M: Peripheral nerve disorders in Lyme-Borreliosis: Nerve biopsy studies from eight cases. Acta Neuropathol 79:271–278, 1989.
184. May EF, Jabbari B: Stroke in Neuroborreliosis. Stroke 21:1232–1235, 1990.
185. Pachner AR, Duray P, Steere AC: Central nervous system manifestations of Lyme disease. Arch Neurol 46:790–795, 1989.
186. Feder HM, Zalneraitis EL, Reik L Jr: Lyme disease: acute focal mening-oencephalitis in a child. Pediatrics 82:931–934, 1988.
186a. Luft BJ, Steinman CR, Neimark HC et al. Invasion of the central nervous system by borrelia burgdorferi in acute disseminated infection. JAMA 267:1364–1367, 1992.
187. Logigian EL, Kaplan RF, Steere AC: Chronic neurologic manifestations of Lyme disease. N Eng J Med 323:1438–1444, 1990.

188. Jacobs JC, Rosen JM, Szer IS: Lyme myocarditis diagnosed by gallium scan. J Pediatr 105:950–952, 1984.

189. Rienzo RJ, Morel DE, Prager D, et al.: Gallium avid Lyme myocarditis. Clin Nucl Med 12:475–476, 1987.

190. Olson LJ, Okafor EC, Clements IP: Cardiac involvement in Lyme disease: Manifestations and management. Mayo Clin Proc 61:745–749, 1986.

191. Marcus LC, Steere AC, Duray PH, et al.: Fatal pancarditis in a patient with coexistent Lyme disease and babesiosis: demonstration of spirochetes in the myocardium. Ann Intern Med 103:374–376, 1985.

192. Reznick JW, Braunstein DB, Walsh RL, et al.: Lyme carditis: electrophysiologic and histopathologic study. Am J Med 81:923–927, 1986.

193. Stanek G, Klein J, Bittner R, Glogar D: Isolation of Borrelia burgdorferi from the mycardium of a patient with longstanding cardiomyopathy. N Eng J Med 322:249–252, 1990.

194. Kishaba RG, Weinhouse E, Chusid MJ, Nudel DB: Lyme disease presenting as heart block. Clin Pediatr 27:291–293, 1988.

195. McAlister HF, Klementowicz PT, Andrews C, et al.: Lyme carditis: an important cause of reversible heart block. Ann Intern Med 110:339–345, 1989.

196. van der Linde MR, Crijns JGM, de Koning J, et al.: Range of atrioventricular conduction distrubances in Lyme borreliosis: A report of four cases and review of other published reports. Br Heart J 63:162–168, 1990.

197. Kimball SA, Janson PA, LaRaia PJ: Complete heart block as the sole presentation of Lyme disease. Arch Intern Med 149:1897–1898, 1989.

198. Baylac-Domengetroy F, Vieyres C, Barraine R: Complete heart block as the sole presentation of Lyme disease. Arch Intern Med 151:1240, 1991.

199. Artigao R, Torres G, Guerrero A, et al.: Irreversible complete heart block in Lyme disease. Am J Med 90:531–533, 1991.

200. Atlas E, Novak SN, Duray PH, Steere AC: Lyme myositis: muscle invasion by Borrelia burgdorferi. Ann Intern Med 103:245–246, 1988.

201. Reimers CD, Pongratz DE, Neubert U, et al.: Myositis caused by Borrelia burgdorferi: report of four cases. J Neurol Sci 91:215–226, 1989.

202. Szer IS, Taylor E, Steere AC: The clinical course and long-term follow-up of children with lyme arthritis. N Eng J Med 325:159–163, 1991.

203. Logigian EL, Kaplan RF, Steere AC: Chronic neurologic manifestations of Lyme disease. N Eng J Med 323:1438–1444, 1990.

204. Arnett FC: The Lyme spirochete: another cause of Reiter's syndrome? Arthritis Rheum 32:1182–1184, 1989.

205. Kaell AT, Volkman DJ, Gorevic PD, Dattwyler RJ: Positive Lyme serology in subacute bacterial endocarditis. A study of four patients. JAMA 2916–2918, 1990.

205a. Feder HM Jr, Shapiro ED, Gerber MA, Hunt M: Common problems in the diagnosis and management of Lyme disease. Pediatr Res 31(#4,Pt.2):122A, 1992.

206. Gerber MA, Shapiro ED: Diagnosis of Lyme disease in children. J Pediatr 121:157–162, 1992.

207. Schutzer SS, Coyle PK, Belman AL, et al.: Sequestration of antibody to Borrelia burgdorferi in immune complexes in serongegative Lyme disease. Lancet 1:312–315, 1990.

208. Hardin JA, Steere AC, Malawista SE: Immune complexes and the evolution of Lyme arthritis N Engl J Med 301:1358–1363, 1979.

209. Hedberg CW, Osterholm MT: Serologic tests for antibody to Borrelia burgdorferi: Another Pandora's box for medicine? Arch Intern Med 150:732–733, 1990.

210. Rose CD, Fawcett PT, Singsen BH, et al.: Use of western blot and enzyme-linked immunosorbent assays to assist in the diagnosis of lyme disease. Pediatrics 33:465–70, 1991.

211. Krause A, Brade V, Schoerner C, et al.: T cell proliferation induced by Borrelia burgdorferi in patients with Lyme borreliosis. Arthritis Rheum 34:393–402, 1991.

211a. Salazar J, Gerber M, Goff C. Long-term outcome of children with early Lyme disease. Pediatr Res 31 (#4,Pt.2):178A, 1992.

212. Rahn DW, Malawista SE: Clinical judgment in Lyme disease. Hospital Practice pp. 39–56, March 30, 1990.

213. Sigal LH: Summary of the first 100 patients seen at a Lyme disease referral center. Am J Med 88:577–581, 1990.

214. Cooper JD, Schoen RT: Epidemiology, clinical features, and diagnosis of Lyme disease. Curr Opin Rheum 4:520–528, 1992.

215. Wrenn K: Ceftriazone versus cefuroxime for meningitis in children. N Eng J Med 322:1821, 1990.

216. Snydman DR, Schenkein DP, Berardi VP, et al.: Borrelia burgdorferi in joint fluid in chronic lyme arthritis. Ann Intern Med 104:798–800, 1986.

217. Schoen RT, Aversa JM, Rahn DW, Steere AC: Treatment of refractory chronic lyme arthritis with arthroscopic synovectomy. Arthritis Rheum 34:1056–60, 1991.

218. Steere AC, Dwyer E, Winchester R: Association of chronic Lyme arthritis with HLA-DR2 alleles. N Eng J Med 323:219–223, 1990.

219. Yoshinari NH, Reinhardt BN, Steere AC: T cell responses to polypeptide Fractions of Borrelia burgdorferi in patients with Lyme arthritis. Arthritis Rheum 34:707–713, 1991.

220. Schlesinger PA, Burke BA, Stillman T: Maternal-fetal transmission of the Lyme disease spirochete, Borrelia burgdorferi. Ann Intern Med 103:67–68, 1985.

221. MacDonald AB, Benach JL, Burgodorfer W: Stillbirth following maternal Lyme disease. NYS J Med 87:615–616, 1987.

222. Levo Y, Nashif M: Musculosekeletal manifestations of bacterial endocarditis. Clin Exp Rheumatol 1:49–52, 1983.

223. Pinals RS, Tunnessen WW: Shunt arthritis. J Pediatr 91:681, 1977.

224. ter Bory EJ, Van Rijswijk MH, Kallenberg CGM: Transient arthritis with positive tests for rheumatoid factor as presenting sign of shunt nephritis. Ann Rheum Dis 50:182–183, 1991.

225. Knitzer PH, Needleman BW: Musculoskeletal syndromes associated with acne. Semin Arthritis Rheum 20:247–255, 1991.

226. Rosner IA, Richter DE, Huettner TL, et al.: Spondyloarthropathy associated with hidradenitis suppurative and acne conglobata. Annals Intern Med 97:520–525, 1982.

227. Wands JR, Lamont JT, Mann E, et al.: Arthritis associated with intestinal bypass procedure for morbid obesity. N Engl J Med 294:121–124, 1976.

228. Utsinger PD: Bypass disease: A bacterial antigen-antibody systemic immune complex disease. Arthritis Rheum 23:758, 1980.

229. Jorizzo JL, Apisarnthanarax P, Subrt P, et al.: Bowel-bypass syndrome without bowel bypass. Arch Intern Med 143:457–461, 1983.

230. LeVine ME, Dobbins WO III: Joint changes in Whipple's disease. Semin Arthritis Rheum 3:79–93, 1973.
231. Fleming JL, Wiesner RH, Shorter RG: Whipple's disease: Clinical, biochemical and histopathologic features and assessment of treatment in 29 patients. Mayo Clin Proc 63:539–551, 1988.
232. Southern JF, Moscicki RA, Magro C, et al.: Lymphedema, lymphocytic myocarditis, and sarcoidlike granulomatosis: Manifestations of Whipple's disease. JAMA 261:1467–1470, 1989.
233. MacCarthy J, O'Brien N: Phalangeal microgeodic syndrome of infancy. Arch Dis Child 51:472–474, 1976.
234. Kaibara N, Masuda S, Katsuki I, et al.: Phalangeal microgeodic syndrome in childhood: report of seven cases and review of the literature. Eur J Pediatr 136:41–46, 1981.
235. Winchester R: AIDS and the rheumatic diseases. Bull Rheum Dis (Arthritis Foundation) Vol. 39, No. 5, pp. 1–10, 1990.
236. Nordstrom DM, Petropolis AA, Giorno R, et al.: Inflammatory myopathy and acquired immunodeficiency syndrome. Arthritis Rheum 32:475–479, 1989 (see also correspondence 33:298, 1990).
237. Walter EB, Drucker RP, McKinney RE, Wilfert CM: Myopathy in human immunodeficiency virus-infected children receiving long-term Zidovudine therapy. J Pediatr 119:152–155, 1991.
238. D'Agati V, Seigle R: Coexistence of AIDS and lupus nephritis: a case report. Am J Nephrol 10:243–247, 1990.
239. Sculerati N, Borkowsky W: Pediatric human immunodeficiency virus infection: an otolaryngologist's perspective. J Otolaryngol 19:182–188, 1990.
240. Soberman N, Leonidas JC, Berdon WE, et al.: Sonographic observations of parotid enlargement in 10 HIV positive children. AJR 157:553–556, 1991.
241. Yancey WB Jr, Dolson LH, Oblon D, et al.: HTLV-1-associated adult T-cell leukemia/lymphoma presenting with nodular synovial masses. Am J Med 89:676–683, 1990.
242. Lohr KM: Rheumatic manifestations of diseases associated with substance abuse. Semin Arthritis Rheum 17:90–111, 1987.
243. Kaye BR, Fainstat M: Cerebral vasculitis associated with Cocaine abuse. JAMA 258:2104–2106, 1987.
243a. Daggett RB, Haghighi P, Terkeltaub RA: Nasal cocaine abuse causing an aggressive midline intranasal and pharyngeal destructive process mimicking midline reticulosis and limited Wegener's Granulomatosis. J Rheumatol 17:838–840, 1990.
243b. Lam M, Ballou SP. Reversible scleroderma renal crisis after cocaine use. NEJM 326:1435, 1992.
244. Haueisen DC, Weiner DS, Weiner SD: The characterization of "transient synovitis of the hip" in children. J Pediatr Orthop 6:11–17, 1986.
245. Bickerstaff DR, Neal LM, Brennan PO, Bell MJ: An investigation into etiology of irritable hip. Clin Pediatr 30:353–356, 1991.
246. Lindsley CB. Schaller JG: Arthritis associated with inflammatory bowel disease in children. J Pediatr 84:16–20, 1974.
247. Burbige EJ, Huang SS, Bayless TM: Clinical manifestations of Crohn's disease in children and adolescents. Pediatrics 55:866–871, 1975.
248. Passo MH, Fitzgerald JF, Brandt KD: Arthritis associated with inflammatory bowel disease. Dig Dis Cl 31:492–497, 1986.

249. Orholm M, Munkholm P, Langholz E, et al.: Familial occurrence of inflammatory bowel disease. N Eng J Med 324:84–88, 1991.
250. Heyman MB, Perman JA, Ferrell LD, Thaler MM: Chronic nonspecific inflammatory bowel disease of the cecum and proximal colon in children with grossly normal-appearing colonic mucosa: diagnosis by colonoscopic biopsies. Pediatrics 80:255–261, 1987.
251. Al-Hadidi, Khatib G, Chhatwal P, Khatib R: Granulomatous arthritis in Crohn's disease. Arthritis Rheum 27:1061–1062, 1984.
252. Dver NH, Dawson AM, Verbov JL., et al.: Cutaneous polyarteritis nodosa associated with Crohn's disease. Lancet 1:648–650, 1970.
253. Thompson DG, Lennard-Jones JE, Swarbrick ET, et al.: Pericarditis and inflammatory bowel disease. Q J Med 189:93–97, 1979.
254. Dawes PT, Atherton ST: Coeliac disease presenting as recurrent pericarditis. Lancet 1:1021–1022, 1981.
255. Sohar E, Gafni J, Pras M, Heller H: Familial Mediterranean fever. Am J Med 43:227–253, 1967.
256. Lehman TJA, Peters RS, Hanson V, Schwabe AD: Long-term colchicine therapy of familial Mediterranean fever. J Pediatr 93:876–878, 1978.
257. Majeed HA, Carroll JE, Khuffash FA, Hijazi Z: Long-term colchicine prophylaxis in children with familial Mediterranean fever (recurrent hereditary polyserositis). J Pediatr 116:997–999, 1990.
258. Matzner Y, Ayesh SK, Hochner-Celniker D, et al.: Proposed mechanism of the inflammatory attacks in familial Mediterranean fever. Arch Intern Med 150:1289–1291, 1990.
258a Ozyilkan E, Simsek H, Telatar H. Tumor necrosis factor in familial Mediterranean fever. Am J Med 92:579–580, 1992.
258b Pras E, Aksentijevich I, Gruberg L, et al. Mapping of a gene causing familial Mediterranean fever to the short arm of chromosome 16. NEJM 326:1509–1513, 1992.
259. Majeed HA, Baraket M: Familial Mediterranean fever (recurrent hereditary polyserositis) in children: analysis of 88 cases. Eur J Pediatr 148:636–641, 1989.
260. Zemer D, Pras M, Sohar E, et al.: Colchicine in the prevention and treatment of the amyloidosis of familial Mediterreanean fever. N Eng J Med 314:1001–1005, 1986.
261. Schwabe AD, Monroe JB: Meningitis in familial Mediterranean fever. Am J Med 85:715–717, 1988.
262. Majeed HA, Quabazard Z, Hijazi Z, et al.: The Cutaneous manifestations in children with familial Mediterranean fever (Recurrent hereditary polyserositis). A six-year study. Q J Med 278:607–616, 1990.
263. Heller H, Gafni J, Michaeli D, et al.: The arthritis of familial Mediterranean fever. Arthritis Rheum 9:1–17, 1966.
264. Simon G, Marbach JJ: Familial Mediterranean fever with temporomandibular joint arthritis. Pediatrics 57:801–812, 1976.
265. Lehman TJA, Hanson V, Kornreich H, et al.: HLA-B27 negative sacroilitis: A manifestation of familial Mediterranean fever in childhood. Pediatrics 61:423–426, 1978.
266. Cohen AS: Amyloidosis. Bull Rheum Dis (Arthritis Foundation) 40: No. 2 pp. 1–12, 1991.
267. Bakir F, Murtadha M, Issa N: Amyloidosis and periodic peritonitis (familial Mediterranean fever). West J Med 131:193–195, 1979.

268. Pras M, Gafni J, Jacob ET, et al.: Recent advances in familial Mediterranean fever. In Yearbook of Medicine. Year Book Medical Publishers, pp. 261–270, 1984.

269. Wallace SL: Colchicine. Semin Arthritis Rheum 3:369–381, 1974.

270. Kuncl RW, Duncan G, Watson D, et al. Colchicine myopathy and neuropathy. N Engl J Med 316:1562–1568, 1987.

271. Chang Yi Han: Mechanism of action of colchicine. Arthritis Rheum 18:493–496, 1975.

272. Kilburn HL: Solitary mastocytoma of infancy. Clin Pediatr 13:60–62, 1974.

273. Marshall J, Walker J, Lurie HI, et al.: Solitary mastocytoma and the mastocytoses. S Afr Med J 31:867–876, 1957.

274. Demis DJ: The mastocytosis syndrome: Clinical and biological studies. Ann Intern Med 59:194–206, 1963.

275. Lindsley CB, Miner PB Jr: Seronegative juvenile rheumatoid arthritis and mast cell-associated gastritis. Arthritis Rheum 34:106–109, 1991.

276. Melamed I, Feanny SJ, Sherman PM, Roifman CM: Benefit of Ketotifen in patients with eosinophilic gastroenteritis. Am J Med 90:310–314, 1991.

277. McAdam LP, O'Hanlan MA, Bluestone R, Pearson CM: Relapsing polychondritis. Medicine 55:193–215, 1976.

278. Isaak BL, Liesegang TJ, Michet CJ: Ocular and systemic findings in relapsing polychondritis. Ophthalmology 93:681–689, 1986.

279. O'Hanlon M, McAdam LP, Bluestone R, Pearson CM: The arthropathy of relapsing polychondritis. Arthritis Rheum 19:191–194, 1976.

280. Hashimoto K, Arkin CR, Kang HA: Relapsing polychondritis: An ultrastructural study. Arthritis Rheum 20:91–97, 1977.

281. Arundell FW, Haserick JR: Familial chronic atrophic polychondritis. Arch Dermatol 82:439–440, 1960.

282. Blau EB: Relapsing polychondritis and retropertioneal fibrosis in an 8-year-old boy. Am J Dis Child 130:1149–1152, 1976.

283. Muckle TJ: The 'Muckle-Wells' syndrome. J Dermatol 100:87–92, 1979.

284. Darranco VP, Minor DB, Solomon H: Treatment of relapsing polychondritis with dapsone. Arch Dermatol 112:1286–1288, 1976.

285. Bowness P, Hawley IC, Morris T, et al.: Complete heart block and severe aortic incompetence in relapsing polychondritis: clinicopathologic findings. Arthritis Rheum 34:97–100, 1991.

286. Goldbloom RB, Stein PB, Eisen A, et al.: Idiopathic periosteal hyperostosis with dysproteinemia. A new clinical entity. N Engl J Med 274:873–878, 1966 (see also Goldbloom RB: Commentary. In: Gellis SS (ed.) Yearbook of Pediatrics, Yearbook Medical Pub., Chicago, 1977, p. 308).

287. Cameron BJ, Laxer RM, Wilmot DM, et al.: Idiopathic periosteal hyperostosis with dysproteinema (Goldbloom's syndrome): case report and review of the literature. Arthritis Rheum 30:1307–1312, 1987.

288. Goldsmith DP, Rose CD, Sharrar WC, et al.: Idiopathic multifocal periostitis (IMP)—a rare entity simulating JRA. Arthritis Rheum 33:S89, 1990.

289. Gerscovich EO, Greenspan A, Lehman WB: Idiopathic periosteal hyperostosis with dysproteinemia-Goldbloom's syndrome. Pediatr Radiol 20:208–211, 1990.

290. Ringel RE, Haney PJ, Brenner JI, et al.: Periosteal changes secondary to prostaglandin administration. J Pediatr 103:251–253, 1983.

291. Dupont AG, Verbeelen DL, Six RO: Weber-Christian panniculitis with mem-

branous glomerulonephritis. Am J Med 75:527–528, 1983.

292. Case records of the Massachusetts General Hospital. Case 21-1984. N Eng J Med 310:1374–1381, 1984.

293. Sorenson RU, Abramowsky CR, Stern RC: Ten-year course of early-onset Weber-Christian syndrome with recurrent pneumonia: a suggestion for pathogenesis. Pediatrics 78:115–120, 1986.

294. Lemley DE, Chun B, Cupps TR: Sterile splenic abscesses in systemic Weber-Christian disease. Unique source of abdominal pain. Am J Med 83:567–570, 1987.

295. Buck BE, Yang LC, Caleb MH, et al.: Measles virus panniculitis subsequent to vaccine administration. J Pediatr 101:366–373, 1982.

296. Ilowite, N. Personal Communication.

297. Marhaug G, Havidsten D: Arthritis complicating acute pancreatitis—a rare but important condition to be distinguished from juvenile rheumatoid arthritis. Scand J Rheumatol 17:397–399, 1988.

298. Jakobiec FA, Mottow L: Pediatric orbital pseudotumor. In: Jakobiec FA (ed.) Ocular and Adnexal Tumors. Aesculapius Press, Birmingham, AL, 1978, pp. 644–658.

299. Saul RA, Lee WH, Stevenson RE: Caffey's disease revisited: further evidence for autosomal dominant inheritance with incomplete penetrance. Am J Dis Child 136:56–60, 1982.

300. Heyman E, Laver J, Beer S: Prostaglandin synthetase inhibitor in Caffey disease. (Letter) J Pediatr 101:314, 1982.

301. Parker S, Griffiths HJ: Prostaglandin induced cortical hyperostosis. Orthopedics 13:243–244, 1990.

302. Younge D, Drummond D, Herring J, Cruess RL: Melorheostosis in children: clinical features and natural history. J Bone Joint Surg 61-B:415, 1979.

303. Dimar JR, Campion TS: Melorheostosis: Two case presentations and review of the literature. Orthop Rev 16:615–621, 1987.

304. Abdul-Karim FW, Carter JR, Makley JT, et al.: Intramedullary osteosclerosis. A report of the clinicopathologic features a five cases. Orthopedics 11:1667–1676, 1988.

305. Furia JP, Schwartz HS: Hereditary multiple diaphyseal sclerosis: A tumor simulator. Orthopedics 13:1267–1274, 1990.

306. Hoover DL, Khan JA, Giangiacomo J: Pediatric ocular sarcoidosis. Surv Ophthalmol 30:215–228, 1986.

307. Pattishall EN, Strope GL, Spinola SM, Denny FW: Childhood sarcoidosis. J Pediatr 108:169–177, 1986.

308. Lindsley CB, Godfrey WA: Childhood sarcoidosis manifesting as juvenile rheumatoid arthritis. Pediatrics 76:765–768, 1985.

308a. Sahn EE, Hampton MT, Garen PD, et al.: Preschool sarcoidosis masquerading as juvenile rheumatoid arthritis: Two case reports and a review of the literature. Pediatr Dermatol 7:208–13, 1990.

309. Gross KR, Malleson PN, Culham G, et al.: Vasculopathy with renal artery stenosis in a child with sarcoidosis. J Pediatr 109:387, 1986.

310. Jabs DA, Houk JL, Bias WB, Arnett FC: Familial granulomatous synovitis, uveitis, and cranial neuropathies. Am J Med 78:801–804, 1985.

311. Miller JJ: Early-onset "sarcoidosis" and "familial granulomatous arthritis (arteritis)": The same disease. J Pediatr 109:387, 1986.

312. Pastores GM, Michels VV, Stickler GB, et al.: Autosomal dominant granulomatous arthritis, uveitis, skin rash, and synovial cysts. J Pediatr 117:403–408, 1990.

313. Rose CD, Eichenfield AH, Goldsmith DP, Athreya BH: Early onset sarcoidosis with aortitis—"juvenile systemic granulomatosis?" J Rheumatol 17:102–106, 1990.

313a. Shaikh S, Soubani AO, Rumore P et al.: Lytic osseous destruction in vertebral sarcoidosis. NYS J Med 92:213–218, 1992 (Also see Editorial, pp. 177–178).

314. Simons FER, Schaller JG: Benign rheumatoid nodules. Pediatrics 56:29–33, 1975.

315. Rao NA, Font RL: Pseudorheumatoid nodules of the ocular adnexa. Am J Ophthalmol 79:471–478, 1975.

316. Knigh PJ, Reiner CB: Superficial lumps in children. Pediatrics 72:147–153, 1983.

317. Rush PJ, Bernstein BH, Smith CR, Shore A: Chronic arthritis following benign rheumatoid nodules of childhood. Arthritis Rheum 28:1175–1178, 1985.

318. Kaye BR, Kaye RL, Bobrove A: Rheumatoid nodules: Review of the spectrum of associated conditions and proposal of a new classification, with a report of four seronegative cases. Am J Med 76:279–292, 1984.

319. Jacobs JC: JRA and hyperphosphatasemia. J Pediatr 107:828–829, 1985.

320. Schonau E, Herzog KH, Bohles HJ: Transient hyperphosphatasaemia of infancy. Eur J Pediatr 148:264–266, 1988.

321. Kurzrock R, Cohen PR: Erythromelalgia: Review of clinical characteristics and pathophysiology. Am J Med 91:416–422, 1991 (See also 93:111–114, 1992).

322. Rush PJ, Shore A, Coblentz C, Wilmot D, Corey M, Levison H: The musculoskeletal manifestations of cystic fibrosis. Semin Arthritis Rheum 15:213–225, 1986.

323. Petty RE, Cassidy JT, Heyn R, et al.: Secondary hypertrophic osteoarthropathy. An unusual cause of arthritis in childhood. Arthritis Rheum 19:902–906, 1976.

324. Schaller J: Arthritis as a presenting manifestation of malignancy in children. J Pediatr 81:793–797, 1972.

325. Fink CW, Windmiller J, Sartain P: Arthritis as the presenting feature of childhood leukemia. Arthritis Rheum 15:347–349, 1972.

326. Lopez-Enriquez E, Morales AP, Robert F: Effect of atropine sulfate in pulmonary hypertrophic osteoarthropathy. Arthritis Rheum 23:822–824, 1980.

327. Sagransky DM, Greenwald JD: Seropositive rheumatoid arthritis in a patient with cystic fibrosis. Am J Dis Child 134:318–319, 1980.

328. Schidlow DV, Goldsmith DP, Palmer J, Huang NN: Arthritis in cystic fibrosis. Dis Child 59:377–379, 1984.

329. Dixey J, Redington AN, Butler RC, et al.: The arthropathy of cystic fibrosis. Ann Rheum Dis 47:218–233, 1988.

330. Cohen AM, Yulish BS, Wasser KB, et al.: Evaluation of pulmonary hypertrophic osteoarthropathy in cystic fibrosis. Am J Dis Child 140:74–77, 1986.

331. Maki M, Hallstrom O, Verronen P, et al.: Reticulin antibody, arthritis, and coeliac disease in children. Lancet 1:479–480, 1988.

332. Riely CA: Familial intrahepatic cholestasis: an overview. In: Walker WA, Durie PR, Hamilton JR, et al. (eds.) Pediatric Gastrointestinal Disease. B.C. Decker, Philadelphia, 1990, pp. 1025–1332.

333. Baker DH, Harris RC: Congenital absence of the intrahepatic bile ducts. Am J

Roent 91:875–884, 1964.

334. Rogalsky RJ, Black GB, Reed MH: Orthopaedic manifestations of leukemia in children. J Bone Joint Surg 68A:494–501, 1986.

335. Musiej-Nowakowska E, Rostropowicz-Denisiewicz K: Differential diagnosis of neoplastic and rheumatic diseases in children. Scand J Rheum 15:124–128, 1986.

336. Berkelbach JW, Sprenkel VD, Timmermans AJM, et al.: Polyarthritis as the presenting symptom of a malignant fibrous histiocytoma of the heart. Arthritis Rheum 28:944–947, 1985.

337. Jonsson OG, Sartain P, Ducore JM, Buchanan GR: Bone pain as an initial symptom of childhood acute lymphoblastic leukemia: association with nearly normal hematologic indexes. J Pediatr 117:233–237, 1990.

338. Case records of the Massachusetts General Hospital: Case 14-1986. N Eng J Med 314:973–981, 1986.

339. Ruzal-Shapiro C, Berdon WE, Cohen MD, Abramson SJ: MR imaging of diffuse bone marrow replacement in pediatric patients with cancer. Radiology 181:587–589, 1991.

340. Boumpas DT, Wheby MS, Jaffe ES, et al.: Synovitis in angioimmunoblastic lymphadenopathy with dysproteinemia simulating rheumatoid arthritis. Arthritis Rheum 33:578–582, 1990.

340a. Kaiser BA, Mochon M, Chadarevian, J-P de: Eleven-year-old girl with acute renal failure, arthritis, hyperuricemia, and family history of rheumatic disorders. J Pediatr 121:317–322, 1992.

341. Martinez-Lavin M, Pineda C, Valdez T, et al.: Primary hypertrophic osteoarthropathy. Semin J Arthritis Rheum 17:156–162, 1988.

341a. Cooper RG, Freemont AJ, Riley M, et al.: Bone abnormalities and severe arthritis in pachydermoperiostosis. Ann Rheum Dis 51:416–419, 1992.

342. Rosen PR, Micheli LJ, Treves S: Early scintigraphic disgnosis of bone stress and fractures in athletic adolesecents. Pediatrics 70:11–15, 1982.

343. Engh CA, Robinson RA, Milgram J: Stress fractures in children. Trauma 10:532–541, 1970.

344. Devas M: Stress Fractures. Churchill Livingstone, Edinburgh, 1975.

345. Beals RK, Cook RD: Stress Fractures of the Anterior Tibial Diaphysis. Orthopedics 14:869–875, 1991.

346. Cruess RI: The pathology of acute necrosis of cartilage in slipping of the capital femoral epiphysis. J Bone Joint Surg 45A:1013–1024, 1963.

347. Bleck EE: Idiopathic chondrolysis of the hip. J Bone Joint Surg 65A:1266–1275, 1983.

348. Taillard W, Grasset E: La coxite laminaire juvenile. Revue Chir Orthop 50:159–181. 1964.

349. Bernstein B, Forrester D, Singsen B, King KK, Kornreich H, Hanson V: Hip joint restoration in juvenile rheumatoid arthritis. Arthritis Rheum 20:1099–1104, 1977.

350. Ippolito E, Bellocci, Santori FS, Ghera S: Idiopathic chondrolysis of the hip: An ultrastructural study of the articular cartilage of the femoral head. Orthopedics 9:1383–1387, 1986.

351. Valenzuela F, Aris H, Jacobelli S: Transient osteoporosis of the hip. J Rheum 4:59–64. 1977.

352. Hongladarom T, Anderson DW: Transient painful osteoporosis of the hip. Contemp Orthop 2:148–154, 1980.

352a. Goldenstein-Shainberg, Cossermelli W, Chu L et al. Arthritis as a manifestation of self-mutilation. J Rheum 19:174–176, 1992.

353. Nellhaus G: Neurogenic arthropathies (Charcot's joints) in children. Clin Pediatr 14:647–653, 1975.

354. Dreyfuss JR, Glimcher MJ: Epiphyseal injury following frostbite. N Engl J Med 253:1065–1068, 1955.

355. Carrera GF, Kozin F, McCarty DJ: Arthritis after frostbite injury in children Arthritis Rheum 22:1082–1087, 1979.

356. Brown JP, Rola-Pleszczynski M, Menard H-A: Eosinophilic synovitis: clinical observations on a newly recognized subset of patients with dermatographism. Arthritis Rheum 29:1147–1151, 1986.

357. Campbell AN, Freedman MH, McClure PD: Autoerythrocyte sensitization. J Pediatr 103:157–160, 1983.

358. Clark GD, Key JD, Rutherford P, Bithoney WG: Munchausen's syndrome by proxy (child abuse) presenting as apparent autoerythrocyte sensitization syndrome: An unusual presentation of Polle syndrome. Pediatrics 74:1100–1102, 1984.

359. Sugai S, Yasuda Y, Shimizu S, et al.: DNA autosensitivity in two Japanese sisters. Arthritis Rheum 33:287–292, 1990.

360. Ficat RP, Arlet J, Hungerford DS (eds.) Ischemia and Necrosis of Bone. Williams & Wilkins, Baltimore, 1980, pp. 1–196.

361. Roy DR: Perthes-like changes caused by acquired hypothyroidism. Orthopedics 14:901–904, 1991.

362. Editorial: Perthe's disease. Lancet 1:895–896, 1986.

363. Lowe TG: Scheuermann Disease. J Bone Joint Surg 72A:940–945, 1990.

364. Siemsen JK, Brook J, Meister L: Lupus erythematosus and avascular bone necrosis. Arthritis Rheum 5:492–501, 1962.

365. Fisher DE, Bickel WH: Corticosteroid-induced avascular necrosis. J Bone Joint Surg 53A:813–859, 1971.

366. Editorial: crackling joints. Lancet 2:649, 1971.

367. Chondromalacia patellae. Lancet 1:558–559, 1985.

368. Bourne MH, Hazel WA Jr, Scott SG, Sim FH: Anterior knee pain. Mayo Clin Proc 63:482–491, 1988.

369. Arcoman JP, Kamhi E, Karas S, Moriarty VJ: Transchondral fracture and osteochonditis dessicans of talas. NYS J Med 78:2183–2189, 1978.

370. Robinson RP, Franck WA, Carey EJ, Goldberg EB: Familial polyarticular osteochondritis dessicans masquerading as JRA. J Rheum 5:190–194, 1978.

370a. Ledwith CA, Fleisher GR: Slipped capital femoral epiphysis without hip pain leads to missed diagnosis, Pediatrics 89:660–662, 1992.

371. Knowlton RG, Katzenstein PL, Moskowitz RW, et al.: Genetic linkage of a osteoarthritis associated with mild chondrodyplasia. N Eng J Med 322:526–530, 1990.

372. Brink SJ: Limited joint mobility as a risk factor for complications in youngsters with insulin-dependent diabetes mellitus. In: Pediatric and Adolescent Diabetes Mellitus. Chicago, Year Book, 1987, pp. 305–312.

373. Kapoor A, Sibbitt WL: Contractures in diabetes millitus: The syndrome of limited joint mobility. Semin Arthritis Rheum 18:168–180, 1989.

374. Sherry DD, Rothstein RRL, Petty RE: Joint contractures preceding insulin-dependent diabetes mellitus. Arthritis Rheum 25:1362–1364, 1982.

375. Costello PB, Tambar PK, Green FA: The prevalence and possible prognostic importance of arthropathy in childhood diabetes. J Rheumatol 11:62–65, 1984.
376. Rosenbloom AL, Silverstein JH, Lezotte DC, et al.: Limited joint mobility in childhood diabetes mellitus indicates increased risk for microvascular disease. N Engl J Med 305:191–194, 1981 (see also editorial, pp. 217–219).
377. Rudolf MJC, Genel M, Tamborlane WV, et al.: Juvenile rheumatoid arthritis in children with diabetes mellitus. J Pediatr 99:519–524, 1981.
378. Avioli LV, Krane SM: Metabolic Bone Disease. Vols. 1 and 2. Academic Press, New York, 1978.
379. Brenton DP, Dent CE: Idiopathic juvenile osteoporosis. In: Bickel H, Stern J (eds.) Inborn Errors of Calcium and Bone Metabolism University Park Press, Baltimore, 1976, pp. 222–238.
380. Smith R: Idiopathic juvenile osteoporosis. Am J Dis Child 133:889–891, 1979.
381. Teotia M, Teotia SPS, Singh RK: Idiopathic juvenile osteoporosis. Am J Dis Child 133:894–900, 1979.
382. Hoekman K, Papapoulos SE, Peters ACB, et al.: Characteristics and biphosphonate treatment of a patient with juvenile osteoporosis. J Clin Endocrinol Metab 61:952–956, 1985.
383. Marder HK, Tsang RC, Hug G, Crawford AC: Calcitriol deficiency in idiopathic juvenile osteoporosis. Am J Dis Child 136:914–917, 1982.
384. Cornelis F, Bardin T, Faller B, et al.; Rheumatic syndromes and β_2 microglobulid amyloidosis in patients receiving long-term peritioneal dialysis. Arthritis Rheum 32:785–788, 1989.
385. Bywaters EGL, Dixon ASTJ, Scott JT: Joint lesions of hyperparathyroidism. Ann Rheum Dis 22:171–187, 1963.
386. Hunt PA, Wu-Chen ML, Handal NJ, et al.: Bone disease induced by anticonvulsant therapy and treatment with calcitriol (1,25-dihydroxyvitamin D3) Am J Dis Child 140:715–718, 1986.
387. Siris ES, Clemens TL, Dempster DW, et al.: Tumor-induced osteomalacia. Kinetics of calcium, phosphorus, and vitamin D metabolism and characteristics of bone histomorphometry. Am J Med 82:307–312, 1987.
388. Pollack JA, Schiller AL, Crawford JD: Rickets and myopathy cured by removal of a non-ossifying fibroma of bone. Pediatrics 52:364–371, 1973.
389. Ryan EA, Reiss E: Oncogenous osteomalacia: review of the world literature of 42 cases and report of two new cases. Am J Med 77:501–512, 1984.
390. Asnes RS, Berdon WE, Bassett CA: Hypophosphatemic rickets in an adolescent cured by excision of a non-ossifying fibroma. Clin Pediatr 20:646–648, 1981.
391. Carey DE, Drezner MK, Hamdan JA, et al.: Hypophosphatemic rickets/osteomalacia in linear sebaceous nevus syndrome: A variant of tumor induced osteomalacia. J Pediatr 109:944–1000, 1986.
392. Silverton SF, Hadded JG: Medical reversal of acquired hypophosphatemic osteomalacia. Am J Med 82:1077–1081, 1987.
393. Bland JH, Frymoyer JW: Rheumatic syndromes of myxedema. N Engl J Med 282:1171–1173, 1970.
394. Hunter T, Chalmers IM, Dube WJ, et al.: Episodic polyarthralgia associated with Hashimoto's thryroiditis. Arthritis Rheum 31:303, 1988.
395. LeRiche NGH, Bell DA; Hashimoto's thyroiditis and polyarthritis: A possible subset of seronegative polyarthritis. Ann Rheum Dis 43:594–598, 1984.
396. Farbman K, Wheeler MF, Glick SR: Arthritis induced by antithyroid medica-

tion. NY State J Med 69:826–831, 1969.

397. Thomas J, Collipp PJ, Sharma RK: Thyroid acropachy. Am J Dis Child 125:745–746, 1973.

398. Kingsley GH, Hickling P: Polyarthropathy associated with Cushing disease. Br Med J 292:1363, 1986.

399. Calabrese, LH, White, CS: Musculoskeletal manifestations of Addison's disease. Arthritis Rheum 22:558, 1979.

400. Levy EN, Ramsey-Goldman R, Kahl LE: Adrenal insufficiency in two women with anticardiolipin antibodies. Cause and Effect? Arthritis Rheum 33:1842–1846, 1990.

401. Pittsley RA, Yoder FW: Retinoid hyperostosis: skeletal toxicity associated with long-term administration of 13-cis-Retinoic acid for refractory ichthyosis. N Eng J Med 308:1012–1017, 1983 (see also editorial pp. 1024–1025).

402. Lippe B, Hensen L, Mendoza G, et al.: Chronic vitamin A intoxication. Am J Dis Child 125:634–636, 1981.

403. DiGiovanna JJ, Helfgott RK, Gerber LH, Peck GL: Extraspinal tendon and ligament calcification associated with long-term therapy with etretinate. N Eng J Med 315:1177–1182, 1986.

404. James MB, Leonard JC, Fraser JJ, Stuemky JH: Hypervitaminosis A: A Case Report. Pediatrics 69:112–115, 1982.

405. Teotia M, Teotia SPS, Kunwar KB: Endemic skeletal fluorosis. Arch Dis Child 46:686–691, 1971.

406. Bhussry BR, et al.: Toxic effects of larger doses of fluoride. in: Fluorides and Human Health. World Health Organization, Geneva, 1970, pp. 225–271.

407. Waldbott GL: Fluoride intoxication. JAMA 244:331, 1980.

408. Christie DP: The spectrum of radiographic bone changes in children with fluorosis. Radiology 136:85–90, 1980.

409. Fisher RL: Medcalf TW, Henderson MC: Endemic fluorosis with spinal cord compression. A case report and review. Arch Intern Med 149:697–700, 1989.

410. Mason JO: A message to health professionals about fluorosis. JAMA 265:2939, 1991.

411. Shapiro JR, Fallat RW, Tsang RC: Achilles tendinitis and tenosynovitis: a diagnostic manifestation of familial type II hyperlipoproteinemia in children. Am J Dis Child 128:486–490, 1974.

412. Buckingham RB, Bde GG, Bassett DR: Polyarthritis associated with type IV hyper-lipoproteinemia. Arch Intern Med 135:286-290, 1975.

413. Bjorkhem I, Skrede S: Familial diseases with more storage of sterols than cholesterol: cerebrotendinous xanthomatosis and phytosterolemia. In Scriver CR, Beaudet AL, Sly WS, Valle D (eds.) The Metabolic Basis of Inherited Disease, 6th ed. McGraw-Hill, 1989, pp. 724–730.

414. Belamarich PF, Deckelbaum RJ, Starc TJ, et al.: Response to diet and cholestyramine in a boy with sitosterolemia. Pediatrics 86:977–981, 1990.

415. Stapleton FB, Nyhan WL, Borden M, Kaufman IA: Renal pathogenesis of familial hyperuricemia: studies in two kindreds. Pediatr Res 15:1447–1453, 1981.

416. Middlemiss JH, Braband H: Juvenile gout. Clin Radiol 13:149–152, 1962.

417. Decker JL, Vandeman PR: Renal calculi preceding gouty arthritis in a child. Am J Med 32:805–810, 1962.

418. Vora S: Isozymes of phosphofructokinase. Isozymes: current topics in biological

and medical research. 6:119–167, 1982.

419. Liberman UA, Samuel R, Halabe A, el al.: Juvenile metabolic gout caused by chronic compensated hemolytic syndrome. Arthritis Rheum 25:1264–1266, 1982.

420. Harlan WR, Cornoni-Huntley J, Leaverton PE: Physiologic determinants of serum urate levels in adolescence. Pediatrics 63:569–575, 1979.

421. Boss GR, Seegmiller JE: Hyperuricemia and gout: Classification, complications and management. N Engl Med 300:1459–1468, 1979.

422. Kelley WN: Hyperuricemia. In Kelley WN, Harris ED Jr, Ruddy S, Sledge CB (eds.) Textbook of Rheumatology. Saunders, Philadelphia, 1989, pp. 1395–1436.

423. Rosenblatt D, Homes LB: Development of arthritis in Lowe's syndrome. J Pediatr 85:924–925, 1974.

424. Athreya BH, Schumacher HR, Getz HD, et al.: Arthropathy of Lowe's (oculocerebrorenal) syndrome. Arthritis Rheum 26:728–736, 1983.

425. Kaplan P, Kitschner M, Watters G, Costa MT: Contractures in patients with Williams syndrome. Pediatrics 84:895–899, 1989.

426. Bensen WG, Laskin CA, Little HA, et al.: Hemochromatoric arthropathy mimicking rheumatoid arthritis. Arthritis Rheum 21:844–848, 1978.

427. Goldschmidt H, Spiera H, Schumacher HR, Zaroulis CG: Idiopathic hemochromatosis presenting as amenorrhea and arthritis. Am J Med 82:1057–1059, 1987.

428. Kidd KK: Genetic linkage and hemochromatosis. New Engl J Med 301:209–210, 1979.

429. Nesterov AI: The clinical course of Kashin-Beck disease. Arthritis Rheum 7:29–40, 1964.

430. Takamori T: Kaschin-Beck's disease. The Professor Tokio Takamori Foundation, Gifu University School of Medicine, Japan, 1968 (2 vols).

431. Sokoloff L: The history of Kashin-Beck disease. NYS J Med 89:343–351, 1989.

432. Mseleni Joint Disease. Editorial. Lancet 2:483–484, 1985.

433. Reginato AJ: Articular chondrocalcinosis in the Chiloe Islanders. Arthritis Rheum 19:395–404, 1976.

434. Mirahmadi KS, Coburn JW, Bluestone R: Calcific periarthritis and hemodialysis. JAMA 223:548–549, 1973.

435. Diggs LW: Bone and joint lesions in sickle cell disease. Clin Orthop 52:119–143, 1976.

436. Duthie RB, Rizza CR: Rheumatologic manifestations of the hemophilias. Clin Rheum Dis 1:53–93, 1975.

437. Johnson CR, Corrigan JJ, Gall EP: Treatment of hemophilia arthritis with D-penicillamine. Arthritis Rheum 33:S111, 1990.

438. Klofkorn RW, Lightsey AL: Hemarthrosis associated with Glanzmann's thrombastenia. Arthritis Rheum 22:1390–1393, 1979.

439. Wilfert CM, Buckley RH, Mohanakumar T, et al.: Persistent and fatal central nervous system echovirus infections in patients with agammaglobulinemia. N Engl J Med 296:1485–1489, 1977.

440. Ammann AJ, Wara DW, Pillarisetty RJ, Talal N: The prevalence of autoantibodies in T-cell, B-cell, and phagocytic immunodeficiency disorders. Clin Immunol Immunopathol 14:456–466, 1979.

441. Fraser KJ, Clarris BJ, Muirden KD, et al.: A persistent adenovirus type 1

infection in synovial tissue from an immunodeficient patient with chronic, rheumatoid-like polyarthritis. Arthritis Rheum 28:455–458, 1985.

442. Case records of the Massachusetts General Hospital: Case 34-1988. N Eng J Med 319:495–509, 1988.

443. Cassidy JT, Petty RE, Sullivan DB: Occurrence of selective IgA deficiency in children with JRA. Arthritis Rheum 20:181–183, 1977.

444. Pelkonen P, Savilahti E, Makela A-L: Persistent and transient IgA deficiency in juvenile rheumatoid arthritis. Scand J Rheumatol 12:273–279, 1983.

445. Levitt D, Cooper M: Immunoregulatory defects in a family with selective IgA deficiency. J Pediatr 98:52–58, 1981.

446. Schopfer K, Feldges A, Baerlocher K, et al.: Systemic lupus erythematosus in Staphylococcus aureus hyperimmunoglobulinemia E syndrome. Br Med J 287:524–526, 1983.

447. Rodney GE, Park BH, Ford D, et al.: Defective bactericidal activity of peripheral blood leukocytes in lipochrome histiocytosis. Am J Med 49:322–327, 1970.

448. Schaller JG: Arthritis and immunodeficiency. Arthritis Rheum 20:443–445, 1979.

449. Manzi S, Urbach AH, McCune AB, et al.: Systemic lupus erythematosus in a boy with chronic granulomatosus disease: case report and review of the literature. Arthritis Rheum 34:101–105, 1991.

450. Jacobs JC, Goetzl EJ: "Streaking leukocyte factor," arthritis and pyoderma gangrenosum. Pediatrics 56:570–578, 1975.

451. Abu-Elmagd K, Jegasothy BV, Ackerman CD, et al.: Efficacy of FK 506 in the treatment of recalcitrant pyoderma gangrenosum. Transplant Proc 23:3328–3329, 1991.

451a. Elgart G, Stover P, Larson K et al. Treatment of pyoderma gangrenosum with cyclosporine: Results in seven patients. J Am Acad Dermatol 24:83–86, 1991.

452. Jacobs JC: Hypergammaglobulinemic purpura in a child. J Pediatr 87:91–93, 1975.

453. Ferreiro JE, Pasarin G, Quesada R, Gould E: Benign hypergammaglobulinemic purpura of Waldenstrom associated with Sjogren's syndrome. Am J Med 81:734–740, 1986.

454. Sim TC, Grant JA: Hereditary angioedema: its diagnostic and management perspectives. Am J Med 88:656–664, 1990.

455. Stoppa-Lyonnet D, Tosi M, Laurent J, et al.: Altered C1 inhibitor genes in type 1 hereditary angioedema. N Eng J Med 317:1–6, 1987 (see also pp. 43–44: editorials).

456. Ley SJ, Williams RC Jr: A family with hereditary angioedema and multiple immunologic disorders. Am J Med 82:1046–1051, 1987.

457. Pan CC, Ward MK, Spitzer R, et al.: Non-SLE glomerulonephritis associated with hereditary angioedema: long-term follow-up. Pediatr Res 27 # 2:335A, 1990.

458. Frigas E: Angiedema with acquired deficiency of the C1 inhibitor: a constellation of syndromes. Mayo Clin Proc 64:1269–1275, 1989.

459. Alsenz J, Bork K Loos M: Autoantibody-mediated acquired deficiency of C1 Inhibitor. N Eng J Med 316:1360–1366, 1987.

460. Brown JP, Rola-Pleszczynski M, Menard H-A: Eosinophilic synovitis: clinical observations on a newly recognized subset of patients with dermatographism. Arthritis Rheum 29:1147–1151, 1986.

461. Grandel KE, Farr RS, Wanderer AA, et al.: Association of platelet-activating factor with primary acquired cold urticaria. N Eng J Med 313:405–409, 1985.

462. Ireland TA, Werner DA, Rietschel RL, et al.: Cutaneous lesins in cryofibrinogenemia. J Pediatr 105:67–70, 1984.

463. Ratner D, Eshel E, Vigder K: Juvenile rheumatoid arthritis and milk allergy. J R Soc Med 78:410–413, 1985.

464. Brady JE: Rheumatoid arthritis and food allergy: a review of the scientific literature. Food Allergy Update Newsletter 6:1–8, 1989.

465. Panush RS: Food induced ("allergic") arthritis: clinical and serologic studies. 17:291–294, 1990.

466. Beri D, Malaviya AN, Shandilya R, Singh RR: Effect of dietary restrictions on disease activity in rheumatoid arthritis. Ann Intern Med 47:69–72, 1988.

467. Bowen J, Boudoulas H, Wooley CF: Cardiovascular disease of connective tissue origin. Am J Med 82:481–488, 1990.

468. Boucek RJ, Noble NL, Gunja-Smith Z, et al.: The Marfan syndrome: A deficiency in chemically stable collagen cross-links. N Engl J Med 305:988–991, 1981.

469. Gott VL, Pyertiz RE, Magovern GJ, et al.: Surgical treatment of aneursyms of the ascending aorta in the Marfan syndrome. N Eng J Med 314:1070–1074, 1986.

470. Brody JE: Personal health. The New York Times. March 12, 1986.

471. McKusick VM: Heritable Disorders of Connective Tissue, 4th ed. Mosby, St. Louis, 1972.

472. Byers PH, Holbrook KA: Molecular basis of clinical heterogeneity in the Ehlers-Danlos Syndrome. Ann NY Acad Sci 460:298–310, 1985.

473. Hollister D: Heritable disorders of connective tissue: Ehlers-Danlos syndrome. Pediatr Clin North Am 25:575–591, 1978.

473a. Bertin PH, Treves R, Julia A, et al.: Ehlers-Danlos syndrome, clotting disorder and muscular dystrophy. Ann Rheum Dis 48:953–956, 1989.

474. Wenstrup RJ, Murad S, Pinnell SR: Ehlers-Danlos syndrome type VI: Clinical manifestations of collagen lysyl hydroxylase deficiency. J Pediatr 115:405–409, 1989.

475. Beighton P, Grahama R, Bird H: Hypermobility of joints. Springer-Velag, Berlin, Heidelberg, pp. 1–178, 1983.

476. Byers PH, Siegel RC, Holbrook KA, et al.: X-linked cutis laxa. Defective cross-link formation in collagen due to decreased lysyl oxidase activity. New Engl J Med 303:61–65, 1980.

477. Bowen J, Boudulas H, Wooley CF: Cardiovascular disease of connective tissue origin. Am J Med 82:481–488, 1990.

478. Glesby MJ, Pyeritz RE: Association of mitral valve prolapse and systemic abnormalities of connective tissue. A phenotypic continuum. JAMA 262:523–528, 1989.

479. Harinstein D, Buckingham RB, Braun T, et al.: Systemic joint laxity (the hypermobile joint syndrome) is associated with temporomandibular joint dysfunction. Ann Rheum Dis 47:254, 1988.

480. Lewkonia RM, Ansell BM: Articular hypermobility simulating chronic rheumatic disease. Arch Dis Child 58:988–992, 1983.

481. Biro F, Gewanter HL, Baum J: The hypermobility syndrome. Pediatrics 72:701–706, 1983.

482. Holzberg M, Hewan-Lowe KO, Olansky AJ: The Ehlers-Danlos syndrome: Recognition, characterization, and importance of a milder variant of the classic form. J Ma Acad Dermatol 19:656–666, 1988.
483. Arroyo IL, Brewer EJ, Giannini EH: Arthritis/arthralgia and hypermobility of the joints in school children. J Rheumatol 15:978–980, 1988.
484. Gedalia A, Press J. Articular symptoms in hypermobile schoolchildren: A prospective study. J Pediatr 119:944–946, 1991.
485a. Grana WA, Moretz JA: Ligamentous laxity in secondary school athletes. JAMA 240:1975–1976, 1978.
485b Jessee EF, Owen DS Jr., Sagar KB: The benign hypermobile joint syndrome. Arthritis Rheum 23:1053–1056, 1980.
486. Dacre JE, Huskisson EC: Arthritis in Down's syndrome. Ann Rheum Dis 47:254–255, 1988.
487. Yancey CL, Smijewski C, Athreya BH, Doughty RA: Arthropathy of Down's syndrome. Arthritis Rheum 27:929–934, 1984.
488. Olson JC, Bender JC, Levinson JE, et al.: Arthropathy of Down syndrome. Pediatrics 86:931–936, 1990.
489. Petty RE, Malleson P, Kalousek DK: Chronic arthritis in two children with partial deletion of chromosome 18. J Rheumatol 14:586–587, 1987.
490. Balestrazzi P, Gerraccioli GF, Ambanelli U, Giovannelli G: Juvenile rheumatoid arthritis in Turner's syndrome. Clin Exp Rheumatol 4:61–62, 1986.
491. Beighton P: Inherited Disorders of the Skeleton. Churchill Livingstone, New York, 1978.
492. Beighton P, De Paepe A, Dawks D, et al.: International nosology of heritable conditions of connective tissue. Am J Med Genet 29:581–594, 1988.
493. Valduea AF: The nail-patella syndrome. J Bone Joint Surg 55B:145–162, 1973.
494. Letts M: Hereditary onycho-osteodysplasia (nail-patella syndrome). A three-generation familial study. Orthopaed Rev 20:267–272, 1991.
495. Petajan JH, Momberger GL, Aase J, et al.: Arthrogryposis syndrome (Kuskokwim disease) in the eskimo. JAMA 209:1481–1486, 1969.
496. Jones KL: The fetal alcohol syndrome. Addictive Diseases 2:79–88, 1975.
497. Mirise RT, Shear S: Congenital contractual arachnodactyly. Arthritis Rheum 22:542–546, 1979.
498. Ardinger HH, Hanson JW, Harrod MJE, et al.: Further delineation of Weaver Syndrome. J Pediatr 108:228–235, 1986.
499. Abe K, Niikawa N, Sasaki H: Zollinger-Ellison syndrome with Marden-Walker syndrome. Am J Dis Child 133:735–738, 1979.
500. Esterly NB, McKusick VA: Stiff skin syndrome. Pediatrics 47:360–369, 1971.
501. Solimena M, Folli F, Denis-Donino S, et al.: Autoantibodies to glutamic acid decardoxylase in a patient with stiff-man syndrome, epilepsy, and type 1 diabetes mellitus. N Eng J Med 318:1012–1220, 1988 (see also editorial pp. 1060–1061).
502. Liberfarb RM, Hirose T, Holmes LB: The Wagner-Stickler syndrome: a study of 22 families. J Pediatr 99:394–399, 1981.
503. Omdal R, Laerdal A, Kjellwvold KH: Milticentric reticulohistiocytosis in a 9-year-old boy. Arthritis Rheum 31:1588–1590, 1988.
504. Raphael SA, Cowdery SL, Faerber EN, et al.: Multicentric reticulohistiocytosis in a child. J Pediatr 266–269, 1989.
505. Zayid I, Farraj J: Familial histocytic dermatoarthritis. Am J Med 54:793–800, 1973.

506. Stowens DW, Teitelbaum SL, Kahn AJ, Barranger JA: Skeletal complications of Gaucher disease. Medicine 64:310–322, 1985.
507. Nightingale SL: Alglucerase approved for Gaucher's disease. JAMA 265:2934, 1991.
507a.Katz K, Cohen JI, Zib N, et al.: Fractures in children who have Gaucher disease. J Bone Joint Surg 69A:1361–1370, 1987.
508. Sheth KJ, Bernhard GC: The arthropathy of Fabry disease. Arthritis Rheum 22:781–783, 1979.
509. von Scheidt W, Eng CM, Fitzmaurice TF, et al.: An atypical variant of Fabry's disease with manifestations confined to the myocardium. N Eng J Med 324:395–399, 1991.
510. Abul-Haj SK, Martz DG, Douglas WF, et al.: Farber's disease: Report of a case with observations on its histogenesis and notes on the nature of the stored material. J Pediatr 61:221–232, 1962.
511. Moser HW: Ceramidase deficiency: Farber's lipogranulomatosis. In Stanbury JB, Wyngaarden JB, Frederickson DS (eds.) The Metabolic Basis Inherited Disease, 4th ed. McGraw Hill, New York, 1989, pp. 1645–1653.
512. Ben-Yoseph Y, Gagne R, Parvathy MR, et al.: Diagnosis and carrier detection of Farber disease (ceramidase deficiency) in plasma and leukocytes. Pediatr Res 255:139A, 1989.
513. Katzenstein PL, Malemud CJ, Pathria M, et al.: Early-onset primary osteoarthritis and mild chondrodysplasia: radiographic and pathologic studies with an analysis of cartilage proteoglycans. Arthritis Rheum 33:674–684, 1990.
514. Spranger JW, Langer LO, Wiedermann MD: Bone Dysplasias. Saunders, Philadelphia, 1974.
514a.Spranger J, Albert C, Schilling F et al. Progressive pseudorheumatoid arthritis of childhood. Eur J Pediatr 140:34–40, 1983.
515. Wynne-Davis R, Gormley J: the prevalence of skeletal dysplasias: an estimate of the minimum frequency and the number of patients requiring orthopedic care. J Bone Joint Surg 67B:133–137, 1985.
516. Patrone NA, Kredich DW: Arthritis in children with multiple epiphyseal dysplasia. J Rheumatol 12:145–149, 1985.
517. Knowlton RG, Katzenstein PL, Moskowitz RW, et al.: Genetic linkage of a polymorphism in the type II procollagen gene (COL2A1) to primary osteoarthritis associated with mild chondrodyplasia. N Eng J Med 322:526–530, 1990.
518. Morris L, Kozlowski K, McNaught P, Silink M: Tricho-rhino-phalangeal syndrome I. Australas Radiol 29:167–173, 1985.
519. Stearns ZR, Lacassie Y, MacEwen GD: Perthes-like disease and the tricho-rhino-phalangeal syndromes: The first black patient. Orthopedics 13:468–473, 1990.
520. McGuire RA Jr., Reinert CM: Hereditary multiple exostosis. Orthop Rev 16:29–34, 1985.
521. Lackman RS, Cohen A, Hollister D, et al.: Metachrondromatosis. In: Skeletal Dysplasias. Birth Defects 10:171–178, 1974.
522. Gorham LW, Stout AP: Massive osteolysis (acute spontaneous absorption of bone, phantom bone, disappearing bone). Its relation to hemangiomatosis. J Bone Joint Surg 37A:985–1004, 1955.
523. Erickson CM, Hirschbever M, Stickler GB: Carpal-tarsal osteolysis. J Pediatr 93:779–782, 1978.

524. Udell J, Schumacher HR, Kaplan F, Fallon MD: Idiopathic familial acroosteo-lysis: Histomorphometric study of bone and literature review of the Hajdu-Cheney Syndrome. Arthritis Rheum 29:1032–1038, 1986.

525. Shurtieff DB, Sparkes RS, Clawson K, et al.: Hereditary osteolysis with hyper-tension and nephropathy. JAMA 188:363–368, 1964.

526. Hollister DW, Rimoin DL, Lachman RS, et al.: The Winchester syndrome: A non-lysosomal connective tissue disease. J Pediatr 84:701–709, 1974.

527. Prieur AM, Griscelli C, Lampert F, et al.: A chronic, infantile, neurological, cutaneous and articular (CINCA) syndrome. J Rheumatol 66:57–68, 1987.

528. Brueton LA, Sanderson IR, Jadresic L, et al.: An infant with chronic articular and cutaneous manifestations: a new syndrome? Proc Roy Soc 82:223–225, 1989.

529. Glover MT, Lake BD, Atherton DJ: Infantile systemic hyalinosis: Newly recog-nized disorder of collagen? Pediatrics 87:228–234, 1991.

530. Jacobs JC, Downey JA: Juvenile rheumatoid arthritis. In: Downey JA, Low NL (eds.) The Child with Disabling Illness. Saunders, Philadelphia, 1974, pp. 5–24.

531. Jacobs JC, Phillips PE, Johnston AD: Needle biopsy of the synovium of chil-dren. Pediatrics 57:696–701, 1976.

532. Athreya BH, Schumacher HR: Pathologic features of a familial arthropathy associated with congential flexion contractures of fingers. Arthritis Rheum 21:429–437, 1978.

533. Schubiner JM, Simon MA: Primary bone tumors in children. Ortho Cl NA 18:577–595, 1987.

534. Aprin H: Benign Chondroblastoma. Orthopedics 4:1134–1140, 1981.

535. Altman B, Ruby LK: Plexiform neurofibroma presenting as wrist synovitis. A case report. Orthopedics 5:1333–1335, 1982.

536. Orlowski JP, Mercer RD: Osteoid osteoma in children and young adults. Pediatrics 59:526–532, 1977.

537. Saville PD: A medical option for the treatment of osteoid osteoma. J Pediatr 66:1409–1411, 1980.

538. Cohen MD, Harrington TM, Ginsburg WW: Osteoid osteoma: 95 cases and a review of the literature. Semin Arthritis Rheum 12:265–281, 1983.

539. Haueisen DC, Weiner DS, Weiner SD: The characterization of "transient syno-vitis of the hip" in children. J Pediatr Orthop 6:11–17, 1986.

540. Osteoid osteoma: elements of diagnosis and treatment. Contemp Orthopaed 18:461–467, 1989.

541. Voto SJ, Cook AJ, Ewing JW, Weiner DS: CT-guided excision as a treatment for osteoid osteoma. Surg Rounds Orthopaed, pp. 31–36, February 1990.

542. Gerber NJ, Dixon St J: Synovial cysts and juxta-articular bone cysts (geodes). Semin Arthritis Rheum 3:323–348, 1974.

543. Medical World News, February 11, 1972, p. 50E.

544. O'Dell JR, Andersen PA, Hollister JR, West SG: Anterior tibial mass: an un-usual complication of popliteal cysts. Arthritis Rheum 27:113–115, 1984.

545. Lewis RC, Coventry MB, Soule EH: Hemangioma of the synovial membrane. J Bone Joint Surg 41A:264–271, 1959.

546. Moon NF: Synovial hemangioma of the knee joint. Clin Orthop 90:183–190, 1973.

547. Linsons MA: Synovial hemangioma as a cause of recurrent knee effusions.

JAMA 242:2214–2215, 1979.

548. Visuri T: Recurrent spontaneous haemarthrosis of the knee associated with a synovial and juxta-articular haemangiohamartoma. Ann Rheum Dis 49:554–556, 1990.

549. Docken WP: Pigmented villonodular synovitis: A review with illustrative case reports. Semin Arthritis Rheum 9:1–22, 1979.

550. Flandry F, Hughston JC: Pigmented villonodular synovitis. J Bone Joint Surg 69A:942–949, 1987.

551. Hajdu SI: Differential diagnosis of soft tissue and bone tumors. Philadelphia, Lea & Febiger, 1986.

552. Ladisch S, Jaffe ES. The histiocytoses. In Pizzo P, Poplack DG (eds) Pediatric Oncology. Philadelphia: J. B. Lippincott, 1988, pp. 491–504.

553. Israels SJ, Chan HL, Daneman A, Weitzman SS: Synovial sarcoma in childhood. AJR 142:803–806, 1984.

554. Case records of the Massachusetts General Hospital: Case 10-1990. N Eng J Med 683–690, 1990.

554a. Menendez LR, Brien E, Brien WW. Synovial sarcoma. Orthop Rev 21:465–471, 1992.

555. Rosenberg AM: Analysis of a pediatric rheumatology clinic population. J Rheumatol 17:827–830, 1990.

556. Ehrlich EL, Fisher RL: Orthopedic conversion reactions in children and adolescents. Conn Med 41:681–683, 1977.

557. Maisami M, Freeman JM. Conversion reactions as body language. Pediatrics 80:46–52, 1987.

558. Sills EM: "Rheumatic" syndromes of obscure origin. (Editorial.) J Pediatr 120:675, 1988.

559. Sherry DD, McGuire T, Mellins E, et al.: Psychosomatic musculoskeletal pain in childhood: Clinical and psychological analyses of 100 children. Pediatrics 88:1093–1099, 1991.

560. Maisami M, Freeman JM: Conversion reactions in children as body language: a combined child psychiatry/neurology team approach to the management of functional neurologic disorders in children. Pediatrics 80:46–52, 1987.

561. Libow JA, Schreier HA: Three forms of factitious illness in children: When is it Munchausen syndrome by proxy? Am J Orthopsychiat 56:602–611, 1986.

562. Block SR: Fibrositis and the concept of generalized rheumatism: the confessions of an unrepentant lumper. Occupational Problems in Medical Practice 5 (#3):1–6, 1990.

563. Thompson JM: Tension myalgia as a diagnosis at the Mayo Clinic and its relationship to fibrositis, fibromyalgia, and myofascial pain syndrome. Mayo Clin Proc 65:1237–1248, 1990.

564. Wolfe F, Smythe HA, Yunus MB, et al.: The American College of Rheumatology 1990 Criteria for the Classification of Fibromyalgia. Report of the Multicenter Criteria Committee. Arthritis Rheum 33:160–171, 1990.

565. Hadler NM: A critical reappraisal of the fibrositis concept. In Bennett RM (ed.) The fibrositis/fibromyalgia syndrome. Current issues and perspectives. Am J Med 81: Suppl. 3A:1–115, 1986.

566. Hadler NM: The plight of the patient whose illness is labeled as fibrositis or a related paralogism. Occupational Problems in Medical Practice 5 (#3):6–8, 1990.

567. Bernstein BH, Singsen BH, Kent JT, et al.: Reflex neurovascular dystrophy in childhood. J Pediatr 93:211–215, 1978.
568. Gold S: Diagnosis and management of hysterical contracture in children. Br Med J 1:21–23, 1965.
569. Goldsmith DP, Vivino FB, Eichenfield AH, et al.: Nuclear imaging and clinical features of childhood reflex neurovascular dystrophy: Comparison with adults. Arthritis Rheum 32:480–485, 1989.
570. Sherry DD, Weisman R: Psychologic aspects of childhood reflex neurovascular dystrophy. Pediatrics 81:572–578, 1988.
571. Hyler SE, Sussman N: Chronic factitious disorder with physical symptoms (the Munchausen syndrome). Psychiatric Clin North Am 4:365–377, 1981.
572. Batshaw ML, Wachtel RC, Deckel AW, et al.: Munchausen's syndrome simulating torsion dystonia. N Eng J Med 312:1437–1439, 1985.
573. Lane TJ, Manu P, Matthews DA: Depression and somatization in the chronic fatigue syndrome. Am J Med 91:335–344, 1991.
574. Katz BZ, Andiman WA: Chronic fatigue syndrome. Current literature and clinical issues. J Pediatr 113:944–947, 1988.
575. Gold R, Sixbey J, et al.: Chronic fatigue: a prospective clinical and virologic study. JAMA 264:48–53, 1990.
576. Shafran SD: The chronic fatigue syndrome. Am J Med 90:730–739, 1991.
577. Paperny D, Hicks R, Hammar SL: Munchausen's syndrome. Am J Dis Child 134:794–795, 1980.
578. Aduan RP, Fauci AS, Dale DC, et al.: Factitious fever and self-induced infection. Ann Intern Med 90:230–242, 1979.
579. Reich P, Gottfried LA: Factitious disorders in a teaching hospital. Ann Intern Med 99:240–247, 1983.
580. Meadow R: Factitious illness—the hinterland of child abuse. In Recent Advances in Pediatrics, No. 7, Churchill Livingston, New York, 1984, pp. 217–232.
581. Zitelli BJ, Seltman MF, Shannon RM: Munchausen's syndrome by proxy and its professional participants. Am J Dis Child 141:1099–1102, 1987.

3

Juvenile Rheumatoid Arthritis

Diagnostic Criteria

Juvenile rheumatoid arthritis (JRA) (JA) has been the diagnostic label applied to any child whose arthritis is of unknown origin, begins under age 16, and persists for a minimum of 6 weeks.[1,2] Arthritis is defined as swelling or both pain and limitation of motion in at least one joint. "Unknown origin" means that the physician has considered and excluded all other diseases, both common and unusual, that may cause or be associated with arthritis (Table 3.1). These "classification" criteria, adopted by a panel of experts (the JRA Criteria Subcommittee of the American Rheumatism Association—ARA, now the American College of Rheumatology—ACR), were extraordinarily successful in helping physicians distinguish arthritic disorders from other disorders in childhood. After 5 years, only 3% of children diagnosed as JRA by these criteria turned out to have some other disease. Interest in childhood arthritis was stimulated by publication of these criteria, and they helped to bring about the end of an era in which children with arthritis were frequently misdiagnosed and subjected to long hospitalizations, unnecessary surgery, harmful immobilization, and inadequate or inappropriate drug therapy.

Subtypes of JRA

During the past decade, it has become apparent that these criteria actually identify a consortium of different disorders, a panache with different genetic susceptibility determinants, environmental offsets, pathology, prognoses, and clinical patterns (Table 3.2).[2-10] As a result, these criteria failed to provide a strong relationship between diagnosis and prognosis in a given pa-

231

Table 3.1. Clues to Some Unsual Causes of Arthritis in Children

Clue	Diagnosis	Diagnostic Procedure
Strong family history of hip replacements in young individuals with degenerative hip disease	Spondyloepiphyseal dysplasia	Lateral spine x-ray
Pain in foot with atrophy of extremity	Osteoid osteoma	Bone scan, CT Scan
Recurrent brief attacks of severe monarticular arthritis with slight ecchymosis	Synovial hemangioma	CT scan, Phlebolith on x-ray (late)
Recurrent brief attacks with rash overlying affected joints	Familial Mediterranean fever	Observation of rash and attack
Punched-out lytic lesions in metacarpals and multiple bones	Child abuse with traumatic pancreatitis	Serum amylase/lipase Bone scan for hidden lesions
Initial onset of hip pain while doing a split	Acute chondrolysis or transient demineralization of the hip	Repeat hip x-rays
Thick hyperostotic erythematous proximal phalanges with periostitis and bone chards	Child abuse—beating across fingers with a ruler	X-ray
Exposure to plant thorns shortly before the onset of monarticular arthritis	Plant-thorn synovitis	Joint exploration
Bizarre (traumatic) lesions of fingers and toes with family history of "extraordinary brave deeds"	Congenital indifference to pain	History
Low-grade pain in the upper tibia in young boys with appearance of periosteal new bone	Stress fracture	X-ray, bone scan
Recurrent episodes of arthritis with chickenpoxlike rash	Mucha-Habermann disease	Lesion biopsy
with painful plaque rash and fever	Sweet's syndrome	Lesion biopsy

Table 3.1. Clues to Some Unusual Causes of Arthritis in Children* (*Continued*)

Clue	Diagnosis	Diagnostic Procedure
Recurrent episodes of arthritis:		
with fever and erysipeloid rash of lower extremities	Familial Mediterranean fever	History; trial of colchicine
with erythema nodosum or pyoderma	Inflammatory bowel disease	GI radiographs, colonoscopy
Pauciarticular arthritis with history of unusual skin lesion ("bug bite") the month before	Lyme arthritis	History Serology; Western Blot
Arthritis with large postauricular lymph nodes	2° syphilis	Serology; dark field of mucous membrane lesions
Arthritis with embolic skin lesions and tenosynovitis	Gonorrhea	Cervical/urethral/ synovial fluid cultures
Arthritis with intermittent refusal to bear weight, severe pain, anemia, transient episodes of severe bone pain	Leukemia or other malignancy	Bone marrow, abdominal ultrasound; chest x-ray; MRI; catecholamines
Arthritis that starts with bent thumbs within a few months of birth	Familial hypertrophic synovitis	Family history, biopsy
Arthritis with pyoderma gangrenosum and no systemic disease	"Streaking leukocyte factor"	Serum enhancement of WBC random mobility
Arthritis with rash appearing in newborn period	Congenital arthropathy with rash	History; skin or liver biopsy
Bizarre posturing of hand or foot	Reflex sympathetic (neurovascular) dystrophy	Physical examination
Monarticular arthritis with night pain at rest, exquisite response to aspirin	Osteoid osteoma	Bone scan; CT scan
Sudden episodes of flushing and fever in an infant	Solitary mastocytoma	Physical examination

* See Chapter 2 for detailed discussion.

Table 3.2. The Spectrum of Childhood Arthritis

	Systemic		*Polyarticular*	
Type of onset	Spiking fever Rheumatoid rash Hepatosplenomegaly Lymphadenopathy Polyserositis Myalgia, arthralgia Leukocytosis, anemia		Symmetrical arthritis	
Pattern of joint symptoms	Same as pauciarticular JRA (40% of systemic onset patients)	Same as polyarticular JRA (60% of systemic onset patients)	Arthritis involving upper and lower extremities; both small and large joints (wrists, hands, elbows, shoulders, hips, knees, ankles, feet, jaw, and neck); but not lumbodorsal spine	
Rheumatoid factor	Negative	Negative	Negative	Positive
Course of joint disease	Remitting–40%	Remitting with scarring—35% Severe, unremitting and destructive—25%	Remitting May "burn out"	Persistent chronic and destructive
Age at onset (median)	5 years	5 years	3 years	12 years
Sex ratio	M = F	M = F	F>>M	F>>>M
Antinuclear antibody	Absent	Absent	+ in 25%	+ in 75%
HLA-associated	?	?	DPw3	DR4
Uveitis	Rare	Rare	Rare	Absent
Comments	Systemic manifestations usually ultimately remit even if arthritis continues		Extra-articular manifestations generally mild	Childhood onset of classical adult RA Subcutaneous rheumatoid nodules common

(Modified with permission from Wedgwood and Schaller, *Hosp Prac*, June 1977.)

Table 3.2. The Spectrum of Childhood Arthritis (*Continued*)

Pauciarticular		
Asymmetrial arthritis		
Onset in knee only in 50% of cases. Monarticular in 74%	Few joints at onset (average 2): severe periarticular inflammation; periostitis; enthesopathy; SI joints, low back and first MTP joint; primarily lower extremity. Strong familial pattern	Few joint involved; typically knee, hip, ankle; occasionally spotty involvement of other joints as well
Negative	Negative	Negative
Joint destruction rare but some chronic knee damage	Remitting—occasional rapid destruction, especially of hips; calcification of the inflamed entheses (heel spurs) follows lytic lesions in heel entheses	Remitting; mild enthesopathy; no joint destruction, no calcification of the enthesis
2 years	10 years	6 years
F >>>> M	M >> F	F > M
+ in 50%	Occasionally transiently positive at onset	+ in 25%
DR5 (6, 8)	B27	None (? many subsets)
+ in 40% Subacute and chronic	8% in childhood 25% in lifetime (acute, subacute, and chronic)	Rare
Total blindness in 17% in the past was the major disability. Average number of joints at onset = 1.3	May progress to ankylosing spondylitis; may begin with Reiter's syndrome. Average number of joints at onset = 2.5	Not a well-defined group

tient. It had been noted by Still in 1896[11] and was reemphasized by Green in 1940[12] and many subsequent authors[2-10] that there were great differences between children who had spiking fever to 106°F daily, those children who had severe polyarticular disease but no systemic manifestations, and those whose arthritis was limited to one or a few joints. Accordingly, in 1977, the ARA-JRA diagnostic criteria were modified to divide patients with JRA into three onset subtypes: systemic (prolonged high fever), polyarticular (five or more affected joints; all cervical spine and all carpal or tarsal joints on one hand or foot count as only one each), and pauciarticular (four or fewer joints).[13] By general agreement, the onset subtype is determined 6 months after the beginning of disease. Several studies have shown that 75–85% of children will either remit or remain in that subset 5 years later. Onset subtypes are convenient for study and for clinical trials, but they have less significance for the individual patient than the current pattern of disease and its course.[14]

It has also become apparent that all forms of "childhood" arthritis may begin at any age.[15] The rarity of the rheumatoid-factor-positive ("seropositive") adult form of rheumatoid arthritis (RA) in childhood has merely served to cast the subsets of seronegative arthritis in sharper focus in the population of arthritic children. New understandings from the study of arthritis in childhood may be extended to seronegative arthritis in adults and vice versa.[16] Subsets created by age, sex, or counting joints are only a temporary way of separating out various arthritic diseases. If diagnostic criteria are not subject to constant modification, they may serve to inhibit rather than to foster scientific progress.

Recent studies indicate that at least some of these clinical constellations are not accidentally derived but are predetermined by heritable susceptibility factors.[10,17-19] While much remains to be done, it appears inevitable that more intense study of arthritic subsets identified by genetic markers will lead to better understanding of both the pathogenesis and clinical manifestations of the various arthritic diseases. Neither the clinical subsets nor the genetic markers exist in isolation relative to each other. At this moment it seems to the author that pursuit of new information is most likely to be successful if groups are defined by genetic markers rather than by overlapping clinical characteristics. However, at the time of this writing, adequate information is not available to enable us to do so in this chapter. Thus, with the exception of the HLA-B27 group, we continue to divide patients into the officially recognized onset subtypes: systemic, polyarticular, and pauciarticular.

Laboratory Studies

The ARA-JRA diagnostic criteria do not include laboratory, histologic, or radiographic items.[13,14,16] The diagnosis of JRA is made by physical examination. Laboratory studies are performed to help in excluding other dis-

Table 3.3. Disorders Associated with the Presence of Rheumatoid Factor

Rheumatic diseases: RA, SLE, scleroderma, MCTD, Sjögren's syndrome
Acute viral infections: mononucleosis; hepatitis; others, including recent
    immunizations
Parasitic infections: malaria, schistosomiasis, etc.
Chronic infections and inflammatory disorders: SBE, Tbc, syphillis, salmonellosis,
    sarcoid, chronic liver disease, etc.
Immune-complex diseases; Waldenström's hypergammaglobulinemia purpura,
    cryoglobulinemia

orders that have specific laboratory abnormalities, to aid in identification of those subsets of JRA associated with specific serologic or immunologic markers, and to provide a measure of the extent of the inflammation and its systemic effects (see Table 1.6). It will perhaps surprise the nonpediatric rheumatologist that ESR and CRP are often normal in nonsystemic forms of JRA.[20,21] Extraordinarily high ferritin levels are found in older-age onset systemic JRA.[21a]

It is important to remember that rheumatoid factors are not specific for RA (Table 3.3). In childhood, most common causes of a positive test for rheumatoid factor are laboratory error (overly sensitive slide tests) or recent viral illness. The overwhelming majority of cases of childhood arthritis are not associated with the presence of rheumatoid factor, and the diagnosis of RA is always obvious in the subset of childhood arthritis that is characterized by the presence of consistently high titers of rheumatoid factor.[22] The test for rheumatoid factor is, therefore, not performed to help in the diagnosis of JRA but to identify that subset of children whose disease is most likely to resemble early onset severe adult RA. Tests for rheumatoid factor are also commonly positive in children with SLE and in both localized scleroderma and progressive systemic sclerosis.

Antinuclear antibodies (ANAs) are present in about 60% of arthritic children, with highest frequency in little girls with pauciarticular disease and big girls with classic adult RA.[23] Speckled and homogenous patterns predominate but all staining patterns may be seen and all are associated with increased risk for iridocyclitis as initially reported by Schaller.[24] Antihistone ANAs are common in pauciarticular patients and are found in higher titer in those with a history of iritis.[25]

Many other antibodies and immunologic abnormalities have been described in JRA but their significance in the evolution of the disease remains obscure.[26–35]

Synovial fluid is examined to exclude bacterial infection in monarticular disease at its onset or in polyarticular disease in which septic infection seems a diagnostic consideration[36,37] (see Chapter 2 under Acute and Chronic Infections of the Bones and Joints). Synovial biopsy is obtained only if the tuberculin test is positive. Needle biopsy of the knee in children has been a

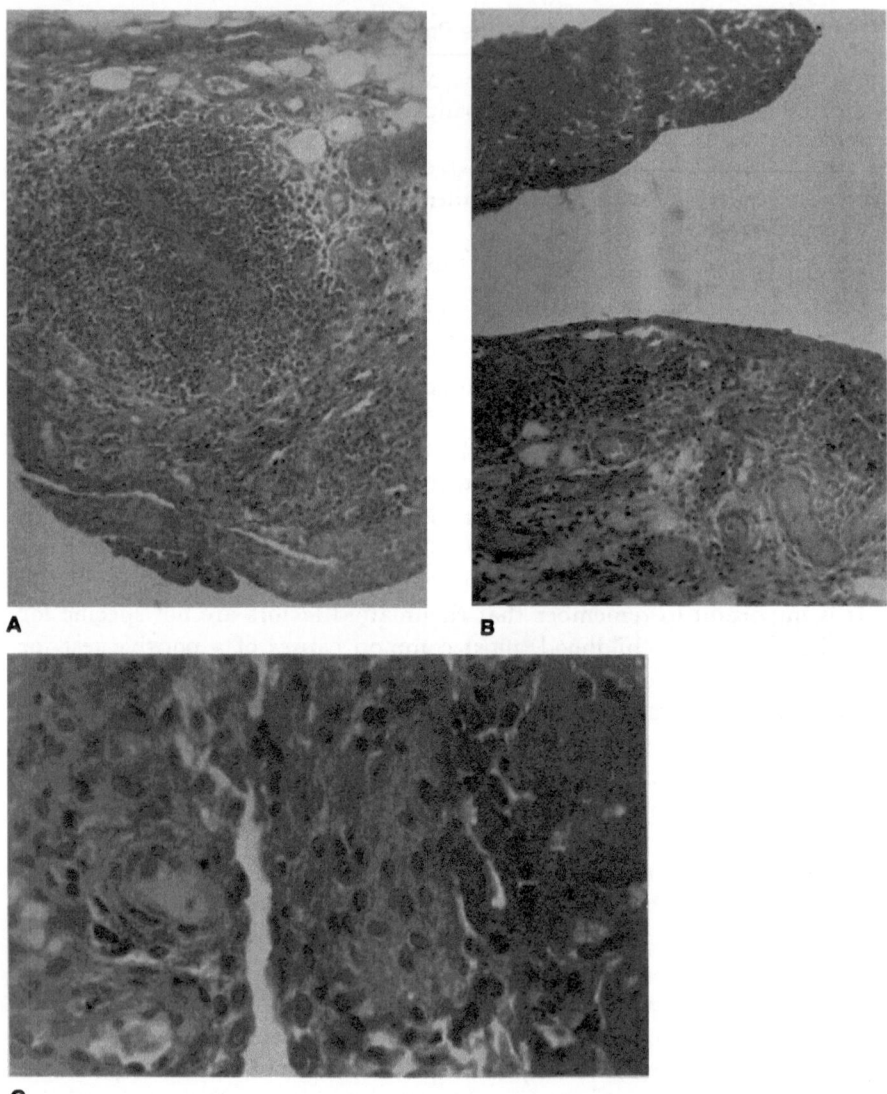

Figure 3.1. Three patterns of rheumatoid synovitis in one needle biopsy. (**A**) A lymphocytic (Allison-Ghormley) nodule in the center field is surrounded by a more diffuse infiltrate of "round" (plasma) cells. (**B**) Necrotic villi (*top left*); hypervascular sublining tissues with a diffuse "round cell" (lymphocytic and plasma cell) infiltrate. (**C**) Fibrinoid necrosis (*right margin*) and hypertrophic synovial histiocytes lining villi. (**A** and **B**) ×200; (**C**) ×640. (Reprinted with permission from Jacobs et al., ref 38. Copyright by the American Academy of Pediatrics.)

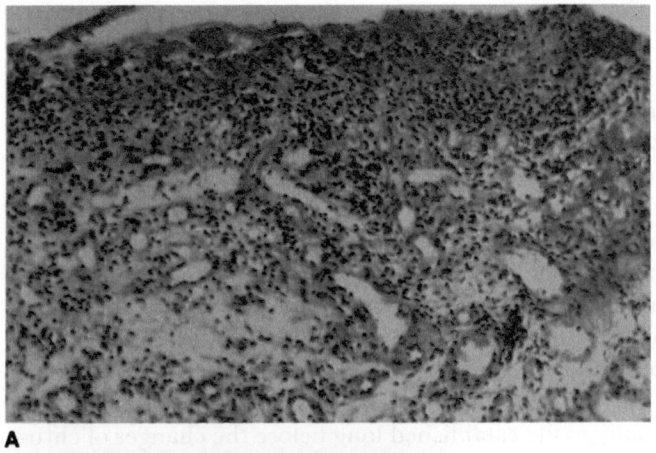

A

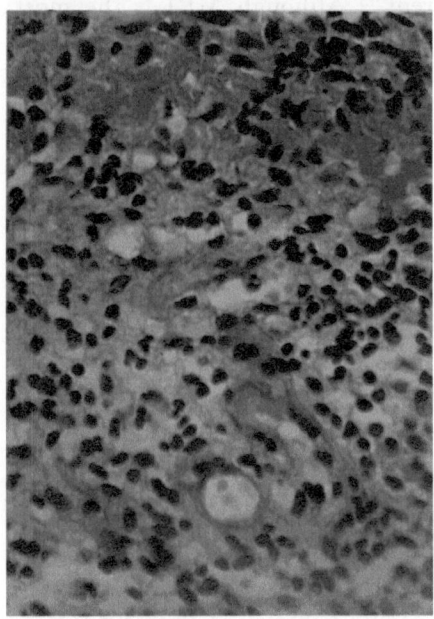

B

Figure 3.2. Rheumatoid synovitis mimicking septic synovitis. (**A**) The synovial surface is marked by granulation tissue comprising a dense capillary network and a cellular inflammatory exudate. (**B**) The exudate is largely lymphocytic but interpersed with occasional neutrophils. The surface is lined with necrotic fibrinoid material entrapping reactive cells. (**A**) ×200; (**B**) ×640. (Reprinted with permission from Jacobs et al., ref. 38. Copyright by the American Academy of Pediatrics.)

satisfactory technique in our clinic (Fig. 3.1).[38] However, while biopsy findings may be compatible with RA, the diagnosis cannot be established on the basis of a biopsy (Fig. 3.2).[39–41] Therefore, pathologic examination is of no value unless it shows a specific nonrheumatoid disease process. While open biopsy should be a harmless procedure, it has generally been followed by immobilization and/or disuse of the joint by the child, with resultant frequent permanent severe loss of function. The yield from open biopsies is so small and the risk so high that we have essentially abandoned doing them except in most unusual cases.[38,42] Arthroscopic biopsy can be performed if needle biopsy fails, but it has a higher complication rate.

Radiographic Studies

There are no radiographic findings that are characteristic of early JRA. Periarticular demineralization, bandlike areas of metaphyseal rarefaction identical to those of leukemia, and dense "growth-arrest" lines are all non-specific findings that cannot be interpreted as diagnostic of JRA.[42,43] Periosteal new-bone formation, especially in the fingers, described as an early finding in JRA, is rarely seen in our clinic. We suspect many previously reported cases really represented spondyloarthritis with sausage digits.

Radiographs, ultrasound, CT, bone and gallium scans, and MRI are obtained solely to exclude other disorders that may be confused with JRA. Rarely, a bone scan performed for possible osteomyelitis shows other subclinically involved joints and suggests the diagnosis of childhood arthritis. The diagnosis of JRA is usually easily established long before the changes of chronic arthritis are radiographically apparent.[43] Although MRI is the most sensitive technique for detecting subtle synovial and cartilage changes, its use in JRA is limited by motion in small children, inability to examine multiple joints, and expense.[44–47]

Epidemiology of Arthritis in Childhood

Arthritis is not rare in pediatric practice: in a year, one in 100 children will have joint pain requiring evaluation, and about one in 10,000 will develop chronic arthritis.[48,49] Although studies of childhood arthritis, using differing survey methods and diagnostic criteria, have shown varying prevalence,[50] a study from upper New York State showing a prevalence of 1.1 per 1000 in school-age children is probably the most accurate published estimate.[51] Minor transient musculoskeletal complaints of rheumatic origin are probably even more frequent.

Studies of the age of onset of childhood arthritis all show a peak incidence in the second year of life and a bimodal curve with a second rise later in the first decade.[42,50,52] Recent studies show that these curves are an amalgam of the varying age-incidence patterns of specific subsets; rheumatoid-factor-positive early onset adult RA and HLA-B27-associated spondyloarthritis contribute to the late-onset peak; the other subsets all have an unusually high incidence between 1 and 4 years of age (Table 3.2).[5–9,50]

More females than males have arthritis at any age. Females are more frequently clinically affected in all subsets other than the systemic (equal) and HLA-B27-associated (males 2:1). Extrapolation of data from several studies suggests that the early onset pauciarticular and polyarticular groups may have as high as 7:1 female preponderance (Table 3.2).[5,8,42]

The relative incidence of the various-onset subsets of JRA depends on the referral patterns to the reporting clinic. In our own clinic, at present, the overwhelming majority of new patients have pauciarticular disease (Table

Table 3.4. Mode of Onset of Juvenile Rheumatoid Arthritis

Author	Years	Number of Cases	Systemic (%)	Polyarticular (%)	Pauciarticular (%)
Calabro et al.[79]	1960–1977	200	20	49	31
Stillman and Barry[6]	1923–1977	204	19	41	40
Schaller[5]	1967–1977	112	20	30	50
Fink[7]	1970–1977	151	23	18	59
Hanson et al.[8]	1955–1977	563	43	23	34
Levinson et al.[9]	1958–1977	156	20	33	47
Jacobs	1978–1981	260	9	16	75

3.4). In older-reported series, polyarticular disease was the most common subset.[53]

Familial Incidence

Siblings are at increased risk—the answer to a question frequently asked by parents—but the exact additional risk is unknown.[54] The risk in families with affected individuals carrying HLA-B27 or HLA-DR4 markers is not inconsequential. Our experience and that in the literature suggest that in every 350 cases (after exclusion of spondyloarthritis and seropositive patients) one sibling pair will be observed. Since the prevalence of childhood arthritis is thought to be 1:1000 children, the risk to siblings appears to be two or three times higher than would be expected. The familial risk is further enhanced by the presence of iritis and HLA-DR5[54] and DR8.[55] Most parents find this risk inconsequential, all the more so since almost all familial cases are pauciarticular.

Nevertheless, there is evidence that parents of young-onset JRA patients have fewer subsequent children, suggesting some voluntary limiting of fertility.[56] While there seem to be inherited predispositions to at least some forms of childhood arthritis, the genetic effect is complex (polygenic) and weakly penetrant.[57,58]

Systemic JRA (Still's Disease)

Children with this form of JRA usually begin their illness with high spiking fever (>103°F daily), a typical rash, lymphadenopathy, hepatosplenomegaly, abdominal pain, myalgia, and arthralgia (Fig. 3.3). Sometimes pleurisy, pericarditis, and myocarditis are the predominant manifestations. Arthritis is often relatively inapparent at the onset of the illness.[59] Uveitis is uncommon in this form of JRA but does occur occasionally. The first clear descrip-

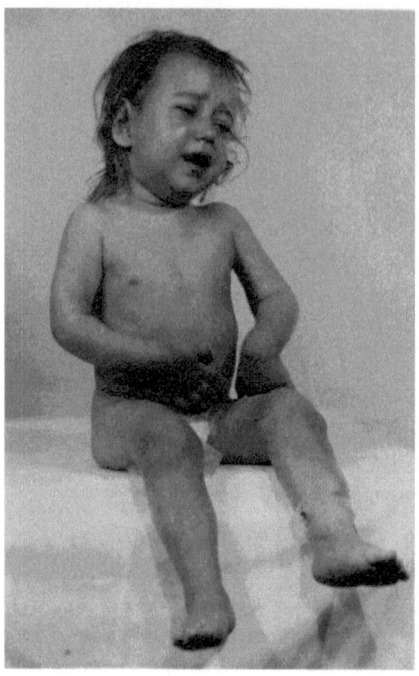

Figure 3.3. Systemic JRA that had its onset at age 5 months.

tion of this form of JRA was by Still in 1896.[11] Systemic-onset disease accounts for 9% of new childhood arthritis patients registered in our clinic (Table 3.4).

Differential Diagnosis

JRA is an important consideration in the differential diagnosis of unexplained fever. However, popularization of the notion of JRA as a cause of most unexplained fevers in childhood has unfortunately resulted in considerable diagnostic error. Physicians sometimes forget that a definite diagnosis of JRA requires *arthritis*, persistent for at least 6 weeks, *plus exclusion* of all other disorders that could conceivably cause the fever and arthritis.[13] Experienced pediatric rheumatologists are well aware that many children for whom this diagnosis is considered on the basis of fever alone will have some other disorder (Table 3.5).[60-62] The differential diagnosis of arthritis in childhood is discussed in Chapter 2 and in the chapters on the other specific connective-tissue syndromes. However, the three groups of disorders most frequently mistaken for systemic JRA are infection, inflammatory bowel disease, and malignancy; these entities account for 50–73% of children with prolonged "fever of unknown origin." The infections tend to be osteomyelitis or hidden

Table 3.5. Causes of Prolonged Fever of Unknown Origin in Childhood

Ultimate Diagnosis (%)	McClung[62]	Lahr and Hendley[61]	Pizzo et al.[60] Under Age 6	Over Age 6	Adults*
Infection	29	33	65	40	31/23
JRA	6	13	6	15	4/3
Inflammatory bowel disease	3	6		9	2/2
Malignancy	8	13	8	4	31/7
SLE	3			6	
Familial Mediterranean fever	4				1/1
Factitious fever (parent- or child-induced)	9	4			3/4
Other causes**	17	12	15	6	16/34
Never diagnosed	21	19	6	20	12/26

*Adult data from Larson, *Medicine* 61:269–292, 1982 and Knockaert, *Arch Intern Med* 152:51–55, 1992.
**Includes anhidrotic ectodermal dysplasia.[64]

abscess, most often in the abdomen or pelvis. The most common malignancies are leukemia, lymphomas, and neuroblastoma. Weight loss, fever, and arthralgia are common presenting manifestations of these malignant disorders.[63] Bone pain out of proportion to visible arthritis or accompanied by refusal to walk suggests malignancy rather than JRA. Even after exclusion of malignancy and infection, only 10–20% of children with unexplained fever turn out to have JRA (Table 3.5).

There is no way to avoid an extensive workup for children who are thought to have systemic JRA but who do not fulfill the diagnostic criteria. As we have emphasized, even in those with arthritis, other causes must be excluded. For those *without obvious arthritis*, a presumptive diagnosis of JRA may be made only after the most thorough study excludes the common mimics. Such a workup routinely includes chest and skeletal radiographic surveys, abdominal ultrasound, technetium bone scan, gallium scan, bone-marrow examination, and, when appropriate, a small-bowel series, colonoscopy, barium enema, and CT and MRI scans.[65] If lymphadenopathy is present, a lymph node biopsy may also be necessary.[66] The entire workup can be completed in a few days. If all of these studies are normal, a child with hectic fever, in the absence of arthritis, may be considered to probably have JRA and may be *managed as if he does*. The diagnosis, however, remains *tentative*, and it is appropriate to remain alert to missed clues to other diagnostic possibilities.

Table 3.6. Manifestations of Systemic JRA

Hectic fever
Salmon-pink evanescent rash
Arthritis and torticollis
Myalgia
Hepatosplenomegaly and Iymphadenopathy
Tenosynovitis
Pericarditis and myocarditis
Pleurisy and lung infiltrates
Abdominal pain
Irritability, drowsiness, meningismus
Acute laryngeal stridor
Anemia, leukocytosis, thrombocytosis, greatly elevated ESR and interleukin-6[77]

Epidemiology

The most common age at onset is between the first and fourth birthday.[42,50,67,68] However, both adults and children at any age may be affected.[15,69–72] Our youngest patient was 6 weeks old. Up to one-third of cases begin in teenagers or adults.[4,50] Males and females are equally frequently affected. Onset is uncommon in winter.[73]

Manifestations (Table 3.6)

Fever. A typical fever pattern has been described (quotidian) as one or two daily hectic spikes, sometimes to 105°F, and then a return to 98.6°F or below.[59,74] Our experience suggests that return to subnormal temperature (<98°F) usually occurs only in those given aspirin or NSAIDs at the time of the peak.[74] Children given no medication at the height of the spike tend to have hectic fever without return to below normal (Fig. 3.4). The fever spikes often take place late in the afternoon or in early evening and may be accompanied by shaking chills. Children who do not have pleurisy, pericarditis, or

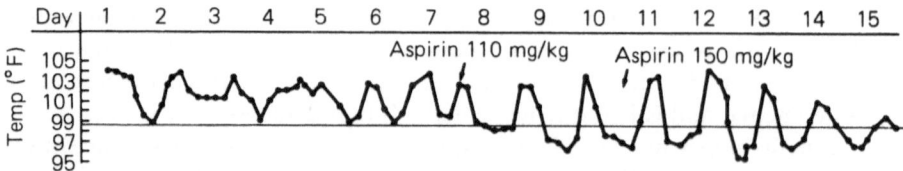

Figure 3.4. Typical hectic fever pattern of systemic JRA (patient pictured in Fig. 3.5). The temperature does not generally fall below 98.6° unless aspirin is given, as shown during the week of observation without therapy. Some response is noted soon after aspirin is begun, but satisfactory control of fever is dependent on achieving a therapeutic level of salicylate. Steady-state salicylate levels are not achieved until about the ninth day of therapy.

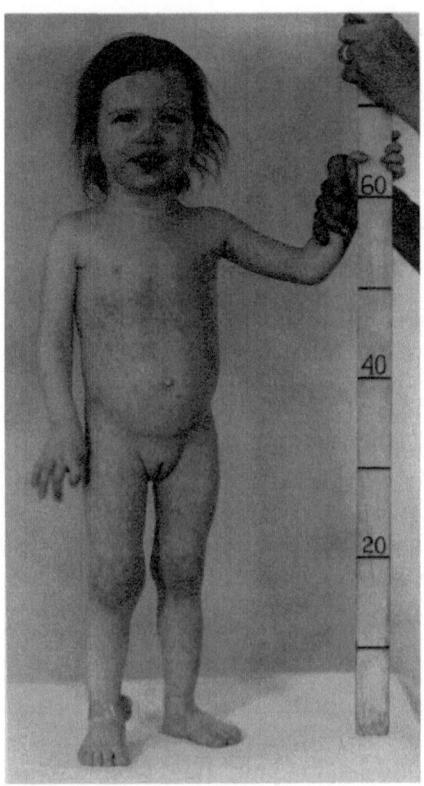

Figure 3.5. Typical rheumatoid rash in 2 year-old dwarfed child who had a year of fever and rash before arthritis was apparent. The Koebner phenomenon is apparent where she has scratched the abdomen. On the thighs, the rash is associated with a livedo reticularis pattern.

myocarditis often look surprisingly well at the time they are febrile as compared to children febrile with acute disorders.

Rash. A distinctive evanescent salmon-pink macular or maculopapular rash, most commonly on the trunk or overlying joints, occurs in most children with systemic JRA (Fig. 3.5).[75,76] As one looks at the rash, it seems to change slightly, with new spots appearing while others disappear. Rubbing or scratching the skin may elicit the rash (Koebner phenomenon); in about 25% of cases, the rash itches. If one is sufficiently familiar with the rash, a presumptive diagnosis can be made on the basis of the rash and fever alone. However, occasionally, catecholamine-secreting tumors or other disorders may present with a similar rash. Thus the presence of typical rash does not relieve the physician from the need to exclude other diagnostic possibilities.

The rash of JRA is often most pronounced at the time of the fever spikes. If these are limited to evenings, it may he worthwhile for the physician to reexamine the child at that time, as the fleeting rash may not have been noticed by the family or hospital staff. The rash of JRA may come and go during the course of treatment even though fever and arthritis are controlled with medication.

Biopsy of the rash is not necessary since it is the clinical characteristics rather than the pathologic features that are useful to the physician. Where biopsies have been performed for academic study, the primary finding has been edema, as in urticaria. In florid cases, mild perivascular infiltrates of lymphocytes or polymorphonuclear cells may be seen in the loose connective tissue of the subepithelial layer.[76,78] When fever and arthritis are accompanied by a rash suggesting impetigo or psoriasis, Reiter's syndrome is the most likely diagnosis (see Chapter 4).

Arthritis. Children with systemic JRA fall into two groups: (1) those with obvious severe, unremitting polyarticular disease who have a rather poor prognosis for ultimate joint function and who account for the major crippling and death in JRA and (2) those with arthralgia without much arthritis who have an excellent prognosis for future joint function and often must represent a different disorder from the severe polyarticular systemics.[42,79,79a] While the severe polyarticular systemic-onset JRA population represents a discouraging challenge to the pediatric rheumatologist and a fearful prospect to parents of children diagnosed as JRA, it constitutes a very small percentage of children with arthritis, perhaps 2% of those registered in our consultation clinic.

Torticollis. During the acute attack, more than half the children have neck pain and torticollis. Neck pain is often the most prominent arthritic manifestation in systemic-onset patients.[6] Cervical-spine pain, therefore, may be a good clue to diagnosis in children with relatively little visible arthritis. On the other hand, patients with torticollis have been referred to us who had eosinophilic granuloma, craniopharyngioma, and unrecognized rotatory cervical subluxations;[80] osteomyelitis of a first rib can also cause torticollis.[81]

Myalgia. Myalgia is often a prominent symptom in Still's disease, especially in children with little arthritis.[82] Elevations of creatinine phosphokinase are generally mild, if present at all.[83] The severity and quality of the muscle pain in systemic JRA resemble the degree seen in adult polymyalgia rheumatica and this presumably is a manifestation of vasculitis in muscle. Lumbar, cervical, and thigh muscles are most commonly affected. Muscle weakness is not seen. Muscle biopsies are obtained only in children thought to have polyarteritis nodosa or some other form of systemic vasculitis. In Still's disease, biopsies have usually been normal, but occasionally a perivascular accumulation of round cells has been found in connective tissues surrounding muscle, especially in adults.[69,84]

Hepatosplenomegaly. Systemic JRA is frequently accompanied by enlargement of the liver and spleen. Minor abnormalities in SGOT and SGPT are common.[83] Sometimes the hepatomegaly is alarming, extending 10 cm below the costal margin. When liver biopsies have been obtained, only nonspecific inflammation in the periportal areas has been seen.[85]

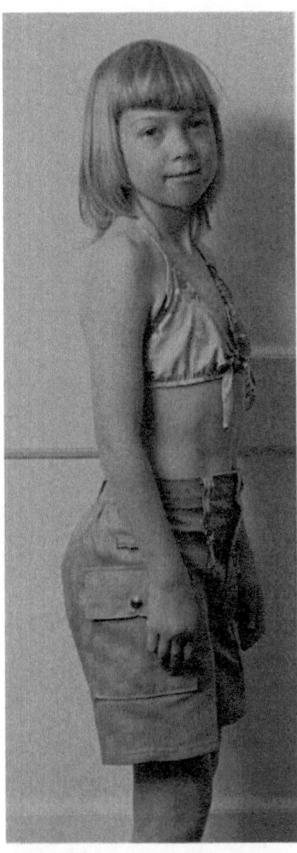

Figure 3.6. Proliferative polyarticular JRA with cystic "synovial pouches" at the wrists and shoulders. Stance indicates flexion contracture at the elbow with limited supination, often an early but unrecognized arthritic manifestation in children. The accentuated lordotic posture is a clue to disease in the hips and is accommodated by standing with the knee bent. Some of these girls do not complain of pain (as initially observed by Still[11] and emphasized by Grokoest et al.[42]), and an early diagnosis may not be made at the time of routine pediatric examiniation unless the joints are carefully examined.

Lympadenopathy. Nondiagnostic lymphoid reactive follicular hyperplasia is also most always present in systemic JRA: at times, the nontender and freely movable lymph nodes may reach 5 cm in diameter.[86] Nuclear debris with phagocytosis by histiocytes (necrotizing lymphadenitis) is seen occasionally.[87]

Tenosynovitis. Proliferative inflammation about the wrist commonly creates dorsal synovial pouches (Fig. 3.6). Sometimes these "masses" are mistaken for "tumors." Synovial pouches are also occasionally seen in other joints (Fig. 3.7). An unusual manifestation of tenosynovitis that we have seen in two children with systemic JRA is tenovaginitis of the superior oblique tendon of the eye, resulting in Brown's syndrome. This syndrome is characterized by intermittent vertical diplopia and a clicking sensation on trying to move the eye up and inward; the click is followed by resumption of normal vision. This syndrome has also been reported in adults with arthritis.[88]

Pericarditis and Myocarditis. About one-half of children with systemic JRA have pericarditis during the initial attack often with pleuritis and sometimes

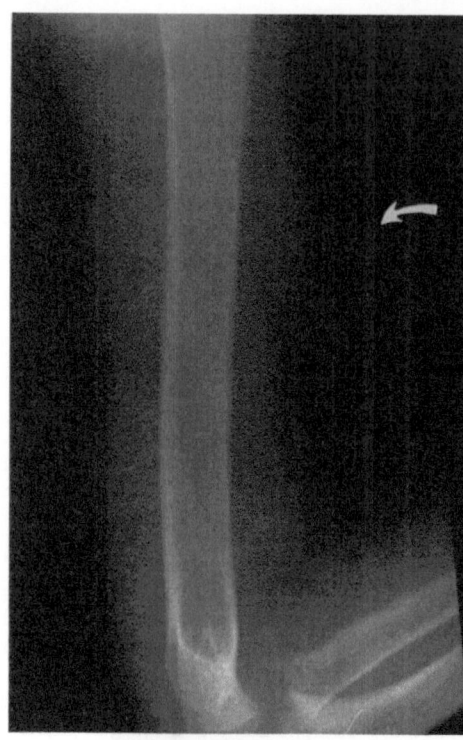

A

Figure 3.7. Shoulder effusion dissecting into biceps muscle creating a synovial cyst seen on plain radiograph (**A**) where it was thought to represent biceps tendon rupture. Ultrasound (**B**) indicated a cyst which disappeared spontaneously. Patient had same problem on opposite side on another occasion. Similar cystic dissections may be seen below the knee in the gastrocnemius muscle.

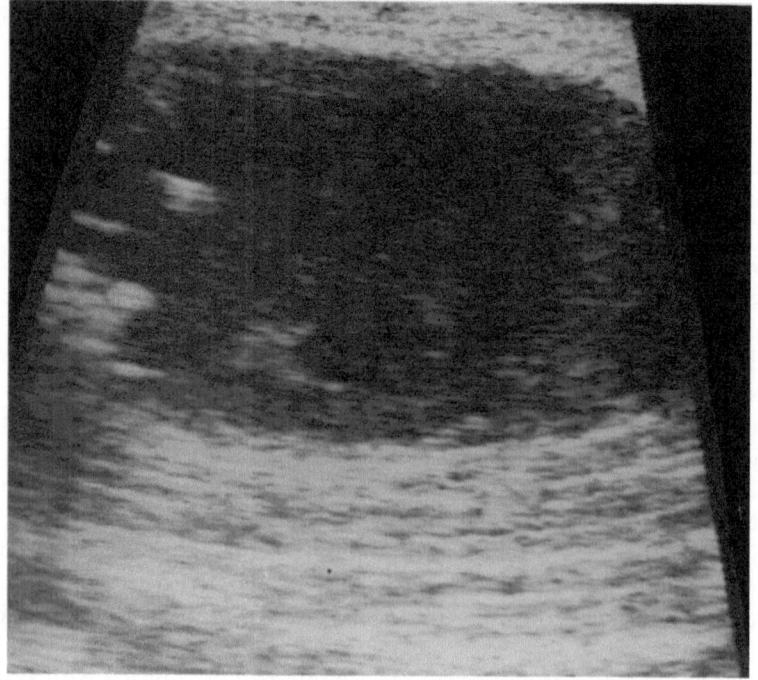

B

a triad including pneumonitis.[89] Usually, the pericarditis is asymptomatic or manifested only by minimal chest pain, and diagnosis depends on the demonstration of echocardiographic, radiographic, and electrocardiographic abnormalities (Fig. 3.8). Occasionally, the pericarditis is associated with myocarditis, cardiac tamponade, and severe congestive heart failure (Fig. 3.9).[90–92] Attacks of pericarditis and myocarditis usually last between 1 and 15 weeks, with an average of 2 months. However, some patients tend to have recurrent attacks.[93–96] These patients resemble patients with recurrent Coxsackie B viral pericarditis and myocarditis.[95,96] In one adult with this syndrome, Coxsackie B3 virus could still be demonstrated in the pericardial fluid 1½ years after the first of many recurrent episodes.[97] Adenovirus has also been demonstrated in the pericardial fluid of one child at the onset of systemic JRA,[98] and we are aware of adenovirus isolation from bone marrow and pleural fluid in two other patients at the onset of systemic JRA. A similar vasculitis syndrome has also been associated with the demonstration of high titers of hepatitis B virus antigen in pericardial fluid.[99] Two cases of hemophagocytic syndrome, characterized by systemic proliferation of benign hemophagocytic histiocytes, resulting in fever, hepatosplenomegaly, and cytopenia,[100] suggesting viral infection at the time of onset of systemic JRA have been reported,[101,102] and elevations of antibody titers to Coxsackie virus have occasionally been noted.[103,104] An immunodeficient individual has had arthritis as a manifestation of persistent adenovirus infection in the synovium, analogous to the dermatomyositislike syndrome seen in agammaglobulinemic children with persistent viral infection of the central nervous system.[105] These are isolated cases, however, and in most patients with pericarditis the pathogenesis of the episode is unknown and there is little to support a viral etiology for JRA.[106]

Although symptomatic constrictive pericarditis has not been reported in childhood JRA, adhesive pericarditis is a common finding in the select population of children with JRA who are examined postmortem.[11,93,94] Myocarditis that was not recognized during life may be demonstrated at postmortem examination (Figs. 3.8 and 3.9).

Valvulitis. Rheumatoid nodules on the heart valves and chordae tendineae have not been reported in children, but we have seen one child with seropositive RA associated with tuberculosis in whom rheumatoid nodules were demonstrated in the lung, heart, and meninges at the time of postmortem examination (Fig. 3.10). These findings were analogous to those seen in the animal model of arthritis called "adjuvant arthritis". Aortic insufficiency occasionally occurs in polyarticular disease.[107]

Pleurisy and Lung Infiltrates. One-third of children with systemic-onset JRA have radiographic evidence of pleural effusions during the acute episode. These are often associated with pericarditis and are sometimes also accompanied by transient lung infiltrates that disappear along with the pericarditis and pleurisy as the disease comes under control.[4] Still's disease is an

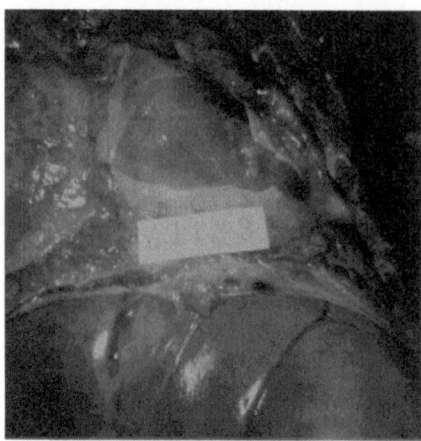

Figure 3.8. Fibrinous pericarditis was found at autopsy in a child with systemic JRA who died following the second injection of gold (see Fig. 3.43). The pericarditis was clinically silent and unrecognized.

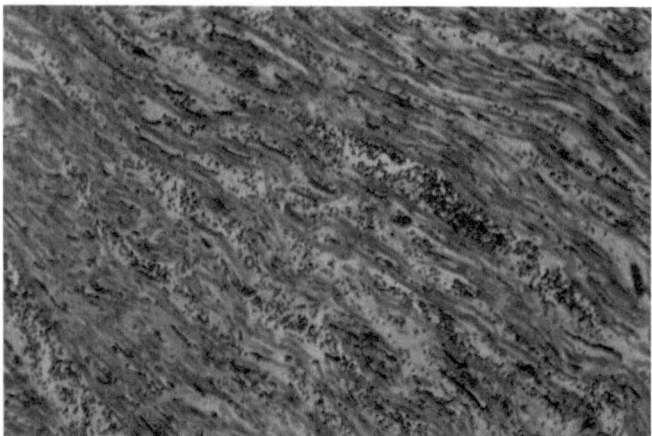

Figure 3.9. Flagrant myocarditis noted in the same patient (Fig. 3.8) was also "silent."

important consideration in the differential diagnosis of the syndrome of recurrent pleurisy and pericarditis in childhood. Occasional cases of fibrosing alveolitis, lymphoid interstitial pneumonia, rheumatoid nodules in the lung, and recurrent episodes of pulmonary hemorrhage have been seen in children with arthritis.[108–111] Subclinical abnormalities of pulmonary function may be common in JRA.[112] One case of primary pulmonary hypertension has been reported.[113]

Abdominal Pain. Diffuse abdominal pain suggestive of serositis is a prominent symptom in about 10% of children with systemic JRA.[86]

Laryngeal Stridor. Systemic JRA occasionally presents with stridor as the most apparent symptom, a result of life-threatening acute cricoarytenoid

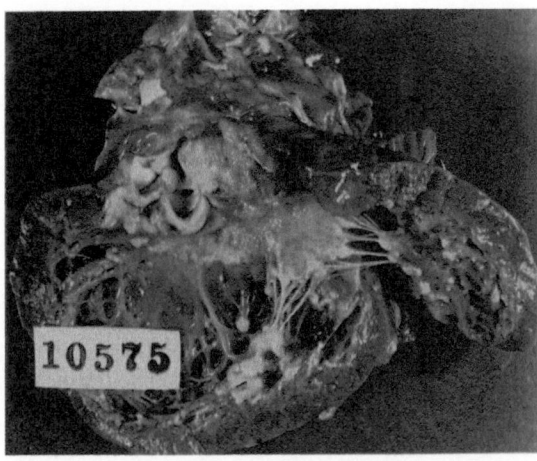

Figure 3.10. Endocardial rheumatoid nodules found at autopsy in a 6-year-old girl with seropositive JRA who died of congestive heart failure. Left ventricle, mitral, and aortic valve granulomas caused stiff valves and extended to the chordae tendineae and the endocardium of the papillary muscles, trabeculae carneae, and adjacent ventricular endocardium. Patient also had arrested tuberculosis. Today one could study the role of microbial superantigens and heat shock proteins in the creation of such a disease process, and of receptor-targeted immunotherapy (See: Bull Rheum Dis 41#3, 1992).

arthritis.[78,114] Although arthritis may also be demonstrable elsewhere, it is usually not noted in the context of caring for the child with a compromised airway.

Cerebral Manifestations. Irritability, drowsiness, meningismus, and nonspecific electroencephalographic changes are all frequently observed in systemic JRA.[115] An episode of cerebral vasculitis has been documented by cerebral angiogram in one child with JRA.[116] O'Connor reported one child with hemiparesis, and we have had one patient with a transient hemiparesis.[117] Occasional children have been reported with either febrile or afebrile seizures. Perivascular mononuclear-cell inflltrates in the brain and mononuclear inflammation of the meninges were demonstrated in all patients whose brains were examined in a postmortem study.[117] Immune complexes were found in the spinal fluid of one of those children. Central nervous system (CNS) involvement is probably more frequent than has been previously recognized in Still's disease. However, it is not as frequent as suggested by postmortem material, which reflects the incidence only in the most severely ill patients at the time of death.

Renal Disease. Significant renal pathology is not a part of JRA except in those few children who develop amyloidosis. However, transient albuminuria, leukocyturia, erythrocyturia, hypercalcuria, and decreased creatinine clearance are reported to occur in about one-third of especially carefully followed patients if repeated examinations were performed looking for these abnormalities.[118–120] Minor changes may also be seen on renal-biopsy specimens.[118] While some of the renal findings must be a result of damage by drugs[121] (see below); it also seems likely that some may be a manifestation of the disease itself, albeit generally a manifestation of seemingly little consequence.[122]

Amyloidosis. Amyloidosis may be a complication of any chronic disease and in the past accounted for up to 50% of deaths from childhood arthritis.[42,123,124,125] Transient proteinuria is the first manifestation, but the diagnosis is usually not suspected until more persistent proteinuria occurs. Associated symptoms include nephrotic edema, hypertension, hepatosplenomegaly, abdominal pain, diarrhea, and congestive heart failure. Diagnosis is usually achieved by aspiration of abdominal fat,[126] but scintigraphy with ^{123}I serum amyloid P component may be the best way of diagnosing, locating, and monitoring the extent of systemic amyloidosis.[127,127a] Amyloidosis is very rare in children in the United States; the reason for the increased incidence in European pediatric rheumatology clinics is unknown but may be related to the tendency of such clinics to serve disproportionate numbers of severely affected and immunologically deficient individuals.[128]

Amyloidosis has been reported in equal numbers of male and female arthritic children and is not limited to those with systemic disease.[121,124] One might suspect from this observation that there is at least equal risk of amyloidosis in severely affected childhood-onset male spondyloarthritis, although data to confirm such a hypothesis are not available at present. Colchicine may prevent amyloidosis or cause it to regress.[129]

Renal Papillary Necrosis. Renal papillary necrosis (RPN), a known complication of analgesic use, has not been associated with the use of aspirin alone in JRA.[130] Wortmann et al. reported RPN in three severe JRA patients treated with many drugs.[131] The children had unexplained hypertension or hematuria; IVPs demonstrated filling of an entire papillary region, typical of RPN. The authors emphasized that all of their patients were chronically dehydrated, which may cause RPN and which would certainly increase the risk of RPN with anti-inflammatory drug therapy. Care should be taken to avoid chronic dehydration in children receiving analgesic therapy. However, Allen et al. recently observed RPN in five children treated with NSAID who had only pauciarticular disease.[132]

Anemia. Hemoglobin of less than 10 grams (g) has been reported to occur in 39% of children with JRA at some time during their course.[86] The anemia seems to be a result of a combination of factors, including iron deficiency[133] (poor diet, increased losses as a result of medications, malabsorption of oral iron,[134,135] impaired release of iron stores), shortened life-span of red blood cells, impaired release of erythrocytes from a hyperplastic bone marrow,[86] blunted erythropoietin production,[136] and interleukin I–mediated serum suppression of erythropoeisis.[137,138] Erythroid hypoplasia has also been reported in one child,[139] and we have seen one child with generalized marrow hypoplasia in our clinic.

Case Report

A 3-year-old boy was admitted to the Babies Hospital in April 1972 with a 2-week history of fever and polyarthritis. A diagnosis of JRA was made, and treatment was begun with aspirin with only partial control of his symptoms. His hemoglobin fell to 5.6 g, his WBC to 1400/mm^3, and his platelet count to 52,000. The bone marrow was hypoplastic. His symptoms were controlled with the addition of tiny doses of prednisone (3 mg daily) to his aspirin regimen, and the hematologic parameters returned to normal as his symptoms subsided. Four months later, he had an exacerbation of symptoms while receiving a lowered dose of aspirin. Three weeks later, he was readmitted with pancytopenia (hemoglobin, 6.3 g; WBC, 800; platelet count, 32,000). At this time, he was found to have pneumococcal bacteremia. He was treated with appropriate antibiotics, blood and platelet transfusions, and, after control of the infection, with prednisone, 30 mg daily. Aspirin treatment was subsequently reinstituted and prednisone gradually withdrawn without ill effect. After 2 years, his arthritis remitted, and aspirin treatment was discontinued. However, 2 years later, he again developed high spiking fever and polyarthritis. Although the arthritic symptoms responded to aspirin, he again developed pancytopenia with a severely hypoplastic marrow, which again responded to prednisone therapy. Manifestations of systemic JRA persisted for many years, requiring treatment with prednisone as well as many other antirheumatic medications, including choline salicylate. He remained somewhat anemic, but his WBC and platelet count were normal.

Although children with G6PD deficiency are generally instructed not to take salicylates, studies suggest that a therapeutic level of salicylate in G6PD-deficient individuals does not produce hemolysis.[140]

It is often impossible to utilize ordinary laboratory methods to document iron deficiency in children with severe JRA. Serum iron and iron-binding-capacity determinations are altered by chronic disease. Serum ferritin and transferrin are often elevated in children with active arthritis even if they are iron deficient, and so cannot be used as a guide to iron deficiency.[141] Bone-marrow stains for iron are a satisfactory method of proving iron deficiency but are impractical except in special circumstances. Although a therapeutic trial of iron therapy is not the ideal method of diagnosing iron deficiency, it is often the only practical approach in children with JRA.[133] In a recent study of adults with classic RA the combination of low MCV and very high serum ferritin and transferrin always indicated iron deficiency.[142]

Other nutritional anemias have not been documented in JRA.[143] However, some nutritional anemias may be drug induced, and all deficiency anemias may be intertwined biochemically and pathologically.[144] Further study of the possible role of deficiencies of vitamins and minerals in these children is needed.

That part of the anemia that is due to iron deficiency generally responds to proper oral iron administration. However, occasionally oral iron is not absorbed and parenteral iron administration is required.[134,139] We have seen no adverse reactions to intramuscular iron but intravenous iron-dextran infusions may exacerbate arthritis.[145] Severe anemia unresponsive to iron therapy is sometimes a major manifestation of the systemically ill patient. When systemic disease is controlled, anemia often disappears. Occasionally, very ill patients will require alternate-day prednisone or methotrexate therapy to control otherwise-intolerable anemia. It remains to be determined whether recombinant human erythropoeitin is of value.[146,146a]

Disturbances of Linear Growth (Dwarfing). Somatic growth arrest was reported as an important feature of systemic or severe polyarticular JRA by Still,[11] and was reemphasized by Kuhns and Swain,[147] by Coss and Boots (Fig. 3.5),[148] Ansell and Bywaters,[149] and Bernstein et al.[150] Growth-arrest lines in the metaphyses of ill children are a reflection of the cessation of growth due to end-organ inability of the bones to respond to growth hormone and/or a direct inhibitory effect of illness on growing cartilage. Growth-hormone deficiency is not a part of JRA,[151,152] and remission or control of the disease is associated with prompt catch-up growth (Fig. 3.11).[149] Permanent dwarfing results only from disease that begins early and is uncontrolled throughout childhood or from steroid therapy (Fig. 3.11).[149,153] We will soon know whether these non–growth-hormone-deficient children can respond to

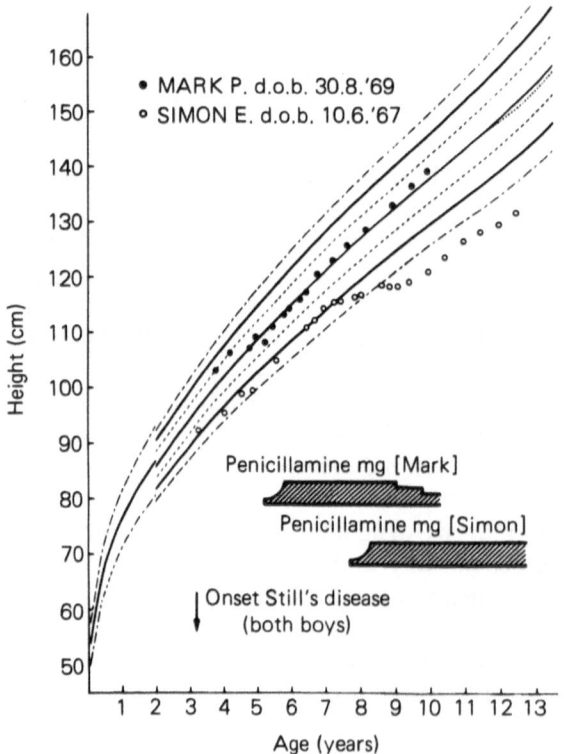

Figure 3.11. Fall-off in linear growth associated with poorly controlled JRA. Patient Mark P. had quick resumption of growth as his disease came under control but will not quite achieve his original anticipated adult height. Patient Simon E., with an inadequate response to drug therapy, will remain dwarfed despite recent control of disease. (Reprinted with permission from Ansell and Hall, ref. 376.)

exogenous growth hormone and achieve near-normal height.[154] If so, it will probably require six injections weekly for many years. There may be potential hazards to the growth plates,[155] and while growth hormone may combat steroid catabolism of protein it enhances the adverse effects on carbohydrate metabolism and increases glomerular filtration rate, which may alter drug excretion, so there my be problems with long-term use in arthritic children. While large daily doses of corticosteroids may result in some irreversible stunting of growth, morning alternate-day steroid or corticotropin therapy may actually foster linear growth if the systemic manifestations associated with growth failure are controlled by a dose of corticosteroids that does not inhibit growth.[153,156–158] Height may also be adversely affected by collapse of vertebral bodies secondary to steroid therapy and immobility, and by flexion contractures at the hips and knees.[149,150]

Other causes of growth failure, including hypothyroidism and autoimmune polyendocrinopathy, have been reported in association with JRA and must be excluded in arthritic children with growth failure.[159–161]

Ectopic Ossification. Occasionally, children with severe long-standing JRA develop new-bone formation in tissues that do not normally ossify.[42,51,162] This occurs most often in subcutaneous tissues adjacent to affected large joints or in areas subject to pressure from splints or shoes but has also been noted in the eye, brain, and spinal cord. Spurlike calcifications in ligaments, previously reported as a feature of JRA, were more likely manifestations of spondyloarthritis, and most of these children with ectopic calcification may represent examples of severe spondyloarthritis.[162]

The Course of Still's Disease

Children with systemic-onset disease separate themselves into two categories. In one group (about 40% of systemic JRA), there is very little arthritis. Therapy tends to completely control the arthritis, which disappears when the febrile episode subsides. While severe, the illness has a relatively brief course. Febrile episodes rarely last more than 6 months at a time but frequently recur at least once.[4,74,79] These patients usually ultimately recover without sequelae or with minimal joint dysfunction.

A second group of patients develops arthritis that does not remit when the systemic symptoms are controlled. This includes the 25% of systemic-onset patients who develop incessant intractable polyarticular disease that is progressively destructive; permanent handicap is inevitable. In most older-published series, this group was selectively overrepresented and equaled about 5% of the total childhood arthritis population. Recent registrations in our clinic indicate that most arthritis in childhood is pauciarticular, and the proportion of these terribly ill, unremitting crippled children has decreased to less than 2% of all arthritis in children. The remaining 35% of systemic-onset patients tend to have a spectrum of polyarticular disease that may ultimately remit, leaving some scars but a normally functioning adult. Forty percent of patients with recurrent attacks requiring steroid therapy require hip prosthesis in a series followed for an average of 23 years.[163]

Death in Still's Disease

The incidence of death has progressively decreased from 7% reported in earlier series[42] to 5%[164] to 2%.[165] Since almost all deaths in the United States now are in the systemic polyarticular group, however, the incidence of death in that population in the 20 years prior to the last decade seems to have been around 14%.[8,165] The most common causes of death have been amyloidosis, infection, intractable heart failure, and accidents.[124,164,165] Some accidents are related to the presence of arthritis.

Death rates from all causes are diminishing in all pediatric rheumatology clinics.[124] In our own hospital, during the decade 1961–1970, there were five deaths. In the next decade, despite a greatly increased number of patients, there were only two deaths, one septic (gold neutropenia) and one arthritis-related accident. Both deaths were theoretically avoidable. During the last decade there were no deaths, but death has on occasion been narrowly averted; these threatened patients have had disseminated intravascular coagulation (DIC), probably the most common cause of death now in arthritic children.

Prevention of Death

Recognition of DIC in JRA. It has been said that all children with systemic JRA have "low-grade" DIC;[166,167] if so, it is certainly not reflected in low fibrinogen levels or low platelet counts. On the contrary, systemic disease almost always is characterized by very high platelet counts and fibrinogen levels. If as a child becomes more ill the platelet count and fibrinogen fall to normal levels that child is endangered.[168] Although we first recognized precipitation of this life-threatening syndrome by the second injection of gold,[169] it has become apparent that it may follow introduction of any medication and on occasion be a complication of viral illness.[170–172] Although not recognized as DIC, cases were first reported by Kornreich in 1971,[173] and in that report one may find the features which we now recognize as characteristic: (1) a new rash—not typical of JRA, (2) lymphadenopathy and hepatosplenomegaly, (3) elevation of SGOT/PT and, in some cases, bilirubin, (4) thrombopenia, (5) lowering of ESR, and (6) paucity of arthritis. Other features seen in some patients include diarrhea; adult respiratory distress syndrome (ARDS);[174] rhabdomyolysis with elevation of CPK, myoglobinuria, and renal manifestations; drowsiness; and coma.[175] Even in highly specialized centers 7/11 of these patients have died. Our experience and that of others suggest that prompt recognition and vigorous management of this syndrome results in (almost) 100% survival.[176] Management includes (1) stopping all medications, (2) high-dose intravenous steroid,[170,177,178] (3) providing vitamin K and coagulation factors (fresh-frozen plasma), and (4) intensive care. Some patients recover from this syndrome spontaneously. However, if death is to be avoided altogether, probably all patients with this syndrome will have to be treated vigorously. Once intractible GI bleeding or intracranial bleeding has occurred, treatment is likely to be ineffective.

We have seen one patient with dysfibrinogenemia without thrombopenia which resulted from aspirin treatment of a child with JRA and an unrecognized choledochal cyst.[179] Erythrophagocytic syndromes[100–102] and angioimmunoblastic lymphadenopathy with dysproteinemia[180,181] are similar to this coagulopathy.

Prevention of Addisonian Crisis. Patients taking corticosteroids required steroid support for surgery, in case of accident, or for the stress of serious infection. Missed doses due to vomiting in stress situations and forgetting to provide parenteral steroids in stress continue to be an avoidable cause of death.

Treatment of Still's Disease

Treatment of Fever and Arthritis. Salicylates were obtained from plants and used as antipyretics and for analgesia by Hippocrates over 2000 years ago.[182] Easily dissolved palatable 81-mg tablets are available and very convenient for parents of infants and young children. Ordinary 325-mg generic aspirin tablets provide the cheapest nonsteroidal anti-inflammatory therapy (Table 3.7). Buffering often prevents the achievement of constant therapeutic salicylate levels (Fig. 3.12)[183] and has not been shown to prevent gastric erosion.[184]

The mechanisms of action of aspirin remain a great mystery. In 1971, Vane reported that aspirin inhibits the synthesis of prostaglandins, hormonelike substances that can cause redness, swelling, and fever.[185] Other anti-inflammatory actions of aspirin are probably directed at lymphokine action on target cells or lymphokine production by lymphocytes.[186] It is unlikely that any one action accounts for the total response.

The anti-inflammatory effects of aspirin in arthritis are only demonstrable at high dosage.[187] In adults, 4 g daily is required; similar studies have not been performed in children. Analgesia is achieved by considerably lower doses.

Aspirin remains a commonly used treatment in Still's disease and is usually only effective in controlling fever and arthritis after a salicylate level of between 25 and 30 mg/dl is achieved. A few patients require and tolerate slightly higher levels (Figs. 3.13 and 3.14).[188,189] In systemically ill patients,

Table 3.7. Relative Cost of Antirheumatic Drugs

Drug	Size (mg)	Cost per 100 ($)	Daily Dose (40 kg)	Daily Cost to Patient
Salicylates				
Aspirin	325	2.10	9	.19
Bayer timed-release aspirin	650	10.00	4	.40
Ecotrin	325	7.90	8	.63
Bufferin	325	9.70	8+	.78*
Baby aspirin	81	7.00	35	2.45
Trilisate	500/tsp	31.06 (240 cc)	5 tsp	2.59
NSAIDs				
Naprosyn susp.	125mg/tsp	52.27 (480 cc)	4 tsp	2.17
Indocin	25	50.35	3	1.51
Naprosyn	250	74.55	2	1.49
Clinoril	150	91.25	2	1.83
Nalfon	300	56.85	5	2.84
Motrin	400	11.35	4	.45
Meclomen	50	64.30	4	2.57
Tolectin	200	51.95	6	3.11
Orudis	50	92.15	3	1.86
Ansaid	50	71.80	3	2.15
Feldene	10	129.70	1	1.30
Voltaren	50	88.65	3	2.57
Dolobid	250	52.75	3	1.58

*Rapid excretion may result in the need for increased dosage.

Table 3.8. Doses of Drugs and Frequency of Administration Required to Control Fever in Systemic JRA

Regimen	Alone	With Prednisone (0.6–1.0 kg q.o.d.)	Usual Recommended Dose
Aspirin*	130–150 mg/kg/day (6 doses)	110–180 mg/kg/day (Higher dose on "off-prednisone" day)**	90–110 mg/kg
Tolmetin	30 mg kg day (5 doses)	40 mg/kg	20–30 mg/kg
Naproxen	20 kg/day (3 doses)	25 mg/kg	10–15 mg/kg

*Success depended on patient's ability to tolerate 130–150 mg/kg/day with salicylate levels 25–39 in 6 doses (day and night).
**Subsequent patient has required the higher dose on the "on-prednisone" day.
(Reprinted with permission from Jacobs, ref. 198.)

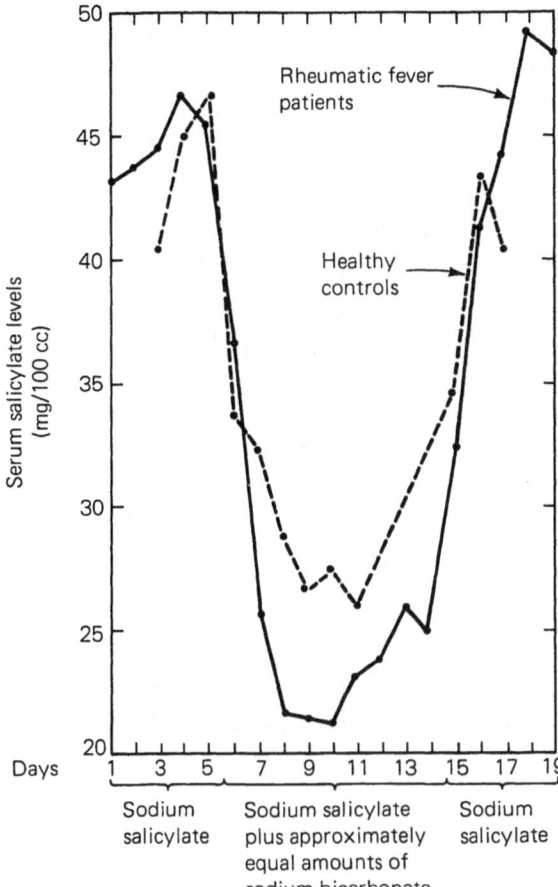

Figure 3.12. Dramatic decrease in salicylate levels caused by buffering with equal amounts of sodium bicarbonate. (Based on data of Smull et al., JAMA 125:1173–1174, 1944. From Gross M, Greenberg LA: *The Salicylates: A Critical Bibliographic Review.* Hillhouse Press, New Haven, 1948.)

these levels are rarely if ever obtained with less than 110 mg/kg/day, which is the customary starting dose (up to 3.6 g daily). Often a higher per-kilogram dose is required in young children. Some systemically ill children require and tolerate much higher doses to achieve a therapeutic level (Tables 3.8, 3.9); this is especially true in children receiving concomitant prednisone therapy (Fig. 3.15). One of our sickest patients with malabsorption and concomitant steroid therapy required 300 mg/kg/day; some children require six doses daily for control of fever.

In patients who tolerate an average dose without adverse symptoms and whose disease is controlled with that dose, salicylate levels need not be measured. However, in patients requiring dosage regulation to achieve control of the disease or in those who develop signs of salicylism, blood levels are measured[190,191] and the dose is adjusted. Salicylate levels reach their peak 9 days after the initiation of steady-dose therapy and tend to fall off slightly

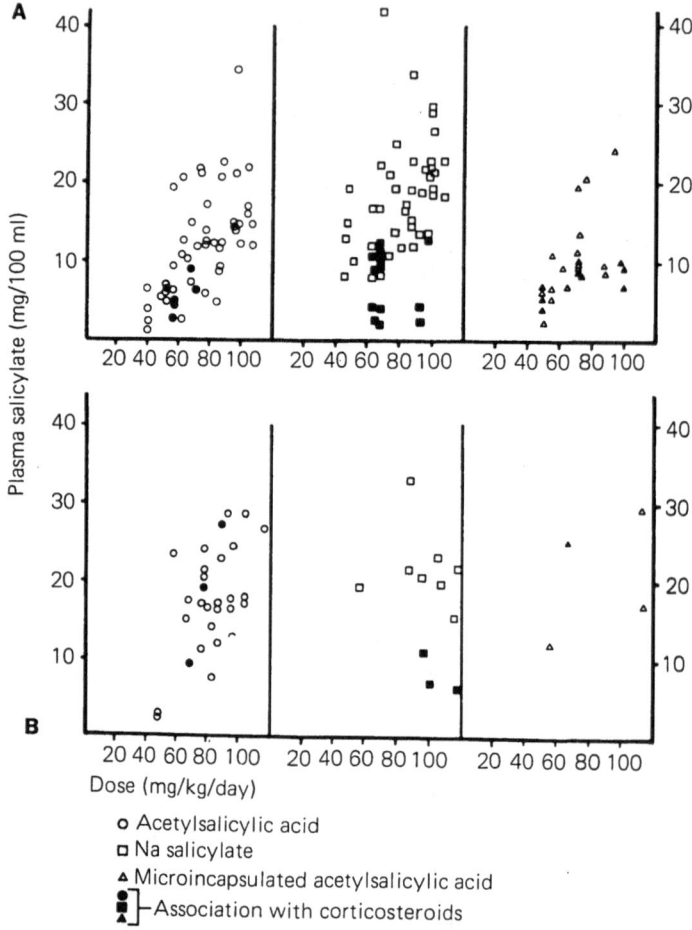

Figure 3.13. Great interindividual variability of plasma salicylate levels is shown in children receiving the same dose, both as outpatients (**A**) and inpatients (**B**). For example, in 14 patients taking sodium salicylate as outpatients, a daily dose between 99 and 106 mg/kg (mean, 101 mg) yielded plasma salicylate concentrations ranging from 15 to 30 mg/dl in different individuals; similarly, a daily dose of acetylsalicylic acid (ASA) between 78 and 83 mg/kg (mean, 80 mg) in outpatients gave plasma salicylate levels varying from 6 to 24 mg/dl in different children. Note lowering of levels caused by additions of corticosteroids. (Reprinted with permission from Bardare et al.[191])

thereafter.[192] At high serum levels, small-dosage increments may result in considerable increases in serum levels.[193] We generally increase by no more than 10% at one time. Similarly, if toxicity occurs, a reduction in dosage of 10% is often adequate to reach a tolerable therapeutic level (Table 3.9). Levels vary widely in the same patients,[191,193] often related to activity. More activity seems to reduce the serum level in a given individual.[194] Noncom

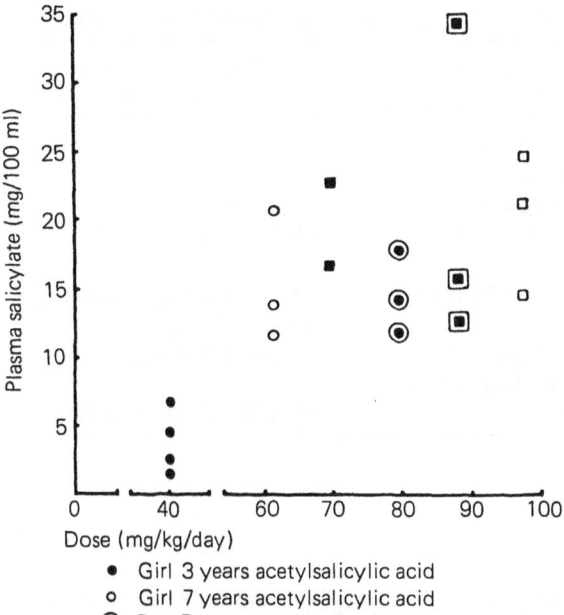

Figure 3.14. Daily plasma salicylate levels differ greatly in the same individual receiving the same dose as shown; in a 3-year-old boy, the level varied from 12 to 34 mg/dl despite steady dosing with 90 mg/kg and obtaining specimens under identical circumstances regarding time after last dose. (From Bardare et al.,[191] Reproduced with permission of the authors and the editor of *Archives of Disease in Childhood.*)

● Girl 3 years acetylsalicylic acid
○ Girl 7 years acetylsalicylic acid
◉ Boy 5 years acetylsalicylic acid
□ Boy 4 years acetylsalicylic acid
■ Girl 2 years Na salicylate
▣ Boy 3 years Na salicylate

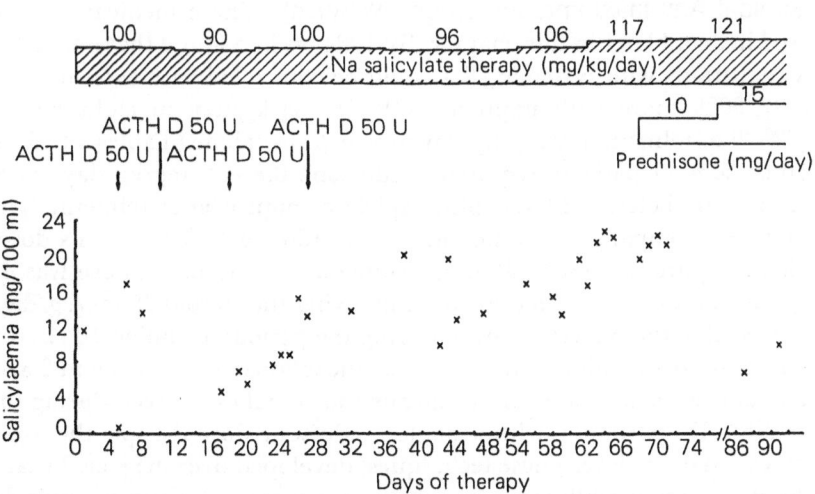

Figure 3.15. The addition of corticosteroids causes a prompt reduction in plasma salicylate levels. In a patient receiving daily prednisone, a high dose of salicylate (121 mg/kg/day) yields only a very low salicylate level (9 mg/dl). It is impossible to prescribe appropriate amounts of salicylate to patients receiving concomitant corticosteroid therapy without measuring the salicylate level until the patient is receiving a steady dose of both drugs. (Reprinted with permission from Bardare et al.[191])

Table 3.9. Regimens Used to Control Fever in Systemic JRA (10 new patients)

Regimen	Number of children controlled with this regimen	Regimens which failed in these patients
Aspirin	2 (sal level 25–39; 130–150 kg; 6 doses)	
Tolmetin.	1 (30 kg; 5 doses)	ASA, Tol 20/kg
Naproxen	2 (9–20kg; 3 doses)	ASA, Tol 20–40/kg
Tolmetin + Prednisone q.o.d.	3 (40 kg; 0.6–1/kg q.o.d.)	ASA, Nap 23/kg; Tol 30/kg
Naproxen + Prednisone q.o.d.	1 (25kg; 1/kg q.o.d.)	ASA, Tol 20 kg + Pred 2/kg q.o.d.
Aspirin + Prednisone q.o.d.	1 (110–180 alt kg; 0.8 kg q.o.d.)	ASA, Tol 32 kg, Nap 20/kg

From Jacobs, ref. 198, with permission.

pliance is also a common cause of variable levels.[86] Tinnitus is not a reliable guide to salicylate levels.[195] Careful regulation of salicylate levels protects the child from unnecessary exposure to more toxic agents. The important pharmacokinetic considerations for achieving optimal salicylate dosage are listed in Table 3.10.

Nonsteroidal Anti-Inflammatory Drugs (NSAIDs). These medications are discussed in detail later in this chapter. By 1984 we had found that only 20% of new registrants with systemic JRA could be controlled with aspirin alone and only 30% more with naproxen (19–25 mg/kg/day in eight hourly doses)[196,197] or tolmetin (30 mg/kg/day in five doses) alone (Tables 3.8, 3.9). The other 50% of patients required prednisone 0.6–1.0 mg/kg/day every second morning before 7:30 A.M. plus aspirin or naproxen or tolmetin. The aspirin dose accompanying the steroid *averaged* 150 mg/kg/day and six doses were often required on the "off"-prednisone day; the tolmetin dose was 40 mg/kg/day and the naproxen dose accompanying the steroid 25 mg/kg/day. Sometimes all of the NSAID is given during the period beginning 10 P.M. on the night of steroid administration or 6 A.M. the following morning and 2 A.M. the "on" day; for some patients this means the actual dose given during the 24 h of NSAID alternating with a single prednisone dose is triple the usual recommended daily dose. These techniques, developed over the past 7 years, have been extremely helpful to us in achieving control of patients without the need for daily steroids.

Slower-acting Agents. If despite maximally tolerated salicylate or NSAID treatment, a patient cannot attend school or lead a relatively normal life, corticosteroids are necessary (Fig. 3.16). Standard "slower-acting" agents,

Table 3.10. Important Pharmacokinetic Considerations for Achieving Optimal Salicylate Dosage

Pharmacokinetic studies show half-life varies with tissue saturation.
  High-dose steady state not achieved for 7–9 days.
  At high levels, small dosage changes cause large variations in serum levels.

Urinary excretion varies greatly with small changes in urine pH.
  Scrum levels are greatly increased by small decreases in urine pH.
  Serum levels are greatly decreased by small increases in urine pH.

Great interindividual variation in dose is required to achieve the same level.
Great intraindividual variation in serum levels occurs at different times in the same
  patient on the same dose.
Great variation in tolerated and effective levels in different children.

Addition of corticosteroids to therapeutic regimen causes reduction in the salicylate
  level and requires considerable increase in salicylate dose to achieve prior level.
Removal of corticosteroids from the therapeutic regimen causes increase in the salicylate level and poisoning if not carefully monitored.

Systemically ill and anemic patients often require high doses due to malabsorption
  and/or altered metabolism of salicylate.

Note: Salicylate increases blood alcohol concentrations.[200]

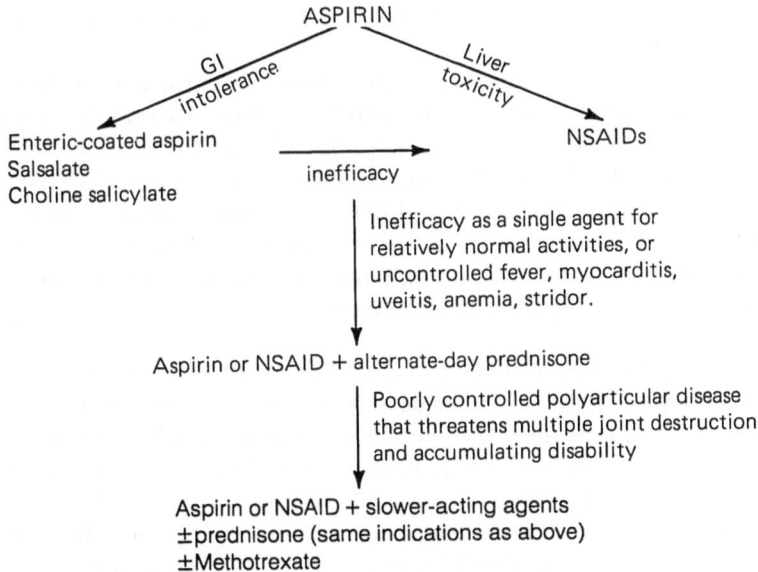

Figure 3.16. Treatment module for childhood arthritis.

Table 3.11. Indications for Systemic Corticosteroid Therapy in JRA

Fever that cannot be controlled with any NSAID
Myocarditis
Tamponade not controlled with intrapericardial steroid injection
Uveitis not controlled with local steroids
Intolerable anemia
Inability to ambulate
Disseminated intravasular coagulation (DIC)
Acute laryngeal stridor

discussed in the section on polyarticular disease, may also help in the control of arthritis in systemic-onset patients,[199] but not generally during the acute phase.

Corticosteroids. When fever and polyarthritis cannot be controlled with maximum regimens of nonsteroidal anti-inflammatory agents, it may be necessary to add prednisone to the regimen (Tables 3.9 and 3.11). It is always preferable and usually possible to use an alternate-day regimen. Most children with disease that requires steroids can be adequately managed with full doses of aspirin or another NSAID and a "boost" of a small dose of prednisone every second morning (10–15 mg god). Very sick children who cannot be controlled with ordinary alternate-day steroid supplements usually will respond to surprisingly large alternate-day doses of prednisome (3 mg/kg/dose) or whatever dose is required to control their unimaginable pain, fever, and anemia. The regimen must be individualized for each child. Monitoring of prednisone blood levels is complicated and not yet generally available.[201]

The adverse effects of long-term glucocorticoid therapy are well known to the clinician (Table 3.12).[202] Alternate-day steroid therapy has provided the physician with the ability to slow progression of the disease and avoid bed-chair crippling with an acceptable amount of steroid toxicity. Even "astronomically" high alternate-day doses are better tolerated than daily steroids.[203–206] Corticosteroids, therefore, if administered skillfully, are the tool that avoids bed-chair crippling, whereas if misused, these same drugs can cause increased crippling or even death.

Alterations in Salicylate Dosage Required after Introduction of Supplemental Corticosteroids. It has been repeatedly demonstrated that salicylate levels fall after the introduction of corticosteroids to the therapeutic regimen (Figs. 3.13, 3.15, and 3.17). Even a single injection of steroids into a joint lowers salicylate levels dramatically for up to 5 days.[209] Therefore, when adding prednisone, it is necessary to redetermine the salicylate level and increase the dose of salicylates to maintain maximum-tolerated serum level.[191,210] If the physician is not alert to this phenomenon, there may be a

Table 3.12. Adverse Effects of Glucocorticoid Therapy

Metabolic
  Central obesity
  Glucose intolerance
  Hyperosmolar nonketotic coma
  Hyperlipidemia
Endocrine
  Hypothalamic-pituitary-adrenal axis suppression
  Growth failure in children
  Menstrual irregularities
Musculoskeletal
  Osteoporosis
  Aseptic necrosis of bone
  Myopathy acutely worsened by pancuronium bromide
    (Pavulon)[207]
Cutaneous
  Thin, fragile skin
  Purpura
  Striae
  Acne
  Hirsutism
  Impaired wound healing
Ocular
  Posterior subcapsular cataracts
  Glaucoma
Central nervous system
  Psychiatric disorders
  Pseudotumor cerebri
Cardiovascular-renal
  Sodium and water retention
  Hypokalemic alkalosis
  Hypertension
  Premature atherosclerosis[208]
Gastrointestinal
  Pancreatitis
  Peptic ulcer
  Intestinal perforation
Impaired immune response
  Bacterial, viral, fungal, and parasitic infections

(Modified with permission from Nelson and Conn, ref. 202, p. 766.)

tendency to continuously increase the prednisone dosage, resulting in further lowering of the salicylate level and the need for more prednisone. Although this principle has been repeatedly emphasized, our experience suggests that it is repeatedly neglected even by experienced rheumatologists.

It is equally important to be alert to the potential for salicylate poisoning

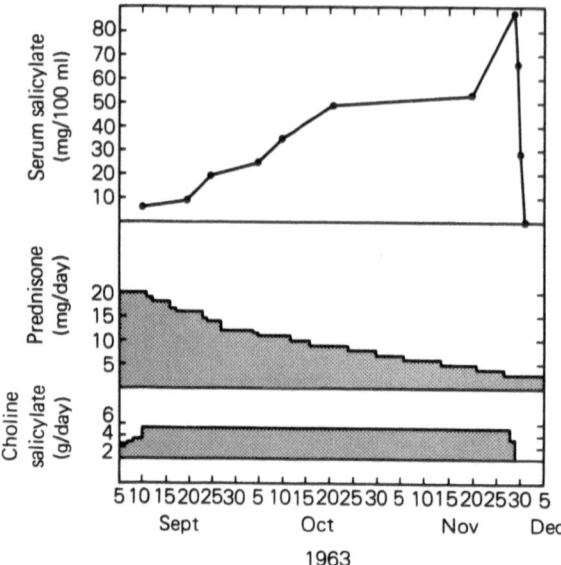

Figure 3.17. Dramatic progressive salicylate poisoning of a 5-year-old boy with JRA produced by gradual withdrawal of prednisone while maintaining a steady dose of salicylate. Note that initially, while receiving prednisone (1 mg/kg/day), a salicylate level of only 10 mg/dl was achieved despite the administration of about 250 mg of salicylate/kg/day. (Reprinted with permission from Klinenberg and Miller, ref. 210. Copyright 1965, American Medical Association.)

when lowering the dose of prednisone administered to children also receiving aspirin. In this circumstance, salicylate levels rise, and the dose of aspirin may have to be adjusted downward to avoid poisoning (Fig. 3.17).[191,210] We teach these principles to the parents of our patients, who can then determine when to measure the levels and are often able to make the necessary adjustments in dosage without instructions from the physician.

Salicylate Toxicity. Flavored tablets must be dissolved (not chewed) and ingestion must be followed by liquid to avoid dental carries.[211] Children tolerate aspirin well, and dyspepsia is rare. However, for many children with systemic and polyarticular disease, effective treatment demands a salicylate level close to toxicity.[188–190]

If adequate control of a child's arthritis requires maximum-tolerated doses of aspirin, it goes without saying that the parent must be aware of the signs of salicylate poisoning. Contrary to medical folklore, tinnitus does not correlate well with salicylate levels.[195] When aspirin treatment is begun, we advise the parent of the three cardinal signs of too much aspirin (Table 3.13):

1. *Change in personality for the worse.* In general, after institution of aspirin therapy in the arthritic child, there is improvement in disposition with relief of pain and inflammation. After a week, if aspirin levels increase to toxic proportions, there will be a behavioral regression, with irritability and emotional lability, requiring measurement of the level, prompt report (2 h), and reduction in dosage.
2. *Fast breathing.* Although all children with high salicylate levels breathe more rapidly than normal, a greatly increased respiratory rate simulating

Table 3.13. Cardinal Signs of Salicylate Toxicity

Change in personality for the worse (irritability, lability, depression, withdrawal)
Fast breathing ("croup")
Nausea (anorexia) or vomiting

dyspnea or croup should be assumed, in these children, to represent salicylate poisoning, requiring prompt measurement of the serum level prior to any further salicylate administration.

3. *Nausea and vomiting.* Most children with systemic JRA requiring maximum salicylate levels will have improved appetites as fever and pain are controlled. However, if the salicylate level then climbs to toxic proportions, the improvement in appetite will be replaced by anorexia followed by nausea and, if the dosage is not then reduced, by repetitive vomiting. Sometimes a child vomits only occasionally, usually shortly after taking the medicine, as the sole manifestation of too much aspirin, presumably because levels are too high only intermittently. Parents and physicians can be alert to this potential by recognizing that any vomiting requires measurement of the salicylate level. Parents often assume vomiting to be a result of a viral illness. No such assumption is permissible unless the salicylate level has been measured and demonstrated to be nontoxic. Viral illnesses are common in children and may result in lowering of salicylate levels due to vomiting of medications or increases in levels due to relative dehydration from the illness; we cannot distinguish one from the other without the salicylate level. Our office and hospital staff is trained to obtain these levels at any time at the request of any of our patients (without formality) and to promptly provide the results in our absence to the parents, who are aware of the desired therapeutic levels and the technique of dosage omission and regulation. In order to care for arthritic children adequately, salicylate levels must be available 24 h/day with 2-h reporting. Less than this will result in increased use of more toxic secondary agents in these children. A technique for microsalicylate determinations ensures greater patient/parent compliance in toddlers.[190]

Reye's Syndrome. Almost everyone interprets the available data as supporting an increased risk of Reye's syndrome in children taking aspirin and, perhaps, nonaspirin salicylates.[212] In certain centers caring for arthritic children, Reye's syndrome occurs in frightening numbers of their patients;[213,214] in other centers, such as our own, there have been no cases despite 30 years of high-dose aspirin administration to large numbers of patients. This remains an enigma.

Parents now stop aspirin when they know their children are exposed to varicella. Influenza may be asymptomatic in more than 50% of cases and children are frequently exposed to others with viral illnesses which could be influenza; stopping medication with each viral exposure is impractical, and there is no evidence at all that stopping the aspirin at the time of exposure reduces the risk. The need to administer influenza vaccine to arthritic children yearly, sometimes with considerable adverse reaction and always with inconvenience and expense of yet another needle, discourages most parents in New York from choosing aspirin as the drug of choice for their arthritic children though it may be the safest agent.[215]

Bleeding as Result of Salicylate Administration. This particular toxic side effect of aspirin administration deserves special consideration. Tiny doses of aspirin have long been recognized to have the potential to cause bleeding in those with hemophilia.[216] Occasionally, patients with bleeding disorders secondary to abnormalities of platelet aggregation report bleeding with aspirin.[217] What was not initially recognized was that this might be paradoxically dose-related. Recent evidence suggests that this effect may not be seen in patients receiving high doses of aspirin.[218] Bleeding time may also not be further increased in such patients by the nonacetylated salicylate preparations, salicylsalicylic acid (salsalate; Disalcid), and choline magnesium salicylate (Trilisate; see below).[219]

Easy bruisability may result from prolongation of the prothrombin time in children receiving chronic aspirin therapy.[220] Even in children in whom the determination of prothrombin time is normal, vitamin K, 5 mg orally daily, may be reported by patients to reduce bruisability and nosebleeds.

Significant gastrointestinal hemorrhage is a rare complication of aspirin administration in children. Controversy exists over whether such hemorrhage occurs only in those with primary coagulation defects or whether it can occur in normals as well.[221,222] When such hemorrhage occurs in children treated with aspirin alone, it is generally a result of gastric bleeding.

Salicylates and the Liver. When the SGOT/SGPT tests became available, it was observed that patients with rheumatic fever being treated with large doses of aspirin frequently had elevated levels of these "liver" enzymes. No harmful effects were reported associated with these chance laboratory observations.[223] Subsequent studies in arthritic children, coincident with the institution of machine determinations of multiple blood chemistries, revealed that unrecognized asymptomatic elevations of "liver" enzyme (below 400 units) occurred with aspirin therapy in 25% of children with arthritis, were often dose-related, tended to disappear with reduction of dose or with time alone, and generally seemed to have no pathologic consequences.[224] Nevertheless, it remains possible that subtle symptoms or liver damage might occur in such children.[225] It seems reasonable not to discontinue aspirin and institute more toxic agents solely because of chance laboratory observations, but if equal control of the arthritis can be achieved with agents of equal or less toxicity without these abnormalities, it would seem the prudent course to change to those agents. Thus, only in the case of severe life-threatening elevations in enzymes would it be worth instituting daily corticosteroids as an alternative to aspirin, but at even lower levels of enzyme abnormality, consideration should be given to trying other nonsteroidal anti-inflammatory agents that do not raise the level of SGOT/SGPT. These drugs may be instituted on the same day the aspirin is withdrawn, and the liver enzyme abnormalities, if caused by aspirin, generally are eliminated within a few days.[226]

A small number of children develop symptomatic hepatotoxic effects of salicylate with elevations of SGOT/SGPT over 1000 units, tender hepatomegaly, vomiting, and a prolonged prothrombin time. Continuation of aspirin therapy may result in serious, even fatal, hepatotoxicity. In most studies, this intolerance occurs more frequently in systemically ill patients, especially those with little or no arthritis, who may represent a different subset with more primary hepatic involvement.

It is our policy to measure SGOT/SGPT in all patients prior to instituting therapy and during the period of dosage regulation. These enzymes are also measured in patients with abdominal pain or malaise and in those manifesting symptoms of salicylate toxicity.

Occasionally, using choline salicylate in lieu of other salicylate preparation results in less hepatotoxicity.[189] In some children who cannot tolerate salicylates, other nonsteroidal anti-inflammatory agents can be substituted successfully without hepatoxicity. However, while these agents are rarely hepatotoxic, the same patients who cannot tolerate salicylates sometimes cannot tolerate these agents, either. In other children, adequate control of fever is not achieved with these agents, at least with currently accepted dosage and with our inability to measure serum levels to identify those who might require a higher dose to achieve a meaningful serum level (due to altered absorption, metabolism, or excretion). A stratagem that we generally find effective in very difficult situations in which serious salicylate hepatotoxicity occurs and no other agent provides adequate control is the use of alternate-day steroids plus aspirin. Some children will tolerate a required and otherwise intolerable salicylate level when taking relatively small doses (1 mg/kg) of alternate-day prednisone in addition to salicylate. The mechanism by which the prednisone protects the liver in this situation is speculative.

Gastritis and Ulcers. Within a few minutes of aspirin ingestion, gastric acidity increases, presumably as a result of back-diffusion of hydrogen ions in the mucosa. Whether salicylate administered systemically has a similar effect is controversial.[227] Animal experiments suggest that the mucosa develops some resistance to this effect with chronic administration.[222]

The weight of evidence suggests that gastric and duodenal ulcers are associated with heavy aspirin usage.[222,227a] There is some evidence of increased susceptibility to ulcers in patients with RA even without salicylate treatment. In our experience, duodenal ulcers are not uncommon in arthritic children. While the role of aspirin in the causation of these ulcers may be controversial, there is no question that patients with peptic or duodenal ulcer disease are less tolerant of aspirin than normal and suffer from worse dyspepsia than others.[222]

We have seen no instance of major gastrointestinal bleeding from duodenal ulcer in an arthritic child treated with aspirin alone; the same cannot be said for combinations of aspirin with corticosteroids and indomethacin, which have in one instance each resulted in uncontrollable hemorrhage requiring gastrectomy in two children under the age of 5. These experiences have sensitized us so that we treat ulcer symptoms by changing to enteric-coated aspirin and providing frequent milk feeds, sucralfate, and antacids if there is nocturnal ulcer pain. In the presence of documented ulcers H2 blockers are also administered. Misoprostol, a protaglandin E1 analog prescribed for the prophylaxis and healing of peptic ulceration associated with NSAID use, has not been studied in children but may be useful.[228]

The toxic effects of salicylates have been overemphasized when compared to their therapeutic benefits and the billions of tablets consumed each year.[222] Aspirin has been accused of causing analgesic nephropathy, but there is no proof of a single case in a child receiving aspirin alone.[130,131,229] Although hearing may be temporarily reduced, especially at high frequencies, there is no evidence that permanent hearing loss results from chronic aspirin administration. There are a great many other metabolic, endocrinologic, hematologic, and immunologic effects of aspirin administration that are adequately reviewed elsewhere.[182,230]

Special Aspirin Preparations. There is increasing evidence that enteric-coated aspirin produces fewer gastroduodenal erosions.[231] Some children with dyspepsia who cannot tolerate regular aspirin will tolerate enteric-coated aspirin and absorb it well, attaining adequate and reliably constant salicylate levels.[232] In these youngsters, there is no reason not to use enteric-coated tablets.[233] Not all enteric-coated tablets are equally well absorbed.[234,235] In one study, Ecotrin was best absorbed, and this and Easprin (975 mg) are the sole enteric-coated tablets in use in our clinic. We have sometimes seen even these tablets undigested and whole in the stool of our patients.

Sustained-Release Aspirin. These tablets are constructed so as to provide sustained release over an 8-h period, presumably providing better nighttime and early morning blood levels and fewer peaks and troughs. This is achieved by partial absorption in the stomach and the rest in the small intestine.[236] Controversy exists as to whether sustained serum salicylate levels are really better achieved during chronic administration of these costly tablets. However, some patients with dyspepsia who do not absorb enteric-coated tablets will do well with sustained-release tablets.

Older children hate to take medicines in school both because the other children will "see" and because many schools require the children to go to the nurse's office to have their medicine administered to them. These antiquated countertherapeutic school regulations infantilize and isolate our handicapped children, who we wish to become responsible for their own care and self-sufficient despite their handicaps. American Academy of Pediatrics policy for school health advocates children being permitted to take their own medications in school.[237]

Any medication with a long-enough half-life or a sustained-release tablet which allows teenagers to avoid taking medicines in school may be advantageous and worth considerable additional expense. In adults, better compliance has been shown to be achieved with less frequent dosage schedules, resulting in better control of arthritis by drugs with a long half-life when compared with equipotent medications that require more frequent administration.[238]

Other Forms of Salicylate. Salsalate and choline magnesium trisalicylate are hydrolyzed in vivo to salicylic acid and so presumably have comparable activity to aspirin. They are nonacetylated and therefore presumably do not affect platelet aggregation.[219] Salicylate levels can be determined and regulated just as when aspirin is administered, providing a mechanism to determine compliance and optimal dosage. These preparations are much more expensive than aspirin (Table 3.7) but have provided control of disease in some children who could not take aspirin.

Salsalate (salicylsalicylic acid), marketed in the United States under the trade name Disalcid, is available only in nondissolvable tablet form, with each tablet equal to 500 mg of salicylate. Dosage regulation is the same as for aspirin; presumably, medication can be administered at 8-h intervals. Salsalate commonly produces abnormalities in routine thyroid function tests similar to those found in central hypothyroidism.[238a]

Choline salicylate is also available in tablet form as choline magnesium trisalicylate. This product (Trilisate) is reported to be useful in some patients who cannot tolerate aspirin but has not been tested in children. Tablets (500 mg, 750 mg, and 1000 mg of active ingredient) contain more than half of the salicylate as the magnesium salt, which might cause diarrhea in some children. A palatable syrup (500 mg/tsp) is available.

While choline salicylate liquid has been very useful in pediatric rheumatologic practice, its presence in the household is akin to the threat of oil of wintergreen, another potent salicylate liquid that has resulted in death as a result of toddler ingestion. We tend not to prescribe choline salicylate when there are toddlers in the home who may accidentally ingest it and are careful to warn parents to keep it locked up at all times.

Treatment of Pericarditis and Myocarditis

Mild pericarditis can often be successfully treated with aspirin alone.[86,88,90,91,93] Colchicine may also be helpful.[239] However, when pericar-

Look for Beck's Triad

Distended neck veins
(or high CVP, venous
hypertension)

Distant heart sounds

Arterial hypotension

Also note:

Cyanosis, air hunger
(Patient may be disturbed,
anxious, or wildly agitated;
in later stages, CNS de-
pression, coma, cardiac
arrest)

Possible increased area
of cardiac dullness out-
side the apical point of
maximal impulse

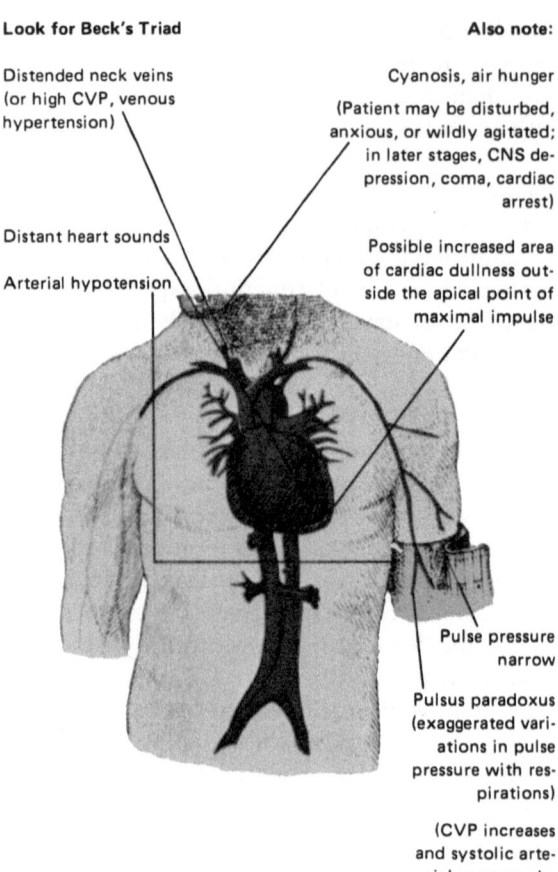

Pulse pressure
narrow

Pulsus paradoxus
(exaggerated vari-
ations in pulse
pressure with res-
pirations)

(CVP increases
and systolic arte-
rial pressure de-
creases during
inspiration)

Figure 3.18. Pericardial tamponade may occur in children
with systemic JRA and de-
mands prompt diagnosis and
therapy. Of 80 patients with
tamponade reported by
Shoemaker, 87% had one or
more signs of Beck's triad, but
only 35% showed all three.
These findings may occur
rather late in the course. If
treatment is delayed until all
the classic signs of the triad
are present, cardiac arrest is
likely to intervene. (Reprinted
with permission from *Hospital
Medicine*, November 1978,
copyright by Hospital Publications, Inc.)

ditis and myocarditis are life-threatening (Fig. 3.18), prednisone should be instituted promptly (2 mg/kg/day in four divided doses).[86,88,90–92,94]

When steroids are to be administered to patients in congestive heart failure, it is useful to give an injection of furosemide 1 h prior to the first dose of steroid. This helps avoid further fluid overload. Potassium losses may be increased by both diuretics and steroids. Supplemental potassium may be given if necessary. Miller has suggested that death may result from digitalis-induced arrhythmia in these children.[91] Patients with myocarditis are very prone to arrhythmia, and digitalis should, therefore, be avoided.[240]

Aspirin is not given initially to these patients because of the risk of increasing cardiac failure due to the increased metabolic rate induced by aspirin. After congestive heart failure has been controlled with prednisone, aspirin therapy is instituted. During concomitant steroid therapy, large doses of aspirin may be required to achieve an adequate salicylate level. The change to alternate-day prednisone (usually 150 mg qod) is then made. The salicylate dosage may have to be gradually reduced if, due to reduction in steroid dosage (see above), serum salicylate begins to rise to toxic levels. This regimen allows rather prompt discharge from the hospital with gradual reduction of alternate-day prednisone (maintaining steady serum salicylate levels) over a period of several months, avoiding rebound exacerbations.

We have experience so far with only one case treated with intrapericardial injection of corticosteroids as the sole treatment for pericardial tamponade in an arthritic child but have also used this regimen as an emergency supplement. This technique was reported initially by Scharf et al. in 1976[241] and is based on considerable reported experience in adults with tamponade associated with renal dialysis.[242,243] In our case, we injected 200 mg of triamcinolone hexacetonide (Aristospan 20 mg/cc) at the time of tamponade, continuing high-dose oral aspirin but giving no systemic steroids. Removal of fluid at the time of the pericardiocentesis relieved the immediate problem; following the injection of steroids, there was no reaccumulation of fluid (Fig. 3.19). Had there been reaccumulation, we were prepared to offer a second injection. While this treatment is unusual, it does seem to offer a simple, safe, and effective bedside procedure in place of months of oral prednisone administration. We have used this approach in Kawasaki disease and the postpericardectomy syndrome and are determined to use it as our first approach to all children with tamponade from JRA provide the fluid is anterior so the procedure can be safely accomplished.

Treatment of Laryngeal Stridor

When systemic JRA presents with airway (cricoarytenoid) obstruction, corticosteroids should be promptly administered. After the obstruction has been relieved, salicylates are introduced and steroids gradually weaned away.[114]

Polyarticular Juvenile Rheumatoid Arthritis

All forms of arthritis may be polyarticular both in onset or course. The real significance of "polyarticular" is the implication of symmetrical destructive disease in many joints (Fig. 3.20). Later age of onset and involvement of many joints of the fingers, hands, and wrists are associated with poorer prognosis than polyarticular disease primarily limited to the lower extremities.[244,245] These prognostic determinants are the same in JRA and in young adult arthritics.[246]

Adverse prognosis in polyarticular JRA is most closely correlated with the *consistent* presence of *significant amounts* of rheumatoid factor.[57] It is thus useful to subdivide polyarticular-onset JRA into "seropositive" and "seronegative" subsets.

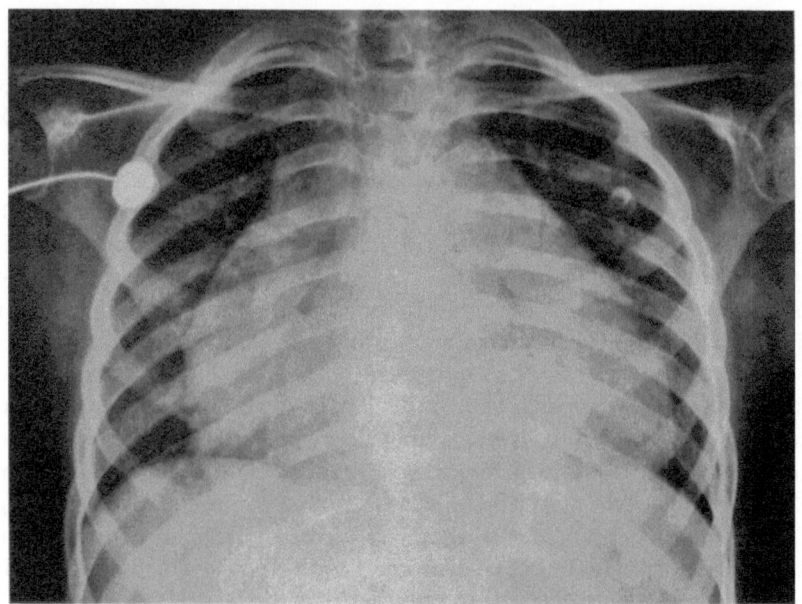

A

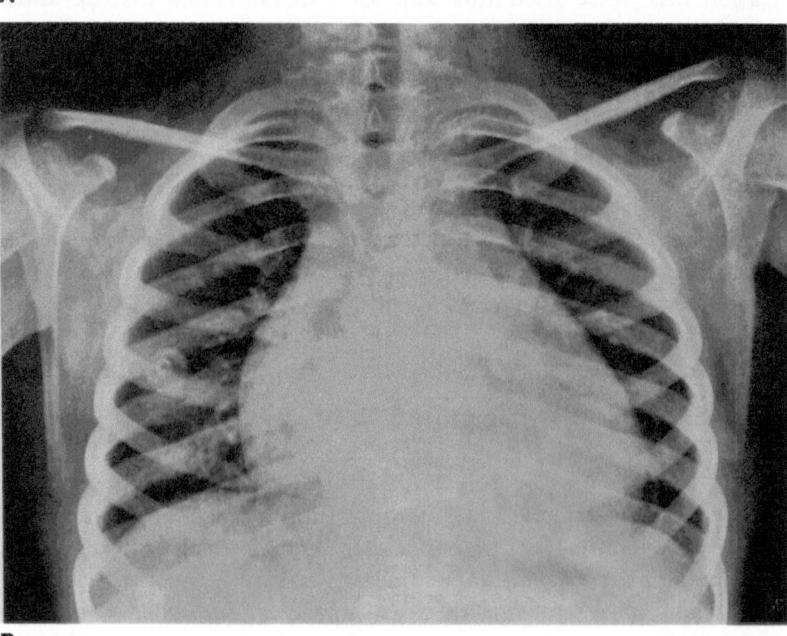

B

Figure 3.19. (A) Severe cardiomegaly shown in a chest film of a child with systemic JRA with pericarditis and tamponade despite aspirin therapy. **(B)** Repeat film 2 days later, after injection of depot steroids into the pericardial sac. No other treatment was necessary; the patient continued to receive aspirin, and all evidence of pericarditis gradually disappeared.

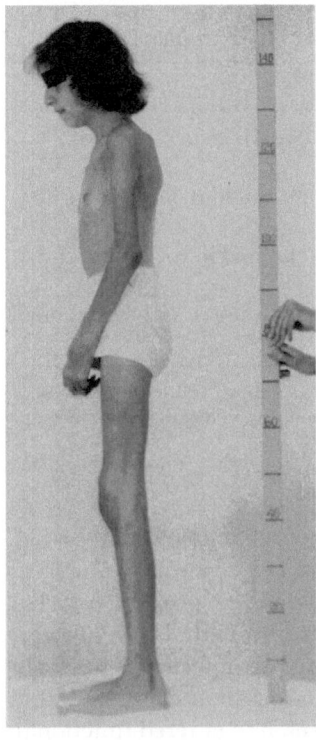

Figure 3.20. Poorly controlled polyarticular JRA affecting essentially all joints symmetrically and causing depression, delayed puberty, and dwarfing of this 13-year-old girl.

Epidemiology and Prognosis

Polyarticular Seropositive JRA. (Childhood Onset Classic Adult RA).[16] Most arthritic children with consistently significantly positive tests for rheumatoid factor are girls, have the onset of disease after age 8, have rheumatoid nodules, do not remit,[248] and have severe progressive disease with extensive radiographic changes. In one series, after an average of less than 5 years, 50% had reached class III or IV disability[5] (Table 3.14). The childhood early onset of this adult form of RA is thus associated with a very poor functional prognosis, indicating that girls affected this early have a special propensity for the disorder. This group represents less than 7% of the total JRA population in older reports and less than 3% of arthritic children currently being registered in our clinic. In both adults and children this subset of RA has been associated with HLA-DR4,[249] and severity correlates with levels of both IgM and IgG rheumatoid factor.[250] Aggressive therapy is necessary from the moment of onset.[251]

Polyarticular Seronegative JRA. Previously reported series of seronegative polyarticular JRA include some patients who have what we would now term

Table 3.14. Classification of Functional Status in Rheumatoid Arthritis (ACR)*[247]

Class	Characteristics
I	Completely able to perform usual acitivities of daily living (self-care, vocational, and avocational)
II	Able to perform usual self-care and vocational activities, but limited in avocational activities
III	Able to perform usual self-care activities, but limited in vocational and avocational activities
IV	Limited in ability to perform usual self-care, vocational, and avocational activities

*Usual self-care activities include dressing, feeding, bathing, grooming, and toileting. Avocational (recreational and/or leisure) and vocational (work, school, homemaking) activities are patient-desired and age- and sex-specific.

HLA-B27-associated spondyloarthritis with more joints involved than usual (see Chapter 4) and some patients with slightly more severe forms of pauciarticular JRA. However, we mean primarily to include in this group a population whose disease most resembles seropositive early onset adult RA but who do not have rheumatoid factor. Girls are more frequently affected. The ANA test is positive in 25% of these patients. Rheumatoid nodules are rare. After an average of 7 years of disease, 15% of these children had entered functional class III or IV as a result of very severe joint destruction.[5] While the prognosis is not good for the children, it is much better than that of the seropositive group.

Clinical Features

Onset. By the time they get to the rheumatologist, most of these youngsters have obvious arthritis. However, prior to diagnosis, there is often a period of months during which arthritis is present but not recognized, although the physician knows they are ill with low-grade fever, lethargy, weight loss, and morning stiffness. In addition to symmetrical involvement of many large joints, especially the wrists, these children almost always have distal small-joint symmetrical arthritis involving the proximal interphalangeal (PIP) and metacarpophalangeal (MCP) joints. Other frequently affected joints include the interphalangeal toe joints, cervical spine, and temporomandibular joints. Synovial outpocketings or pouches are frequently seen overlying the wrists (tenosynovitis) (Fig. 3.6). Joints are frequently warm but usually not tender. Effusions are easily demonstrated, and limitation of extension is apparent in many joints. Occasionally, patients have "dry" arthritis without effusions or warmth but with progressive flexion contractures. If routine pediatric examinations do not include examining the range of motion of joints, the diagnosis may be missed for years. Some of these patients, primarily girls, do not complain of pain despite obvious arthritis.[42,246,252]

Rheumatoid Nodules. Subcutaneous nodules near the olecranon process at the elbow are frequently palpable in seropositive arthritic children (Fig. 3.40B). Microscopic examination shows central necrosis and palisading fibroblasts, identical to the pathology in seropositive adult nodules (Fig. 3.21). Polyarticular arthritic children also sometimes have transient nodules over the interphalangeal joints of the fingers and toes. These tend to come and go with exacerbations of the disease. Some authors indicate slight pathologic differences between these nodules and those of adult RA.[253,254]

Course

Structure of the Joints. Rheumatoid arthritis primarily affects the synovial joints which are diarthroses; that is, a joint resembling a hinge, with a cavity and free movement.[255] The articulating bones are covered by a hyaline (glasslike) lining, the articular cartilage. The marginal nonarticulating connective tissue is called the synovial membrane (Fig. 3.22). This membrane provides the substances necessary for metabolism of articular cartilage and is the source of synovial fluid.

The joint is surrounded by a fibrous capsule. The bone is lined by a thin connective tissue membrane—the periosteum. Ligaments secure opposing bone surfaces and may attach to bone inside or outside the capsule. Tendons attach muscle to bone inside the capsule. The site of attachment of a ligament or tendon to bone is called an enthesis. The motion of tendons and muscles over bony prominences is facilitated by bursae, closed sacs lined with a protruding bursal (synovial) membrane. There are at least 156 bursae in the body.

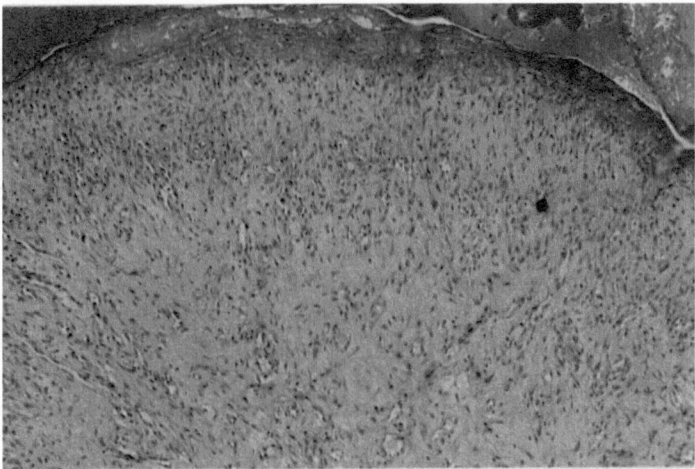

Figure 3.21. Rheumatoid nodule showing typical palisading granuloma. The patient was a 16-year-old boy with cystic fibrosis of the pancreas who developed seropositive rheumatoid arthritis.

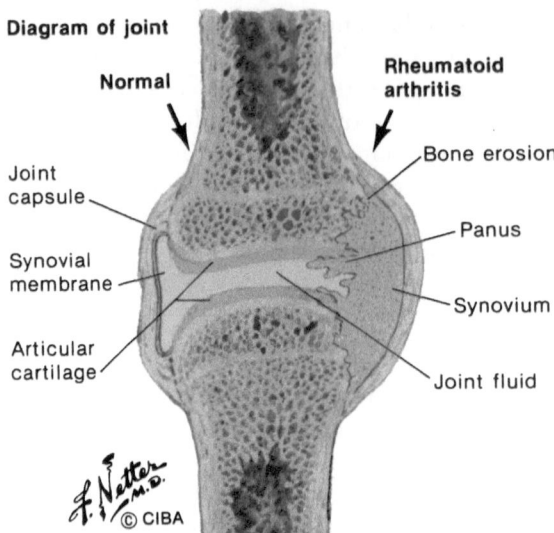

Figure 3.22. Diagrammatic representation of joint in rheumatoid arthritis. (Reprinted with permission from *Clinical Symposia* 31(4):23, 1979. Copyright by CIBA Laboratories.)

All of these structures may become inflamed and contribute to pathology in and around the joints.[254] Although the potential exists for varying types of inflammation to constitute different forms of arthritis, sorting out these differences remains to be accomplished. However, the recognition of the importance of the more frequent, severe, and calcifying inflammation at the enthesis in HLA-B27-associated spondyloarthritis provides a clue indicating that immunogenetic techniques may help in identifying different pathophysiologic processes now grouped under one umbrella (JRA or RA) (see Chapter 4).

Pathologic Considerations

The diverse group of diseases we call JRA, induced by a variety of genetically controlled responses to different environmental stimuli, all have in common inflammation in and around the joint. This inflammation seems to be perpetuated by immunologic events rather than by continued active infection.[256]

Synovium. The inflammatory reaction in the synovium begins with congestion and edema (Table 3.15). This is followed by cellular infiltration, at first with polymorphonuclear leukocytes, then with small lymphocytes, and in advanced cases with plasma cells and multinucleated giant cells. The synovial lining cells multiply, elongate, and palisade. Lymphoid follicles with germinal centers (Allison-Gormley nodules) form in some cases. Blood vessels proliferate and form granulation tissue. The synovium thickens in a villous fashion (Figs. 3.1, 3.22).

Articular Cartilage. In more severe cases, the inflammation extends from the synovium into the articular cartilage. A mantle of granulation tissue, a pan-

Table 3.15. Synovitis

Characteristics	Effects
Proliferation of synovial lining cells	Stretching of the capsule, ligaments, tendons
Infiltration of synovium by inflammatory cells	Granulomatous proliferation and villus formation
Effusion of fluid containing inflammatory cells	Invasion of tendons, cartilage, and bone by pannus and destruction by proteolytic enzymes
	Increased connective tissue producing stiffness and reduced range of motion
	Either capsuloligamentous laxity and hypermobility or fibrous ankylosis and ultimately bony ankylosis

nus, forms covering the bone and connecting the inflamed cartilage to the inflamed synovium (Fig. 3.22).

Destruction of cartilage by this inflammation leads to bony erosions. If the pannus continues to grow, the cartilage may be continually eroded until it disappears altogether.

Subchondral Bone. Continuous with the inflammation in the synovial tissue is osteitis, inflammation in the bone itself. Periarticular demineralization (osteolysis) is common in epiphyseal bone. If the epiphyseal plate is involved, growth is retarded, and dwarfism may result. Erosions and cystlike areas of destruction may be apparent. Osteoporosis also occurs from disuse.

Periosteum. The synovial recesses in the phalanges are large and extend for long distances along the phalanges. Therefore, synovitis in the proximal interphalangeal joints may be associated with concomitant periostitis in the immediately adjacent bone shaft. Periostitis without synovitis is not characteristic of JRA, although it may be seen in a variety of other disorders including syphilis and HLA-B27-associated spondyloarthritis. Periostitis is rare in JRA.

Ankylosis. Newly formed connective tissue, which constitutes the scar resulting from granulation tissue in and around the joints, may form fibrous contractures and articulations or may rarely even calcify, producing bony ankylosis.

Joint Deformities

Detailed description of the pathomechanics in each joint are beyond the scope of this monograph. In every joint, a balance exists between the muscles and tendons and the bones through which they exert their action. At first, capsular distension and bulging of the synovium may initiate deformity. If the invasive inflammatory synovium grows into the cartilage, tendons, and ligaments, the capsular and ligamentous supports weaken. Inflamed tendons may contract or rupture. Articular surfaces remodel under the forces of abnormal muscle pull. The healthy balance of forces is lost. Soft tissues contract, and there is fibrosis involving the capsule and periarticular tissues, resulting in loss of mobility of the joint. Subluxation may occur in severe disease (Figs. 3.23 and 3.24).

Bone Deformities

Unique deformities may occur in the growing skeleton. Chronic hyperemia may result in accelerated growth in affected growth centers (Fig. 3.25). An extremity or appendage may be elongated (Figs. 3.26 and 3.27). In the short bones, growth arrest may occur, resulting in permanent underdevelopment of a bone. If accelerated maturity results in asymmetric premature fusion of an epiphysis, the extremity may ultimately be shortened (Fig. 3.40B).

Systemic disease of all sorts inhibits growth, presumably as a result of

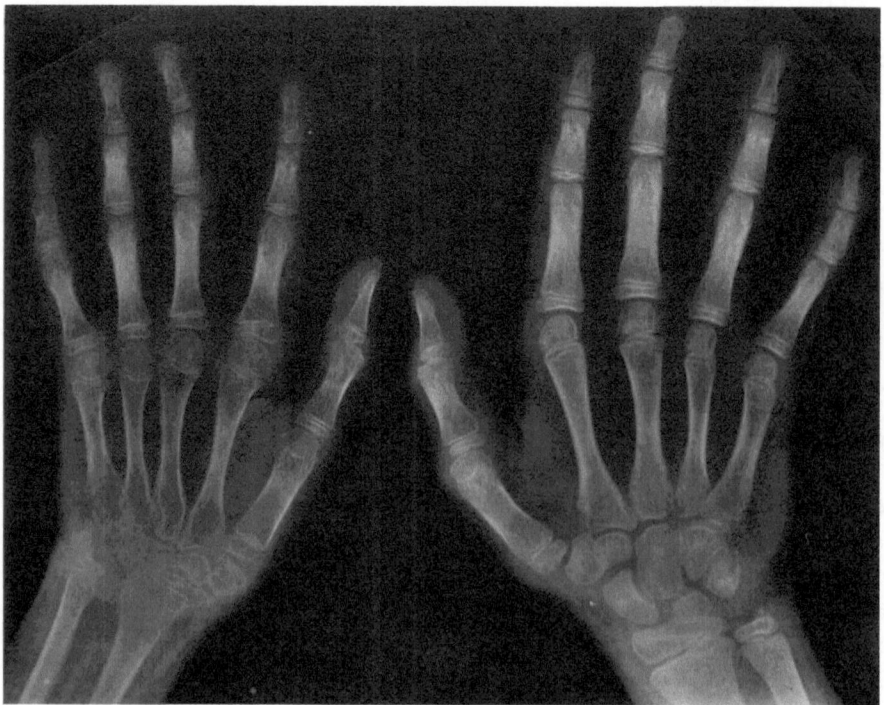

Figure 3.23. Severe arthritis of the left wrist in a 9-year-old girl with onset of pauciarticular seronegative, B27-negative arthritis at age 2 years.

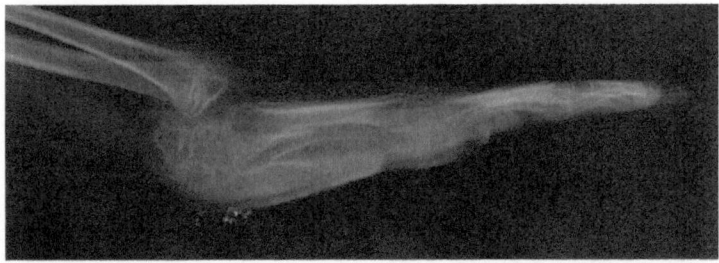

Figure 3.24. Lateral view of wrist shown in Fig. 3.23. This child, with minimal disease elsewhere, has "disappearing bones" (the "opera-glass hand") with severe subluxation.

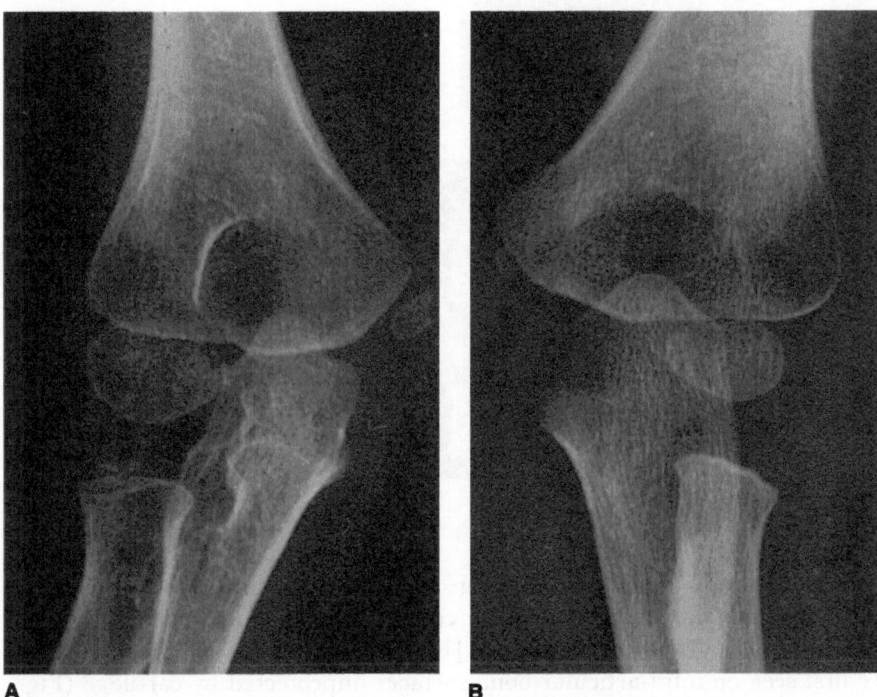

A   **B**

Figure 3.25. Growth disturbance in JRA with advanced skeletal maturation on the involved side and retarded maturation on the opposite side. Patient is a female, aged 3 years 9 months. Involved elbow (**A**) shows advanced skeletal maturation, 5 years, in involved areas. Uninvolved elbow (**B**) shows retardation in skeletal maturation, 2 years 8 months, in corresponding areas without local disease. (Reprinted with permission from Grokoest et al., ref. 42.)

end-organ inability to respond to growth hormone. Inflammation at the growth plate and deformities may also contribute to short stature. The administration of daily corticosteroids also arrests growth, presumably by a suppressive effect on cell proliferation in peripheral tissues. Large doses of

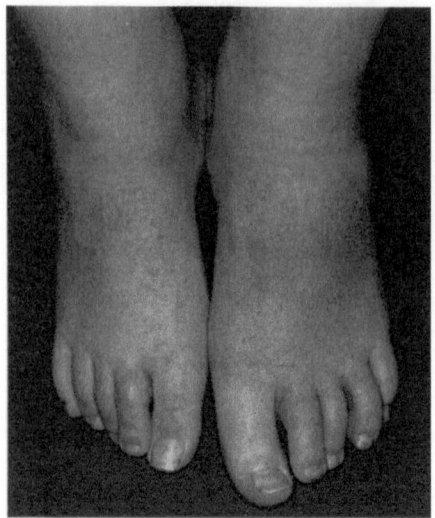

Figure 3.26. Enlargement and accelerated growth of the left foot in JRA.

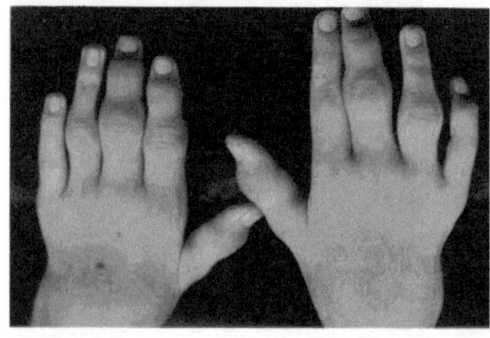

Figure 3.27. The right second finger has linear overgrowth, the left fifth finger is foreshortened.

alternate-morning steroids ($>$1 mg/kg/day) may also stunt growth, whereas small doses may accelerate growth by controlling systemic disease.

Bone erosions are a late finding in JRA, resemble those of adult RA, and are first seen on intra-articular bone surfaces unprotected by cartilage (Fig. 3.28). Joint narrowing and fibrous and bony ankylosis are seen in severe cases (Fig. 3.23).

Specific Joint Involvement

Temporomandibular Joint. Temporomandibular joint (TMJ) disease is common in all forms of childhood arthritis but most severe in girls with progressive disease.[257] It may be asymptomatic and overlooked on routine examination. Interference with the normal growth pattern in the mandible results in a shortened ramus. In rare patients, the mandibular dysplasia is asymmetric.

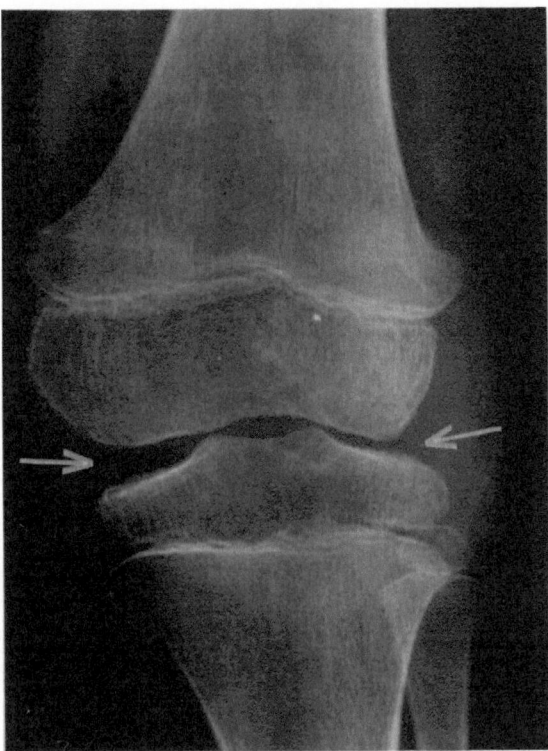

Figure 3.28. Knee in severe systemic polyarticular JRA (age 7 years; onset at age 3 years) showing erosions and narrowed joint space (*arrow*) (see also Fig. 3. 44).

The soft-tissue profile of the face is determined by the triad of nose, lips, and chin. Although the chin is only a part of the mandible, it is the most conspicuous frontal component in man. A pleasing and harmonious profile is often lost in JRA (Fig. 3.29A).[42,258]

The micrognathia of JRA is also often associated with gross dental malocclusion. There may be difficulty in chewing food, and the patient may speak with a lisp. Only the second molar teeth may contact when the patient closes her mouth. Tendinous insertions of the lateral pterygoid muscles may be destroyed along with the condyle, which is flattened, eroded, and rarefied. The mouth is then opened as if it were a hinge, with little or no gliding motion.

Elongation osteotomy of the body of the mandible and restoration of the contour of the jaw by iliac bone grafting or silicone implant may result in great cosmetic improvement[259] and contribute to the psychological well-being of the arthritic teenager (Fig. 3.29B). In rare instances, the interincisal opening decreases to a dangerously small orifice due to ankylosis of the TMJ. A vitallium plate may then be inserted to restore joint motion to normal.

Cervical Spine. Cervical spine involvement is common in all subsets and torticollis may be the sole presenting symptom of childhood arthritis. Loss

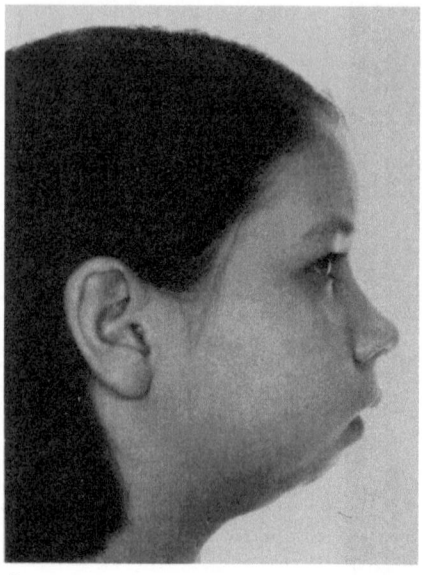
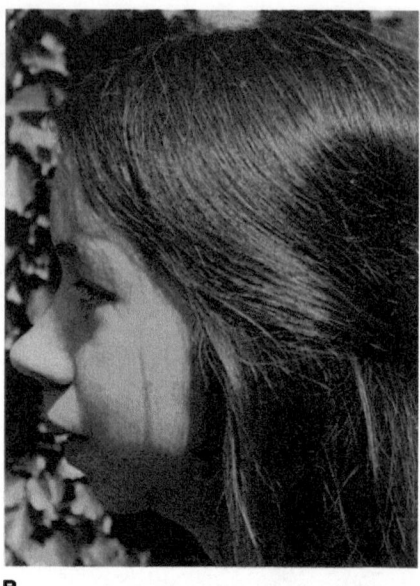

A   **B**

Figure 3.29. (A) Mandibular dysplasia (HLA-B27-associated spondyloarthritis) also shown in polyarticular JRA in Fig. 3.41. **(B)** Bone-graft reconstruction of the chin produced an obvious change in affect.

of the sharp margins of the articular facets of the C-2–C-3 apophyseal joint may first be seen radiologically after years of clinical disease (see Fig. 4.28).[42,43,260] If the disease progresses, erosions occur, followed in even more severe cases by bony bridging and fusion of the cervical segments. Intervertebral disk spaces may be narrowed and the stature and anterior-posterior diameter of the vertebral bodies may be diminished.

Growth deformities in the cervical spine result in a short neck with increased cervical lordosis, dorsal kyphosis, and compensatory overgrowth of the lumbar vertebrae (Figs. 3.20 and 3.30).[260] Although cervical spine involvement almost always starts at the C-2–C-3 level, it may occasionally extend down to the thoracic spine (Figs. 3.31 and 3.32).[42,43] Subluxation of the atlas on the axis, as is seen in severe adult RA, may occur in the worst cases but rarely causes a clinical problem.[261,262] Spinal-cord compression may rather occur in the thoracic area as a complication of steroid-induced epidural lipomatosis.[263]

Anesthesiologists must be aware of potential difficulty with intubation and of the additional hazards (dislocation, fracture, and cord injuries) that may occur during anesthesia.[264] In patients who develop laryngospasm and cannot be intubated tracheostomy may be necessary.[259] Spinal or local anesthesia should be used whenever possible.[265]

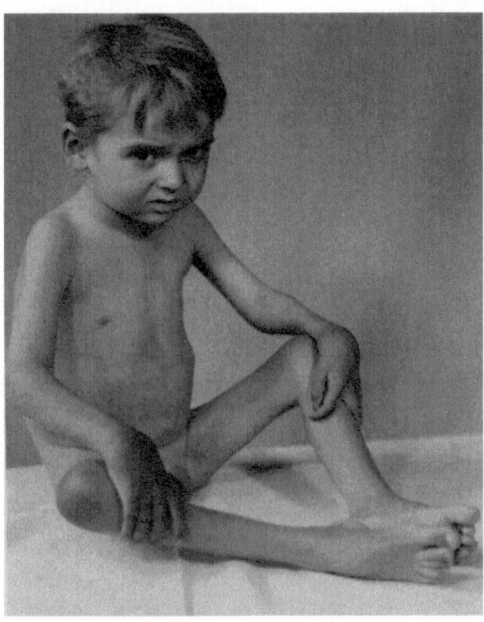

Figure 3.30. Growth deformities in the cervical spine result in a short neck with increased cervical lordosis and dorsal kyphosis (see also Fig. 3.20).

Cricoarytenoid Arthritis. Schlesinger first called attention to laryngeal arthritis causing stridor, dyspnea, and cyanosis in JRA. Occasionally, life-threatening stridor is the presenting manifestation of systemic-onset JRA.[78,114] Tracheostomy may be avoided by prompt institution of prednisone therapy, which can usually subsequently be weaned away after adequate salicylates have been administered. Some cases may respond to periodic oral beclomethasone diproprionate (BDP) inhalation.[266] The acute swelling that produces the dramatic initial symptom subsides without apparent significant residua. Hoarseness may result from chronic laryngeal arthritis in polyarticular patients. Laryngeal ankylosis has not been reported in childhood, but fibrosis can make intubation for surgery difficult in older children.[264]

Peripheral Joint Manifestations. A detailed description of the combined results of inflammation and destruction of each individual joint of the growing child is available elsewhere[268] and is beyond the scope of this monograph. Articular and periarticular pain and swelling are followed promptly by juxta-articular demineralization. Muscular wasting is soon apparent in affected areas. Overgrowth of the epiphyses may produce gross enlargement of the rapidly developing ends of the long bones, while the shafts may be thinned. Small bones may be underdeveloped. Specific radiographic and clinical findings may include:[42,43,268]

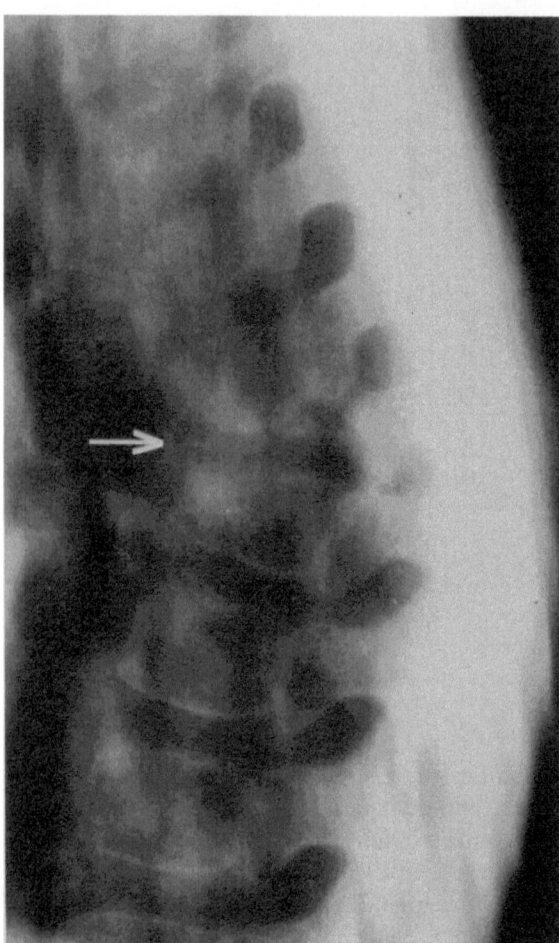

Figure 3.31. Complete destruction of mid-dorsal vertebra with gibbus deformity resembling tuberculosis in a 9-year-old boy with severe systemic polyarticular JRA. Needle biopsy demonstrated "rheumatoid inflammation" (Fig. 3.32). Vertebral destruction by rheumatoid inflammation is rarely reported.[267]

Hands and Wrists.[269] Altered length and width of digits and individual bones, crenation, crowding and fusion of carpal and carpometacarpal joints and bones into solid masses, proximal interphalangeal joint contractures and fusion, and spindle and pencil-tip appearance of the fingers. In the hand and wrist, there is normally a complicated balance between the forces of a multitude of tendons and ligaments. As this is lost, collapse deformities occur with hyperextension of one joint and compensatory flexion of another. Classic deformities include "swan neck" and "boutonnière" deformities of the fingers, palmar subluxation, and radial or ulnar deviation of the MCP joints (Fig. 3.33). Use of the hand in activities of daily living may accentuate the deformity, and a vicious cycle of deforming forces may be established.

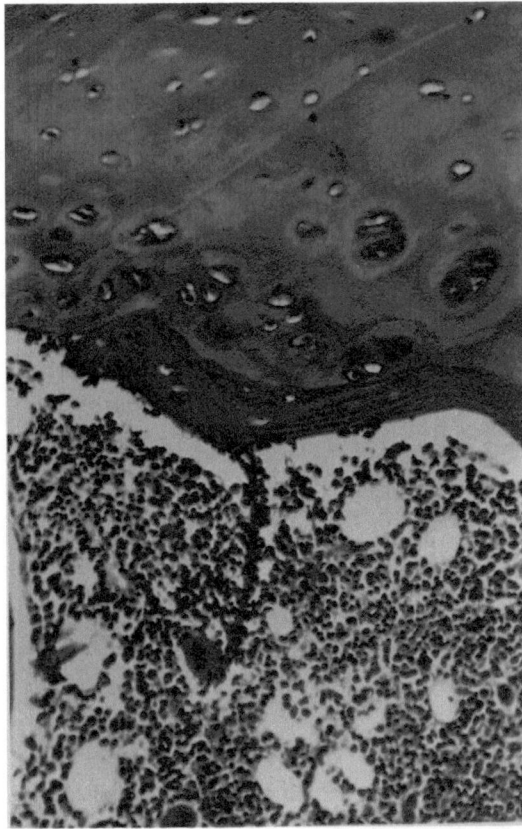

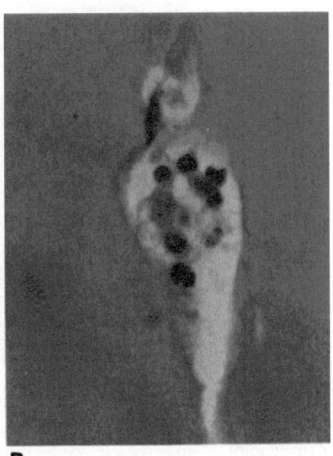

Figure 3.32. Needle biopsy of the apophyseal joint (T-7) in patient (Fig. 3.31) showing chondromucinous changes in the deeper layers of articular cartilage (**A**), causing destruction (hyperplastic bone marrow below); in a high-power view (**B**) lymphocytes can be seen invading a bone lacuna in articular cartilage. (**A**) × 40; (**B**) × 128.

Knees. Flexion contracture at the knee is common (Fig. 3.34). In addition to all of the usual manifestations of arthritic inflammation at the knee, children often develop an impressive valgus deformity. This may result from overgrowth of the leg at the knee, requiring the child to assume the valgus position to walk with less limp (Fig. 3.35).[270] However, it may also result from hip disease when limitation of external rotation of the hip causes assumption of the valgus position at the knee. Since we have adopted a policy of providing both lifts to the short leg and vigorous physiotherapy aimed at correcting limited hip rotation, we have not had to do stapling procedures and only in one case osteotomies to correct the knee valgus.

Hips. Hip involvement is common in all forms of childhood arthritis and is characterized by both a flexion contracture and by simultaneous limitation of full flexion, abduction, and rotation (Fig. 3.34). Some of the findings are a result of iliopsoas and adductor spasm. The hip pathology is sometimes

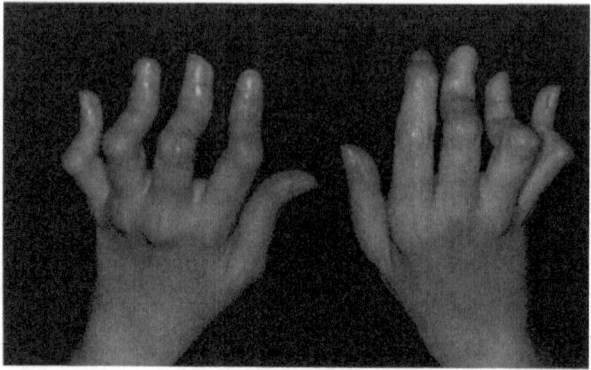

Figure 3.33. "Boutonnière" deformities (left, 2–5; right 3–5) chacterized by flexion deformities of the proximal interphalangeal joints and extension deformities of the distal interphalangeal joint. "Swan-neck" deformities consisting of hyperextension of the proximal interphalangeal joint and flexion of the distal interphalangeal joint are also developing in the right second finger. Patient had the onset of polyarticular seropositive JRA at age 9, without multisystem disease but with positive antinuclear antibodies, low serum total hemolytic complement, and elevated anti-DNA antibodies. Now age 32, she continues to have destructive arthritis as her only symptom. The deformities resemble those seen in the "lupus hand" but are not correctable and are accompanied by radiologic evidence of severe destructive changes. More common finger abnormalities in severe long-standing JRA are shown in Figure 3.27.

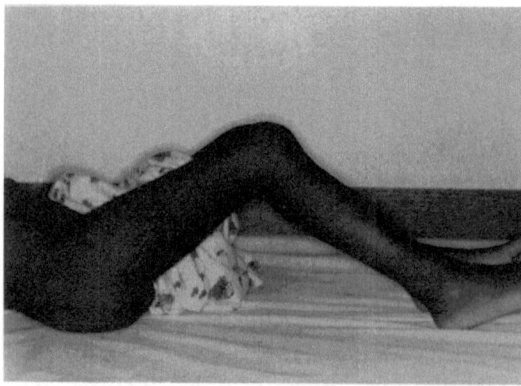

Figure 3.34. Hip and knee contractures typical of the child allowed to become wheelchairbound; the child sits all day with the knees and hips flexed. Rehabilitation requires surgical release of iliotibial bands and other soft-tissue contractures about the hips and knees with a vigorous immediate postoperative exercise program and prohibition of the wheelchair.

masked by a typical compensatory increased lumbar lordosis, which, if noted, provides a clue to its existence (Figs. 3.6, 3.41).

There is loss of substance and broadening of the femoral head. The neck is often poorly developed, and cystic changes appear in the head and neck. Later, marked narrowing of the joint space may be accompanied by secondary degenerative changes and aseptic necrosis of the femoral head. Acetabular destruction and protrusio, coxa magna, and dislocation may occur (Figs. 3.36, 3.51, 3.54, and 3.56).

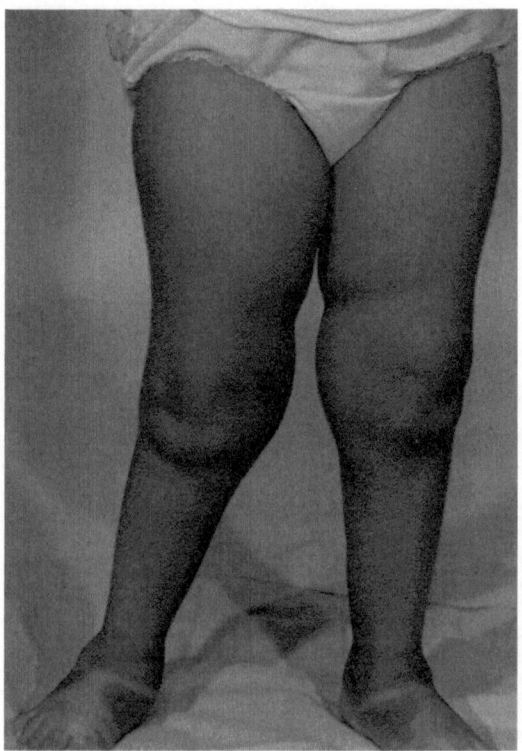

Figure 3.35. Although the patient has bilateral knee (and ankle) effusions, the right leg has overgrown, resulting in the child's having to stand with the knee in valgus; the deformity is progressive. Surgical correction (stapling or osteotomy) is avoided by lifting the opposite (good) heel by building up the oppposite shoe. This deformlty is also caused by nip disease resulting in limited external rotation of the hip with compensatory assumption of the valgus knee posture to walk; this may be treated with physical therapy to maximize external rotation at the diseased hip.

Feet. Although the knee is the most frequently involved joint in all forms of childhood arthritis, significant scarring is more frequent at the ankle and tarsus (Fig. 3.37). The foot is a complex articulation involving many joints in several planes. In addition to the many synovial joints, many bursae and tendon sheaths may be diseased, just as in the hand (Fig. 3.38). Fibrous, cartilaginous, or bony fusion of tarsal bones (tarsal coalition) may be mistaken for a congenital anomaly. Displacement of the talus by effusion may simulate "vertical talus" (Fig. 3.39) and be the presenting manifestation of JRA.

Deformities of the hips and knees may also cause compensatory deformities in the feet. Valgus deformity is more common than varus, but both may occur. Valgus foot deformities are sometimes compensatory for valgus knee deformities.

Elbows. Limitation of supination of the elbow is one of the most common and subtle diagnostic signs of childhood arthritis and may occur without flexion contracture. Most severely affected arthritic children have limitation of both extension and supination (Fig. 3.40).

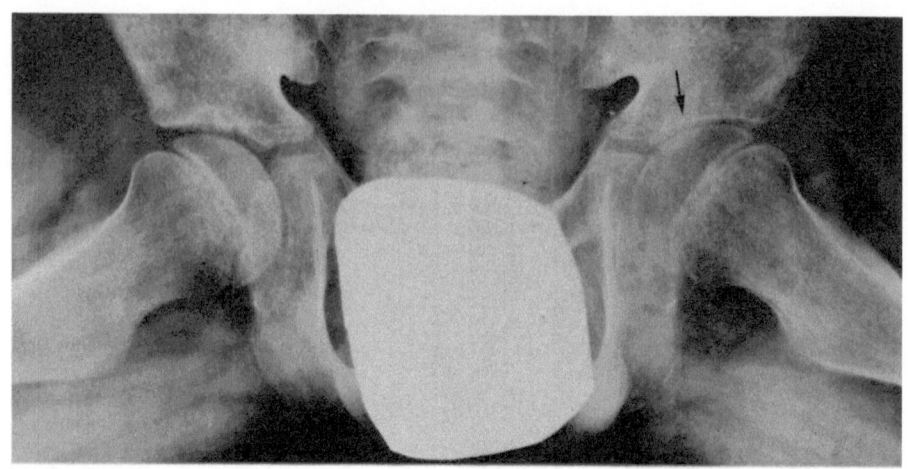

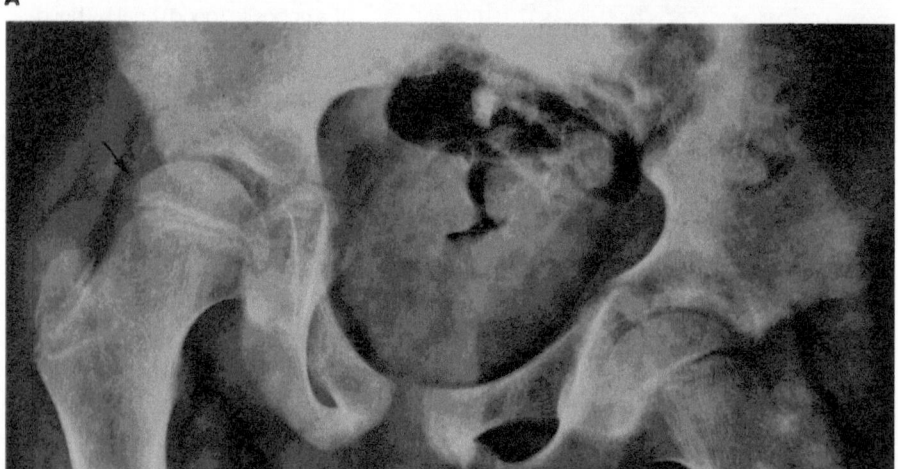

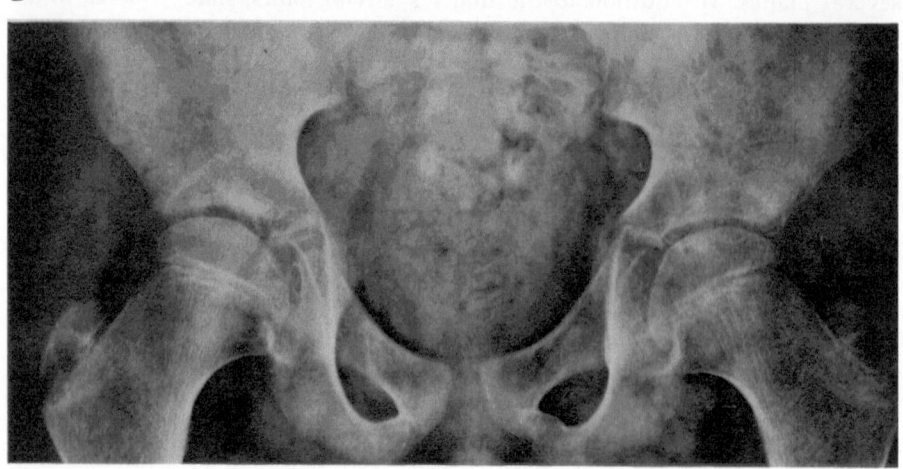

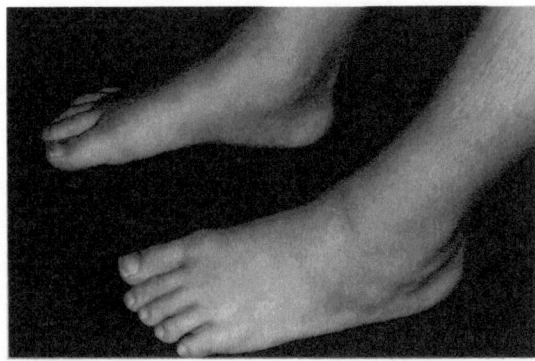

Figure 3.37. Inability to dorsiflex the ankles and limited eversion are common findings in polyarticular JRA.

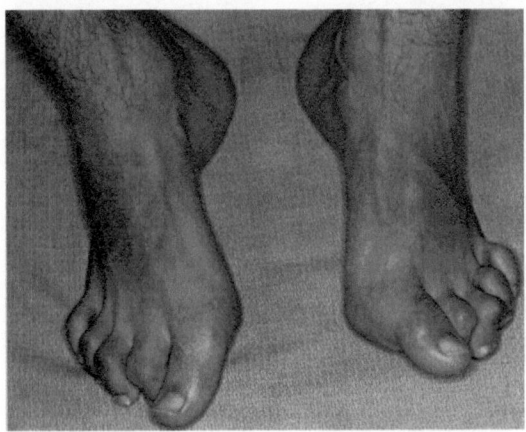

Figure 3.38. Hallux valgus and flexion contractures of the toes in a teenage boy with polyarticular JRA. The toe abnormalities are the same as those seen in the fingers. Cavus feet and/or bunions may be the presenting manifestations of childhood arthritis.

Shoulders. The shoulders are frequently affected in severe polyarticular disease. Both the acromioclavicular joint and the glenohumeral joint may be affected; the latter may be accompanied by necrosis of the humeral head and growth disturbances in the humerus. Severe disease may produce painful swelling of the joint and all the surrounding bursae (Fig. 3.40).

◁————————————————————————

Figure 3.36. Bilateral hip disease in an 8-year-old boy with systemic JRA (onset at age 3). **(A)** Following a jump into the swimming pool, there was acute chondrolysis of the left hip, illustrated here by sudden joint-space narrowing (*arrow*) not seen previously (see Chapter 2, Acute Chondrolysis of the Hip, and Fig. 2.56). **(B)** Six weeks later joint-space restoration is apparent in the left hip (similar to that seen in patients without arthritis who suffer acute lamellar coxitis, Fig. 2.56) but the right hip is seen to be subluxed, apparently as a compensation for the painful left hip. Without treatment (other than continuing aspirin), the subluxation disappeared on the right side, and the joint space in the left hip returned to normal **(C)**. The patient has continued to have severe arthritis and, following a flare of systemic manifestations at age 15, had accelerated bilateral destruction of the hip joints that frequired surgical replacement at age 16.

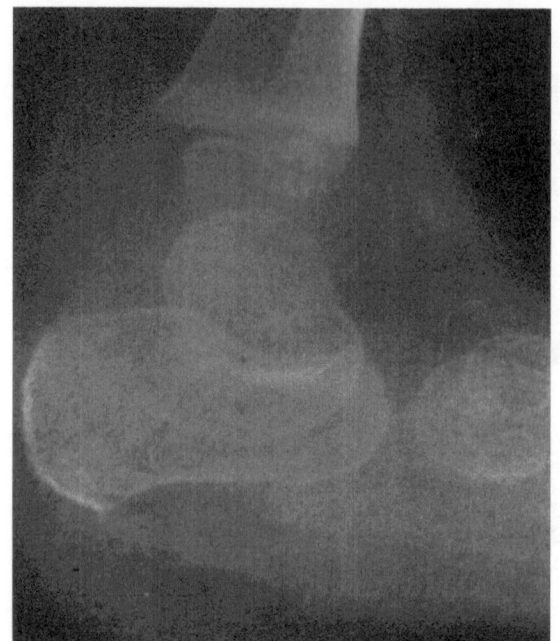

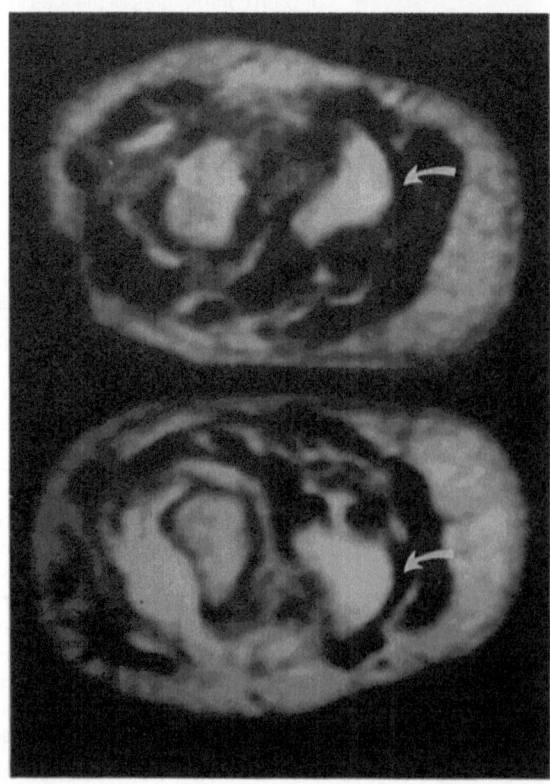

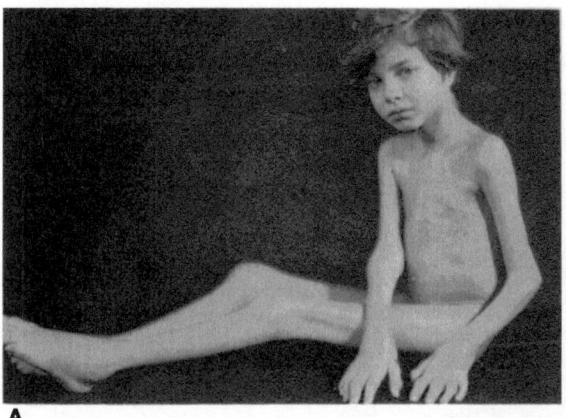

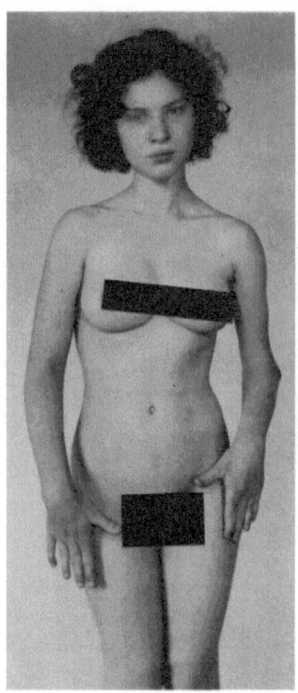

Figure 3.40. (**A**) At age 9, this youngster with extensive seropositive polyarticular disease has apparently equal arm length. However, by age 15 (**B**) the entire left upper extremity is seen to be foreshortened. A rheumatoid nodule is visible below the left elbow. Flexion contractures are visible in many joints.

Treatment of Polyarticular JRA

Drugs are only one part of the prescription for children with rheumatic disease. Drugs are important, however, and talented prescribing indicates knowledge and competence. Physical and occupational therapy help to maintain strength and function. The attitudes of the prescriber and the therapeutic team may determine compliance, maintain morale of the child and family, and enable growth and development to proceed despite the soulsapping nature of chronic sickness. The physician and the patient/parent become partners in control of the disease. A sense of control, albeit less control than one would wish, is ego rewarding and helps combat depression. Part of prescribing for these children involves teaching the parent and eventually the child the purposes of each medication, its potential benefits and side effects, and the methods used to regulate the dose so as to achieve maximum benefit and minimum side effects. The maximum potential benefit from drugs can only be achieved with such teamwork (Fig. 3.41).

Figure 3.39. (**A**) JRA presenting as ankle effusion displacing talus to simulate vertical talus. (**B**) MRI performed for evaluation of apparent vertical talus shows effusions (*arrows*) displacing talus. Correct interpretation avoids surgery.

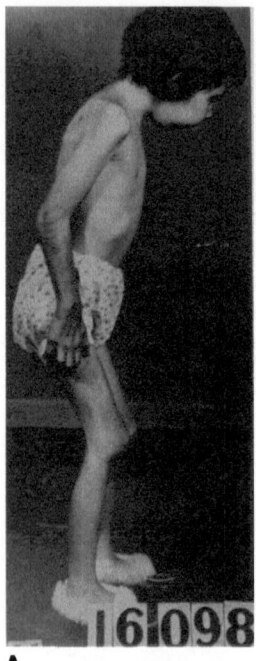 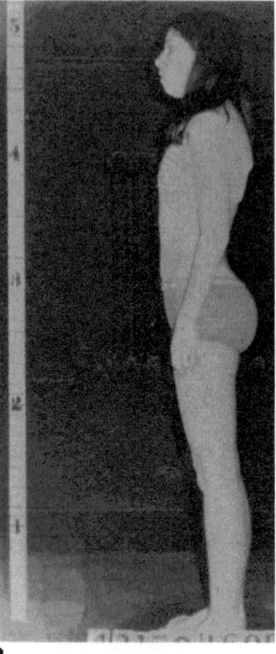

A   **B**

Figure 3.41. Example of the accomplishments of a therapeutic team in the care of a child with severe polyarticular JRA. At age 6, both hips were said to be dislocated (**A**). Nine years later, although she still had severe arthritis with delayed puberty and short stature, she could function in normal teenage society (**B**). (Reprinted from the *Arthritis Reporter*, Spring 1972, with permission of the Arthritis Foundation, New York Chapter, and Dr. J.S. Stillman.)

Anti-inflammatory Drugs

Salicylates. Aspirin is no longer the primary therapeutic agent in JRA even though it is generally equally effective and much cheaper than any currently available, equally safe alternative therapy.[271] Most parents and some doctors fear aspirin and choose the risks of other NSAIDs in preference to aspirin.[272] As a result we now have extensive experience with the newer nonsteroidal anti-inflammatory agents in children. The principles and techniques of therapy have already been discussed in the section on systemic JRA.

Other Nonsteroidal Anti-inflammatory Drugs (NSAIDs). The salicylate radical has been chemically modified to produce an ever-increasing number of agents that have as their goal better efficacy and fewer side effects (Table 3.16).[273] The average daily cost is 10–15 times that of ordinary aspirin. More than 50 antirheumatic compounds are reported to be currently under investigation. None have been proved to retard the rate of cartilage destruction in humans[274] or to induce remission of disease. So far, no one agent has proved to be superior for all patients.[271,273] In general, however, indomethacin, tolmetin, naproxen, and sulindac appear to be more effective in HLA-B27–associated spondyloarthritis.[271,275,276] Agents with a long half-life such as naproxen, which requires administration only twice daily, achieve better

Table 3.16. Drugs Used for the Treatment of Arthritis in Children

Nonsteroidal Anti-inflammatory Agents: Salicylate Preparations

Aspirin, 325-mg or 81-mg tablets

Enteric-coated aspirin, 325-mg, 500-mg, 975-mg tablets

Sustained-release aspirin, 650-mg tablets

Choline magnesium trisalicylate, 1 tsp = 500-mg equivalent, 500- 750-mg and 1000-mg tablets

Salsalate (salicylsalicylic acid), 500-mg, 750-mg tablets

80 + mg/kg/day—salicylate level measured to achieve efficacy or maximum tolerated level (4–6)

Nonsalicylate NSAIDs Labeled by U.S. FDA for Use in Children

Tolmetin (Tolectin), 20–30 mg/kg/day (4); 1800-mg max dose

Naproxen (Naprosyn), 10–15 mg/kg/day (2); 1500-mg max dose

Ibuprofen (Motrin), 40–50 mg/kg/day (4); 2400-mg max dose

NSAIDs Not Yet Labeled by U.S. FDA for Use in Children

Indomethacin (Indocin),* 1–3 mg/kg/day (3–4); 200-mg max dose

Fenoprofen (Nalfon), 40–50 mg/kg/day (4); 3200-mg max dose

Ketoprofen (Orudis), 3–5 mg/kg/day (4); 300-mg max dose

Meclofenamate (Meclomen),† 4–7 mg/kg/day (3); 300-mg max dose

Sulindac (Clinoril), 4–6 mg/kg/day (2); 400-mg max dose

Flurbiprofen (Ansaid), 3–4 mg/kg/day, (3–4), 300-mg max dose

Piroxicam (Feldene), 0.3 mg/kg/day single daily dose

Diclofenac (Voltaren), 2–3 mg/kg/day (3–4), 200-mg max dose

Diflunisal (Dolobid), 7–21 mg/kg/day (2–3), 1500-mg max dose

Slower-Acting Antirheumatic Drugs

Hydroxychloroquine, 7 mg/kg/day; 300-mg max dose

Gold (injectable), 0.5–1 mg/kg/week; 50-mg max dose

Gold (oral), 0.1 mg/kg/day; 9-mg max dose

Penicillamine, 5–10 mg/kg/day; 500-mg max dose

Immunosuppressive agents

Methotrexate, 10 mg/mm^2/once weekly

*Labeled for use in resistant cases.

†Preliminary trials in children showed excessive toxicity.

Numbers in parentheses indicate usual number of daily doses.

compliance and may be more effective on this basis alone in all forms of arthritis.[238,277] Objective comparisons of efficacy and tolerance of all these agents and their comparison to aspirin and the other salicylates have been handicapped by the general lack of availability of serum levels. Therapeutic trials have been conducted with arbitrary dosage, making no allowance for differences in individual absorption, metabolism, and excretion.[196] Pharmacokinetic principles, which had led to improvement in the care of asthmatic and epileptic children, have not yet been applied to the use of these agents in children.[278]

A paucity of clinics with sufficient numbers of patients and staff to conduct controlled clinical trials has also delayed the accumulation of knowledge about these drugs in children. Most tests with adults have included primarily seropositive patients; the number of children to whom the conclusions are directly applicable is small. The few reported studies in children have made no effort to separately determine efficacy among the various subsets of childhood arthritis.[226] In the United States, at the time of this writing, only three of these agents (tolmetin, ibuprofen, and naproxen) have been tested sufficiently to satisfy the requirements of the Food and Drug Administration (FDA) for labeling for general use in arthritic children. This dilemma is not easily solved. On the one hand, it is well established that the results of drug studies in adults should not be applied to children without testing in children. On the other hand, some sick children are being deprived of medications that would undoubtedly be of benefit to them and are available to adults with identical conditions. Both the children and the drugs are thus "orphaned."

Availability of these agents has led to a new approach in our management of older arthritic children. We often have the youngster try a number of different agents briefly. Within a few days, many youngsters can report their individual preference based on subjective relief of symptoms and tolerance of side effects (Table 3.17). Maximum benefit, however, is not seen in some children until after 12 weeks of administration of relatively high doses.[279]

Tolmetin Sodium. The U.S. JRA Cooperative Drug Study Group demonstrated, within the limitations stated above, that tolmetin sodium, 20–30 mg/kg/day in three or four divided doses, was equal or better than aspirin, 80–100 mg/kg/day in four doses, in terms of anti-inflammatory effect and was slightly better tolerated than aspirin.[226] Studies suggest a half-life in adults of 4–6 h and peak serum levels 40 min after single doses.[280] In adult nonarticular rheumatism and soft-tissue disease, common in pauciarticular JRA, tolmetin surpassed aspirin in efficacy. We find it very useful in spondyloarthritic children. In the pediatric clinical trial, liver enzyme abnormalities related to aspirin therapy promptly returned to normal.[226] Licensing of the drug in the United States includes children, so informed consent and therapeutic trial protocols are not required, and the drug may be used in children by general physicians. It is available only in bad-tasting 200-mg tablets that must be divided and disguised for children who cannot swallow tablets. It is about 10 times as expensive as ordinary aspirin but only twice as expensive as flavored soluble "baby" aspirin tablets administered in similarly efficacious dosage.

Naproxen. Although not tested in the United States, experience in Europe showed sufficient efficacy and tolerance in children to warrant FDA labeling of pills and syrup for children in the United States.[281–283] A long half-life of 13 h has been confirmed in children, providing greatly increased con-

Table 3.17. Adverse Reactions Associated with the Use of Nonsteroidal Anti-inflammatory Drugs.

Incidence Generally Greater than 1%	*Incidence Generally Less than 1%*
Gastrointestinal	*Gastrointestinal*
Gastrointestinal pain (10%)	Gastritis or gastroenteritis
Dyspepsia*	Peptic ulcer
Nausea* with or without vomiting	Gastrointestinal bleeding
Diarrhea*	GI perforation
Constipation*	Liver function abnormalitis
Flatulence	Jaundice, sometimes with fever
Anorexia	Cholestasis
Gastrointestinal cramps	Hepatitis
	Pancreatitis
Dermatologic	
Rash*	*Dermatologic*
Pruritus*	Stomatitis
	Sore or dry mucous membranes
Central Nervous System	Erythema multiforme
Dizziness*	Toxic epidermal necrolysis
Headache*	Stevens-Johnson syndrome
Nervousness	
Drowsiness*	*Cardiovascular*
	Congestive heart failure in patients with
Special Senses	marginal cardiac function
Tinnitus*	Arrhythmia
Renal	*Hematologic*
Edema*	Thrombocytopenia
Hematuria*	Leukopenia, thrombocytopenia
Proteinuria*	Increased prothrombin time in patients
	on oral anticoagulants
Hematologic	Hemolytic anemia
Hematocrit lowered more than 10%[†]	
	Central Nervous System
Cardiovascular	Vertigo
Palpitation	Altered mental state
	Special Senses
	Blurred vision, diplopia, deafness
	Hypersensitivity Reactions
	Anaphylaxis
	Angioneurotic edema
	Hypersensitivity syndrome consisting
	of some or all of the following: fever,
	lung infiltrates,[287a] chills, skin rash,
	changes in liver function, jaundice,
	leukopenia, and eosinophilia; rarely,
	fatalities have been reported
	Renal
	Acute renal failure, interstitial nephritis,
	nephrotic syndrome

* Incidence generally between 3 and 9%. (Those reactions occurring in less than 3% of patients are unmarked.)
† Incidence generally 42% in children.

venience, better compliance, and perhaps improved control of disease. In adults with RA, preference was expressed for naproxen and other anti-inflammatory drugs compared with aspirin, but this effect was entirely explained by better compliance.[238] However, in ankylosing spondylitis (AS), naproxen was a considerably better agent than aspirin and was even slightly preferred over indomethacin, the agent previously found to be more effective in AS.[238] I have found it generally well tolerated and an excellent agent for use in teenagers with spondyloarthritis, both HLA-B27–positive and –negative.[275] In small children, it has been tested at 10–15 mg/kg/day in two divided doses.[281–285] We use the larger dose and find it to be well tolerated. In teenagers, we generally start with 250 mg twice daily and increase the evening dose to 375 or 500 mg as needed and tolerated. Some children cannot tolerate naproxen due to lethargy or psychic effects ("like being on a trip"), and one youngster who was greatly benefited could not tolerate the palpatations it occasionally produces. Bullous photosensitive rashes are frequent in those with "little Orphan Annie" complexion.[286,287]

Ibuprofen. Ibuprofen, 20 mg/kg/day, has been shown to be safe and efficacious in children, but the half-life is short and divided doses are necessary.[288] The drug is extremely well tolerated, is available as a syrup, and has sometimes been helpful in children who could not tolerate other drugs (Fig. 3.42). However, liver enzyme abnormalities seen with aspirin therapy may or may not return to normal with ibuprofen. Higher doses are generally required for control of fever in children with systemic JRA (40 mg/kg/day).

Indomethacin. Indomethacin, 2 mg/kg/day in four divided doses, has been used safely in children with control of fever and arthritis.[188] There is great variability in half-life; twice-a-day dosage, advocated in adults, has not been reported in children. This drug was better than aspirin in most trials involving patients with AS and related disorders.[238,239] However, naproxen is preferred by many patients who cannot tolerate the headaches, dizziness, and fatigue caused by indomethacin. Higher-than-recommended doses have been reported in association with death from liver disease and infection in children[290] and aplastic anemia seems to be more frequently associated with indomethacin than other NSAIDS.[291] The drug seems reasonably safe in proper dosage and is, in some patients with HLA-B27–associated spondyloarthritis, preferred to all others. Oral suspension is available; indomethacin is FDA labeled for use in children resistant to alternative NSAIDS.

Other NSAIDs not FDA labeled for use in children but studied by the Pediatric Rheumatology Collaborative Drug Study Group and found safe and efficacious include *fenoprofen* (40 mg/kg/day),[292] *flurbiprofen* (4 mg/kg/day),[293] *ketoprofen* (4mg/kg/day),[294] *proquazone* (20 mg/kg/day),[295] *meclofenamate* (7.5 mg/kg/day),[296] and *pirprofen* (15 mg/kg/day).[297] European studies report safety and efficacy of *piroxicam* (0.3 mg/kg/day in a single dose),[284] *sulindac* (2.5 mg/kg/day in two doses),[298] and *diclofenac* (2–3 mg/kg/

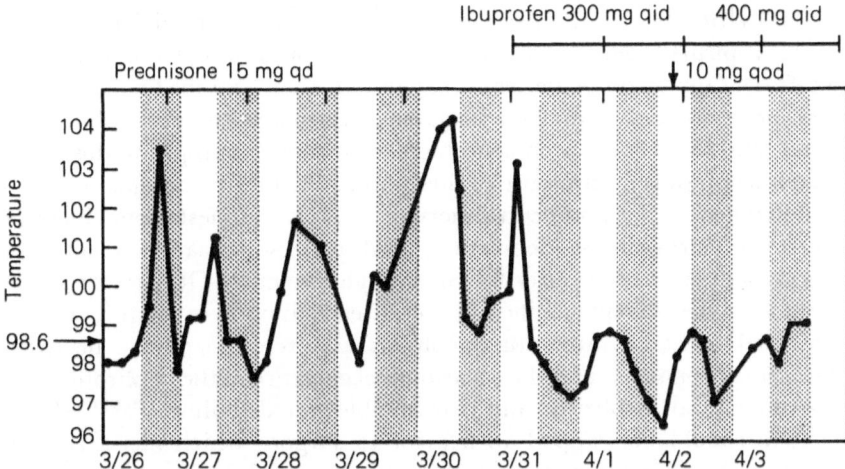

Figure 3.42. Steroid-sparing effect of NSAIDs. Nonsteroidal anti-inflammatory drugs, such as ibuprofen, may be used to control fever in children with systemic JRA who are unable to tolerate salicylates. NSAIDs may be used together with alternate-day steroids in patients whose fever cannot be controlled with NSAIDs alone. Alternate-day prednisone plus an NSAID may be more effective in controlling fever than daily prednisone alone, as shown in this illustration. (Reprinted with permission from Brewer EJ: Nonsteroidal antiinflammatory agents. *Arthritis Rheum* 20:513–525, 1977; copyright by American Rheumatism Association.)

day).[285,299] It is unclear whether the risk of hepatotoxicity is greater with diclofenac than with other NSAIDs.[300] Rash from meclofenamate is so frequent that it is probably a poor choice for children.[296] Phenylbutazone may cause death from aplastic anemia and is not used in children.[291,301]

NSAIDs may result in disappearance of phenotypically activated circulating T cells and functionally activated B cells along with improvement in ESR and rheumatoid factor in responsive patients.[302] Absorption may be delayed but is not ultimately impaired by simultaneous administration of sucralfate an agent which we frequently administer to children with GI intolerance of NSAIDs, which often relieves that problem.[303] H_2 blocking agents may reduce blood levels of NSAIDs.[304] Efficacy and safety of misoprostol in children have not been established.[305,306] Fortunately children not exposed to alcohol and tobacco are at lower risk of serious GI bleeding than are adults.

Studies of interactions between NSAIDs have produced conflicting results.[271,307] To avoid interference and a lower net effect, only one anti-inflammatory drug is generally used at one time in any patient. In a few special circumstances, the combination of aspirin and another NSAID such as indomethacin or naproxen seems to have been helpful to our patients. However, such combinations may increase the risk of analgesic nephropathy.[130]

Hazards of NSAIDs. These new drugs have all of the potential toxic side effects of aspirin[271] plus a higher incidence of anaphylactic-type reactions.[307a,b] Our early experience suggested that extraordinarily high doses of indomethacin might be associated with increased susceptibility to infection, but this has not been a problem with more appropriate doses.[290] The major symptoms limiting use of these drugs in children are gastrointestinal intolerance[308–310b] and central-nervous-system manifestations, including headache, drowsiness, depression, and depersonalization reactions. These reactions may occur after taking a single tablet.[311] Other worrisome problems with these agents include the reported reduction in renal function, the potential to cause interstitial nephritis and renal papillary necrosis (analgesic nephropathy), and the occasional occurrence of the nephrotic syndrome, interstitial nephritis and irreversible renal failure.[130,271,312–324] Medication should be stopped 48 h prior to surgery which has a risk of hemorrhage.[324a,b] Children are at less risk than adults for renal complications.[325]

Slower-Acting Antirheumatic Drugs. Sulfasalazine, gold, chloroquine, and penicillamine, the drugs included in this category, do not have the standard laboratory properties of anti-inflammatory drugs and generally are rather specific for rheumatic diseases. Weeks to months of therapy are required before a beneficial effect may be expected. While it is possible they may in some cases induce remission of the disease and inhibit cartilage destruction, they have not been proved to do so.[326–331] They are generally not effective or tolerated during the years of systemic illness in systemic JRA;[332] injectable gold and sulfasalazine have been associated with life-threatening systemic reactions.

The indication for use of the slower-acting drugs is generally considered to be persistently poorly controlled polyarticular disease that threatens multiple joint destruction and accumulating disability (Fig. 3.16). Potential therapeutic benefits must be balanced against the potentially serious side effects of treatment with these agents. The number of children requiring these medications is small, their potential toxicity is great, and considerable clinical experience is necessary for their safe and effective use. The care of such children should be either in or supervised by pediatric rheumatology clinics.

Sulfasalazine. This combination of sulfapyridine and 5 aminosalicylic acid, long used in children with inflammatory bowel disease, has recently become a favored second-line agent for both children and adults with arthritis.[333–344] Very little of the salicylate and almost all of the sulfa are absorbed.[338] The mechanisms of action are unknown but seem to be antibacterial and anti-inflammatory. In our experience a dose of 30 mg/kg/day is well tolerated by most children and produces add-on or better benefit in terms of reduction in effusions, joint contractures, and number of affected joints in 60% of arthritic children on NSAIDs who can continue this medication for 3 months.[337] Evidence of efficacy is confirmed by return of ESR to normal within 3 months in 80% of those children in whom it was elevated. Good results were seen in all forms of childhood arthritis except systemic JRA patients who in the preliminary trial did not tolerate it.[337,342–344] Within 3 months the medication had to be stopped for allergic rashes/serum sickness (12%), GI complaints (6%), or neutropenia (4%) in almost one-quarter of the children; a pair of twins who responded well subsequently had to stop the medication because of pronounced and persistent elevations of SGOT/PT partially caused by insecticide spray, but then definitely worsened by sulfasalazine.

Although double-blind randomized trials of efficacy have not yet been carried out in children, studies in adults suggest that sulfasalazine is more efficacious than hydroxychloroquine and equal to parenteral gold in preventing erosions at 1 year provided that the agent was started early in the course of the illness.[334,335] A recent comparative review found little difference in efficacy between methotrexate, injectable gold, penicillamine, and sulfasalazine, with sulfasalazine most efficacious in lowering ESR.[345]

In addition to the well-recognized gastrointestinal, hematologic, and allergic complications, most of which occur during the first month or 3 months of therapy, rare pulmonary, hepatic, cardiac, and neurologic side effects may occur, and drug-induced lupus may also occur.[346–351] Nevertheless, the risk/ benefit ratio favors sulfasalazine over other second-line agents and we now offer it to any non-systemic JRA patient whose arthritis is not completely controlled with NSAIDs.

Chrysotherapy. We no longer administer parenteral gold to children.[352] Gold evolved as a therapeutic agent for RA as a result of Koch's demonstration that the in vitro growth of tubercle bacilli was inhibited by gold and Forestier's erroneous assumption that tuberculosis was related to RA. Despite a multitude of studies, the mechanism of action of gold in RA remains unknown.[353]

Chrysotherapy was in wide use for 30 years before the controlled study of the Empire Rheumatism Council managed to demonstrate that it was more effective than placebo; the difference in effect was not overwhelming, and the advantage of 20 weeks of parenteral gold therapy was lost at the time of 2-year follow-up.[354,355] No similar study has been performed in children. However, many experienced physicians have reported the efficacy of gold in some pediatric cases and the need for continued maintenance therapy to maintain the clinical effect.[199,356] Scientific studies do not prove the commonly stated clinical dictum that gold has the capability of inducing a remission. Naturally, in any disease characterized by exacerbations and remissions, any long-term therapy will coincide on occasion with remission.

Fifteen to thirty percent of children started on parenteral gold therapy must discontinue treatment because of adverse side effects.[357] Gold salts are reported to be 10 times more toxic than any other therapy used in Great Britain and over a 7-year period accounted for 16 deaths in the U.K.[358,358a]

Death is most commonly from narrow aplasia and its complications, especially overwhelming sepsis. Other side effects include severe mucocutaneous reactions, autoimmune thrombocytopenia, and membranous nephropathy. We have seen one child with fatal disseminated intravascular coagulation and reviewed the record of another (not fatal) after the *second* test-dose injection of gold and are now aware of many other similar cases (Fig. 3.43).[169,170,178]

Some toxic reactions to gold seem to be immunologically mediated. For example, proteinuria is 32 times more common in patients with HLA-DR3 and so seems to be genetically controlled.[359]

When the decision to give parenteral gold is made, a complete blood count, platelet count, blood chemistry determination, and urinalysis are obtained, and a test dose of gold is given as soon as the results are available. The total weekly dose is calculated as 0.5–1 mg/kg/dose (50-mg maximum for adults).[199] Patients are started with a test dose equal to one-fifth the weekly dose which is increased one-fifth weekly so that the full dose is achieved on the fifth injection. A complete blood count, platelet count, and urinalysis are obtained on the day of each dose, and the gold is not given until the results are checked by the physician. The injection is omitted if there is any rash or laboratory abnormality. Unexplained fever early in the course of gold therapy suggests the possibility of sepsis due to neutropenia and requires immediate evaluation. Serum gold levels are generally unavailable and have not yet been proved to be useful.

To avoid long waits in the clinic, we taught responsible parents to give the intramuscular injections at home after our telephone approval indicating that the laboratory studies that day were normal.[360] With this system, they had the blood and urine studies in their own neighborhoods, and some of the inconvenience of gold injections was removed. So long as the child was improving, we continued the gold weekly, usually for a period of 1 year. If the

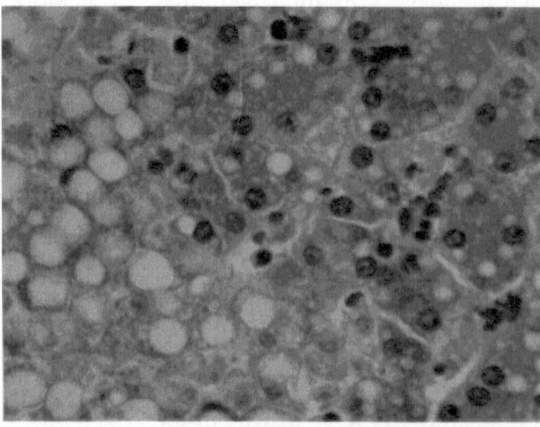

Figure 3.43. Disseminated intravascular coagulation (clogging blood vessels with red blood cells) with necrosis and fatty metamorphosis of the liver following the second injection of gold.

youngster was in remission, we gradually reduced the gold injections to every 2, 3, and then 4 weeks and, if still in remission, discontinued the injections after about 2 years. If there was no improvement with gold, we gave up the therapy after 6–9 months. If the arthritis worsened soon after reducing the frequency of gold administration, we resumed the weekly injections. A number of different intramuscular gold preparations are marketed. There are no clear-cut distinctions between them. Most of the injected gold is excreted via the kidneys and some goes through the gastrointestinal tract.[361,362] However, with time, there are increasing deposits in all tissues, which remain for years after cessation of therapy. A controlled trial showed oral gold to be safe and modestly efficacious in children.[363] Injectable gold is probably only marginally, if at all, better than oral second-line agents in children.[345,363]

Oral Gold (Auranofin). In a well-conducted multi-institutional collaborative study comparing placebo with auranofin over a 6-month period there was only marginal (p = 0.24) benefit of oral gold over placebo at 6 months.[364] There is some suggestion that early treated patients do better than children first treated after 2 years. Although oral gold has the potential to cause all of the same side effects as parenteral gold they seem to occur in lower frequency.[365,366] Diarrhea limits the dose usually to 0.15 mg/kg/day with a maximum of 9 mg daily. Careful monitoring for adverse side effects is carried out monthly. Steady-state blood levels are achieved after 3 months of therapy.[367] Although only about 13% of children treated with oral gold for years are still taking it after 5 years, even though 83% of that series still had signs of active arthritis,[368] possible efficacy and reasonable safety may make trials of auranofin worthwhile in severely affected children whose disease is not controlled by NSAIDs and sulfasalazine.[369]

Penicillamine. Penicillamine was initially found to be of use in Wilson's disease and has been used in lead poisoning and cystinuria in children. The discovery that penicillamine helps some adults with RA resulted from a trial by Jaffe in a patient with high-titer rheumatoid factor.[370] Based on laboratory evidence that the drug could dissociate human macroglobulins in vitro, he hypothesized that penicillamine would cause intravascular dissociation of IgM rheumatoid factor. The patient apparently benefited, and the level of rheumatoid factor was reduced, but for unknown reasons. Despite a great many studies, the mechanism leading to improvement remains unknown. Unlike gold, whose efficacy can be demonstrated in experimental models of arthritis such as adjuvant disease, penicillamine is ineffective in any such model. About all that can be said is that based on the extraordinarily wide range of serious drug-induced "autoimmune" disorders penicillamine can produce as side effects of its use,[371] it must act on some very basic immunologic mechanism(s).[370]

Multicenter controlled trials with penicillamine in adults have demonstrated statistically significant improvement in such measures of arthritic activity as grip strength, hemoglobin, and ESR. The results were not all that impressive. For example, in one such study, the average ESR in the treated group was reduced from 53 mm/h to 46 mm/h.[372] Twenty-six percent of the patients had to discontinue the therapy because of side effects. However, some experienced clinicians were enthusiastic about penicillamine as a therapeutic agent in severe active RA inadequately responsive to conventional therapy.[373,374] The drug has been used in a few hundred children with polyarthritis without systemic manifestations and is said to be about as effective as gold, equally toxic to gold, but preferred because it can be taken orally.[375,376] In an uncontrolled series using a dose of 15–30 mg/kg/day, 69% of children receiving the drug as their first slow-acting agent were said to benefit; 53% of children being treated with penicillamine after receiving gold without benefit were said to benefit from penicillamine.[376] A US multicenter collaborative controlled trial failed to show benefit from 10 mg kg/day[377] but children in France did a little better.[378–380]

Side effects of penicillamine administration may include thrombocytopenia, agranulocytosis, aplastic or hemolytic anemia; membranous nephropathy with nephrotic syndrome,[381] rapidly progressive glomerulonephritis; Goodpasture's syndrome; cholestatic hepatitis; serious rashes including pemphigus; myasthenia gravis; polymyositis,[382] thyroiditis; and lupus erythematosus.[370,371] Vitamin B_6 deficiency may be combated by simultaneous administration of 25 mg of vitamin B_6 daily at a different time than the medication.[383] No harmful effects of coincident heavy-metal chelation have been noted, but they could be unrecognized, as could other effects of its lathyrogenic and collagen basement-membrane-altering properties. Serious proteinuria is more likely to occur in the same patients who develop proteinuria with gold, especially those with HLA-DR3.[359] Insulin antibodies may also occur.[384]

Dosage regulation of penicillamine cannot be based on serum levels, which are not available. In adults, increased side effects and few benefits have been achieved with doses in excess of 600 mg daily. A complete blood count, platelet count, urinalysis, and chemistries are obtained prior to each increase and monthly thereafter. Urinary protein determination with filter-paper strips can be done more frequently by the parent at home. The reported incidence of side effects requiring withdrawal of medications varies from 10 to 30%. Other antirheumatic medications have to be continued since a beneficial effect may not be noted for months. A favorable response is unlikely if improvement has not occurred within 6 months.[385]

Hydroxychloroquine. This antimalarial compound has been reported to be equally effective as gold in adults with RA but fell into disfavor when irreversible retinal toxicity was reported.[386,387] Despite lack of efficacy in a large multicenter collaborative trial[377] pediatric centers have continued to use it and consider it to be an effective agent with greater ease of administration and less toxicity than gold or penicillamine.[388–390] At a dosage of 5–7 mg/kg/day (maximum 200 mg daily) given as a single dose, the most frequent side effect is reported to be corneal deposition, which is reversible and said to be dose-related. The most worrisome side effect is macular degeneration, which may progress after the drug is withdrawn.[391] Patients with known familial tendency to macular degeneration may be at higher risk. With careful, frequent ocular monitoring and drug withdrawal, the incidence of significant retinopathy threatening vision may be kept to 1%.[390–392a] Glucose-6-phosphate dehydrogenase (G6PD) deficiency, once thought to be a contraindication, rarely if ever causes hemolysis in patients treated with hydroxychloroquine.[393] The lack of popularity of this drug represents doubts about efficacy in the face of this ocular hazard in a disorder with increased ocular risk from uveitis. If a controlled trial showed efficacy, this agent would be more widely used and has the potential for combined use with penicillamine or gold, sulfasalazine, and methotrexate. Hydroxychloroquine appears to reduce the severity of hepatotoxicity of salicylates and methotrexate.[394]

When hydroxychloroquine is used with success, the drug is generally continued in full dosage for 6 months and then gradually reduced over a 2-year period. Chloroquine must be kept locked in the medicine cabinet. Death has been reported after childhood ingestion of as little as 0.8 gram.[395] Myopathy, cardiomyopathy, and neuropathy may occur in addition to hematologic and dermatologic side effects.[396,397]

Combination of Drugs. In severely affected children it is our present practice to use combinations of drugs: (1) salicylate or other NSAID; (2) oral gold or penicillamine; (3) hydroxychloroquine; (4) sulfasalazine and, in refractory cases, all of these plus methotrexate. Our clinical impression is that this approach works better than our previous method, which was to withdraw any agent whose value did not seem proven within 6 months. At present there is no documented study which supports our approach,[251] although a recent report of efficacy of methotrexate in refractory childhood arthritis may, at least in part, reflect the benefits of such polypharmacy,[398] and other anecdotal reports indicate a similar approach elsewhere.[399–401a] Prompt therapy is also most essential for the group with rheumatoid-factor-positive childhood onset of adult RA. There appears to be a "window of opportunity" during which aggressive therapy may be disease modifying; scars cannot be benefitted by dangerous medications.[402–402a]

Corticosteroid Treatment of Severe Polyarticular JRA

If properly used in JRA, corticosteroids may prevent blindness; enable function as opposed to the alternative of a bed-chair existence with all that implies for the child and family; and prevent death from overwhelming myopericarditis. With improper use, they may foster crippling or death.

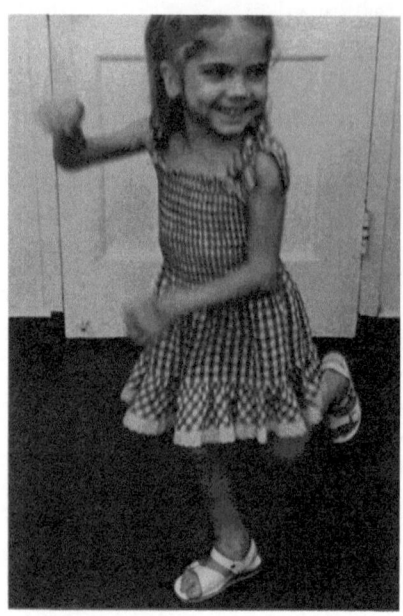

Figure 3.44. Severe systemic JRA (age 9 years, onset at age 3 years). Patient has large effusions in all joints and requires 3.9 grams of aspirin daily plus 17 mg of prednisone on alternate mornings for control of fever and arthritis. She has had a cerebrovascular accident from which she has fully recovered and required a gastrectomy for uncontrollable hemorrhage caused by a penetrating duodenal ulcer at a time when she was receiving indomethacin, aspirin, and steroids. She has failed to be helped by hydroxychloroquine, gold, pencillamine, or plasmapheresis. The alternate-day steroids enabled her to attend school and summer camp and to lead an almost normal life despite progressive joint destruction (see Fig. 3.28). At college 10 years later she is taking methotrexate.

For some severely affected children, a small dose of prednisone on alternate mornings (together with their nonsteroidal drug and slow-acting agent) may make the difference between going to school and a reasonably normal life or becoming a bed-chair cripple (Fig. 3.44).[157,403–405] The risks of alternate-day prednisone are small when weighed against the alternatives.[406] Animal studies and clinical evidence in these children indicate that loss of weight bearing is associated with worse cartilage destruction (see Figs. 3.51 and 3.52).[407–411] Occasionally, we see the rare child who comes to us already wheelchair-bound, demineralized and weak, and with crush fractures and characteristic absence of cartilage at the knees and hips out of proportion to anything we ever see in our own most severely affected children (see Fig. 3.51).[412,413] Much of this is secondary to entering the wheelchair. All of our patients attend regular school daily and none are ever allowed in a wheelchair. In our opinion, if prednisone is required to achieve that goal, it is well used for that purpose.

Small divided doses of prednisone can also be used in very severe polyarticular JRA (1 mg four times daily). However, we have not used daily prednisone except in systemic JRA for many years and have found alternate-day regimens to be preferable. While we try to use the smallest dose possible on alternate days (10 mg), we use whatever is needed for continued ambulation. Rifampin increases plasma clearance of prednisone, resulting in reduced efficacy.[414] Pharmacologic maneuvers to minimize osteoporosis in steroid-treated children have not yet been adequately studied but nasal calcitonin may have promise in this regard[415] and deflazacort may be bone sparing when compared with prednisone.[416]

Pulse Corticosteroid Therapy. Massive intravenous doses of corticosteroids administered over a short period of time ("pulse" therapy) have been reported to sometimes be helpful in renal graft rejection reactions, SLE, and other rheumatic diseases.[417] Experience with a few arthritic children suggests that this technique may be helpful on rare occasions but that in general too-frequent injections are required. Doses of 20–30 mg/kg of methylprednisone have general been used.[418,419]

Intravenous Gamma Globulin. A controlled trial is underway in systemic JRA and soon to begin in polyarticular JRA. Extensive experience in Kawasaki disease has shown the agent to be relatively safe, very expensive, and difficult to administer in institutions not equipped for long outpatient IV therapy. Preliminary studies[420] and our experience show that there is short-lived improvement in systemic features including fever and anemia and some improvement in arthritis. Infusions in most, but not all, patients (2 g/kg) given every 4 weeks may reduce the need for prednisone by 80% but significantly reduce effusions and number of actively inflamed joints in only half the children. Nevertheless, gamma globulin may be a useful emergency treatment at times of drug reactions or in certain selected patients.[421,422] Placenta-eluted gamma globulins are also being studied.[423]

Immunosuppressive Agents. The incidence of death from JRA is about 7% in reported series.[125] While this is probably an overestimate, based on disproportionately severe cases being seen in large referral centers, it constitutes an underestimate for the select group in which almost all deaths occur: the severe polyarticular group characterized by persistent unremitting disease. It seems reasonable to suppose that these agents, despite their potential for early or late significant or even fatal side effects, might be appropriate for the treatment of those youngsters who are potentially threatened with severe and permanent wheelchair crippling or death, or with becoming "twisted wreckage."[402,424,425]

Methotrexate. Although methotrexate is an old drug not used in childhood arthritis despite its availability for more than 30 years, it is currently in wide use for refractory childhood arthritis.[426,427] This reflects the poor efficacy and presumably equal toxicity[428] of gold, penicillamine, and hydroxychloroquine and azathioprine[429] in a disease which, while only occasionally life-threatening and usually remitting without meaningful sequelae with or without therapy, is awful in its worst forms. After methotrexate was documented to be relatively safe and efficacious in adults with RA[430,431] it was tried in children and reported to be reasonably safe and efficacious if

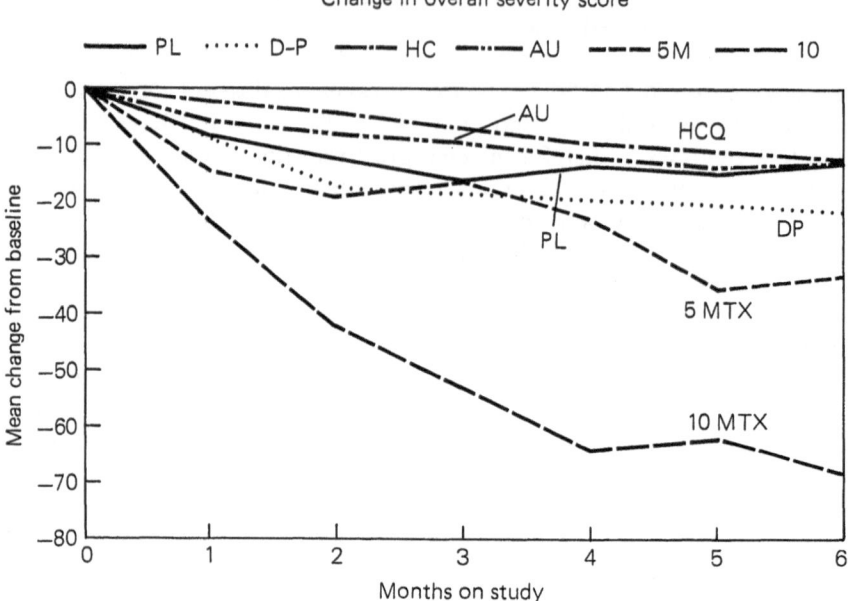

Figure 3.45. Meta-analysis of antirheumatic drug trials in juvenile rheumatoid arthritis carried out by the Pediatric Rheumatology Collaborative Drug Study Group (PRCSG). PL = placebo; DP = D-penicillamine; HC = hydroxychloroquine; AU = auranofin; 5M = methotrexate (5 mg/mm²/week); 10 = methotrexate (10 mg/mm²/week). Only 10 mg/mm²/week methotrexate was distinguishable from placebo with respect to efficacy. (Kindly supplied by Dr. E.H. Giannini, PRCSG.)

given in a dose of 10 mg/mm²/week.[432–434] Some authors measure serum levels and adjust doses upward for those who have poor absorption of drug; for these studies the medication is given with water after an 8-h fast and the fasting blood level is determined 1 h later.[426] Levels less than 0.6 μg tended to be associated with less than optimal results and higher levels, achieved with doses as high as 1.1 mg/kg/week, were sometimes effective and tolerated when lower doses had failed.[436,437] Salicylates, NSAIDs, and sulfonamides may increase levels and, therefore, both efficacy and toxicity.[438,439] Growth hormone may hasten excretion of all medications.

While methotrexate may slow radiologic progression of disease, it does not prevent it.[440–441a] Severe flare-ups in disease may be expected following withdrawal.[442,443] In adults, cumulative toxicity over 5 years amounts to 54%.[444] Most liver injury is mild and clinically insignificant[445–449a] but occasionally severe injury occurs (cirrhosis).[450–452a] Five percent of adults have severe pulmonary toxicity.[453] Stomatitis, leukocytoclastic vasculitis, central-nervous-system dysfunction, xylose malabsorption with jejunal histologic changes, and bone-marrow suppression may occur.[453–456] Osteopathy, delayed fracture healing, and increased risk of postsurgical complications are important considerations in children requiring scoliosis or other surgery.[457,458]

Methotrexate improves quality of life for some patients (29%)[459] and is a useful agent, better than and perhaps better tolerated than gold or penicillamine[460] (Fig. 3.45). However, it is not the ultimate agent: anemia was improved in only 43% of children, number of swollen joints reduced by only 46%, swelling in joints with persistent swelling reduced by only 52%, and corticosteroid dosage reduced in only one-third children who required steroids.[427] Results are better if it is introduced early in the course of disease and may be enhanced by sulfasalazine and hydroxychloroquine,[436,437] and possibly by increased or parenteral dosage with leucovorin rescue.[461] Intramuscular injections may be given by patients or parents;[360] subcutaneous injections may be bioequivalent to intramuscular.[437]

Azathioprine. In adults, no difference could be shown between azathioprine 150 mg/day and methotrexate, 15mg, once weekly, at 24 weeks; it is generally thought that methotrexate works faster but this could not be documented in a controlled trial.[462] More than 10% of children treated with 2.5 mg/kg/day in a controlled trial had to be withdrawn due to toxicity, primarily neutropenia/infections, and benefit over placebo was minimal but statistically significant at 16 weeks for subjective total assessment and functional capacity.[463] Despite increased risk of malignancy with long-term usage,[464] and hepatotoxicity and hypersensitivity reactions requiring discontinuation within 1 year in about 12% of patients,[465] azathioprine has a reasonable safety profile[466] if only it were more effective.[465a]

Cyclophosphamide. Cyclophosphamide at 75 mg/day inhibits erosions and relieves symptoms in adult RA but has generally unacceptable risks;[467,468] in life-threatening disease the risks may be acceptable.[469–472] Intravenous pulses (500 mg/mm^2) at 4–6-week intervals provided little improvement and all patients withdrew after 6 months;[473] higher doses, similar to those used in SLE, have not been studied. Combinations of cyclophosphamide, azathioprine, and hydroxychloroquine have been tried in adults.[474]

Chlorambucil. Chlorambucil, 0.01–0.16 mg/kg/day, given to children with JRA-associated amyloidosis, intractible vision-threatening uveitis, or uncontrolled systemic disease, was moderately effective[123,124] but associated with 100% chromosomal injuries,[475] occasional leukemia,[476] and gonadal injury.[477] Melphalan and colchicine might also be worthy of trial in JRA with amyloidosis.[478,479]

Cyclosporine. Adults and one child with arthritis unresponsive to conventional therapy have been treated with cyclosporine. ESR and rheumatoid factor have not been reduced but inflammation and functional symptoms have improved.[480-487] Nephropathy limits dosage to 4 mg/kg, probably the maximum safe dose; close safety monitoring is essential, especially if higher doses are required.[488-493] Children generally require higher doses than adults.[492] In a recent study in adults, cyclosporine was no better than penicillamine,[493] and increases risk of lymphoma.[493a]

Levamisole. This potent antihelminthic has some anti-inflammatory effects at high dosage and has thymominetic effects on T lymphocytes.[494] The beneficial effects in adults with RA are said to be similar to those obtained with gold and penicillamine, but not as good as those found with azathioprine.[495] A high incidence of fatal agranulocytosis, seizures, and coma has prevented adequate study in children and suggests that levamisole is unlikely to be useful in JRA.[496,497] However, unusually high doses were given to some of the children. New agents derived from levamisole or with similar pharmacologic properties and less toxicity may be discovered and be of more use in childhood arthritis.[497]

Plasma Exchange and Lymphocyte Depletion. Reducing the amounts of circulating antibody and immune complexes in antibody- or immune-complex–mediated diseases by plasma exchange is a technique used in Goodpasture's syndrome, SLE, and myasthenia gravis. Initial reports, based on somewhat sketchy evidence, have been enthusiastic. Plasmapheresis, lymphoplasmapheresis, and lymphapheresis have been tried in RA with varying success.[498-500] In one report of plasma exchange in JRA, success was dependent on the simultaneous administration of fresh-frozen plasma and was associated with an accidental death.[501] Apheresis at present must be considered a research procedure rather than an accepted mode of therapy.

Since high titers of rheumatoid factor or significant immune complexes have usually not been demonstrated in JRA, the mode of action of plasma exchange, if it worked, would be entirely unknown. We have tried plasmapheresis in one terribly ill systemic JRA patient. A femoral vein catheter was required. Blood transfusions were also required since the child was too small to provide blood for "priming" of the machine. Prompt improvement was seen in terms of arthritis, serum levels of immune globulins, and ESR. However, within a few weeks, the patient had resumed her prior state. The technical difficulties and repetitive hazards of doing this procedure in this small child outweighed its small benefits.

The use of total body lymphoid irradiation to achieve lymphocyte depletion in adult RA has not provided long-term improvement sufficient to warrant trials in children.[400] Thymopoietin,[502] typrilose,[503] gamma interferon,[504] tetracycline,[505] and fish oil[506] are safer agents being studied in adults. Arthritic children who developed myasthenia gravis and were subjected to thymectomy have had complete remission of their arthritis.[507] A few, but only a few, patients improve when they take birth-control pills[508] or amantadine.[509] Extracorporeal photochemotherapy is now being studied in adults.[510] Parents try many unconventional remedies.[511]

Pauciarticular Juvenile Rheumatoid Arthritis

It has long been recognized that arthritis in childhood frequently affects only one or a few joints.[3,12] In 1977, the ARA-JRA criteria committee agreed to classify children who, at 6 months after onset of arthritis, have disease limited to one to four joints as a pauciarticular subset.[13] This is the most frequent form of arthritis in childhood and accounts for an increasing proportion of patients seen in large childhood arthritis clinics (Table 3.4). Large joints, especially those of the lower extremities, are most frequently affected, and involvement is often asymmetrical and spotty.

The pauciarticular group has a better prognosis than either the systemic or polyarticular groups. Most patients will make a full recovery from the arthritis and have no disability. However, 11–37% of pauciarticular onset children will ultimately have a polyarticular course, and some significant disability in individual joints may occur. Visual impairment from chronic uveitis is also a significant risk in this group.[82]

Just as it has become apparent that it is difficult to make general statements about children with JRA without dividing them into clinical subsets, it has become obvious that what has been called pauciarticular JRA is an amalgam of different disorders. However, no two authorities agree at this moment on how to subdivide this group. Everyone recognizes the need to identify those patients who really have the disorder AS.[82,275,512] In our current schema of subdividing JRA, we have used histocompatibility testing as an aid to subset characterization. For purposes of study and prognosis as well as a useful guide to drug management, we find it most helpful to identify all HLA-B27 patients and consider them a separate disorder. Similar patients have been reported elsewhere as one subset of pauciarticular JRA.[82] HLA-B27-associated arthritis is discussed in Chapter 4.

All authors agree on a second clinical subset of pauciarticular disease, which is often characterized as "little girls with one swollen knee, a positive test for antinuclear antibody, and a high risk of chronic uveitis."[18,82] In one study, 10% of arthritic children belonged to this subset. (Only 65% of these were ANA-positive.)[82] Some authors have included all patients with chronic uveitis as a single subset (i.e., not limited to females). Children with the onset of pauciarticular arthritis prior to age 5 tend to be in this subset. Recent studies in our laboratories and others have shown that HLA-B27-negative, early onset pauciarticular JRA with uveitis is associated with HLA-DR5.[10,18,513] Other HLA-D–region antigens are associated with increased risk of pauciarticular JRA in some populations; a single mechanism (shared epitope) may be responsible for the increased susceptibility.[514]

The characterization of pauciarticular JRA into subsets is not just of clinical interest. With recent evidence suggesting that JRA may represent a series of disorders with T-cell defects, it is reasonable to presume that different patterns of disease may be a reflection of different variations in immunologic function.[515] For purposes of study, we are now dividing the HLA-B27-negative pauciarticular patients into two subsets: DR5-positive and DR5-negative.

HLA-DR5-Associated Pauciarticular JRA

Among 39 pauciarticular-onset patients known to be HLA-B27-negative, we found 23 DR5-positive patients.[10,513] The tested population was not unselected and was weighted for uveitis, so it may not be a totally accurate representation of the constituency of the total B27-negative pauciarticular group. Seven DR5 patients were males; one of these had uveitis. Thus, while males (seven of 23) are not as frequently affected as females (16 of 23), they did not constitute an insignificant part of this population. The number of affected joints at onset averaged only 1.3. In 17 of 23 patients (74%), the onset was monarticular. The knee was most frequently affected (12 of 23), with hip and ankle the other relatively frequently affected joints (five of 23). Elbow, finger, foot, and TMJ were all affected in single instances; in no cases were the wrists or shoulders affected at the time of onset of arthritis in this population. The arthritis tended to be very mild, to respond to aspirin, and to remit relatively quickly. Recurrent attacks were common, however, and two patients developed a polyarticular course.

The age at onset of this arthritis differs in association with the presence or absence of uveitis. The average age at onset in girls with uveitis was 3.8 years (in the single boy, 3 years), while in girls without uveitis, it was 8.2 years, and in boys without uveitis, 7.5 years. The pattern of arthritis did not vary with age.

This association of DR5 with pauciarticular JRA and especially with girls with JRA and uveitis has since been confirmed by Glass et al.[18] After discussion with us, they selected 45 pauciarticular JRA patients, heavily weighted for females (41) and uveitis (24). Of the 45, 28 were HLA-DR5; 17 of 24 with uveitis were HLA-DR5. As expected from prior reports, ANA was found especially frequently in the DR5-positive girls with uveitis. The relationship between DR5 and this subset of childhood arthritis has been found in all populations so far examined. Our preliminary data suggest that other DR associations found only in individual geographic areas may represent population-biased samples. However, further study is required.

Non-B27, non-DR5 Pauciarticular JRA

Of the 39 HLA-B27-negative patients tested, 16 were also DR5-negative; of these, six were boys and 10 were girls. The average age at onset of arthritis was 6.4 years for boys and 5.9 for girls. There were no apparent differences to distinguish the pattern of arthritis in this subset from the total pauciarticular group, but individual patients might most resemble one of the other subsets, that is, HLA-B27-associated disease, DR5-associated disease, or polyarticular seropositive RA associated with DR4.

Prognosis

The overall prognosis for the entire pauciarticular JRA group is good, with relatively little scarring except in the eyes (see below). However, more severe involvement requiring joint replacement occurs in the B27 group (see Chapter 4), and recent studies indicate that the prognosis for the knees of the DR5 uveitis group may not be as good as we had previously thought.[516] While in our short-term follow-up period the prognosis for joint function seemed good, in a larger long-term series of patients with chronic iritis reported by Kanski, 20% of patients had "severe disease" and ultimately required surgical joint replacement.[517] Pauciarticular patients carrying HLA-DR13-DW18 and DQ6-DW18 are more likely to have persistent disease.[518]

Treatment

In most pauciarticular patients, aspirin, 90 mg/kg/day (max. 3.6 g daily) in four divided doses, provides excellent control of the arthritis. A few children respond better to tolmetin or naproxen or tolerate it better, and these agents are now the first choice of most parents. Teenagers may prefer other nonsteroidal anti-inflammatory agents. In our clinic gold, penicillamine, and hydroxychloroquine are not used in the treatment of pauciarticular disease since the toxic hazards of these agents would seem to outweigh their potentia therapeutic promise. We use sulfasalazine extensively in pauciarticular patients.

Antirheumatic medication is continued until the patient has been asymptomatic and has normal laboratory studies for 6 months. Remission is defined by being asymptomatic and having normal laboratory studies for a period of 6 months after cessation of all treatment.

Intra-articular Corticosteroid Injections. Children do not like injections into their joints; general anesthesia may be required for children under age 6.[519] The beneficial effect, if there is any, tends to wear off in days. Intrasynovial injections are occasionally complicated by the introduction of bacteria into the arthritic joint, creating a very difficult diagnostic and therapeutic problem. Experimental evidence suggests hydrocortisone may have a deleterious effect on damaged cartilage in young animals. Repeated injections may foster total joint destruction. Leakage of steroid around the needle tract may cause permanent unattractive atrophy of skin and subcutaneous tissues.[520] Fifty percent of children treated with intra-articular steroids develop calcifications in and around the treated joint, most of which are asymptomatic, but 3/55 develop avascular necrosis, a very serious complication.[521,522] Nevertheless, there are occasions when one injection of long-acting steroid into a single large knee effusion, after removal of fluid, provides great relief of pain, allowing mobilization of the stiff joint and correction of deformity.[13,523,524] The beneficial effect, in some rare instances, may be extremely long-lasting. The risk of a single injection is small, but we do not give repeated injections. Steroids must not be injected at the time of arthroscopy as the risk of infection is high.[525]

Iridocyclitis (Anterior Uveitis)

The association of iritis with arthritis in children; the distinction of this subacute or chronic iritis, which was persistent from the form of iritis that was acute and paroxysmal; and the observation that the parents of children with iritis usually had arthritis were all reported by Jonathan Hutchinson in *Lancet* in 1873,[526] a quarter of a century prior to Still's description of JRA and over a century before we again recognized the heritable tendency.

Subacute or chronic inflammation of the iris and ciliary body occurs in 20% of all children with JRA (Fig. 3.46). Both eyes are ultimately affected in 70% of children with uveitis. Patients tend to have recurrent attacks; in 21% of cases, the duration of eye disease exceeds 10 years.[517] Two percent of arthritic children, or 6% of all with pauciarticular onset seen prior to 1960, were totally blind in 10 years.[42,527,528] Arthritis precedes the onset of uveitis in almost all (92%) cases.[517,529]

The Susceptible Population

If the B27 subset is excluded, about 90% of arthritic children with uveitis are girls. In some series, 60–90% of them have antinuclear antibodies.[529,530] Although the disease is almost always pauciarticular (often monarticular) at onset, it need not remain pauciarticular, and some severely incapacitated patients have uveitis. The mean age at onset of arthritis in the uveitis population is 3.7 years.[517] The knee is the single most commonly affected joint. The arthritic population characterized as little girls with swollen knees and a positive ANA test has a greater than 40% risk of uveitis. In our studies, 90% of arthritic children with subacute or chronic uveitis were of a single HLA-DR type—DR5.[513] Certain DR5 haplotypes predispose more than others.[531] Patients with pauciarticular-onset arthritis remain at risk for uveitis for many years. In 21% of cases, uveitis began more than 5 years after the onset of arthritis.[517]

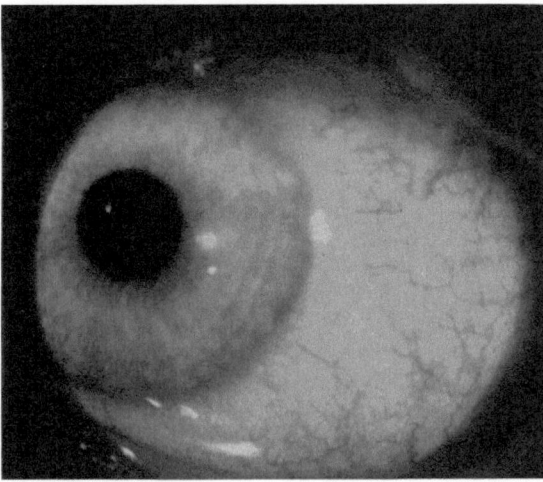

Figure 3.46. Although the subacute or chronic uveitis associated primarily with pauciarticular JRA (especially common in little girls with anti-nuclear antibodies) is generally found only by routine screening slit-lamp examinations, occasionally patients will have a "ciliary-flush" indicating inflammation.

Diagnosis

Most patients are asymptomatic early in the course of their disease, although mild redness of the eye or visual complaints occur occasionally (Fig. 3.46). Thus, early diagnosis depends on routine slit-lamp screening of all arthritic children. This is carried out at 3-month intervals in the most susceptible population. The ophthalmologist notes the number of cells in the anterior chamber and the amount of protein precipitate (flare), using a standard grading system. Fresh keratic precipitates are noted if present. Unfortunately, in published reports, up to 18% of patients already had band keratopathy, and 9% had cataracts at the time of initial diagnosis.[517,532]

Course

If the disease is unilateral when first seen and the second eye becomes involved, it generally is affected within a year. Although attacks of uveitis may be brief, they tend to recur.[517]

All patients are not equally severely affected, and it seems unlikely that all have the same potential for scarring and blindness.[530] Our routine screening procedure identifies some patients with inconsequential disease. However, in the largest published experience (160 cases), Kanski reported some loss of vision in 43% of affected eyes.[517] Twenty-six percent of affected eyes in his series lost all vision or retained only light perception or the ability to count fingers; 17% of affected children were totally blind. It is hoped that with earlier diagnosis and treatment and modern surgical techniques, these figures are a reflection of the past rather than current experience.[528]

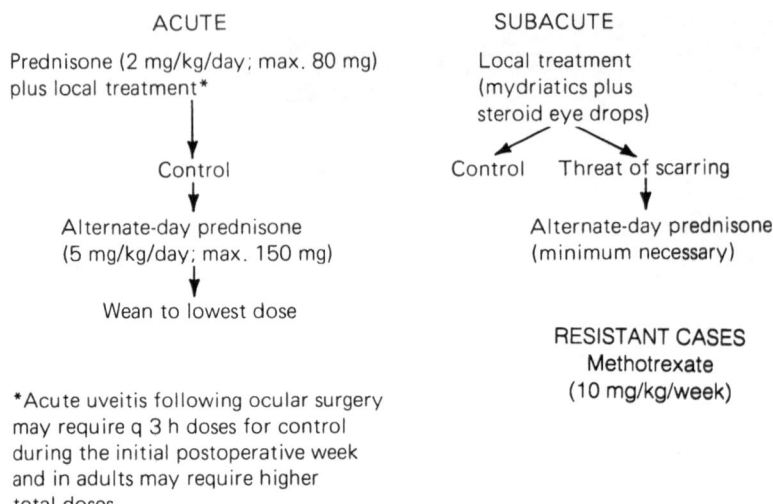

Figure 3.47. Treatment module for uveitis.

Medical Treatment

Most of our patients are already receiving NSAIDs when they develop uveitis.[533] It is not yet known whether sulfasalazine decreases the frequency of iritis.[533a] Uveitis is treated with mydriatics and topical corticosteroid drops administered at frequent intervals.[528,530,534] If a prompt response is not obtained, systemic steroids are instituted (Fig. 3.47). We have not found subtenon injections of steroid a practical approach to therapy and have cared for one child who was blinded as a result of an inadvertent arterial injection.[535] We use prednisone, 1–2 mg/kg/day in divided doses, until the inflammation is completely controlled (usually a few weeks) and then change to an alternate-day regimen (2–5 mg/kg/dose). If the inflammation is controlled, the dose is gradually reduced with careful monitoring of the eyes. The regimen is aimed at preventing visual scars and accepts steroid side effects in an effort to prevent blindness.

This program, together with frequent monitoring of asymptomatic arthritic children, has the potential to prevent blindness totally from late-diagnosed or inadequately controlled uveitis.[528] Nevertheless, we continue to see patients who are blinded by complicated cataracts secondary to inadequately treated uveitis.[536,537]

While in our clinic with this regimen we have had no loss of visual acuity in 86% of children with uveitis in whom the diagnosis was made prior to loss of visual acuity,[529] others have not had similar success and report limited steroid responsiveness.[517] There has been too little experience with immunosuppressive drugs in steroid-resistance uveitis to allow meaningful comment[538–540] but new studies with methotrexate are promising.[540a]

Table 3.18. Results of Cataract Surgery in JRA

Visual Acuity	Smiley and Kanski	Chylack et al.[534]	Key and Kimura	Praeger et al.[543]	Kanski and Crick*	Diamond and Kaplan*,[545]
20/200 or less	8	6	11	4[†]	14	5
20/40–20/120	3	2	9	3	5	2
20/30 or better	1	0	3	13	15	8
Totals	12	8	23	17	34	15

*Acuity groupings slightly different: Kanski and Crick: 20/120 or less, 20/60–20/80, 20/40 or better; Diamond and Kaplan 20/100 or less, 20/70, 20/25, or better.
[†]One failure related to amblyopia exanopsia and three to uncontrolled glaucoma.

Surgery for Band Keratopathy

When vision is obstructed by calcium deposits in the cornea, removal of the band keratopathy by chelation and curretage is a simple and generally successful procedure.[541] Laser surgery may help in resistant cases.

Cataract Surgery in Patients with Uveitis

Until recently, the surgical removal of a complicated cataract in arthritic children was generally followed by blindness (Table 3.18, Fig. 3.48)[541–543] In 1976, we reported a two-phase new approach to these cataracts; removal with the new surgical technique of phacoemulsification and intraoperative and postoperative medical support with daily high-dose steroid therapy.[543] In Dr. Praeger's hands, this technique has now been entirely satisfactory in 13 of 17 cases (Table 3.18, Fig. 3.49). Improved results with new techniques for lensectomy rather than phacoemulsification, but without systemic steroids, have been reported by Kanski and Flynn.[541,542,544] The published results do not equal the combination of phacoemulsification and aggressive steroid therapy. Kaplan and Diamond, after demonstrating that postvitrectomy uveitis in the rabbit was prevented by vigorous steroid therapy, used a steroid regimen similar to ours but with a different surgical procedure (lensectomy with vitrectomy) for patients with complicated cataracts.[545] Their results also do not equal those with phacoemulsification, but their patient population did not include children and may not have been analogous to ours. We have also used our steroid regimen with lensectomy and vitrectomy without phacoemulsification in two children. Both operations were successful in restoring vision, but more steroids seemed to be required than have been required in those cases done with phacoemulsification. Chylack has also reported phacoemulsification to be the procedure of choice in these children.[534] Thus, pending further study, our recommendation would be administration of steroids to completely control inflammation on the day prior to and during

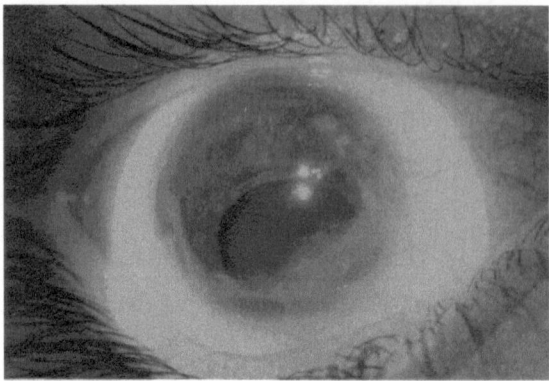

Figure 3.48. Appearance of eye following surgery with old techniques aimed at removing the complicated cataract that results from uveitis. Very few patients we operated on retained useful vision (Table 3.18).

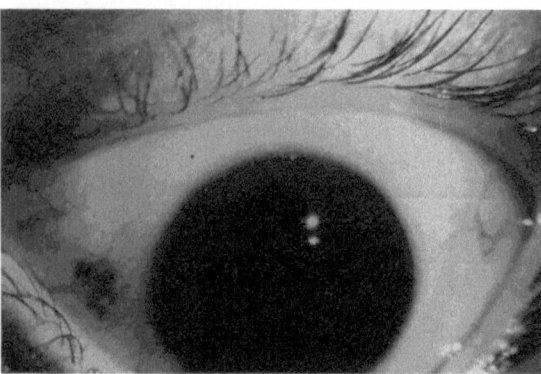

Figure 3.49. Note clear appearance of the eye a few months after surgery using phacoemulsification and high-dose perioperative steroids. Photo shows superior sphincterectomy and inferior iris sphincterotomy with pericentral opacification of intact posterior capsule. Note iris synechia to lens capsule. (Courtesy of Dr. D. Praeger.)

surgery and in sufficient dosage to control inflammation postoperatively with cataract removal by phacoemulsification. The surgical technique and steroid regimen are detailed elsewhere.[543] Unilaterally, blind eyes in young children must be operated on promptly to avoid amblyopia exanopsia. Glaucoma must be adequately treated when present or a blind eye will result despite successful cataract surgery. Trabeculodialysis is said to work best.[541,542]

Arthritis with Psoriasis

All forms of arthritis may occur coincident with psoriasis, but arthritis that mainly involves the distal interphalangeal joints of the hands is most distinctive and is usually called "psoriatic" (Fig. 3.50). Less than half of all arthritic children with psoriasis have this form of arthritis.[546–549] Family history of psoriasis, and nail pitting or onycholysis suggest this subset; dactylitis may be the presenting manifestation. Arthritis with these manifestations in childhood is usually pauciarticular in onset but often progresses to a polyarticular

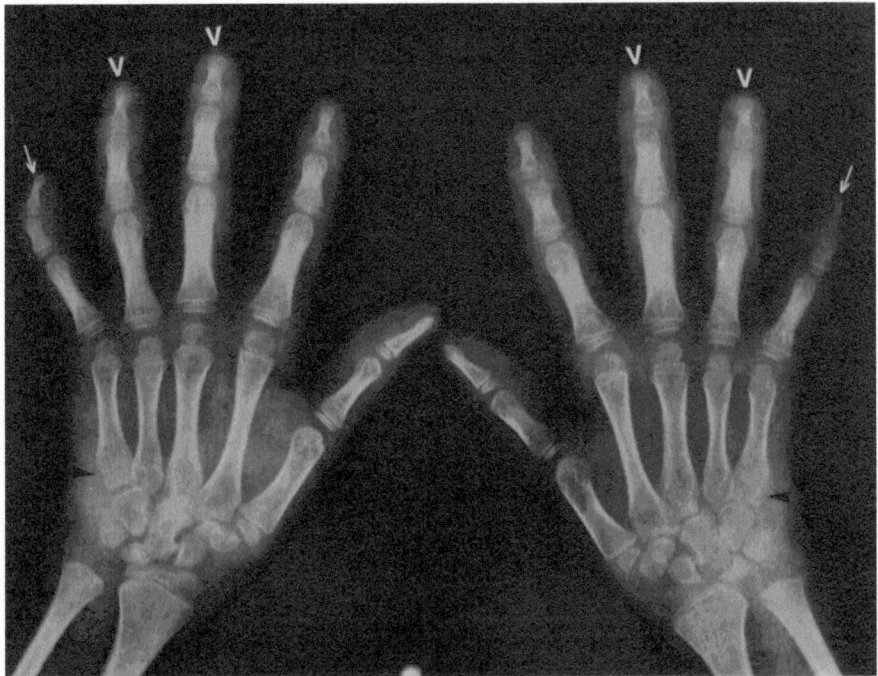

Figure 3.50. Hands of a 9-year-old boy with congenital familiar psoriatic erythroderma, showing loss of soft tissues in the distal finger tufts (*arrowheads*), with beginning loss of bone substance and DIP-joint arthritis in the fifth fingers (*arrows*). There are extensive arthritic changes at the wrists with crenation of the carpal bones and loss of joint space. Note severe erosions visible at the lateral bases of the fifth metacarpal bones (*black arrowheads*). The findings are typical of those seen in other forms of psoriasis.

course.[549] Sacroiliitis occurs in 30% of children with psoriasis and arthritis and, when present, is generally associated with the presence of HLA-B27. Iritis occurs in about 8%.

Females are more commonly affected with arthritis/psoriasis (2.6:1). The mean age of onset is high for childhood arthritis (9–10 years of age). Arthritis usually precedes the appearance of the psoriatic skin lesions. Some authors suggest that synovial-lining cells are less affected, and there is increased inflammation, fibrosis, and thickening of the walls of small and medium-sized synovial arteries when compared with other types of arthritis.[550]

Although psoriatic arthritis in childhood is generally a mild disease, it tends to continue into adult life and, in some cases, is associated with rapid joint destruction. Management is similar to other forms of childhood arthritis and depends on the extent of the joint involvement. Colchicine,[551] cyclosporine,[552] and 1,25-hydroxyvitamin D$_3$[553] may be effective. We have used cyclosporine where all else has failed, with great success; 5 mg/kg/day in two divided doses may be the best starting dose, with close attention to the potential for blood-level alterations caused by drug interactions.[554] Unfortunately, patients' illness may be exacerbated as soon as one tries to withdraw the medication, and the risks increase with long-term use.[554-556]

Exercises as Therapy in Childhood Arthritis

Movement and weight bearing are important in preventing accelerated destruction of cartilage. Evidence from animal studies shows that experimentally damaged cartilage suffers worse destruction if prohibited from weight bearing and exercise.[407,557] Radiographic regrowth of hip cartilage/fibrous tissue allowing improved function has similarly been demonstrated following ambulation of bedridden children with hip destruction from JRA (Fig. 3.51).[411] It is also generally not understood that joint capsular structures and muscle undergo adaptive shortening during immobilization even in the absence of inflammation.[410,558] When combined with inflammation in the synovium and all the periarticular structures, immobilization results in the most aggressive functional impairment of hips and knees, resulting in a bedridden condition (Fig. 3.52). Once bedridden, cartilage destruction and contractures about the joints accelerate.

The reason for the ghastly radiographic appearance of the hips and knees of bedridden JRA patients is not just JRA but the vicious cycle of JRA combined with immobility and lack of weight bearing (Fig. 3.51).[411] Sometimes this cycle is begun by well-meaning physicians who do not understand these physiological mechanisms. The natural tendency is to avoid use of painful joints. It is often hard to convince physicians of the crucial importance of walking on damaged legs in JRA. Convincing parents and children in pain requires a thorough understanding of the critical necessity for ambulation and of the horrendous physical crippling created by immobility in chronic polyarticular JRA.[411]

Complete immobilization of the arthritic joint (as in circular plaster) is never indicated and may result in accelerated loss of muscle strength and prolonged or permanent loss of function. We continue to see children who are put in plaster by orthopedists even though x-rays are normal "just in case" they have missed a fracture. This practice is to be discouraged.

The primary goal of the physical and occupational therapist in JRA is the *maintenance of function* of individual *joints*, of the *child*, and of the *family*. Physical measures to help relieve pain and deformity and to preserve and restore motion and strength are the most-often-emphasized tools of the physicians and allied health personnel in the department of physical medicine and rehabilitation. Their role in the care of these children is greater than the sum of the parts. They exude confidence and show their commitment to function; they emphasize the positive—what the child can do—and fight to minimize

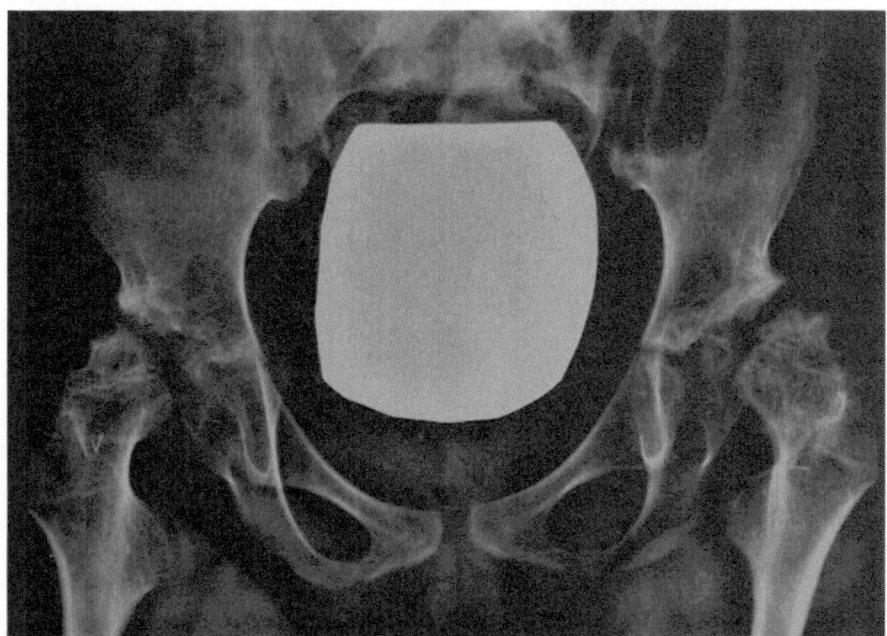

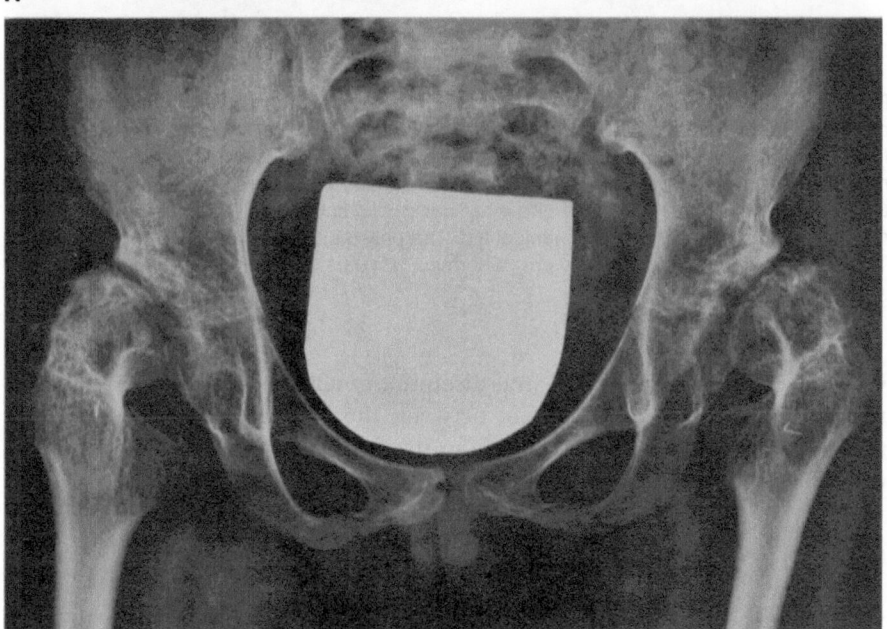

Figure 3.51. Hip radiographs of a 9-year-old Korean girl (Fig. 3 52) brought here for treatment of systemic JRA. The child had been bedridden for 5 years. (**A**) Remineralization and filling-in of bony defects 2 years after patient began to fully bear weight on the joints.[560] (**B**) Metallic objects are broken acupuncture needles. (Reprinted with permission from Jacobs et al., ref. 413.)

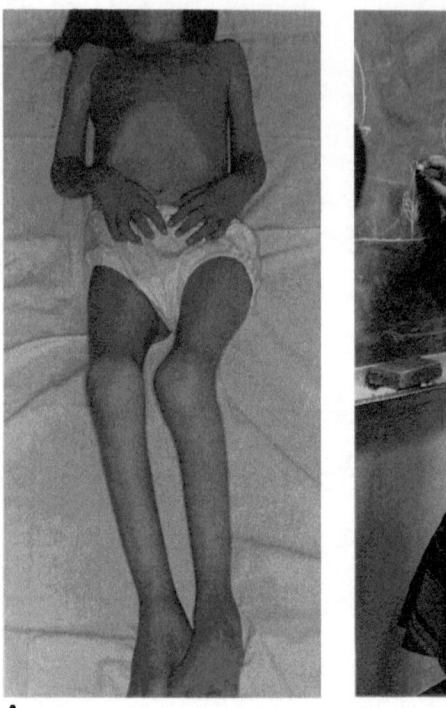 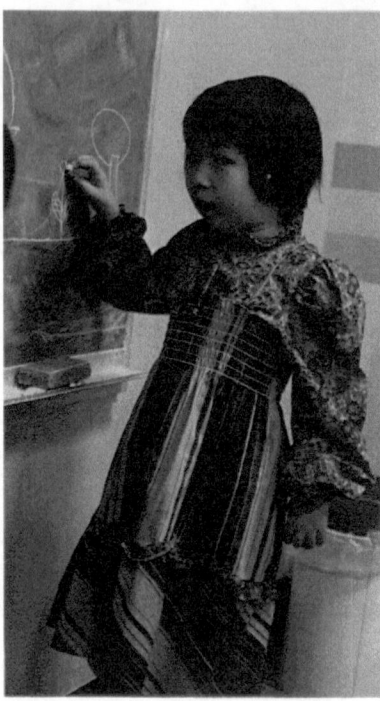

A   **B**

Figure 3.52. Patient at the time she was first seen (**A**) and 3 years later (**B**) following release of iliotibial bands and soft-tissue contractures about the hips and knees (at one operation) followed by 5 h of physical therapy daily for several months. The mother was taught the regimen during the 3-week hospitalization and continued intensive therapy at home. Within 6 months, the child was able to attend a regular public school (despite the language barrier), and to walk without any mechanical aid. The only medicine she received was aspirin. Total hip and knee replacements were performed 10 years later.

what he or she cannot do. The interdisciplinary team exudes optimism, helps to break communication barriers between the primary physician and the family, and contributes, by example to the family, a sense of buoyancy and control over the disease.

Getting Started in the Morning

Gelling and stiffness make early morning one of the worst times of day for the arthritic child. Arising at 6:00 A.M., taking the medicine, then reading in bed or getting a bit more sleep, followed by a warm bath or shower help in getting started. A simple set of limbering-up exercises is performed, and the child assumes straight posture in front of the mirror. Later in the day, the detailed exercise program is continued.

The Specific Exercise Program

If pain is severe, heat in the form of hot baths or local application of towels or soaks may be helpful. The maintenance of motion is achieved by putting every joint of the body, whether involved or uninvolved, through a full range of motion using positions that require as little resistance as possible. The child and parent are shown how to compare normal joint motion with that of affected joints, how to examine the joints, and the visual clues of joint involvement.

A detailed, individually written program is provided to each family as they are taught the exercises. After the program has been taught, it is performed by the child and parent with praise and suggestions from the therapist. This is reviewed and reinforced at several subsequent visits to the rheumatologist. The optimal arrangement is for the physical and occupational therapists to be present in the clinic or office to work with the patients at the regularly scheduled visits or to visit the patients in their homes.[559] We try to avoid separate visits to the therapist.

Although gentle passive stretching exercises are used, active and resistance exercises, especially with resistance applied by the child himself, are more effective. Strength of weak muscles may be improved with muscle-tensing exercises that do not involve joint motion (isometric exercises). Many exercises may be performed while in school or in front of the television.

Gravity is used when possible to prevent or correct deformity. Watching TV in the prone position helps to prevent hip-flexion contractures. Children are also encouraged to sleep in this position.

Sleeping splints may be useful as a means of increasing joint mobility (extension) in the wrists and sometimes the knees. Splints must be adjusted and frequently modified; they meet with a fair amount of resistance from both child and family and are only useful when accepted by both as part of an ego-building program. If physical modes of therapy become a source of conflict between parent and child, either the conflict has to be resolved with a psychological approach or the "therapy" will be unsuccessful or even countertherapeutic.

A heel lift on a short leg (usually the uninvolved leg in asymmetrical disease) will help correct or prevent a flexion contracture in the affected, more rapidly growing knee. Persistent leg length discrepancy may result in relative quadraceps atrophy.[561]

Swimming is an excellent exercise, and our families are encouraged to have pools if possible. The buoyant effect of the water allows large weight-bearing joints to be moved without force; most children enjoy swimming, and the pool attracts friends and is ego-rewarding for our patients. Other coordinated activities such as ball playing or bicycle riding also provide muscle strengthening and ego-rewarding social opportunities. The disease may set limits on the child's performance, but we do not set any limits whatsoever. We also do not prescribe rest; these children naturally rest more than healthy children. Any limitation is inevitably countertherapeutic. Normal childhood is the best therapy. Supplementing normal activities with professionally delivered services can make a great contribution to the patient's welfare; substituting professionally delivered services for being busy with normal activities is relatively useless.[562] Preventing children from doing things for themselves, developing motor skills, and thus achieving independence and autonomy leads to feelings of helplessness and anger that are countertherapeutic. No exercise program can equal the activities of daily living.

Surgery in JRA

Pediatric orthopedic surgery requires special understanding of children and growing bones. Juvenile rheumatoid arthritis creates additional special problems. Prolonged immobilization results in atrophy of bone and muscle. When a child has borderline function, immobilization associated with surgery or with treatment of traumatic fracture from a fall may be enough to make the child a bed-chair invalid. Months or years of effort may be required just to get the child back to where he started.

Thus, surgery is not to be lightly embarked upon and should only be performed by experienced operators in pediatric rheumatology centers. Most reports of surgery in JRA refer to adults who have had JRA since childhood, not to children. The subject of surgery in JRA has been thoroughly reviewed by Arden and Ansell, and the reader is referred to their excellent monograph.[268]

"Prophylactic" Surgery

Synovectomy as a means of preventing rather than relieving disability has been tried and abandoned twice in the history of rheumatology. Its value has not been demonstrated. Synovectomy of the knee often relieves pain but is rarely if ever required for that purpose in children. There are few, if any, benefits[563–564a] and, if performed, they should be done by arthroscopic synovectomy.[565]

Cosmetic Surgery

The small mandible caused by JRA troubles many teenagers and is relatively easily corrected with only a few days of hospitalization (Fig. 3.29). The particular surgical procedures must be individualized by experienced physicians. In very rare cases, temporomandibular joint surgery is needed in youngsters who cannot adequately open the mouth.

Some girls wish cosmetic correction of finger deformities. This can be successfully achieved with relative ease, but function does not improve and may even be somewhat reduced.

Surgery to Relieve Nerve Compression at the Wrist

In rare individuals, extensive tenosynovitis at the wrist may threaten nerve function; simple releases may be performed to prevent serious loss of function. We have not seen children who required wrist surgery to prevent tendon rupture or to relieve flexion contractures in dysfunctional positions, although others report experience with such procedures.

Corrective and Restorative Surgery

Soft-tissue release operations, débridement and therapeutic synovectomy are useful in selected instances in JRA (Fig. 3.52). In our experience, these procedures have only been necessary in children with flexion contractures of the hips and knees, accelerated by sitting in wheelchairs, who were bedridden when we first saw them. In these patients, multiple surgical procedures performed at one time may be an essential part of a massive program aimed at getting the child ambulatory again. This goal can then be achieved with a 7-day-per-week, 5-h-per-day rehabilitation program (Fig. 3.53). However, success requires hard work by a well-coordinated, big-center, experienced pediatric rehabilitation team. Detailed surgical techniques and anesthetic precaution are reviewed elsewhere.[268] Benefits tend to be short-lived.[566]

Total Joint Replacement

Experience with hip replacement in young adults who have had destruction of the hips during childhood has been excellent both in our experience and in other centers.[567-572] The roentgen appearance of the hips should not be used as the criterion for surgery since some patients function well despite an awful radiographic appearance (Figs. 3.54 and 3.55). Replacement of elbows, shoulders, and knees has not yet achieved success equal to hip implants. However, results improve each year.[573,574]

We urge our patients to wait as long as possible before having any joint replacement procedures. The advantage of waiting until the epiphyses close is obvious. In addition, we do not know how long these prosthetic joints are likely to last. Recent experience shows constant technical improvement in implant materials, design, and procedures. Our conservative approach is supported by increasing evidence of potential loss of seemingly fine early prosthetic repair. Early acetabular loosening and radiolucencies predictive of early failure and/or significant heterotopic bone formation are now reported in 15% of hip replacements in young arthritic patients even in the most experienced clinics (Fig. 3.56), and 15-year hip survival is 70%.[568,572] However, we do not allow children to become bed/chair bound; the lives of these youngsters have been transformed by total hip replacement.[570]

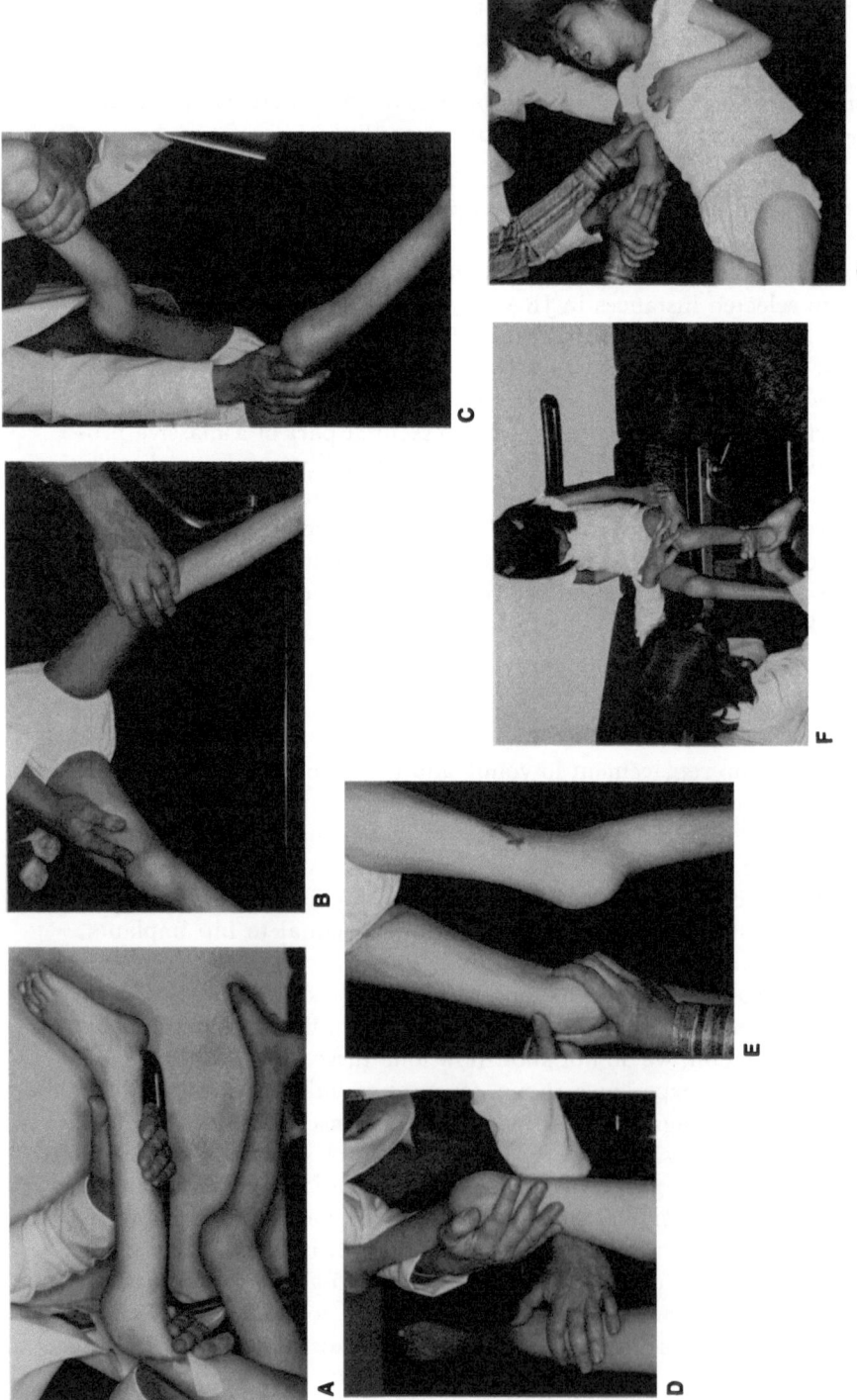

Figure 3.53 An exercise program must include vigorous, active stretching and muscle-strengthening exercise, together with some passive stretching. The parent must carry out the program with the child at home every day, 7 days a week. The therapist provides instruction and encouragement but doesn't actually do the daily exercises. A vigorous physical therapy program was successful in achieving full ambulation in a youngster who had been bedridden for 5 years. The therapy was begun immediately following surgery to release soft-tissue contractures in the iliotibial ligaments and around the

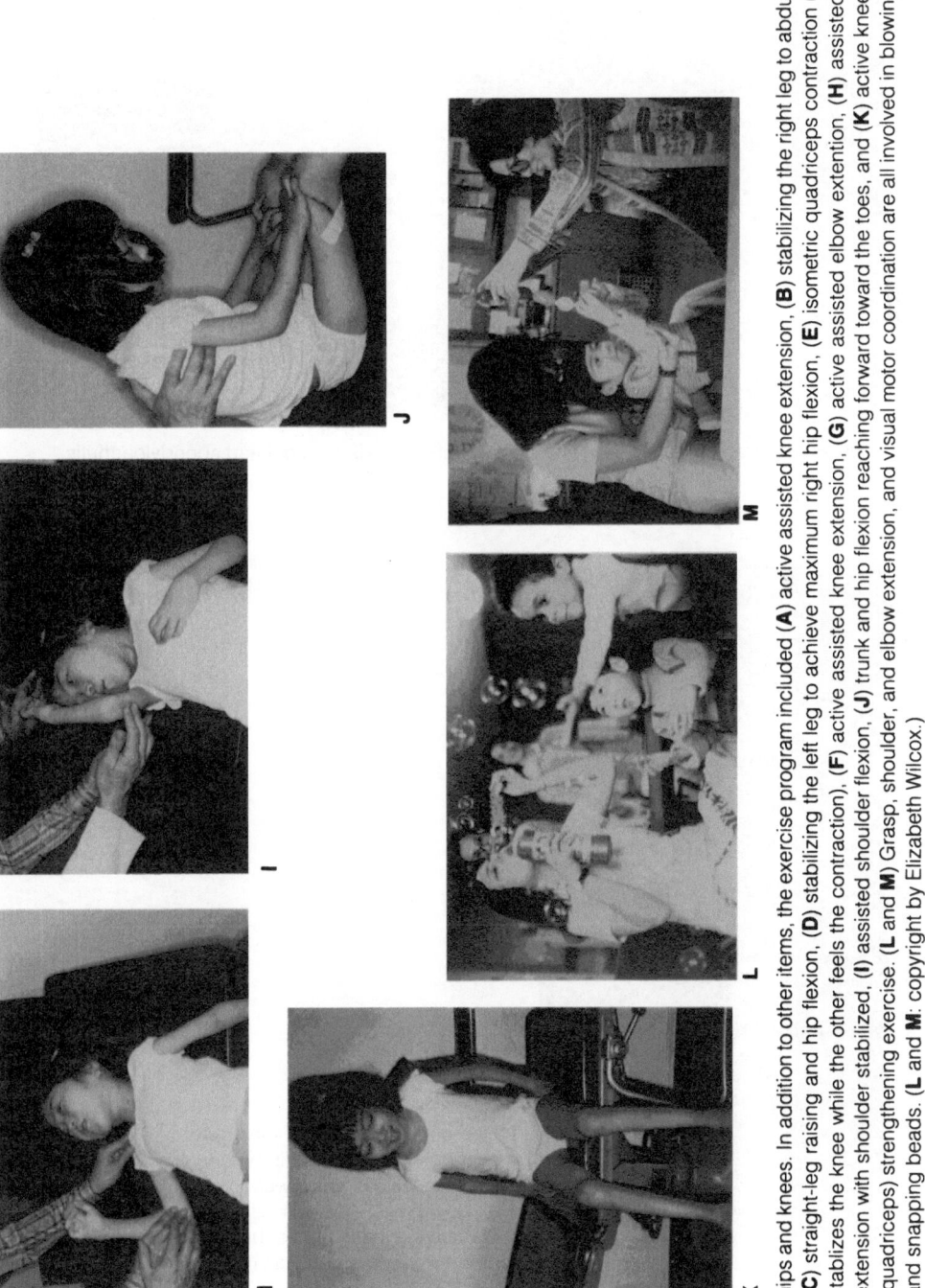

hips and knees. In addition to other items, the exercise program included (**A**) active assisted knee extension, (**B**) stabilizing the right leg to abduct the left, (**C**) straight-leg raising and hip flexion, (**D**) stabilizing the left leg to achieve maximum right hip flexion, (**E**) isometric quadriceps contraction (one hand stabilizes the knee while the other feels the contraction), (**F**) active assisted knee extension, (**G**) active assisted elbow extention, (**H**) assisted shoulder extension with shoulder stabilized, (**I**) assisted shoulder flexion, (**J**) trunk and hip flexion reaching forward toward the toes, and (**K**) active knee-extensor (quadriceps) strengthening exercise. (**L** and **M**) Grasp, shoulder, and elbow extension, and visual motor coordination are all involved in blowing bubbles and snapping beads. (**L** and **M**: copyright by Elizabeth Wilcox.)

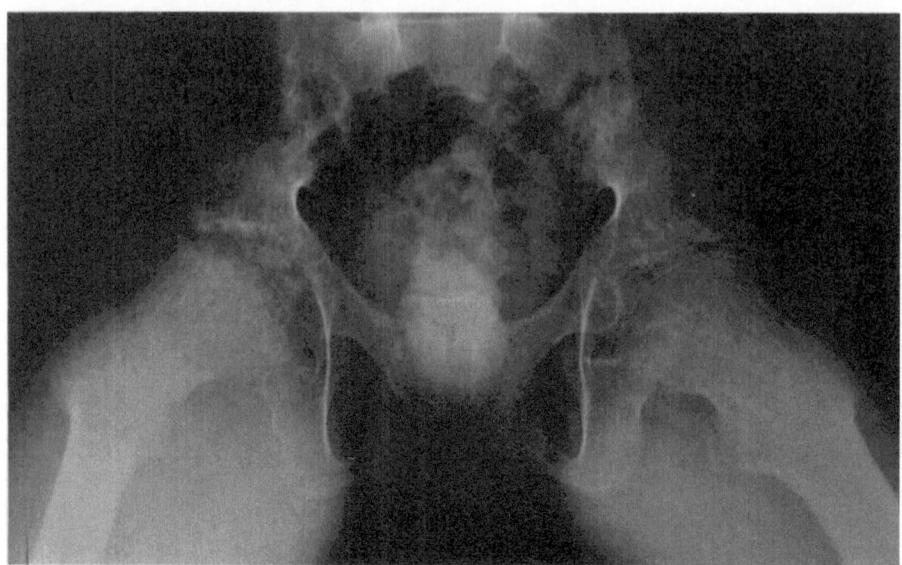

Figure 3.54. Radiograph of the hips in a boy with HLA-B27-associated spondyloarthritis.

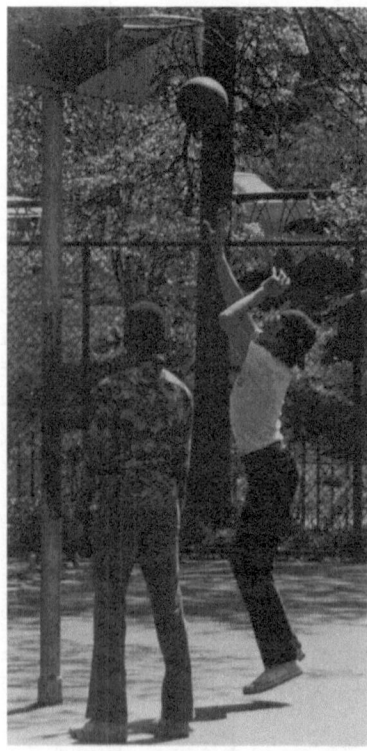

Figure 3.55. Despite the severe radiographic changes (Fig. 3.54), this boy could unexpectedly play basketball and was on his neighborhood team. Although he will ultimately require hip replacement, it has not yet been necessary (5 years after this photograph was taken).

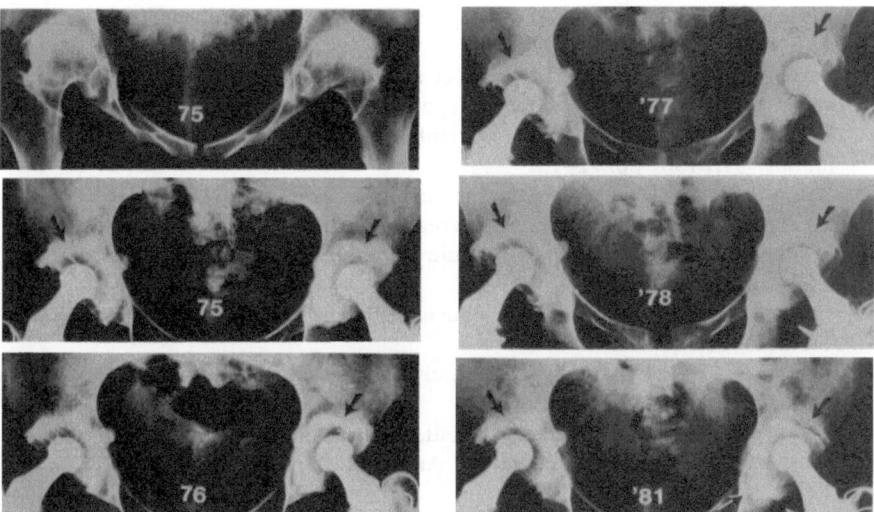

Figure 3.56. Pre- and postoperative radiograph of the hips (*1975*) in a college girl with long-standing JRA who had no hip abduction and desired hip replacement in order to be able to abduct the hips for normal sexual function. Bilateral total hip replacements were well tolerated (in two steps; one hospital admission), and the patient has no pain and is delighted with the result. However, from 1975 to 1981, as shown by the *arrows*, a progressively increasing "lucency" (interface) is seen in the films. This rapid demarcation occurs in 15% of young JRA patients following total hip replacement and may be a permanent obstacle to achieving a permanent fixation of the prosthesis to bone in young individuals. It is thought to be due to hyperelasticity of the bone in young patients.

References

1. JRA Criteria Subcommittee. Criteria for classification of juvenile rheumatoid arthritis. Bull Rheum Dis 25:712–719, 1973.
2. Cassidy JT, Levinson JE, Brewer EJ Jr: The development of classification criteria for children with juvenile rheumatoid arthritis. Bull Rheum Dis 38, #6:1–7, 1989.
3. Calabro JJ, Marchesano JM: The early natural history of juvenile rheumatoid arthritis. Med Clin North Am 52:567–591, 1968.
4. Schaller JG, Wedgwood RJ: Juvenile rheumatoid arthritis: A review. Pediatrics 50:940–953, 1972.
5. Schaller JG: Juvenile rheumatoid arthritis. Arthritis Rheum 20:165–170, 1977.
6. Stillman JS, Barry PE: Juvenile rheumatoid arthritis. Arthritis Rheum 20:171–175, 1977.
7. Fink CW: Patients with JRA: A clinical study. Arthritis Rheum 20:183–184, 1977.
8. Hanson V, Kornreich HK, Bernstein B, et al.: Three subtypes of juvenile rheumatoid arthritis. Arthritis Rheum 20:184–186, 1977.

9. Levinson JE, Balz GP, Hess EV: Report of studies on juvenile arthritis. Arthritis Rheum 20:189–190, 1977.

10. Suciu-Foca N, Jacobs JC, Khan R, et al.: Predisposition to juvenile arthritis: genetic aspects. In Moore T(ed.) Report of the Ross Conference on Pediatric Research. Xanadu, Bahamas, December 3, 1979, Ross Laboratories, Columbus, OH, 1981 pp. 72–75.

11. Baum J, Baum ER: Classics from medical literature: George Frederick Still and his account of childhood arthritis—a reappraisal (with replication of the original monograph On a Form of Chronic Joint Disease in Children). Am J Dis Child 132:192–200, 1978.

12. Green WT: Monarticular and pauciarticular arthritis in children. JAMA 115:2023–2024, 1940.

13. Brewer EJ, Bass J, Baum J, et al.: Current proposed revision of JRA criteria. Arthritis Rheum 20:195–199, 1977.

14. Cassidy JT, Levinson JE, Bass JC, et al.: A study of Classification Criteria for a Diagnosis of Juvenile Rheumatoid Arthritis. Arthritis Rheum 29:274–281, 1986.

15. Bywaters EGL: Still's disease in the adult. Ann Rheum Dis 30:121–133, 1971.

16. Arnett FC, Edworthy SM, Bloch DA, et al.: The American Rheumatism Association 1987 Revised Criteria for the Classification of Rheumatoid Arthritis. Arthritis Rheum 31:315–324, 1988.

17. Stastny P, Fink C: Different HLA-D associations in adult and juvenile rheumatoid arthritis. J Clin Invest 63:124–130, 1979.

18. Glass D, Litvin D, Wallace K, et al.: Early onset pauciarticular juvenile rheumatoid arthritis associated with HLA DRw5, iritis, and antinuclear antibody. J Clin Invest 66:426–429, 1980.

19. van Zeben D, Hazes JMW, Zwinderman AH, et al.: Association of HLA-DR4 with a more progressive disease course in patients with rheumatoid arthritis. Results of a followup study. Arthritis Rheum 34:822–830, 1991.

20. Kunnamo I, Kallio P, Pelkonen P, Hovi T: Clinical signs and laboratory tests in the differential diagonsis of arthritis in children. Am J Dis Child 141:34–40, 1987.

21. Giannini EH, Brewer EJ: Poor correlation between the erythrocyte sedimentation rate and clinical activity in juvenile rheumatoid arthritis. Clin Rheumatol 6:197–201, 1987.

21a.Schwarz-Eywill M, Heilig B, Bauer H, et al.: Evaluation of serum ferritin as a marker for adult Still's disease activity. Ann Rheum Dis 51:683–685, 1992.

22. Eichenfield AH, Athreya BH, Doughty RA, Cebul RD: Utility of rheumatoid factor in the diagonsis of juvenile rheumatoid arthritis. Pediatrics 78:480–484, 1986.

23. Moore TL, Osborn TG, Weiss TD, et al.: Autoantibodies in juvenile arthritis. Semin Arthritis Rheum 13:329–336, 1984.

24. Schaller JG, Johnson GD, Holborow EJ, et al.: The association of antinuclear antibodies with the chronic iridocyclitis of juvenile rheumatoid arthritis (Still's disease). Arthritis Rheum 17:409–416, 1974.

25. Monestier M, Losman JA, Fasy TM, et al.: Antihistone antibodies in antinuclear antibody-positive juvenile arthritis. Arthritis Rheum 33:1836–1841, 1990.

26. Leak AM: Autoantibody profile in juvenile chronic arthritis. Ann Rheum Dis 47:178–182, 1988.

27. Bergroth V, Konttinen YT, Pelkonen P, et al.: Synovial fluid lymphocytes in different subtypes of juvenile rheumatoid arthritis. Arthritis Rheum 31:780–783, 1988.

28. Burdette S, Schwartz RS: Current concepts: immunology idiotypes and idiotypic networks. N. Eng J Med 317:219–224, 1987.

29. Key LL Jr, Hoch S, Cairns L, et al.: Monocyte bone degradation: in vitro analysis of monocyte activity in patients with juvenile rheumatoid arthritis. J Pediatr 108:405–409, 1986.

30. Pauls JD, Silverman E, Laxer RM, Fritzler MJ: Antibodies to histones H1 and H5 in sera of patients with juvenile rheumatoid arthritis. Arthritis Rheum 32:877–83, 1989.

31. Moore TL, Osborn TG, Dorner RW: Cross-reactive antiidiotypic antibodies against human rheumatoid factors from patients with juvenile rheumatoid arthritis. Arthritis Rheum 32:699–705, 1989.

32. Tsokos GC, Inghirami G, Pillemer SR, et al.: Immunoregulatory aberrations in patients with polyarticular juvenile rheumatoid arthritis. Clin Immunol Immunopathol 47:62–74, 1988.

33. Miller JJ III, Olds LC, Silverman ED, et al.: Different patterns of C3 and C4 activation in the varied types of juvenile arthritis. Pediatr Res 20:1332–1337, 1986.

34. Silverman ED, Somma Catherine, Khan MM, et al.: Abnormal T suppressor cell function in juvenile rheumatoid arthritis. Arthritis Rheum 33:205–211, 1990.

35. Moore TL, Osborn TG, Dorner RW: 19S IgM Rheumatoid factor-7S IgG rheumatoid factor immune complexes isolated in sera of patients with juvenile rheumatoid arthritis. Pediatr Res 20:977–981, 1986.

36. Goldenberg DL: Infectious arthritis complicating rheumatoid arthritis and other chronic rheumatic disorders. Arthritis Rheum 32:496–502, 1989.

37. Baldassare AR, Chano F, Zuckner J: Markedly raised synovial fluid leucocyte counts not associated with infectious arthritis in children. Ann Rheum Dis 37:404–409, 1978.

38. Jacobs JC, Philips PE, Johnston AD: Needle biopsy of the synovium of children. Pediatrics 57:696–701, 1976.

39. Sherman MS: The non-specificity of synovial reactions. Bull Hosp Joint Dis 12:110–125, 1951.

40. Wynne-Roberts CR: Anderson CH, Turano AM, Baron M. Light and electron-mircoscopic findings of juvenile rheumatoid arthritis synovium: comparison with normal juvenile synovium. Semin Arthritis Rheum 7:287–302, 1978.

41. Konttinen YT, Bergroth V, Kunnamo I, Haapasaari J: The value of biopsy in patients with monarticular juvenile rheumatoid arthritis of recent onset. Arthritis Rheum 29:47–53, 1986.

42. Grokoest AW, Snyder AI, Schlaeger R: Juvenile Rheumatoid Arthritis, Little, Brown, Boston, 1962.

43. Martel W, Holt JF, Cassidy JT: Roentgenologic manifestations of juvenile rheumatoid arthritis. Am J Roentgenol Radium Ther Nucl Med 88:400–423, 1962.

44. Poznanski AK, Glass RBJ, Feinstein KA, et al.: Magnetic resonance imaging in juvenile rheumatoid arthritis. Int Pediatr 3:304–310, 1988.

45. Senac MO, Deutsch D, Bernstein BH, et al.: MR Imaging in juvenile rheuma-

toid arthritis. AJR 150:873–878, 1988.

46. Stoller DW, Genant HK: Magnetic resonance imaging of the knee and hip. Arthritis Rheum 33:441–449, 1990.

47. Sartoris DJ: Magnetic resonance imaging of the musculoskeletal system. J Musculoskel Med 7:29–45, 1990.

48. Towner SR, Michael CJ Jr, O'Fallon WM, Nelson AM: The epidemiology of juvenile arthritis in Rochester, Minnesota 1960–1979. Arthritis Rheum 26:1208–1213, 1983.

49. Kunnamo I, Kallio P, Pelkonen P: Incidence of arthritis in urban Finnish children: A prospective study. Arthritis Rheum 29:1232–1238, 1986.

50. Petty RE: Epidemiology of juvenile rheumatoid arthritis. In Miller JJ III (ed.) Juvenile Rheumatoid Arthritis. PSG, Littleton, MA 1979, pp. 11–18.

51. Gewanter HL, Roghmann KJ, Baum J: The prevalence of juvenile arthritis Arthritis Rheum 26:599–603, 1983.

52. Laaksonen A: A prognostic study of juvenile rheumatoid arthritis. Acta Paediatr Scand [Suppl.] 166, 1966.

53. Kredich DW: Polyarticular juvenile rheumatoid arthritis. In Miller JJ III (ed.) Juvenile Rheumatoid Arthritis. PSG, Littleton, MA, 1977, pp. 121–134.

54. Clemens LE, Albert E, Ansell BM: Sibling pairs affected by chronic arthritis of children: Evidence for a genetic predisposition. J Rheumatol 12:108–113, 1985.

55. Nepom BS, Malhortra U, Schwarz DA, et al.: HLA and T Cell receptor polymorphisms in pauciarticular-onset juvenile rheumatoid arthritis. Arthritis Rheum 34:1260–1267, 1991.

56. Aaron S, Fraser PA, Jackson JM, et al.: Sex ratio and sibship size in juvenile rheumatoid arthritis kindreds. Arthritis Rheum 28:753–758, 1985.

57. van Kerckhove C, Glass DN: The immunoglobulin supergene family and the polygenic nature of inherited predisposition to rheumatic disease. Arthritis Rheum 30:951–953, 1987.

58. Albert ED, Ansell BM: Immunogenetics of juvenile chronic arthritis. Scand J Rheumatol Suppl. 66:85–91, 1987.

59. Calabro JJ, Marchesano JM: Fever associated with juvenile rheumatoid arthritis. N Engl J Med 276:11–18, 1967.

60. Pizzo PA, Lovejoy FH Jr, Smith DH: Prolonged fever in children: Review of 100 cases. Pediatrics 55:468–473, 1975.

61. Lohr JA, Hendley JO: Prolonged fever of unknown origin. Clin Pediatr 16:768–773, 1977.

62. McClung HJ: Prolonged fever of unknown origin in children. Am J Dis Child 124:544–550, 1972.

63. Schaller J: Arthritis as a presenting manifestation of malignancy in children. J Pediatr 81:793–797, 1972.

64. Estrada R, Schaeffer H, Rosenfeld W, et al.: Anhidrotic ectodermal dysplasia. Fever in a neonate. NYS J Med 81:1791–1793, 1981.

65. Case records of the Massachusetts General Hospital. CASE No. 22:1991. N Eng J Med 324:1575–1584, 1991.

66. Lake AM, Oski FA: Peripheral lymphadenopathy in childhood. Am J Dis Child 132:357–359, 1978.

67. Sullivan DB, Cassidy JT, Petty RE: Pathogenic implications of age of onset in juvenile rheumatoid arthritis. Arthritis Rheum 18:251–254, 1975.

68. Ansell BM, Bywaters EGL: Rheumatoid arthritis (Still's disease). Ped Clin

North Am 10:921–939, 1963.

69. Bujak JS, Aptekar RG, Decker JL, et al.: Juvenile rheumatoid arthritis presenting in the adult as fever of unknown origin. Medicine 52:431–444, 1973.

70. Ohta A, Yamaguchi M, Kaneoka H, et al.: Adult Still's Disease: review of 228 cases from the literature. J Rheumatol 14:1139–1146, 1987.

71. Cush-JJ, Medsger TA Jr, Christy, WC: Adult-onset Still's disease. Clinical course and outcome. Arthritis Rheum 30:186–194, 1987.

72. Reginato AJ, Schumacher HR Jr, Baker DG, et al.: Adult onset Still's disease: experience in 23 patients and literature review with emphasis on organ failure. Semin Arthritis Rheum 17:39–57, 1987.

73. Lindsley CB: Seasonal variation in systemic onset juvenile rheumatoid arthritis. Arthritis Rheum 30:838–839, 1987.

74. Ansell BM, Bywaters EGL: Diagnosis of "probable" Still's disease and its outcome. Ann Rheum Dis 21:253–262, 1962.

75. Isdale IC, Bywaters, EGL: The rash of rheumatiod arthritis and Still's disease. Q J Med 25:377–387, 1956.

76. Calabro JJ, Marchesano JM: Rash associated with juvenile rheumatoid arthritis. J Pediatr 72:611–619, 1968.

77. de Benedetti F, Massa M, Robbioni P, et al.: Correlation of serum interleukin-6 levels with joint involvement and thrombocytosis in systemic juvenile rheumatoid arthritis. Arthritis Rheum 34:1158–1163, 1991.

78. Schlesinger BE, Forsyth CC, White RHR, et al.: Observations on the clinical course and treatment of one hundred cases of Still's disease. Arch Dis Child 36:65–76, 1961.

79. Calabro JJ, Burnstein SL, Staley HL: JRA posing as fever of unknown origin. Arthritis Rheum 20:178–180, 1977.

79a. Schneider R, Lang BA, Reilly BJ, et al.: Prognostic indicators of joint destruction in systemic-onset juvenile rheumatoid arthritis. J Pediatr 120:200–5, 1992

80. Barber FA, Roach JW: Torticollis: A presentation of eosinophilic granuloma: A case report. Orthopedics 9:1237–1239, 1986.

81. Steinberg GG: Osteomyelitis of the rib presenting as painful torticollis: Case report. J Bone Joint Surg 61-A:614–616, 1979.

82. Schaller JG: The diversity of JRA. Arthritis Rheum 20 (Suppl):52–63, 1977.

83. Rachelefsky GS, Kar NC, Coulson A, et al.: Serum enzyme abnormalities in juvenile rheumatoid arthritis. Pediatrics 58:730–736, 1976.

84. Halla JT, Koopman WJ, Fallahi S, et al.: Rheumatoid myositis. Clinical and histologic features and possible pathogenesis. Arthritis Rheum 27:737–743, 1984.

85. Schaller JG, Beckwith B, Wedgwood RJ: Hepatic involvement in juvenile rheumatoid arthritis. J Pediatr 77:203–209, 1970.

86. Brewer EJ, Giannini E, Person D: Juvenile Rheumatoid Arthritis 2nd edition, Saunders, Philadelphia, 1982.

87. Ohta A, Matsumoto Y, Ohta T, et al.: Still's disease associated with necrotizing lymphadenitis (Kikuchi's disease): Report of 3 cases. J Rheumatol 15:981–983, 1988 (see also: Correspondence: 17:568–569, 1990).

88. Wang FM, Wertenbaker C, Behrens MM, Jacobs JC: Acquired Brown's syndrome in children with juvenile rheumatoid arthritis. Ophthalmology 91:23–26, 1984.

89. Yousefzadeh DK, Fishman PA: The triad of pneumonitis, pleuritis, and peri-

carditis in juvenile rheumatoid arthritis. Pediatr Radiol 8:147–150, 1979.

90. Brewer E: Juvenile rheumatoid arthritis-cardiac involvement. Arthritis Rheum 20:231–236, 1977.
91. Miller JJ III: Carditis in JRA. In Miller JJ III (ed.) Juvenile Rheumatoid Arthritis. PSG, Littleton, MA, 1979, pp. 165–173.
92. Yancey CL, Doughty RA, Cohlan BA, Athreya BH: Pericarditis and cardiac tamponade in juvenile rheumatoid arthritis. Pediatrics 68:369–373, 1981.
93. Lietman PS, Bywaters EGL: Pericarditis in juvenile rheumatoid arthritis. Pediatrics 32:855–860, 1963.
94. Svantesson H, Bjorkhem G, Elborgh R: Cardiac involvement in juvenile rheumatoid arthritis: a follow-up study. Acta Paediatr Scand 72:345–350, 1983.
95. Smith WG: Coxsackie B myopericarditis in adults. Am Heart J 80:34–46, 1970.
96. Tilzey AJ, Signy M, Banatvala JE: Persistent coxsackie B virus specific IgM response in patients with recurrent pericarditis. Lancet 1:1491–1492, 1986.
97. Soutar CA: Unusual case of viral pericarditis. Lancet 1:498, 1971.
98. Rahal JJ, Millian SJ, Noriega ER: Coxsackie virus and adenovirus infection: Association with acute febrile and juvenile rheumatoid arthritis. JAMA 235:2496–2501, 1976.
99. Adler R, Takahashi M, Wright HT: Acute pericarditis associated with hepatitis B infection. Pediatrics 61:716–719, 1978.
100. Wong KF, Chan JKC, Chan CH: Psittacosis-Associated hemophagocytic syndrome. Am J Med 91:204–205, 1991.
101. Morris JA, Adamson AR, Holt PJL, Davson J: Still's disease and the virus-associated haemophagocytic syndrome. Ann Rheum Dis 44:349–353, 1985.
102. Heaton DC, Moller PW: Case report: Still's disease associated with Coxsackie infection and haemophagocytic syndrome. Ann Rheum Dis 44:341–344, 1985.
103. Hurst NP, Martkynoga AG, Nuki G, et al.: Coxsackie B infection and arthritis. Br Med J 286:580, 1983.
104. Roberts-Thomson PJ, Ahern MJ, Southwood TR, et al.: Adult onset Still's Disease or Coxsackie Polyarthritis? Aust NZ J Med 16:509–511, 1986.
105. Fraser KJ, Clarris BJ, Muirden KD, et al.: A persistent adenovirs type 1 infection in synovial tissue from an immunodeficient patient with chronic, rheumatoid-like polyarthritis. Arthritis Rheum 28:455–458, 1985.
106. Denman AM: A viral aetiology for juvenile chronic arthritis. J Rheum 27:169–175, 1988.
107. Delgado EA, Petty RE, Malleson PN, et al.: Aortic valve insufficiency and coronary artery narrowing in a child with polyarticular juvenile rheumatoid arthritis. J Rheumatol 15:144–147, 1988.
108. Singleton EB, Wagner ML: Radiographic Atlas of Pulmonary Abnormalities in Children. Saunders, Philadelphia, 1971, p. 240.
109. Athreya BH, Doughty RA, Bookspan M, et al.: Pulmonary manifestations of juvenile rheumatoid arthritis. A report of eight cases and review. Clin Chest Med 1:361–374, 1980.
110. Lovell D, Lindsley C, Langston C: Lymphoid interstitial pneumonia in juvenile rheumatoid arthritis. J Pediatr 105:947–950, 1984.
111. O'Brodovich HM, Way RC, Andrew M, Dent PB: Nonivasive diagnosis of pulmonary hemorrhage in rheumatoid arthritis. Pediatrics 72:720–723, 1983.
112. Wagener JS, Taussig LM, DeBenedetti G, et al.: Pulmonary function in juvenile rheumatoid arthritis. J Pediatr 99:108–110, 1981.

113. Padeh S, Laxer RM, Silver MM, Silverman ED: Primary pulmonary hypertension in a patient with systemic-onset juvenile arthritis. Arthritis Rheum 34:1575–1679, 1991.

114. Jacobs JC, Hui RM: Cricoarytenoid arthritis and airway obstruction in juvenile rheumatoid arthritis. Pediatrics 59:292–294, 1977.

115. Jan JE, Hill RH, Low MD: Cerebral complications in juvenile rheumatoid arthritis. Can Med Assoc J 107:623–625, 1972.

116. Sievers K, Nisshla M, Sievers UM: Cerebral vasculitis visualized by angiography in juvenile rheumatoid arthritis simulating brain tumor. Acta Rheum Scand 14:222–232, 1968.

117. O'Connor D, Bernstein B, Hanson V, et al.: Disease of central nervous system in juvenile rheumatoid arthritis (JRA), abstracted. Arthritis Rheum 23:727, 1980.

118. Anttila R: Renal involvement in juvenile rheumatoid arthritis. A clinical and histopathological study. Acta Paediatr Scand [Suppl.] 227, 1972.

119. Stapleton FB, Hanissian AS, Miller LA: Hypercalciuria in children with juvenile rheumatoid arthritis: association with hematuria. J Pediatr 107:235–239, 1985.

120. Reed A, Haugen M, Pachman LM, Langman CB: Abnormalities in serum osteocalcin values in children with chronic rheumatic diseases. J Pediatr 116:574–580, 1990.

121. Levy M, Prieur A-M, Gubler M-C, et al.: Renal involvement in juvenile chronic arthritis: clinical and pathologic features. Am J Kidney Dis 9:138–146, 1987.

122. Malleson PN, Lockitch G, MacKinnon M, et al.: Renal disease in chronic arthritis of childhood. A study of urinary N-acetyl-8-glucosaminidase and B2-microglobulin excretion. Arthritis Rheum 33:1560–1566, 1990.

123. Schnitzer TJ, Ansell BM: Amyloidosis in juvenile chronic polyarthritis. Arthritis Rheum 20:245–252, 1977.

124. Youyfouka O, David J, Ansell BA, et al.: Mortality and morbidity of a cohort of juvenile arthritis patients with amyloidosis. Arthritis Rheum 335:144, 1990.

125. Baum J. Gutowska G: Death in juvenile rheumatoid arthritis. Arthritis Rheum 20:253–255, 1977.

126. Duston MA, Skinner M, Shirahama T, Cohen AS: Diagnosis of amyloidosis by abdominal fat aspiration: analysis of four years' experience. Am J Med 82:412–414, 1987.

127. Cohen AS, Skinner M: New frontiers in the study of amyloidosis. N Engl J Med 323:542–543, 1990.

127a. Hawkins PN, Richardson S, David J, et al.: Monitoring amyloidosis in juvenile rheumatoid arthritis with serum amyloid P component scintography. Arthritis Rheum 34:S124, 1991.

128. Rostropowicz-Denisiewicz K, Romicka AM, Berkan E, Luft S: The course of amyloidosis in juvenile chronic arthritis with immunoglobulin deficiency. Scand J Rheumatol. Suppl 67:27–29, 1988.

129. Escalante A, Ehresmann GR, Quismorio FP Jr.: Regression of reactive systemic amyloidosis due to ankylosing spondylitis following the administration of colchicine. Arthritis Rheum 34:920–922, 1991.

130. Gall EP, Goldberg M. Editorial. The safety of treating rheumatoid arthritis with aspirin and analgesic nephropathy in 1981: Which drug is responsible? JAMA 247:63–65, 1982.

131. Wortmann DW, Kelsch RC, Kuhns L, et al.: Renal papillary necrosis in juvenile rheumatoid arthritis. J Pediatr 97:37–40, 1980.

132. Allen RC, Petty RE, Lirenman DS, et al.: Renal papillary necrosis in children with chronic arthritis. Am J Dis Child 140:20–22, 1986 (see also editorial pp. 16–17).

133. Koerper MA, Stempel DA, Dallman PR: Anemia in patients with juvenile rheumatoid arthritis. J Pediatr 92:930–933, 1980.

134. Gross SJ, Stuart MJ, Swender PT, et al.: Malabsorption of iron in children with iron deficeincy. J Pediatr 88:795–799, 1976.

135. Vichinsky E: Anemia associated with rhenumatoid arthritis. J Pediatr 94:678, 1979.

136. Hochbery MC, Arnold CM, Hogans BB, Spivak JL: Serum immunoreactive erythropoietin in rheumatoid arthritis: impaired response to anemia. Arthritis Rheum 31:1318–1321, 1988.

137. Maury CPJ, Andersson LC, Teppo A-M, et al.: Mechanism of anaemia in rheumatoid arthritis: demonstration of raised interleukin 1 concentrations in anaemic patients and of interleukin 1 mediated suppression in normal erythropoiesis and proliferation of human erythroleukaemia (HEL) cells in vitro. Ann Rheum Dis 47:972–978, 1988.

138. Dessypris EN, Baer MR, Sergent JS, Krantz SB: Rheumatoid arthritis and pure red cell aplasia. Ann Intern Med 100:202–206, 1984.

139. Rubin RN, Walker BK, Ballas SK, et al.: Erythroid aplasia in juvenile rheumatoid arthritis. Am J Dis Child 132:760–762, 1978.

140. Glader BE: Evaluation of the hemolytic role of aspirin in glucose-6-phosphate dehydrogenase deficiency. J Pediatr 89:1027–1028, 1976.

141. Craft AW, Eastham EJ, Bell JI, et al.: Serum ferritin in juvenile chronic polyarthritis. Ann Rheum Dis 36:271–273, 1977.

142. Vreugdenhil G, Baltus CAM, Van Eijk HG, Swaak AJG: Anaemia of chronic disease: Diagnostic significance of erythrocyte and serological parameters in iron deficient rheumatoid arthritis patients. Br J Rheumatol 29:105–110, 1990.

143. Johansson U, Portinsson S, Akesson A, et al.: Nutritional status in girls with juvenile rheumatoid arthritis. Hum Nutr Clin Nutr 40C:57–67, 1985.

144. Herbert V: The nutritional anemias. Hosp Pract 15(3):65–89, 1980.

145. Winyard PG, Blake DR, Chirico S, et al.: Mechanism of exacerbation of rheumatoid synovitis by total-dose iron-dextran infusion: in-vivo demonstration of iron-promoted oxidant stress. Lancet 1:69–72, 1987 (see also correpondence p. 391).

146. Pincus T, Olsen NJ, Russell IJ, et al.: Multicenter study of recombinant human erythropoietin in correction of anemia in rheumatoid arthritis. Am J Med 89:161–168, 1990.

146a.Fantini F, Gattinara M, Gerloni V, et al.: Severe anemia associated with systemic-onset juvenile rheumatoid arthritis successfully treated with recombinant human erythropoeitin: a pilot study. Arthritis Rheum 35:724–726, 1992.

147. Kuhns JG, Swain LT: Distrubances of growth in chronic arthritis in children. Am J Dis Child 43:1118–1133, 1932.

148. Coss JA Jr, Boots RH: Juvenile rheumatoid arthritis—a study of fifty-six cases with a note on skeletal changes. J Pediatr 29:143–156, 1946.

149. Ansell BM, Bywaters EGL: Growth in Still's disease. Ann Rheum Dis 15:295–319, 1956.

150. Bernstein BH, Stobie D, Singsen BH, et al.: Growth retardation in juvenile rheumatoid arthritis (JRA). Arthritis Rheum 20:212–216, 1977.
151. Bennett AE, Silverman ED, Miller JJ III, Hintz RL: Insulin-like growth factors I and II in children with systemic onset juvenile arthritis. J Rheumatol 15:655–658, 1988.
152. Aitman TJ, Palmer RG, Loftus J, et al.: Serum IGF-I levels and growth failure in juvenile chronic arthritis. Clin Exp Rheumatol 7:557–561, 1989.
153. Sadeghi-Nejad A, Seniro B: Adrenal function, growth and insulin in patients treated with corticoids on alternate days. Pediatrics 43:277–283, 1969.
154. Davies UM, Ansell BM, Woo P: Growth retardation in juvenile chronic arthritis: effect of treatment with biosynthetic human growth hormone. Arthritis Rheum 33:S14, 1990.
155. Rappaport EB, Snoy P, Habig WH, Bright RW: Effects of exogenous growth hormone on growth plate cartilage in rats. Am J Dis Child 141:497–501, 1987.
156. Loeb JN: Corticosteroids and growth. N Engl J Med 295:547–552, 1976.
157. Ansell BM, Bywaters EGL: Alternate-day corticosteriod therapy in juvenile chronic polyarthritis. J Rheum 1:176–186, 1974.
158 Wales JKH, Mllner RDG: Variation in lower leg growth with alternate day steroid treatment. Arch Dis Child 63:981–983, 1988.
159. Richards GE, Pachman LM, Green CC: Symptomatic hypothyroidism in children with collagen disease. J Pediatr 87:82–84, 1975.
160. Collen RJ, Lippe BM, Kaplan SA: Primary ovarian failure, juvenile rheumatoid arthritis, and vitiligo. Am J Dis Child 133:598–600, 1979.
161. Fisher M, Nussbaum M, Abrams CAL, et al.: Diabetes mellitus. Hashimoto's, thyroiditis, and juvenile rheumatoid arthritis. Am J Dis Child 134:93–94, 1980.
162. Pirani CL, Bennett GA: Rheumatoid arthritis: A report of three cases progressing from childhood and emphasizing certain systemic manifestations. Bull Hosp Joint Dis 12:335–367, 1951.
163. Cabane J, Michon A, Ziza J-M, et al.: Comparison of long term evolution of adult onset and juvenile onset Still's disease, both followed up for more than 10 years. Ann Rheum Dis 49:283–285, 1990.
164. Bywaters EGL: Deaths in juvenile chronic polyarthritis. Arthritis Rheum 20:256, 1977.
165. Bernstein B: Death in juvenile rheumatoid arthritis. Arthritis Rheum 20:256–257, 1977.
166. Scott JP, Pachman LM, Gerber PS, et al.: Activation of coagulation in systemic JRA (S-JRA). Arthritis Rheum 26:S57, 1983.
167. Mukamel M, Bernstein BH, Brik R, Lehman TJA: The prevalence of coagulation abormalities in juvenile rheumatoid arthritis. J Rheumatol 14:1147–1149, 1987.
168. Sbarbaro JA, Bennett RM: Aspirin hepatotoxicity and disseminated intravascular coagulation. Ann Intern Med 86:183–185, 1977.
169. Jacobs JC, Gorin LJ, Hanissian AS, Simon JL: Consumption coagulopathy after gold therapy for JRA. J Pediatr 105:674–675, 1984.
170. Silverman ED, Miller JJ III, Bernstein B, Shafai T: Comsumption coagulopathy associated with systemic juvenile rheumatoid arthritis. J Pediatr 103:872–876, 1983.
171. Pinedo HM, Van de Putte BA, Loeliger EA: Salicylate-induced consumption coagulopathy. Ann Rheum Dis 32:66–68, 1973.

172. De Vere-Tyndall A, MacAuley D, Ansell BM: Disseminated intravascular coagulation complicating systemic juvenile chronic arthritis ("Still's disease"). Clin Rheumatol 2:415–418, 1983.
173. Kornreich H, Malouf NN, Hanson V: Acute hepatic dysfunction in juvenile rheumatoid arthritis. J Pediatr 79:27–35, 1971.
174. Lipinski J, Meyer R, Kornetsky C, Cohen BM: Adult respiratory-distress syndrome in salicylate intoxication. Lancet 1:1294–1295, 1979.
175. Case Records of the Massachusetts General Hospital: Case 23-1977. N Eng J Med 296:1337–1346, 1977.
176. Merskey C: DIC: Identification and management. Hosp Pract pp. 83–94, December 1982.
177. Sherry DD, Kredich DW: Transient thrombocytopenia in systemic onset juvenile rheumatoid arthritis. Pediatrics 76:600–603, 1985.
178. Hadchouel M, Prieur A-M, Griscelli C: Acute hemorrhagic, hepatic, and neurologic manifestations in juvenile rheumatoid arthritis: possible relationship to drugs or infection. J Pediatr 106:561–566, 1985.
179. Levy J, Pettei MJ, Weitz JI: Dysfibrinogenemia in obstructive liver disease. J Pediatr Gastroenterol Nutr 6:967–970, 1987.
180. Ohaska A, Saito K, Mori S, et al.: Clinicopathologic and therapeutic aspects of angioimmunoblastic lymphadenopathy-related lesions. Cancer 69:1259–1267, 1992.
181. Steinberg AD, Seldin MF, Jaffe ES, et al.: Angioimmunoblastic lymphadenopathy with dysproteinemia. Ann Intern Med 108:575–584, 1988.
182. Buchanan WW, Rooney RJ, Rennie JAN: Aspirin and the salicylates. Clin Rheum Dis 5:499–539, 1979.
183. Levy G, Leonards JR: Urine pH and salicylate therapy. JAMA 217:81, 1971.
184. Lanza FL, Royer GL Jr, Nelson RS: Endoscopic evaluation of the effects of aspirin, buffered aspirin, and enteric coated aspirin on gastric and duodenal mucosa. N Engl J Med 303:136–138, 1980.
185. Vane JR: Inhibitors of prostaglandin, prostacyclin and thromboxane synthesis. In Coceani F, Olley PJ (eds.) Advances in Prostaglandin Research, Vol. 4 Raven Press, New York, 1978, pp. 27–44.
186. Morley J, Bray MA, Gordon D: The action of anti-inflammatory drugs on the lymphocyte-macrophage axis. In Glynn LE, Schlumberger HD (eds.) Experimental Models of Chronic Inflammatory Disease. Springer-Verlag, Berlin, 1977, pp. 376–390.
187. Boardman PL, Hart FD: Clinical measurement of the anti-inflammatory effects of salicylates in rheumatoid arthritis. Br Med J 4:264–268, 1967.
188. Ansell BM: Juvenile chronic arthritis. In Hart FD (ed.) Drug Treatment of the Rheumatic Diseases. Williams and Wilkins. Sydney, 1987, pp. 196–208.
189. Doughty RA, Giesecke L, Athreya B: Salicylate therapy in juvenile rheumatoid arthritis: dose, serum level, and toxicity. Am J Dis Child 134:461–463, 1980.
190. Jacobs JC, Pesce M: Micro-measurement of plasma salicylate in arthritic children. Arthritis Rheum 21:129–132, 1978.
191. Bardare M, Cislaghi GU, Mandelli M, et al.: Value of monitoring plasma salicylate levels in treating juvenile rheumatoid arthritis. Arch Dis Child 53:381–385, 1978.
192. Levy G: Clinical pharmacokinetics of aspirin. Pediatrics 62:867–872, 1978.
193. Graham GG, Champion GD, Day RD, et al.: Patterns of plasma concentrations and urinary excretion of salicylate in rheumatiod arthritis. Clin Pharmacol Ther

22:410–420, 1977.

194. Wolfe F, Hawley DJ: Remission in rheumatoid arthritis. J Rheumatol 12:245–252, 1985.

195. Halla JT, Hardin JG: Salicylate ototoxicity in rheumatoid arthritis: A controlled study. Ann Rheum Dis 47:134–137, 1988.

196. Day RO, Furst DE, Dromogoole SH, et al.: Relationship of serum naproxen concentration to efficacy in rheumatoid arthritis. Clin Pharmacol Ther 31:733–740, 1982.

197. Wilson JT, Brown RD, Kearns GL, et al.: Single-dose, placebo-controlled comparative study of ibuprofen and acetaminophen antipyresis in children. J Pediatr 119:803–811, 1991.

198. Jacobs JC: New Frontiers in Pediatric Rheumatology. World Health Communications, New York, 1986.

199. Brewer EJ, Giannini EH, Barkley E: Gold therapy in the management of juvenile rheumatoid arthritis. Arthritis Rheum 23:404–411, 1980.

200. Roine R, Gentry T, Hernandez-Munoz R, et al.: Aspirin increases blood alcohol concentrations in humans after ingestion of ethanol. JAMA 264:2406–2408, 1990.

201. Jusko WJ, Rose JQ: Monitoring prednisone and prednisolone, In Tognoni G, Latini R, Jusko WJ (eds.) Frontiers in Therapeutic Drug Monitoring. Raven Press, New York, 1980, pp. 153–161.

202. Nelson AM, Conn DL: Glucocorticoids in rheumatic disease. Mayo Clin Proc 55:758–769, 1980.

203. Byron MA, Jackson J, Ansell BM: Effect of different corticosteroid regimens on hypothalamic-pituitary-adrenal axis and growth in juvenile chronic arthritis. JR Soc Med 76:452–457, 1983.

204. Schurmeyer TH, Tsokos GC, Avgerinos PC, et al.: Pituitary-adrenal responsiveness to corticotropin-releasing hormone in patients receiving chronic, alternate day glucocorticoid therapy. J Clin Endocrinol Metab 61:22, 1985.

205. Moell C, Aronson AS, Selvik G: Growth in rabbits during alternate-day cortisone injections: near normal growth on days without cortisone. Acta Paediatr Scand 77:693–698, 1988.

206. Fauci AS: Corticosteroids in autoimmune disease. Hosp Pract pp. 99–114; October 1983.

207. Kaplan PW, Rocha W, Sanders DB, et al.: Acute steroid-induced tetraplegia following status asthmaticus. Pediatrics 78:121–123, 1986.

208. Nashel DJ: Is atherosclerosis a complication of long-term corticosteroid treatment? Am J Med 80:925–929, 1986.

209. Baer PA, Shore A, Ikeman RL: Transient fall in serum salicylate levels following intraarticular injection of steroid in patients with rheumatoid arthritis. Arthritis Rheum 30:345–347, 1987.

210. Klinenberg JR, Miller R: Effect of corticosteroids on blood salicylate concentrations. JAMA 194:601–604, 1965.

211. Tanchyk AP. Prevention of tooth erosion from salicylate therapy in juvenile rheumatoid arthritis. Gen Dent 34:479–480, 1986.

212. Forsyth BW, Horwitz RI, Acampora D, et al.: New epidemologic evidence confirming that bias does not explain the aspirin/Reye's Syndrome association. JAMA 261:2517–2524, 1989.

213. Remington PL, Shabino CL, McGee H, et al.: Reye syndrome and juvenile rheumatoid arthritis in Michigan. Am J Dis Child 139:870–872, 1985.

214. Rennebohm RM, Heubi JE, Daughtery CC, et al.: Reye syndrome in children receiving salicylate therapy for connective tissue disease. J Pediatr 107:877–880, 1985.

215. Hollister JR: Aspirin in juvenile rheumatoid arthritis. Am J Dis Child 139:866–867, 1985.

216. Kaneshiro MM, Mielke CH Jr, Kasper CK, et al.: Bleeding time after aspirin in disorders of intrinsic clothing. N Engl J Med 281:1039–1042, 1969.

217. Quick AJ: Salicylates and bleeding: the aspirin tolerance test. Am J Med Sci 252:265–269, 1966.

218. Rajah SM, Penny A, Kester R: Aspirin and bleeding time. Lancet 2:1104, 1978.

219. Estes D, Kaplan K: Lack of platelet effect with aspirin analog salsalate. Arthritis Rheum 23:1303–1307, 1980.

220. Goldsweig HG, Kapusta M, Schwartz J: Bleeding, salicylates and prolonged prothrombin time: three case reports and a review of the literature. J Rheum 3:37–42, 1976.

221. Mills DG, Borda IT, Philp RB, et al.: Effects of in viro aspirin on blood platelets of gastrointestinal bleeders. Clin Pharmacol Ther 15:187–192, 1974.

222. Rees WD, Turnberg LA: Reappraisal of the effects of aspirin on the stomach. Lancet 2:410–413, 1980.

223. Manso C, Taranta A, Nydick I. Effects of aspirin administration on serum glutamic oxaloacetic and glutamic pyruvic transaminases in children. Proc Soc Exp Biol Med 93:83–88, 1956.

224. Schaller JG: Chronic salicylate administration in juvenile rheumatoid arthritis: aspirin "hepatitis" and its clinical significance. Pediatrics 62:916–925, 1978.

225. Iancu T, Elian E. Ultrastructural changes in aspirin hepatotoxicity. Am J Clin Pathol 66:570–575, 1976.

226. Levinson JE, Brewer E Jr, Hanson V, et al.: Comparison of tolmetin sodium and aspirin in the treatment of juvenile rheumatoid arthritis. J Pediatr 91:799–804, 1977.

227. Leonards JR, Levy G: Aspirin-induced occult gastrointestinal blood loss: Local versus systemic effects. J Pharm Sci 59:1511–1513, 1970.

227a.Cryer B, Feldman M: Effects of non-steroidal anti-inflammatory drugs on endogenous gastrointestinal prostaglandins and therapeutic strategies for prevention and treatment of non-steroidal anti-inflammatory drug-induced damage. Arch Intern Med 152:1145–1155, 1992.

228. Hopkinson N, Doherty M: NSAID-associated gastropathy—a role for misoprostol? Br J Rheumatol 29:133–136, 1990.

229. Gonwa TA, Hamilton RW, Buckalew VM Jr: Chronic renal failure and end-stage renal disease in northwest North Carolina. Arch Intern Med 141:462–465, 1981.

230. Dixon A, Martin BK, Smith MJ, et al. (eds.): Salicylates, An International Symposium. Churchill Livingstone, London, 1963.

231. Hoftiezer JW, Burks M, Silvoso GR, et al.: Comparison of the effects of regular and enteric-coated aspirin on the gastroduodenal mucosa of man. Lancet 2:609–612, 1980.

232. Orozco-Alcala JJ, Baum J: Regular and enteric-coated aspirin: A re-evaluation. Arthritis Rheum 22:1034–1037, 1979.

233. Baum J: Aspirin in the treatment of juvenile arthritis. Am J Med 74(6A):10–15, 1983.

234. Clark RL, Lasagno L: How reliable are enteric-coated aspirin preparations?

Clin Pharmacol Ther 6:568–574, 1965.
235. McCarty DJ, Csuka M-E: Aspirin in the treatment of chronic inflammatory arthritis. JAMA 257:1331, 1987.
236. Wiseman EH: Plasma salicylate concentrations following chronic administration of aspirin as conventional and sustained release tablets. Curr Ther Res 11:681–688, 1969.
237. American Academy of Pediatrics: Committee on School Health: Administration of medication in school. Pediatrics 74:433, 1984.
238. Wasner C, Britton MC, Kraines RG, et al.: Non-steroidal antiinflammatory agents in rheumatoid arthritis and ankylosing spondylitis. JAMA 246:2168–2172, 1981.
238a. McConnell RJ: Abnormal thyroid function test results in patients taking salsalate. JAMA 267:1242–1243, 1992.
239. Guindo J, Rodriguez de la Serna A, Ramio J, et al.: Recurrent Pericarditis-Relief with colchicine. Cirulation 82:1117–1120, 1990 (See also: Correspondence pp. 1458–1459 and 1830–1831).
240. Goldenbery J, Pessoa AP, Roizenblatt S, et al.: Cardiac tamponade in juvenile chronic arthritis: report of two cases and review of publications. Ann Rheum Dis 49:549–553, 1990.
241. Scharf J, Levy J, Benderly A, et al.: Pericardial tamponade in juvenile rheumatoid arthritis. Arthritis Rheum 19:760–762, 1976.
242. Oakes DD, Light JA, Weidig JC, et al.: Methyl prednisone in uremic pericarditis. Lancet 1:1312–1313, 1977.
243. Buselmeier TJ, Davin TD, Simmons RL, et al.: Treatment of intractable uremic pericardial effusion: avoidance of pericardiectomy with local steroid instillation. JAMA 240:1358–1359, 1978.
244. Feigenbaum SL, Masi AT, Kaplan SB: Prognosis in rheumatoid arthritis. A longitudinal study of newly diagnosed younger adult patients. Am J Med 66:377–384, 1979.
245. Maldonado-Cocco JA, Garica-Morteo O, Spindler AJ, et al.: Carpal ankylosis in juvenile rheumatoid arthritis. Arthritis Rheum 23:1251–1255, 1980.
246. Scott PJ, Ansell BM, Huskisson EG: Measurement of pain in juvenile chronic polyarthritis. Ann Rheum Dis 36:186–187, 1977.
247. Hochberg MC, Chang RW, Dwosh I, et al.: The American College of Rheumatology revised criteria for the classification of global functional status in rheumatoid arthritis. Arthritis Rheum 35:498–502, 1992.
248. Wolfe F, Hawley DJ: Remission in rhuematoid arthritis. J Rheumatol 12:245–252, 1985.
249. Nepom BS, Nepom GT, Mickleson E, et al.: Specific HLA-DR4 associated histo-compatibility molecules characterize patients with seropositive juvenile rheumatoid arthritis. J Clin Invest 76:287–291, 1984.
250. Walker SM, McCurdy DK, Shaham B, et al.: High prevalence of IgA rheumatoid factor in severe polyarticular-onset juvenile rheumatoid arthritis, but not in systemic-onset or pauciarticular-onset disease. Arthritis Rheum 33:199–204, 1990.
251. Harris ED Jr.: Rheumatoid arthritis. Pathophysiology and implications for therapy. N Engl J Med 322:1277–1289, 1990.
252. Sherry DD, Bohnsack J, Salmonson K, et al.: Painless juvenile rheumatoid arthritis. J Pediatr 116:921–923, 1990.
253. Bywaters EGL, Glynn LE, Zeldis A: Subcutaneous nodules of Still's disease.

Ann Rheum Dis 17:278–285, 1958.

254. Hough, AJ Jr, Sokoloff L: The pathology of rheumatoid arthritis and related disorders. In McCarthy DJ (ed.) Arthritis and Allied Conditions, 11th ed. Lea and Febiger, Philadelphia, 1989, pp. 674–697.

255. Gardiner DL: Structure and function of connective tissue and joints. In Scott JT (ed.) Copeman's Textbook of the Rheumatic Diseases, 5th ed. Churchill Livingstone, Edinburgh, 1978, pp. 78–124.

256. Scientific basis for the study of the rheumatic diseases. In McCarty DJ (ed.) Arthritis and Allied Conditions, 11th ed., Section II. Lea and Febiger, Philadelphia, 1989, pp. 189–504.

257. Stabrun AE, Larheim TA, Hoyeraal HM, Rosler M: Reduced mandibular dimensions and asymmetry in juvenile rheumatoid arthritis. Arthritis Rheum 31:602–611, 1988.

258. Engel MB, Richmond J, Brodie AG: Mandibular growth disturbance in rheumatoid arthritis in childhood. Am J Dis Child 78:728–743, 1949.

259. Myall RWT, West RA, Horwitz H, Schaller JG: Jaw deformity caused by juvenile rheumatoid arthritis and its correction. Arthritis Rheum 31:1305–1310, 1988.

260. Espada G, Babini JC, Maldonado-Cocco JA, Garcia-Morteo O: Radiologic review: the cervical spine in juvenile rheumatoid arthritis. Semin Arthritis Rhuem 17:185–195, 1988.

261. Fried JA, Athreya B, Gregg JR, et al.: The cervical spine in juvenile rheumatoid arthritis. Clin Orthop 179:102–106, 1983.

262. Espada G, Babini JC, Maldonado-Cocco JA, Garcia-Morteo O: Radiologic review: The cervical spine in Juvenile rheumatoid arthritis. Semin Arthritis Rheum 17:185–195, 1988.

263. Arroyo IL, Barron KS, Brewer EJ Jr.: Spinal cord compression by epidural lipomatosis in juvenile rheumatoid arthritis. Arthritis Rheum 31:447–451, 1988.

264. D'Arch EJ, Fell RH: Anesthesia in juvenile chronic polyarthritis. In Arden GP, Ansell BM (eds.) Surgical Management of Juvenile Chronic Polyarthritis. Academic Press. London, 1978, pp. 63–74.

265. Scott RD, Sarokhan AJ, Dalziel R: Total hip and total knee arthroplasty in juvenile rheumatoid arthritis. Clin Orthop 182:90–97, 1984.

266. Goldberg J, Kovarsky J: Beclomethasone dipropionate inhalation treatment for chronic hoarseness in rheumatic disease. Arthritis Rheum 26:1412, 1983.

267. Pearson ME, Kosco M, Huffer W, et al.: Rheumatoid nodules of the spine: case report and review of the literature. Arthritis Rheum 30:709–713, 1987.

268. Arden GP, Ansell BM (eds.). Surgical Management of Juvenile Chronic Polyarthritis. Academic Press, London, 1978.

269. Ansell BM: Juvenile arthritis. Clin Rheum Dis 10:657–672, 1984.

270. Vostrejs M, Hollister R: Muscle atrophy and leg length discrepancies in pauciarticular juvenile rheumatoid arthritis. Am J Dis Child 142:343–345, 1988.

271. Stiehm ER: Nonsteroidal anti-inflammatory drugs in pediatric patients. Am J Dis Child 142:1281–1282, 1988.

272. Rosenberg AM: Advanced drug therapy for juvenile rheumatoid arthritis. J Pediatr 114:171–178, 1989.

273. Huskisson EC: Routine drug treatment of rheumatoid arthritis and other rheumatic diseases. Clin Rheum Dis 5:697–706, 1979.

274. Herman JH, Appel AM, Hess EV: Modulation of cartilage destruction by select nonsteroidal antiinflammatory drugs. In vitro effect on the synthesis and activ-

ity of catabolism-inducing cytokines produced by osteoarthritic and rheumatoid synovial tissue. Arthritis Rheum 30:257–265, 1987.

275. Jacobs JC, Berdon WE, Johnston AD: HLA-B27 assoicated spondyloarthritis in childhood: Clinical, pathologic and radiographic observations in 58 patients. J Pediatr 100:521–528, 1982.

276. Hart FD: Ankylosing spondylitis and related disorders. In Hart FD (ed.) Drug Treatment of the Rheumatic Diseases. Williams and Wilkins, Sydney, 1989, pp. 156–161.

277. Luggen ME, Gartside PS, Hess EV: Nonsteroidal antiinflammatory drugs in rheumatoid arthritis: duration of use as a measure of relative value. J Rheumatol 16:1565–1569, 1989.

278. Pippenger CE: Therapeutic drug monitoring: An overview. Therap Drug Monit 1:3–9, 1979.

279. Lovell DJ, Giannini EH, Brewer EJ Jr: Time course of response to non-steroidal antiinflammatory drugs in juvenile rheumatoid arthritis. Arthritis Rheum 27:1433–1437, 1984.

280. Ehrlich GE: Tolmetin sodium: meeting the clinical challenge. Clin Rheum Dis 5:481–497, 1979.

281. Makela AL: Naproxen in the treatment of juvenile rheumatoid arthritis. Scand J Rheumatol 6:193–205, 1977.

282. Ansell BM, Hanna B, Moran H, et al.: Naproxen in juvenile chronic polyarthritis. Eur J Rheum Inflam 2:79–83, 1979.

283. Nicholls A, Hazleman B, Todd RM, et al.: Long-term evaluation of naproxen suspension in juvenile chronic arthritis. Curr Med Res Opin 8:204–207, 1982.

284. Williams PL, Ansell BM, Bell A, et al.: Multicentre study of piroxicam versus naproxen in juvenile chronic arthritis, with special reference to problem areas in clinical trials of nonsteroidal anti-inflammatory drugs in childhood. Br J Rheumatol 25:67–71, 1986.

285. Leak AM, Richter MR, Clemens LE, et al.: A crossover study of naproxen, diclofenac and tolmetin in seronegative juvenile chronic arthritis. Clin Exp Rheumatol 6:157–160, 1988.

286. Suarez SM, Cohen PR, DeLeo VA: Bullous photosensitivity to naproxen: "pseudoporhyria". Arthritis Rheum 33:903–908, 1990.

287. Levy ML, Barron KS, Eichenfield A, Honig PJ: Naproxen-induced pseudoporphyria: a distinctive photodermatitis. J Pediatr 117:660–664, 1990.

287a. Goodwin SD, Glenny RW: Nonsteroidal anti-inflammatory drug-associated infiltrates with eosinophilia. Arch Intern Med 152:1521–1524, 1992.

288. Giannini EH, Brewer EJ, Miller ML, et al.: Ibuprofen suspension in the treatment of juvenile rheumatoid arthritis. J Pediatr 117:645–652, 1990.

289. Rhymer AR, Gengos DC: Indomethacin. Clin Rheum Dis 5:541–552, 1979.

290. Jacobs JC: Sudden death in arthritic children receiving large doses of indomethacin. JAMA 199:932–934, 1967.

291. Editorial. Analgesics, agranulocytosis, and aplastic anaemia: A major case-controlled study. Lancet 2:899–900, 1986.

292. Brewer EJ, Giannini EH, Baum J, et al.: Aspirin and fenoprofen (Nalfon[R]) in the treatment of juvenile rheumatoid arthritis: results of the double blind-trial. A Segment II Study. J Rheumatol 9:123–128, 1982.

293. Bass J, Athreya B, Brandstrup N, et al.: Flurbiprofen in the treatment of juvenile rheumatoid arthritis. J Rheumatol 13:1081–1083, 1986.

294. Brewer EJ, Giannini EH, Baum J, et al.: Ketoprofen (Orudis[R]) in the treatment

of juvenile rheumatoid arthritis. A Segment I Study. J Rheumatol 9:144–148, 1982.

295. Brewer EJ, Giannini EH, Baum J, et al.: Proquazone (Biarsan[R]) in the treatment of juvenile rheumatoid arthritis: A segment I study. J Rheumatol 5:135–139, 1982.

296. Brewer EJ, Giannini EH, Baum J, et al.: Sodium meclofenamate (Meclomen[R]) in the treatment of juvenile rheumatoid arthritis. A segment I Study. J Rheumatol 9:129–134, 1982.

297. Bass JC, Giannini EH, Brewer EJ, et al.: Pirprofen (Rengasil[R]) in the treatment of juvenile rheumatoid arthritis. A segment I study. J Rheumatol 9:140–143, 1982.

298. Bhettay E: Double-blind study of sulindac and aspirin in juvenile chronic arthritis. SAMJ 70:724–726, 1986.

299. Haapasaari J, Wuolijoki E, Ylijoki H: Treatment of juvenile rheumatoid arthritis with diclofenac sodium. Scand J Rheumatol 12:325–330, 1983.

300. Helfgott SM, Sandberg-Cook J, Zakim D, Nestler J: Diclofenac-associated hepatotoxicity. JAMA 264:2660–2662 (see also editiorial pp. 2677–2678).

301. Paulus HE: FDA Arthritis Advisory Committee Meeting: risks of agranulocytosis/aplastic anemia, flank pain, and adverse gastrointestinal effects with use of nonsteroidal antiinflammatory drugs. Arthritis Rheum 30:593–595, 1987.

302. Cush JJ, Jasin HE, Johnson R, Lipsky PE: Relationship between clinical efficacy and laboratory correlates of inflammatory and immunologic activity in rheumatoid arthritis patients treated with nonsteroidal antiinflammatory drugs. Arthritis Rheum 33:623–633, 1990.

303. Caille G, du Souich R, Gervais P, et al.: Effects of concurrent sucralfate administration on pharmacokinetics of naproxen. Am J Med 83 (Suppl 38) 67–73, 1987.

304. Howes CA, Pullar T, Sourindrhin I, et al.: Reduced steady-state plasma concentrations of chlorpromazine and indomethacin in patients receiving cimetidine. Eur J Clin Pharmacol 24:99–102, 1983.

305. Graham DY: Prevention of gastroduodenal injury induced by chronic nonsteroidal antiinflammatory drug therapy. Gastroenterology 96:675–681, 1989.

306. Roth S, Agrawal N, Mahowald M, et al.: Misoprostol heals gastroduodenal injury in patients with rheumatoid arthitis receiving aspirin. Arch intern Med 149:775–779, 1989.

307. Furst DE, Sarkissian E, Blocka K, et al.: Serum concentrations of salicylate and naproxen during concurrent therapy in patients with rheumatoid arthritis. Arthritis Rheum 30:1157–1161, 1987.

307a.O'Brien WM, Bagby GF: Rare adverse reactions to nonsteroidal antiinflammatory drugs. J Rheumatol 12:13–20, 347–353, 562–567, 785–789, 1985.

307b.Hyson CP, Kazakoff MA: A servere multisystem reaction to sulindac. Arch Intern Med 151:387–388, 1991.

308. Barrier CH, Hirschowitz BI: Controversies in the detection and management of nonsteroidal antiinflammatory drug-induced side effects of the upper gastrointestinal tract. Arthritis Rheum 32:926–932, 1989.

309. Langman MJS: Epidemiologic evidence on the association between peptic ulceration and antiinflammatory drug use. Gastroenterology 96:640–646, 1989.

310. Fries JF, Miller SR, Spitz PW, et al.: Toward an epidemiology of gastropathy associated with nonsteroidal antiinflammatory drug use. Gastroenterology 96:647–655, 1989.

310a. Gabriel SE, Bombardier C: NSAID induced ulcers. An emerging epidemic? J Rheumatol 17:1–4, 1990.

310b. Gibson GR, Whitacre EB, Ricotti CA: Colitis induced by nonsteroidal anti-inflammatory drugs. Report of four cases and review of the literature. Arch Intern Med 152:625–632, 1992.

311. Hoppmann RA, Peden JG, Ober SK: Central nervous system side effects of nonsteroidal anti-inflammatory drugs. Aseptic meningitis, psychosis, and cognitive dysfunction. Arch Intern Med 151:1309–1013, 1991.

312. Lindsley CB, Warady BA: Nonsteroidal antiinflammatory drugs: renal toxicity: review of pediatric issues. Clin Pediatr 29:10–113, 1990.

313. Robinson J, Malleson P, Lirenman D, Carter J: Nephrotic syndrome associated with nonsteroidal anti-inflammatory drug use in two children. Pediatrics 85:844–847, 1990.

314. Tietjan DP: Recurrence and specificity of nephrotic syndrome due to tolmetin. Am J Med 87:354–355, 1989.

315. Allen RC, Petty RE, Lirenman DS, et al.: Renal papillary necrosis in children with chronic arthritis. Am J Dis Child 140:20–22, 1986 (see also editorial pp. 16–17).

316. Laxer RM, Silverman ED, Balfe J-W, et al.: Naproxen-associated renal failure in a child with arthritis and inflammatory bowel disease. Pediatrics 80:904–908, 1987.

317. Dunn MJ, Patrono C (eds.): Renal effects of nonsteroidal anti-inflammatory drugs. AJM 81(2B):1–132, 1986.

318. Warren GV, Korbet SM, Schwartz MM, Lewis EJ: Minimal change glomerulopathy associated with nonsteroidal antiinflammatory Drugs. Am J Kidney Dis 13:127–130, 1989.

319. Schwarz A, Krause PH, Keller F, et al.: Granulomatous interstitial nephritis after nonsteroidal anti-inflammatory Drugs. Am J Nephrol 8:410–416, 1988.

320. Stillman MT, Schlesinger PA: Nonsteroidal anti-inflammatory drug nephrotoxicity. Should we be concerned? Arch Intern Med 150:268–270, 1990.

321. Ten RM, Torres VE, Milliner DS, et al.: Acute interstitial nephritis: Immunologic and clinical aspects. Mayo Clin Proc 63:921–930, 1988.

322. Garella S, Matarese RA: Renal effects of prostaglandins and clinical adverse effects of nonsteroidal anti-inflammatory agents. Medicine 63:165–181, 1984.

323. Bender WL, WHelton A, Beschorner WE, et al.: Interstitial nephritis, proteinuria, and renal failure caused by nonsteroidal anti-inflammatory drugs. Immunologic characterization of the inflammatory infiltrate. Am J Med 76:1006–1012, 1984.

324. Clive DM, Stoff JS: Renal syndromes associated with nonsteroidal antiinflammatory drugs. N Eng J Med 310:563–572, 1984.

324a. Cronberg S, Wallmark E, Soderberg I: Effect on platelet aggregation of oral administration of 10 non-steroidal analgesics to humans. Scand J Haematol 33:155–159, 1984.

324b. Connelly CS, Panush RS: Should nonsteroidal anti-inflammatory drugs be stopped before elective surgery? Arch Intern Med 151:1963–1966, 1991.

325. Szer IS, Goldenstein-Schainberg C, Kurtin PS: Paucity of renal complications associated with nonsteroidal antiinflammatory drugs in children with chronic arthritis. J Pediatr 119:815–817, 1991.

326. Iannuzzi L, Dawson N, Zein N, Kushner I: Does drug therapy slow radiologic deterioration in rheumatoid arthritis? N Eng J Med 309:1023–1028, 1983.

327. Scott DL, Symmons DPM, Coulton BL, Popert AJ: Long-term outcome of treating rheumatoid arthritis: results after 20 years. Lancet 1:1108–1111, 1987.
328. Pincus T (ed.) Rheumatoid arthritis: disappointing long-term outcomes despite successful short-term clinical trials. J Clin Epidemiol 41:1037–1041, 1988.
329. Dawes PT, Powler S, Clarke J, et al.: Rheumatoid arthritis: treatment which controls the C-reactive protein and erythrocyte sedimentation rate reduces radiological progression. Br J Rheumatol 25:44–49, 1986.
330. Grondin C, Malleson P, Petty RE: Slow-acting antirheumatic drugs in chronic arthritis of childhood. Semin Arthritis Rheum 18:38–47, 1988.
331. Giannini EH, Brewer EJ, Kuzmina N, et al.: Characteristics of responders and nonresponders to slow-acting antirheumatic drugs in juvenile rheumatoid arthritis. Arthritis Rheum 31:15–20, 1988.
332. Manners PJ, Ansell BM: Slow-acting antirheumatic drug use in systemic onset juvenile chronic arthritis. Pediatrics 77:99–103, 1986.
333. Rosenberg AM: Advanced drug therapy for juvenile rheumatoid arthritis. J Pediatr 114:171–178, 1989.
334. van der Heijde DM, van Riel PL, Nuver-Zwart IH, et al.: Effects of hydroxychloroquine and sulphasalazine on progression of joint damage in rheumatoid arthritis. Lancet 1:1036–1038, 1989.
335. Williams HJ, Ward JR, Dahl SL, et al.: A controlled trial comparing sulfasalazine, gold sodium thiomalate, and placebo in rheumatoid arthritis. Arthritis Rheum 31:702–713, 1988.
336. Ozdogan H, Turunc M, Deringol B, et al.: Sulphasalazine in the treatment of juvenile rheumatoid arthritis: a preliminary open trial. J Rheumatol 13:124–125, 1986.
337. Jacobs JC: Sulphasalazine in the treatment of childhood arthritis: a preliminary report. Arthritis Rheum 33:S145, 1990.
338. Pinals RS: Sulfasalazine in the rheumatic disease. Semin Arthritis Rheum 17:246–259, 1988.
339. Farr M, Kitas G, Waterhouse L, et al.: Sulfasalazine in psoriatic arthritis—A double blind placebo-controlled study. Br J Rheumatol 29:46–49, 1990.
340. Job-Deslandre C, Menkes C-J. Sulphasalazine in the treatment of juvenile spondylarthropathy. Arthritis Rheum 34:S153, 1991.
341. Ansell BM, Hall MA, Woo LP, et al.: A multicentre pilot study of sulphasalazine in juvenile chronic arthritis. Clin Exp Rheumatol 9:201–203, 1991.
342. Ansell BM: Juvenile chronic arthritis and juvenile spondyloarthropathy. Current Opin Rheumatol 3:838–843, 1991.
343. Hertzberger-Ten Cate R, Cats A: Toxicity of sulfasalazine in systemic juvenile chronic arthritis. Clin Exp Rheumatol 9:85–88, 1991.
344. Sherry DD, Wallace CA. Sulfasalazine toxicity in children with systemic onset juvenile rheumatoid arthritis. Arthritis Rheum 34:S153, 1991.
345. Felson DT, Andserson JJ, Meenan RF: The comparative efficacy and toxicity of second-line drugs in rheumatoid arthritis. Results of two metaanalyses. Arthritis Rheum 33:1449–1461, 1990.
346. Taffet SL, Das KM: Sulfasalazine: Adverse effects and desensitization. Dig Dis Sci 28:833–842, 1983.
347. Amos RS, Pullar T, Bax DE, et al.: Sulphasalazine for rheumatoid arthritis: toxicity in 774 patients monitored for one to 11 years. Br Med J 293:420–423, 1986.
348. Marabani M, Madhok R, Capell HA, Hunter JA: Leuocopenia during sulpha-

salazine treatment for rheumatoid arthritis. Ann Rheum Dis 48:505–507, 1989.

349. Farr M, Tunn EJ, Symmons DPM, et al.: Sulphasalazine in rheumatoid arthritis: haematological problems and changes in haematological indices associated with therapy. Br J Rheumatol 28:134–138, 1989.

350. Valcke Y, Pauwels R, van der Straeten M: Bronchoalveolar lavage in acute hypersensitivity pneumonitis caused by sulfasalazine. Chest 92:572–573, 1987.

351. Deboever G, Devogelaere R, Holvoet G: Sulphasalazine-induced lupus-like syndrome with cardiac tamponada in a patient with ulcerative colitis. Am J Gastroenterol 84:85–86, January 1989.

352. Epstein WV: Parental gold therapy for rheumatoid arthritis: A treatment whose time has gone. J Rheumatol 16:1291–1294, 1989.

353. Jessop, JD: Gold in the treatment of rheumatoid arthritis—why, when, how? J Rheum 6(Suppl. 5):12–17, 1979.

354. Empire Rheumatism Council: Gold therapy in rheumatoid arthritis. Final report of a multicenter controlled trial. Ann Rheum Dis 20:315–354, 1961.

355. Epstein WV, Henke CJ, Yelin EH, Katz PP: Effect of parenterally administered gold therapy on the course of adult rheumatoid arthritis. Ann Intern Med 114:437–444, 1991.

356. Levinson JE, Balz GP, Bondi S: Gold therapy. Arthritis Rheum 20:531–535, 1977.

357. Hall MA, Ansell BM, Spencer PE: A comparative study of gold and penicillamine in juvenile chronic arthritis. Presented at the 15th International Congress of Rheumatology, Paris, 1981. Rev Rhum 48(Suppl):, abstract 1290, 1981.

358. Davis P: Undersirable effects of gold salts. J Rheum 6(Suppl. 5):18–24, 1979.

358a. Hansen RM, Varma RR, Hanson, GA: Gold induced hepatitis and pure red cell aplasia. Complete recovery after corticosteroid and N-Acetylcysteinc therapy. J Rheumatol 18:1251–1253, 1991.

359. Wooley PH, Criffin J, Panayi GS, et al.: HLA-DR antigens and toxic reaction to sodium aurothiomalate and D-penicillamine in patients with rheumatoid arthritis. N Engl Med 303:300–302, 1980.

360. Takehara M, Beardmore T: Self administration of parenteral gold and methotrexate in rheumatoid arthritis. Arthritis Rheum 33:S16, 1990.

361. Gottlieb NL: Metabolism and distribution of gold compounds. J Rheum 6(Suppl. 5):2–6, 1979.

362. Gottlieb NL: Gold excretion and retention during auranofin treatment: A preliminary report. J Rheum 6(Suppl. 5):61–67, 1979.

363. Kvien TK, Hoyeraal HM, Sandstad B: Gold sodium thiomalate and D-penicillamine. A controlled, comparative study in patients with pauciarticular and polyarticular juvenile rheumatoid arthritis. Scand J Rheumatol 14:346–354, 1985.

364. Giannini EH, Brewer EJ Jr, Kuzmina N, et al.: Auranofin in the treatment of juvenile rheumatoid arthritis. Results of the USA-USSR double-blind, placebo-controlled trial. Arthritis Rheum 33:466–476, 1990 (see also correspondence 34:934–935, 1991).

365. Katz WA, Blodgett RC Jr., Pietrusko RG: Proteinuria in gold-treated rheumatoid arthritis. Ann Intern Med 101:176–179, 1984.

366. Marcolongo R, Mathieu A, Pala R, et al.: The efficacy and safety of auranofin in the treatment of juvenile rheumatoid arthritis. Arthritis Rheum 31:979–983, 1988.

367. Giannini EH, Brewer EJ, Person DA: Blood gold concentrations in children

with juvenile rheumatoid arthritis undergoing long-term oral gold therapy. Ann Rheum Dis 43:228–231, 1984.

368. Giannini EH, Barron KS, Spencer CH, et al.: Auranofin therapy in juvenile rheumatoid arthritis: results of the five-year open-label extension trial, J Rheumatol 18:1240–1242, 1991.

369. Bombardier C, Ware J, Russell IJ, et al.: Auranofin therapy and quality of life in patients with rheumatoid arthritis. Am J Med 81:565–578, 1986.

370. Jaffe IA: Penicillamine treatment of rheumatoid arthritis—rationale, pattern of clinical response, and clinical pharmacology and toxicology. In Munthe E (ed.) Penicillamine Research Rheumatoid Disease (Penicillamine Symposium). Fabritius, Oslo, Norway, 1976. pp. 11–24.

371. Multz CV: Cholestatic hepatitis caused by penicillamine. JAMA 246:674–675, 1981.

372. Hamilton EDB, Dixon A St J, Davis J, et al.: Multicentre trial with synthetic D-penicillamine in rheumatoid arthritis. JAMA 246:215–218, 1981.

373. Hill HFH: Treatment of rheumatoid arthritis with penicillamine. Semin Arthritis Rheum 6:361–388, 1977.

374. Kean WF, Dwosh IL, Anastassiades TP, et al.: The toxicity pattern of penicillamine therapy. A guide to its use in rheumatoid arthritis. Arthritis Rheum 23:158–164, 1980.

375. Schairer H, Stoeber E: Long-term follow-up of 235 cases of juvenile rheumatoid arthritis treated with D-penicillamine. In Munthe E (ed.) Penicillamine Research in Rheumatoid Disease (Penicillamine Symposium). Fabritius, Oslo, Norway, 1977, pp. 279–281.

376. Ansell BW, Hall MA: Penicillamine in chronic arthritis in childhood. J. Rheum 8(Suppl. 7):112–115, 1981.

377. Brewer EJ, Giannini EH, Kuzmina N, Alekseev L: Penicillamine and hydroxychloroquine in the treatment of severe juvenile rheumatoid arthritis. Results of the U.S.A.-U.S.S.R. double-blind placebo-controlled trial. New Eng J Med 314:1269–1276, 1986 (see also editorial pp. 1312–1314).

378. Prieur AM, Piussan C, P Manigne, et al.: Evaluation of D-penicillamine in juvenile chronic arthritis. A double-blind mutlicentre study. Arthritis Rheum 28:376–382, 1985.

379. Felson DT, Anderson JJ, Meenan RF: Time for changes in the design, analysis, and reporting of rheumatoid arthritis clinical trials. Arthritis Rheum 33:140–149, 1990.

380. Paulus HE, Egger MJ, Ward JR, et al.: Analysis of improvement in individual rheumatoid arthritis patients treated with disease-modifying antirheumatic drugs, based on the findings in patients treated with placebo. Arthritis Rheum 33:477–484, 1990.

381. Hall CL, Jawad S, Harrison PR, et al.: Natural course of penicillamine nephropathy: a long term study of 33 patients. Br Med J 296:1083–1086, 1988.

382. Halla JT, Fallahi S, Koopman WJ: Penicillamine-induced myositis. Observations and unique features in two patients and review of the literature. Am J Med 77:719–722, 1984.

383. Jaffe IA: Adverse effects profile of sulfhydryl compounds in man. Am J Med 80:471–476, 1986.

384. Benson EA, Healey LA, Barron EJ: Insulin antibodies in patients receiving penicillamine. Am J Med 78:857–860, 1985.

385. van Kerckhove C, Giannini EH, Lovell DJ: Temporal patterns of response to D-penicillamine, hydroxychloroquine and placebo in juvenile pheumatoid arthritis. Arthritis Rheum 31:1252–1258, 1988.

386. Huskisson EG: Drugs which apparently affect the rheumatoid disease process. In Hart FD (ed.) Drug Treatment of the Rheumatic Disease. Williams and Wilkins, Sydney, 1987, pp. 65–87.

387. Zvaifler NJ (ed): Update in rheumatology: focus on hydroxychloroquine. Am J Med 85:1–71, 1988.

388. Laaksonen A, Koskiahde V, Juka K: Dosage of antimalarial drugs for children with juvenile rheumatoid arthritis and systemic lupus erythematosus. A clinical study with determination of serum concentration of chloroquine and hydroxychloroquine. Scand J Rheum 3:103–108, 1974.

389. Stillman S: Antimalarials. In Moore TD (ed.) Arthritis in Childhood. Report of the 80th Ross Conference on Pediatric Research. Xanadu, Bahamas, December 2–5, 1979. Ross Laboratories. Columbus, OH, 1981, pp. 125–127.

390. Kvien TK, Hoyeraal HM, Sandstad B: Slow acting antirheumatic drugs in patients with juvenile rheumatoid arthritis—evaluated in a randomized, parallel 50-week clinical trial. J Rheumatol 12:533–539, 1985.

391. Maksymowych W, Russell AS: Antimalarials in rheumatology: efficacy and safety. Semin Arthritis Rheum 16:206–221, 1987.

392. Rynes, RI, Krohel G, Falbo A, et al.: Ophthalmologic safety of long-term hydroxychloroquine treatment. Arthritis Rheum 22:832–836, 1979.

392a. Bernstein HN: Ocular Safety of hydroxychloroquine. Ann Ophthalmol 23:292–296, 1991.

393. Beultler E: Glucose-6-phosphate dehydrogenase deficiency. N Eng J Med 324:169–174, 1991.

394. Fries JF, Singh G, Lenert L, Furst DE: Aspirin, hydroxychloroquine, and hepatic enzyme abnormalities with methotrexate in rheumatoid arthritis. Arthritis Rheum 33:1611–1619, 1990.

395. Jaffe KM, Havens PL, et al.: Childhood chloroquine poisonings—Wisconsin and Washington. JAMA 260:1361, 1988.

396. Ratliff NB, Estes ML, Myles JL, et al.: Diagnosis of chloroquine cardiomyopathy by endomyocardial biopsy. N Eng J Med 316:191–193, 1987.

397. Estes ML, Ewing-Wilson D, Chou SM, et al.: Chloroquine neuromyotoxicity: clinical and pathologic perspective. Am J Med 82:447–455, 1987.

398. Wallace CA, Bleyer WA, Sherry DD, et al.: Toxicity and serum levels of methotrexate in children with juvenile rheumatoid arthritis. Arthritis Rheum 32:677–681, 1989.

399. Shiroky JH, Watts CS, Neville C: Combination methotrexate and sulfasalazine in the management of rheumatoid arthritis: case observations. Arthritis Rheum 32:1160–1164, 1989.

400. Klippel JH, Strober S, Wofsy D: New therapies for the rheumatic diseases. Bull Rheum Dis 38(#4):1–8, 1989.

401. Paulus HE: The use of combinations of disease-modifying antirheumatic agents in rheumatoid arthritis. Arthritis Rheum 33:113–120, 1990.

401a. Williams HJ, Ward JR, Reading JC, et al.: Comparison of auranofin, methotrexate, and the combination of both in the treatment of rheumatoid arthritis. A controlled clinical trial. Arthritis Rheum 35:259–269, 1992.

402. Arthritis Foundation: Challenging the pyramid. A new look at therapeutic

approaches for rheumatoid arthritis. J Rheumatol 17:Suppl 25, Nov. 1990. (See also Editorial, 17:1115–1118, 1990.)

402a. McCarty DJ: Suppress rheumatoid inflammation early and leave the pyramid to the Egyptians. J Rheum 17:1115–1118, 1990.

403. Jacobs JC: Juvenile rheumatoid arthritis. In Downey JA, Low NL (eds.) The Child with Disabling Illness, 2nd ed. Raven Press, New York, 1982, pp. 3–27.

404. Joint Committee of the Medical Research Council and Nuffield Foundation: a comparison of prednisolone with aspirin or other analgesics in the treatment of rheumatoid arthritis. Ann Rheum Dis 18:173, 1959.

405. Harris ED Jr, Emkey RD, Nichols JE, Newberg A: Low dose prednisone therapy in rheumatoid arthritis: a double blind study. J Rheumatol 10:713–721, 1983.

406. Jacobs JC: The arthritic child and the family: Staying in the mainstream. Arthritis Rheum 20:595–597, 1977.

407. De Palma AF, McKeeve CD, Jubin DK: Process of repair of articular cartilage demonstrated by histology and autoradiography with tritiated thymidine. Clin Orthop 48:229–242, 1966.

408. Palmoski M, Perricone E, Brandt KD: Development and reversal of a proteoglycan aggregation defect in normal canine knee cartilage after immobilization. Arthritis Rheum 22:508–517, 1979.

409. Palmoski MJ, Colyer RA, Brandt TKD: Joint motion in the absence of normal loading does not maintain normal articular cartilage. Arthritis Rheum 23:325–334, 1980.

410. Johnson RF: The effect of immobilization on ligaments and ligamentous healing. Contemp Orthop 2:237–241, 1980.

411. Bernstein B, Forrester D, Singsen B, et al.: Hip joint restoration in juvenile rheumatoid arthritis. Arthritis Rheum 20:1099–1104, 1977.

412. Elsasser U, Wilkins B, Hesp R: Bone rarefaction and crush fractures in juvenile chronic arthritis. Arch Dis Child 57:377–380, 1982.

413. Jacobs JC, Dick HM, Downey JA, et al.: Weight bearing as a treatment for damaged hips in juvenile rheumatoid arthritis. N Engl J Med 305:409, 1981.

414. McAllister WAC, Thompson RJ, Al-Habet SM, et al.: Rifampin reduces effectiveness and bioavailability of prednisolone. Br Med J 286:923–925, 1983.

415. Nishioka T, Kurayama H, Yasuda T, et al.: Nasal administration of salmon calcitonin for prevention of glucocorticord-induced osteosporosis in children with nephrosis. J Pediatr 118:703–707, 1991.

416. Loftus J, Allen R, Hesp R, et al.: Randomized, double-blind trial of Deflazacort versus prednisone in juvenile chronic (or rheumatoid) arthritis: A relatively bone-sparing effect of Deflazacort. Pediatrics 88:428–436, 1991.

417. Liebing MR, Leib E, MeLaughlin K, et al.: Pulse methylprednisolone in rheumatoid arthritis. Ann Intern Med 94:21–26, 1981.

418. Miller JJ: Prolonged use of intravenous steroid pulses in the rheumatic diseases of children. Pediatrics 65:980–994, 1980.

419. Barry M: The use of high-dose pulse methylprednisolone in rheumatoid arthritis. Unproved therapy. Arch Intern Med 145:1483–1484, 1985.

420. Silverman ED, Laxer RM, Greenwald M, et al.: Intravenous gamma globulin therapy in systemic juvenile rheumatoid arthritis. Arthritis Rheum 33:1015–1022, 1990.

421. Groothoff JW, van Leeuwen EF: High dose intravenous gammaglobulin in

chronic systemic juvenile arthritis. Br Med J 296:1362–1363, 1988.

422. Becker H, Mitropoulou G, Helmke K: Immunomodulating therapy of rheumatoid arthritis by high-dose intravenous immunoglobulin. Klin Wochenschr 67:286–290, 1980.

423. Combe B, Cosso B, Clot J, et al.: Human placenta-eluted gammaglobulins in immunomodulating treatment of rheumatoid arthritis. Am J Med 78:920–928, 1985.

424. Landsbury J: Quantitation of the activity of rheumatoid arthritis. I. A method for recording its systemic manifestations. Am J Med Sci 231:616–621, 1956.

425. Bunch TW, O'Duffy JD: Disease modifying drugs for progressive rheumatoid arthritis. Mayo Clin Proc 55:161–179, 1980.

426. Wallace CA, Bleyer WA, Sherry DD, et al.: Toxicity and serum levels of methotrexate in children with juvenile rheumatoid arthritis. Arthirits Rheum 32:677–681, 1989.

427. Rose CD, Singsen BH, Eichenfield AH, et al.: Safety and efficacy of methotrexate therapy for juvenile rheumatoid arthritis. J Pediatr 117:653–659, 1990. (See also: Correspondence 119:333–334, 1991.)

428. Singh G, Fries JF, Williams CA, et al.: Toxicity profiles of disease modifying antirheumatic drugs in rheumatoid arthritis. J Rheumatol 18:188–194, 1991.

429. Jeurissen ME, Boerbooms AM, van de Putte LB, et al.: Influence of methotrexate and azathioprine on radiologic progression in rheumatoid arthritis. A randomized double-blind study. Ann Intern Med 114:999–1004, 1991.

430. Kremer JM, Phelps CT: Long-term prospective study of the use of methotrexate in the treatment of rheumatoid arthritis. Update after a mean of 90 months. Arthritis Rheum 35:138–45, 1992.

431. Williams HJ, Willkens RF, Samuelson CO, et al.: Comparison of low-dose oral pulse methotrexate and placebo in the treatment of rheumatoid arthritis. A controlled clinical trial. Arthritis Rheum 28:721–730, 1985.

432. Truckenbrodt H, Hafner R: Methotrexate therapy in juvenile rheumatoid arthritis: a retrospective study. Arthritis Rheum 29:801–807, 1986.

433. Giannini EH, Brewer EJ, Kuzmina N, et al. Methotrexate in resistant juvenile rheumatoid arthritis. NEJM 326:1043–1049, 1992.

434. Graham LD, Myones BL, Rivas-Chacon RF, Pachman LM: Morbidity associated with long-term methotrexate therapy in juvenile rheumatoid arthritis. J Pediatr 120:468–73, 1992.

435. Giannini EH, Shaikov A, Maximov A, et al.: Meta-analysis of antirheumatic drug trials in juvenile rheumatoid arthritis. Arthritis Rheum 34:S152, 1991.

436. Wallace C, Sherry D, Salmonson K: Treatment of juvenile rheumatoid arthritis with higher dose methotrexate. Arthritis Rheum 33:S39, 1990.

437. Jundt JM, Browne BA, Mock D, et al.: Methotrexate pharmacokinetics in rheumatoid arthritis. Arthritis Rheum 33:S61, 1990.

438. Mandel MA: The synergistic effect of salicylates on methotrexate toxicity. Plast Recontruct Surg 57:733–737, 1976.

439. Taylor JR, Halprin KM: Effect of sodium salicylate and indomethacin on methotrexate-serum albumin binding. Arch Dermatol 113:588–591, 1977.

439a. Dupuis LL, Koren G, Shore A, et al.: Methotrexate-Nonsteroidal antiinflamatory drug interaction in children with arthritis. J Rheumatol 17:1469–1473, 1990.

440. Weinblatt ME, Weissman BN, Holdsworth DE, et al.: Long-term prospective

study of methotrexate in the treatment of rheumatoid arthritis. 84-month update. Arthritis Rheum 35:129–37, 1992.

441. Nordstrom DM, West SG, Andersen PA, Sharp JT: Pulse methotrexate therapy in rheumatoid arthritis. Ann Intern Med 107:797–801, 1987.

441a. Rau R, Herborn G, Karger T, Werdier D: Retardation of radiologic progression in rheumatoid arthritis with methotrexate therapy. A controlled study. Arthritis Rheum 84:1236–1244, 1991.

442. Kremer JM, Rynes RI, Bartholomew LE: Severe flare of rheumatoid arthritis after discontinuation of long-term methotrexate therapy. Am J Med 82:781–786, 1987.

443. Flowers MA, Heathcote J, Wanless IR, et al.: Fulminant hepatitis as a consequence of reactivation of hepatitis B virus infection after discontinuation of low-dose methotrexate therapy. Ann Intern Med 112:381–382, 1990.

444. Alarcon GS, Tracy IC, Blackburn WD Jr.: Methotrexate in rheumatoid arthritis. Toxic effects as the major factor in limiting long-term treatment. Arthritis Rheum 32:671–676, 1989.

445. Bjorkman DJ, Hammond EH, Lee RG, et al.: Hepatic ultrastructure after methotrexate therapy for rheumatoid arthritis. Arthritis Rheum 31:1465–1472, 1988.

446. Aponte J, Petrelli M: Histopathologic findings in the liver of rheumatoid arthritis patients treated with long-term bolus methotrexate. Arthritis Rheum 31:1457–1464, 1988.

447. Kremer JM, Lee RG, Tolman KG: Liver histology in rheumatoid arthritis patients receiving long-term methotrexate therapy. Arthritis Rheum 32:121–127, 1989.

448. Shergy WJ, Polisson RP, Caldwell DS, et al.: Methotrexate-associated hepatotoxicity: retrospective analysis of 210 patients with rheumatoid arthritis. Am J Med 85:771–774, 1988.

449. Brick JE, Moreland LW, Al-Kawas F, et al.: Prospective anaylsis of liver biopsies before and after methotrexate therapy in rheumatoid patients. Semin Arthritis Rheum 19:31–44, 1989.

449a. Keim D, Ragadalc C, Heidelberger K, Sullivan D: Hepatic fibrosis with the use of methothexate for juvenile arthritis. J Rheumatol 17:846–848, 1990.

450. Phillips C, Cera P, Mangan T, Newman E: Severe liver disease (SLD) in rheumatoid arthritis (RA) patients on methotrexate (MTX). Arthritis Rheum 33:#5 (Suppl):R15, 1990.

451. Whiting-O'Keefe QE, Fye KH, Sack KD: Methotrexate and histologic hepatic abnormalities: A meta-analysis. Am J Med 90:711–716, 1991.

452. Keim DR, Godoshian-Ragsdale C, Sullivan DB: Liver biopsy with the use of methotrexate for juvenile rheumatoid arthritis. J Pediatr 118:654, 1991.

452a. Hall P ole la M, Ahern MJ, Jarvis LR, et al.: Two methods of assessment of methotrexate hepatotoxicity in patients with rheumatoid arthritis. Ann Rheum Dis 50:471–476, 1991.

453. Carson CW, Cannon GW, Egger MJ, et al.: Pulmonary disease during the treatment of rheumatoid arthritis with low dose pulse methotrexate. Semin Arthritis Rheum 16:186–195, 1987.

454. Furst DE, Kremer JM: Methotrexate in rheumatoid arthritis. Arthritis Rheum 31:305–314, 1988.

455. Wernick R, Smith DL: Central nervous system toxicity associated with weekly

low-dose methotrexate treatment. Arthritis Rheum 32:770–775, 1989.

456. Shupack JL, Webster GF: Pancytopenia following low-dose oral methotrexate therapy for psoriasis. JAMA 259:3594–3596, 1988.

457. Scalone J, Bowen JR: Methotrexate osteopathy: case report. Contemp Orthop 17:46–49, 1988.

458. Lopez-Mendez A, Bridges SL Jr., Han K, et al.: Methotrexate increases risk of post-surgical complications in rheumatoid arthritis patients. Arthritis Rheum 33:#5 (Suppl) R131, 1990.

459. Tugwell P, Bombardier C, Buchanan WW, et al.: Methotrexate in rheumatoid arthritis. Impact on quality of life assessed by traditional standard-item and individualized patient preference health status questionnaires. Arch Intern Med 150:59–62, 1990.

460. Weinblatt ME, Kaplan H, Germain BF, et al.: Low-dose methotrexate compared with auranofin in adult rheumatoid arthritis. A thirty-six week, double-blind trial. Arthritis Rheum 33:330–338, 1990.

461. Shiroky J, Neville C, Esdaile J, Skelton J: High dose methotrexate with leucovorin rescue in the management of rheumatoid arthritis. Arthritis Rheum 33:#5 (Suppl), p. R39, 1990.

462. Hamdy H, McKendry RJR, Mierins E, Liver JA: Low-dose methotrexate compared with azathioprine in the treatment of rheumatoid arthritis. A twenty-four-week controlled clinical trial. Arthritis Rheum 30:361–368, 1987.

463. Kvien TK, Hoyeraal HM, Sandstad B: Azathioprine versus placebo in patients with rheumatoid arthritis: A single center double blind comparative study. J Rheumatol 13:118–123, 1986.

464. Silman AJ, Petrie J, Hazleman B, et al.: Lymphoproliferative cancer and other malignancy in patients with rheumatoid arthritis treated with azathioprine: A 20 year follow up study. Ann Rheum Dis 47:988–992, 1988.

465. Jeurissen MEC, Boerbooms AM Th, van de Putte LBA, Kruijsen MWM: Azathioprine induced fever, chills, rash, and hepatotoxicity in rheumatoid arthritis. Ann Rheum Dis 49:25–27, 1990.

465a. Willkens RF, Urowitz MB, Stablein DM, et al.: Comparison of azathioprine, methotrexate, and the combination of both in the treatment of rheumatoid arthritis. Arthritis Rheum 35:849–856, 1992.

466. Singh G, Fries JF, Spitz P, Williams CA: Toxic effects of azathioprine in rheumatoid arthritis. Arthritis Rheum 32:837–843, 1989.

467. Hardin JG: Cytotoxic-immunosuppressive drugs in the treatment of rheumatoid arthritis. Interm Med 8(12):123–137, 1987.

468. Baker GL, Kehl LE, Zee BC, et al.: Malignancy following treatment of rheumatoid arthritis with cyclophosphamide. Long-term case-control follow-up study. Am J Med 83:1–9, 1987.

469. Parra A, Santos D, Cervantes C, et al.: Plasma gonadotropins and gonadal steroids in children treated with cyclophosphamide. J Pediatr 92:117–124, 1978.

470. Puri HC, Campbell RA: Cyclophosphamide and malignancy. Lancet 1:1306, 1977.

471. Scott DGI, Bacon PA: Intravenous cyclophosphamide plus methylprednisolone in treatment of systemic rheumatoid vasculitis. Am J Med 76:377–383, 1984.

472. Pedersen-Bjergaard J, Ersboll J, Hansen VL, et al.: Carcinoma of the urinary bladder after treatment with cyclophosphamide for non-Hodgkin's lymphoma. N Engl J Med 318:1028–1032, 1988.

473. Arnold MH, Janssen B, Schrieber L, Brooks PM: Prospective pilot study of intravenous pulse cyclophosphamide therapy for refractory rheumatoid arthritis. Arthritis Rheum 32:933–934, 1989.
474. Csuka ME, Carrera GF, McCarty DJ: Treatment of intractable rheumatoid arthritis with combined cyclophosphamide, azathioprine, and hydroxychloroquine. A follow-up study. JAMA 255:2315–2319, 1986.
475. Palmer RG, Varonos S, Dore CJ, et al.: Chlorambucil induced chromosome damage in juvenile chronic arthritis. Arch Dis Child 60:1008–1013, 1985.
476. Palmer RG, Ansell BM: Acute leukaemia related to chlorambucil therapy for juvenile chronic arthritis. Clin Exp Rheumatol 2:81–83, 1984.
477. Callis L, Nieto J, Vila A, et al.: Chlorambucil treatment in minimal lesion nephrotic syndrome: A reappraisal of its gonadal toxicity. J Pediatr 97:653–656, 1980.
478. Cohen AS, Rubinow A, Anderson JJ, et al.: Survival of patients with primary (AL) amyloidosis: colchicine-treated cases from 1978–1983 compared with cases seen in previous years (1961 to 1973). Am J Med 82:1182–1190, 1987.
479. Dhillion V, Woo P, Isenberg D: Amyloidosis in the rheumatic diseases. Ann Rheum Dis 48:696–701, 1989.
480. Shand N, Richardson B: Sandimmun (Cyclosporin A): mode of action and clinical results in rheumatoid arthritis. Scand J Rheumatol 76:265–278, (Suppl) 1988.
481. Bjerkhoel F, Forre O: Cyclosporin treatment of a patient with severe systemic juvenile rheumatoid arthritis. Scand J Rheumatol 17:483–486, 1988.
482. Weinblatt ME, Coblyn JS, Fraser PA, et al.: Cyclosporin A treatment of refractory rheumatoid arthritis. Arthritis Rheum 30:11–17, 1987.
483. Dougados M, Amor B: Cyclosporin A in rheumatoid arthritis: preliminary clinical results of an open trial. Arthritis Rheum 30:83–87, 1987.
484. Forre O, Bjerkhoel F, Salvesen CF, et al.: An open, controlled, randomized comparison of cyclosporine and azathioprine in the treatment of rheumatoid arthritis: a preliminary report. Arthritis Rheum 30:88–92, 1987.
485. Dougados M, Awada H, Amor B: Cyclosporin in rheumatoid arthritis; a double blind, placebo controlled study in 52 patients. Ann Rheum Dis 47:127–133, 1988.
486. Yocum DE, Klippel JH, Wilder RL, et al.: Cyclosporine A in severe treatment-refractory rheumatoid arthritis. Ann Intern Med 109:863–869, 1988.
487. Tugwell P, Bombardier C, Gent M, et al.: Low-dose cyclosporin versus placebo in patients with rheumatoid arthritis. Lancet 335:1051–5555, 1990.
488. Porter GA, Bennett WM, Sheps SG, et al.: Cyclosporine-associated hypertension. Arch Intern Med 150:280–283, 1990.
489. Oates JA, Wood AJJ, Kahan BD: Drug Therapy. Cyclosporine. N Engl J Med 321:1725–1738, 1990 (see also Letters NEJM 322:1530–1531, 1990.)
490. Gupta AK, Rocher LL, Schmaltz SP, et al.: Short-term changes in renal function, blood pressure, and electrolyte levels in patients receiving cyclosporine for dermatologic disorders. Arch Intern Med 151:356–362, 1991.
491. Ost L: Effects of cyclosporin on prednisolone metabolism. Lancent 1:451, 1984.
492. Whitington PF, Emond JC, Whitington SH, et al.: Small-bowel length and the dose of cyclosporine in children after liver transplantation. 322:733–738, 1990.
493. van Rijthoven AWAM, Dukmans BAC, The DHSG, et al.: Comparison of cyclosporine and D-penicillamine for rheumatoid arthritis: A randomized, double blind, multicenter study. J Rheumatol 18:815–820, 1991.

493a. Zijlmans JMJM, van Rijthoven AWAM, Kluin PM, et al. Epstein-Barr virus-associated lymphoma in a patient with rheumatoid arthritis treated with cyclosporine. NEJM 326:1363, 1992.

494. Symoens J, Schuermans Y: Levamisole. Clin Rheum Dis 6(Suppl. 5):603–629, 1979.

495. Horsely K, Petersen K, Bentsen KD, Engstrom-Laurent A, et al.: Serum amino terminal Type III procollagen peptide and serum hyaluronan in rheumatoid arthritis: relation to clinical and serological parameters of inflammation during 8 and 24 months' treatment with levamisole, penicillamine or azathioprine. Ann Rheum Dis 47:116–126, 1988.

496. Editorial: Levamisole, a cautionary note. Lancet 2:291–292, 1979.

497. Prieur AM, Buriot D, Lefur JM: Possible toxicity of levamisole in children with rheumatoid arthritis. J Pediatr 93:304–305, 1978.

498. Wallace DJ, Goldfinger D, Lowe C, et al.: A double-blind, controlled study of lymphoplasmapheresis versus sham apheresis in rheumatoid arthritis. N Eng J Med 306:1406, 1982.

499. Rothwell RS, David P, Gordon PA, et al.: A controlled study of plasma exchange in the treatment of severe rheumatoid arthritis. Arthritis Rheum 23:785–790, 1980.

500. Karsh J, Klippel JH, Plotz PH, et al.: Lymphapheresis in rheumatoid arthritis: A randomized trial. Arthritis Rheum 24:867–873, 1981.

501. Nickleson RW, Brewer EJ, Rossen RD, et al.: Plasma exchange in selected patients with juvenile rheumatoid arthritis. J Pediatr 98:194–200, 1981.

502. Malaise MG, Hauwaert C, Franchimont P, et al.: Treatment of active rheumatoid arthritis with slow intravenous injections of thymopentin. A double-blind placebo-controlled randomized study. Lancet 1:832–836, 1985.

503. Riskin WG, Gillings DB, Scarlett JA: Amiprilose hydrochloride for rheumatoid arthritis. Ann Intern Med 111:455–465, 1989.

504. Cannon GW, Emkey RD, Denes A, et al.: Prospective two-year followup of recombinant interferon-gamma in rheumatoid arthritis. J Rheumatol 17:304–310, 1990.

505. Breedveld FC, Dukmans BAC, Mattie H: Minocycline treatment for rheumatoid arthritis: an open dose finding study. J Rheumatol 17:43–46, 1990.

506. Kremer JM, Jubiz W, Michalek A, et al.: Fish-oil fatty acid supplementation in active rheumatoid arthritis. A double-blinded, controlled, crossover study. Ann Intern Med 106:497–503, 1987.

507. Szobor A: Benefit of thymectomy in immune disease other than myasthenia. Lancet 1:277–278, 1984.

508. van Zeben D, Hazes JMW, Vandenbroucke JP, et al.: Diminished incidence of severe rheumatoid arthritis associated with oral contraceptive use. Arthritis Rheum 33:1462–1465, 1990.

509. Pritchard MH, Munro J: Successful treatment of Juvenile Chronic Arthritis with a specific antiviral agent. Br J Rheumatol 28:521–524, 1989.

510. Malawista SE, Trock DH, Edelson RL: Treatment of rheumatoid arthritis by extracorporeal photochemotherapy. A pilot study. Arthritis Rheum 34:646–654, 1991.

511. Southwood TR, Malleson PN, Roberts-Thomson PJ, Mahy M: Unconventional remedies used for patients with juvenile arthritis. Pediatrics 85:150–154, 1990.

512. Jacobs JC: Arthritis as a manifestation of connective tissue diseases. In Moore TD (ed.) Arthritis in Childhood. Report of the 80th Ross Conference on Pediat-

ric Research. Xanadu, Bahamas, December 2–5, 1979. Ross Laboratories, Columbus, OH, 1981, pp. 18–23.

513. Suciu-Foca N, Jacobs J, Godfrey M, et al.: HLA-DR5 in juvenile rheumatoid arthritis confined to a few joints. Lancet 2:40, 1980.

514. Myers LK, Ball EJ, Nunez G, et al.: HLA-D region epitopes associated with juvenile arthritis. Recognition by alloreactive T call clones and alloantisera. Arthritis Rheum 30:744–751, 1987.

515. Streekawkas AJ, Collery RT, McDowell J, et al.: Direct evidence for loss of human suppressor cells during active autoimmune disease. Proc Natl Acad Sci 75:5150–5154, 1978.

516. Vostrejs M, Hollister R: Muscle atrophy and leg length discrepancies in pauciarticular juvenile rheumatoid arthritis. Am J Dis Child 142:343–345, 1988.

517. Kanski JJ: Screening for uveitis in juvenile chronic arthritis. Br J Opthalmol 73:225–228, 1989.

518. Fernandez-Vina MA, Fink CW, Stastny P. HLA antigens in juvenile arthritis. Arthritis Rheum 33:1787–1784, 1990.

519. Earley A, Cuttica RJ, McCullough CM, Ansell BM: Triamcinolone into the knee joint in juvenile chronic arthritis. Clin Exp Rheumatol 6:153–155, 1988.

520. Balogh K: The histologic appearance of corticosteroid injection sites. Arch Pathol Lab Med 110:1168–1172, 1986.

521. Gilsanz V, Bernstein BH: Joint calcification following intraarticular corticosteroid therapy. Radiology 151:647–649, 1984.

522. Sparling M, Malleson P, Wood B, Petty R: Radiographic followup of joints injected with triamcinolone hexacetonide for the management of childhood arthritis. Arthritis Rheum 33:821–826, 1990.

523. Allen RC, Gross KR, Malleson PN, et al.: Intraarticular triamcinolone hexacetonide in the management of chronic arthritis in children. Arthritis Rheum 29:997–1001, 1986.

524. Huskisson EC: Intraarticular and soft-tissue injections. In Hart FD (ed.) Drug Treatment of the Rheumatic Diseases Williams and Wilkins, Sydney, 1987, pp. 111–116.

525. Montgomery SC, Campbell J: Septic arthritis following arthroscopy and intraarticular steroids. J Bone Joint Surg 71–8:540, 1989.

526. Hutchinson J: On a peculiar form of iritis which occurs in the children of gouty parents. Lancet 1–3, 1873.

527. Calabro JJ, Marchesano JM, Parrino GR: Juvenile rheumatoid arthritis: long-term management and prognosis. J Musculoskeletal Med pp. 17–32, January 1989.

528. Sherry DD, Mellins ED, Wedgwood RJ: Decreasing severity of chronic uveitis in children with pauciarticular arthritis. Am J Dis Child 145:1026–1028. 1991.

529. Spalter HF: The visual prognosis in juvenile rheumatoid arthritis. Trans Am Ophthalmol Soc 73:554–570, 1975.

530. Kanski JJ: Uveitis in juvenile chronic arthritis: incidence, clinical features and prognosis. Eye 2:641–645, 1988.

531. Melin-Aldana H, Giannini EH, Taylor J, et al.: Human leukocyte antigen-DRB1*1104 in the chronic iridocyclitis of pauciarticular juvenile rheumatoid arthritis. J Pediatr 121:56–60, 1992.

532. Rosenberg AM, Oen KG: The relationship between ocular and articular disease

activity in children with juvenile rheumatoid arthritis and associated uveitis. Arthritis Rheum 29:797–800, 1986.

533. Olson NY, Lindsley CB, Godfrey WA: Nonsteriodal anti-inflammatory drug therapy in chronic childhood iridocyclitis. Am J Dis Child 142:1289–1292, 1988.

533a. Dougados M, Berenbaum F, Maetzel A, et al.: The use of sulfasalazine for the prevention of attacks of acute anterior uveitis associated with spondyloarthropathy. Arthritis Rheum 34:S195, 1991.

534. Chylack LT, Dueker DK, Pihlaja DJ: Ocular manifestations of juvenile rheumatoid arthritis: Pathology, florescein iris angiography, and patient care patterns. In Miller JJ III (ed.) Juvenile Rheumatoid Arthritis. PSG, Littleton, MA, 1979.

535. Johns KJ, Chandra SR: Visual loss following intranasal corticosteroid injection. JAMA 261:2413, 1989.

536. Merrimam JC, Chylack LT, Albert DM: Early-onset pauciarticular juvenile rheumatoid arthritis: a histopathologic study. Arch Ophthalmol 101:1085–1092, 1983.

537. Wolf MD, Lichter PR, Ragsdale CG: Prognostic factors in the uveitis of juvenile rheumatoid arthritis. Opththalmology 94:1242–1248, 1987.

538. Herman DC: Endogenous Uveitis: Current concepts of treatment. Mayo Clin Proc 65:671–683, 1990.

539. Palmer RG, Kanski JJ, Ansell BM: Chlorambucil in the treatment of intractable uveitis associated with juvenile chronic arthritis. J Rheumatol 12:967–970, 1985.

540. Palestine AG, Austin HA III, Balow JE, et al.: Renal histopathologic alterations in patients treated with cyclosporine for uveitis. N Engl J Med 314:1293–1298, 1986.

540a. Vawter RL, Macsai M, Fakadej A, et al. Methotrexate for inflammatory eye disease. Arthritis rheum 35 #5S:R12, 1992.

540b. Bridges AJ, Burns RP. Acute iritis associated with primary Sjogren's syndrome and high-titer anti-SS-A/Ro and anti-SS-B-/La antibodies. Athritis Rheum 35:560–563, 1992.

541. Kanski JJ: Juvenile arthritis and uveitis. Surv Ophthalmol 34:253–267, 1990.

542. Kanski JJ, Shun-Shin GA: Systemic uveitis syndromes in childhood: an analysis of 340 cases. Ophthamology 91:1247–1252, 1984.

543. Praeger DL, Schneider HA, Sakowski AD, Jacobs JC: Kelman procedure in the treatment of complicated cataract of uveitis of Still's disease. Trans Ophthalmol Soc UK 96:168–172, 1976.

544. Flynn HW, Davis JL, Culbertson WW, Pars plana lensectomy and vitrectomy for complicated cataracts in juvenile rheumatoid arthritis. Ophthalmology 95:1114–1119, 1988.

545. Diamond JG, Kaplan HJ: Lensectomy and vitrectomy for complicated cataract secondary to uveitis. Arch Ophthalmol 96:1798–1804, 1978.

546. Lambert JR, Ansell BM, Stephenson E, et al.: Psoriatic arthritis in childhood. Clin Rheum Dis 2:339–352, 1976.

547. Sills EM: Psoriatic arthritis in childhood. Johns Hopkins Med J 146:49–53, 1980.

548. Shore A, Ansell BM: Juvenile psoriatic arthritis—an analysis of 60 cases.

J Pediatr 100:529–535, 1982.

549. Southwood TR, Petty RS, Malleson PN, et al.: Psoriatic arthritis in children. Arthritis Rheum 32:1007–1013, 1989.

550. Gerber J, Espinoza LR (eds.) Psoriatic Arthritis. Grune and Stratton, Orlando, 1985.

551. Seideman P, Fjellner B, Johannesson A: Psoriatic arthritis treated with oral colchicine. J Rheumatol 14:777–779, 1987.

552. Steinsson K, Jonsdottir I, Valdimarsson H: Cyclosporin A in psoriatic arthritis: an open study. Ann Rheum Dis 49:603–606, 1990.

553. Huckins D, Felson DT, Holick M: Treatment of psoriatic arthritis with oral 1, 25-dihydroxyvitamin D3: A pilot study. Arthritis Rheum 33:1723–1727, 1990.

554. Ellis CN, Fradin MS, Messana JM, et al.: Cyclosporine for plaque-type psoriasis. Results of a multidose, double-blind trial. N Engl J Med 324:277–294, 1991 (see also correspondence pp. 1894–1985).

555. Randall T: Cyclosporine: vital in today's transplantation, but questions remain about tomorrow. JAMA 264:1794–1797, 1990.

556. van Rijthoven AWAM, Dijkmans BAC, Goei The HS, et al.: Long-term cyclosporine therapy in rheumatoid arthritis. J Rheumatol 18:19–23, 1991.

557. Gay RE, Palmoski MJ, Brandt KD, Gay S: Aspirin causes in vivo synthesis of type I collagen by atrophic articular cartilage. Arthritis Rheum 26:1231–1236, 1983.

558. Williams PE: Effect of intermittent stretch on imobilized muscle. Ann Rheum Dis 47:1014–1016, 1988.

559. Hinojosa J, Anderson J, Strauch C: Pediatric occupational therapy in the home. Am J Occup Ther 42:17–22, 1988.

560. Gallino L, Pountain G, Mitchell N, Ansell BM: Developmental aspects of the hip in juvenile chronic arthritis. A radiologic assessment. Scand J Rhematol 13:310–318, 1984.

561. Vostrejs M, Hollister JR: Muscle atrophy and leg length discrepancies in pauciarticular juvenile rheumatoid arthritis. Am J Dis Child 142:343–345, 1988.

562. Editorial: joint injury and muscle weakness. Lancet 2:381–382, 1984.

563. Jacobsen ST, Levinson JE, Crawford AH: Late results of synovectomy in juvenile rheumatoid arthritis. J Bone Joint Surg 67-A:8–15, 1985.

564. Rydholm U, Elborgh R, Ranstam J, et al.: Synovectomy of the knee in juvenile chronic arthritis: a retrospective, consecutive follow-up study. J Bone Joint Surg 68B:223–228, 1986.

564a. Ovregard T, Hoyeraal HM, Pahle JA, Larsen S. A three-year retrospective study of synovectomies in children. Clin Orthop Rel Res 259:76–82, 1990.

565. Combe B, Krause E, Sany J: Treatment of chronic knee-synovitis with arthroscopic synovectomy after failure of intraarticular injection of radionuclide. Arthritis Rheum 32:10–14, 1989.

566. Mogensen B, Brattstrom H, Svantesson H, Lidgren L: Soft tissue release of the hip in juvenile chronic arthritis. Scand J Rheumatol 12:17–20, 1983.

567. Scott RD, Sarokhan AJ, Dalziel R: Total hip and total knee arthroplasty in juvenile rheumatoid arthritis. Clin Orthop 182:90–97, 1984.

568. Kunec JR: Total hip replacement in patients under thirty-five years of age. Orthopedics 6:1432–1434, 1983.

569. Ruddlesdin C, Ansell BM, Arden GP, Swann M: Total hip replacement in

children with juvenile chronic arthritis. J Bone Joint Surg 68B:218–222, 1986.

570. Arthritis of the hip in children. Lancet 2:260, 1986.

571. Gudmundsson GH, Harving S, Pilgaard S: The Charnley total hip arthroplasty in juvenile rheumatoid arthritis patients. Orthopedics 12:385–388, 1989.

572. Dossick PH, England S, Huo M, et al.: Total hip replacement in juvenile rheumatoid arthritis. Arthritis Rheum 33 #5(Suppl):R40, 1990.

573. Sarokhan AJ, Scott RD, Thomas WH, et al.: Total knee arthroplasty in juvenile rheumatoid arthritis. J Bone Joint Surg 65A:1071–1080, 1983.

574. Nicholas SA, Figgie MP, Alexiades MM, et al.: Total knee replacement in juvenile rheumatoid arthritis. Arthritis Rheum 33 #5(Suppl):R40, 1990.

4

HLA-B27-Associated Spondyloarthritis and Enthesopathy

Spondyloarthritis is a new term that "lumps" patients with a group of interrelated familial arthropathies into one diagnostic category and more definitively differentiates patients with milder manifestations of this form of arthritis from those with RA.[1-8]

In my conceptualization of spondyloarthritis, the prototype of the disease in its most advanced stage is ankylosing spondylitis (AS) with calcification of the spinal ligaments, a stage reached by only a small number of affected individuals.

Reiter's syndrome (RS) is merely a dramatic and historically popularized, albeit uncommon, form of onset.[9-11] Spondyloarthritis usually begins with pauciarticular arthritis or simply with fleeting rheumatic complaints (in children or adults) or with mild inflammatory back pain (in teenagers and adults).[2] Enthesopathy, inflammation of the enthesis, the areas of attachment of connective tissues (ligaments and tendons and fascia) to bone, is an important feature of the disease in most patients and in its most severe form is associated with calcification of the inflamed enthesis.[2,9] Radiologic evidence of erosion or calcification of the sacroiliac (SI) joints is not regarded, as in the past, as the hallmark without which the patient must remain either with no diagnosis or an erroneous one; rather it is looked upon as a midstation on the way from mild forms of spondyloarthritis to AS. Most individuals affected with this disease do not have radiographic changes in the SI joints, and only a proportion of those that do will ever develop ankylosis of the spine (Fig. 4.1). The term *spondyloarthritis*, therefore, does not necessarily imply arthritis of the spine but rather defines a form of arthritis that is pathogenetically related to AS in contradistinction to RA. Arthritis related to AS was formerly thought to be rare in children; most affected children were misdiagnosed as suffering from JRA, acute rheumatic fever, or "growing pains," or were thought to have psychosomatic symptoms without an organic disorder.[4,5] The identification of HLA-B27 as a susceptibility marker for

360

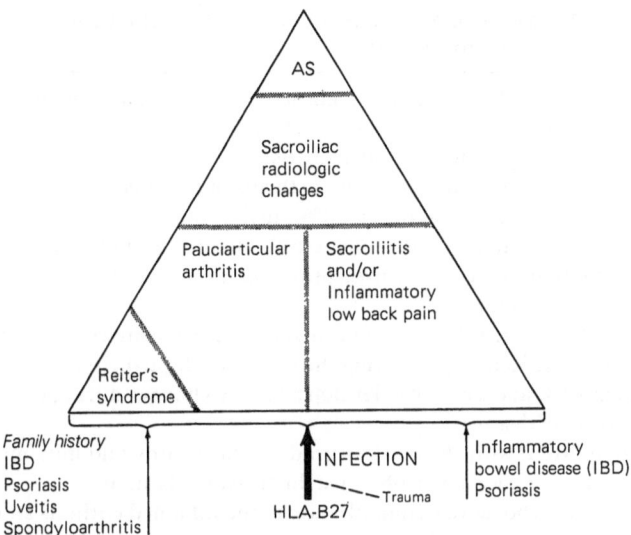

Figure 4.1. The spectrum of HLA-B27–associated spondyloarthritis. Most patients with this form of arthritis have either pauciarticular arthritis and/or sacroiliitis without radiographic changes. Some of these patients go on to develop radiographic changes in the SI joints, and some of those develop ankylosis of the spine. The initial episode of arthritis in some patients is characteristic of RS. (Reprinted with permission from Jacobs J.C.: "Current Concepts in Rheumatology: Spondyloarthritis and enthesopathy." *Arch Intern Med.* 143:103–107, 1983. Copyright by the American Medical Association.)

spondyloarthritis has resulted in recognition of spondyloarthritis as a rather common arthritic disorder in both children and adults (Table 4.1).[3–6] HLA-B27 associated spondyloarthritis and enthesopathy may itself be a prototype of a larger spectrum of arthritic disorders, some of which may be familial.[12]

Historical Considerations*

In 1693–1695 Bernard Connor, an Irish anatomist teaching in France, described an unusual skeleton in which the ilium, sacrum, and the 15 lowest vertebrae and adjoining ribs formed one continuous bone (Fig. 4.2). The first clinical description of the disorder was by Benjamin Travers in 1824. His patient was a 16-year-old girl whose illness started with backache; her entire spine below T-1 was ankylosed within 3 years. At just that time, a young man living on the Isle of Man developed pain in his elbow and knees and within 7½ years, as reported by Lyons, was unable to move anything except his left thumb, right little finger, jaw, and one hip. In 1883, Clutton described a 9-year-old boy whose arthritis began in the first MTP joint and

* As reviewed by Professor Eric Bywaters.[2]

Table 4.1. Characteristics of Childhood-Onset Spondyloarthritis and Enthesopathy Associated with HLA-B27*

Onset in many cases shortly after an undiagnosed, significant, febrile illness; significant skeletal trauma; or bacterial diarrhea

Primarily lower-extremity asymmetrical arthritis

Most frequent onset pattern—monarticular arthritis of the knee

First MTP joint affected in 10% at onset; 20% during course

Enthesopathy (heel pain at insertion of the Achilles tendon and plantar fascia) prominent and sometimes the only presenting manifestation. May be accompanied by tenosynovitis and periostitis

Onset with RS in 10%, but 45% have some associated eye, urinary, or dermatologic manifestations of the Reiter type during the course of the arthritis

Sacroiliac pain in 10% at onset; 20% develop SI x-ray changes during course (after average of 5 years of disease)

Tends to be intermittent with chronic low-grade enthesopathy and inflammation of synarthroses with occasional peripheral arthritic exacerbations

More severe in males who more frequently calcify the inflamed enthesis and may have total destruction of the hips

The risk of developing ankylosis of the spine is relatively small (?2%, ?10%)

Previously was mistaken for JRA, ARF, "growing pains," psychological problems

* Diagnosis is made on the basis of this clinical pattern of symptoms plus the presence of HLA-B27.

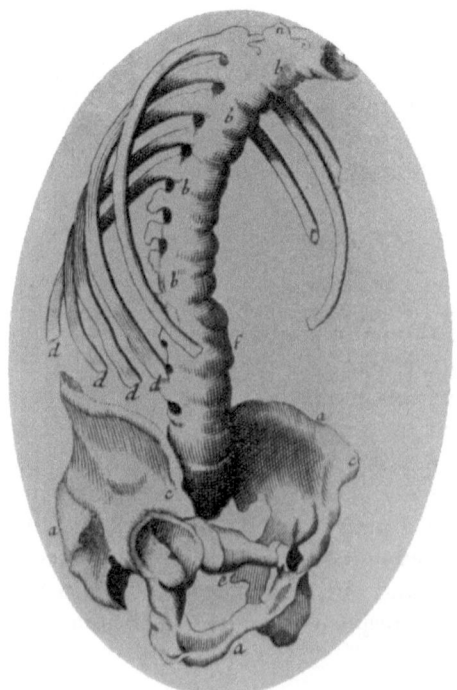

Figure 4.2. The skeletal remains found by Bernard Connor. (Reprinted with permission from Llewellyn-Jones R: *Arthritis Deformans.* Wright, Bristol, England, 1909. Reproduced from Moll J.M.H. (ed.): *Ankylosing Spondylitis.* Churchill Livingstone, Edinburgh, 1980.)

went on to complete ankylosis of the spine and ribs, hip, and a few other peripheral joints over the next 20 years. At the end of the 19th century and during the first years of the 20th, many authors improved on the clinical descriptions of the disease but unfortunately looked upon it as just a special form of RA (which was itself confused with osteoarthritis and sometimes with gout).

Roentgen developed his technique in 1896, and by 1906 Schlayer had described the radiologic features of ankylosis of the spine. However, recognition of radiographic changes in the sacroiliac joints as a diagnostic tool that could predict susceptibility to AS did not occur until Scott popularized this earlier (1932) observation of his in a book published in 1942 entitled *A Monograph on Adolescent Spondylitis or Ankylosing Spondylitis: The Early Diagnosis and its Treatment by Wide-Field X-ray Irradiation.*[13] Scott emphasized that "the onset is insidious extending over a period of five to seven years. . . . It attacks the young . . ." therefore his title "adolescent" to replace "ankylosing" and his keen description of the most important question in his history-taking in his patient: "Did you experience any rheumatism before your back got bad?" to which the majority would say, "I have had 'growing pains' and attacks of wandering rheumatic pains ever since I was a boy." Scott concluded, "A definite percentage of patients under about 25 years of age giving a history of recurrent attacks of wandering pains—often called 'growing pains'— extending over a number of years, might be expected to develop spondylitis sooner or later." He recognized that these youngsters often had no sacroiliac pain and also observed that radiographic changes might appear in the SI joints prior to the development of SI symptoms and almost always appeared prior to radiographic changes in the spine.

Scott's detailed description of the "prespondylitic symptoms" included occasional severe attacks of "growing pains" at night; intermittent attacks of asymmetric peripheral arthritis, primarily of the lower extremities, which come and go; special predisposition for the first MTP joint; and pain at the tendinous insertions in the heel and at the ligamentous attachments at the ribs and shoulders. As cited above, the earliest clinical descriptions by many authors tended to be in children (one a girl), and most emphasized peripheral joint disease as the earliest manifestation (Fig. 4.3).

Unfortunately, Scott did not recognize that most children with the symptom complex he so skillfully observed did not progress to AS. When the hazards of the x-ray therapy he advocated for these children became apparent, many authors stopped citing his work and his cogent observations were lost to an entire generation of children's doctors.

Creation of diagnostic criteria for ankylosing spondylitis caused another great setback in the recognition and understanding of this kind of arthritis in childhood. The criteria proposed in Rome in 1961 (Table 4.2) allowed diagnosis only in the presence of four out of five clinical criteria, including four spinal criteria and iritis or in the presence of one clinical criteria plus x-ray evidence of bilateral sacroiliitis.[2] The more often used criteria that were proposed at a conference in New York in 1968 (Table 4.3) allow a definite

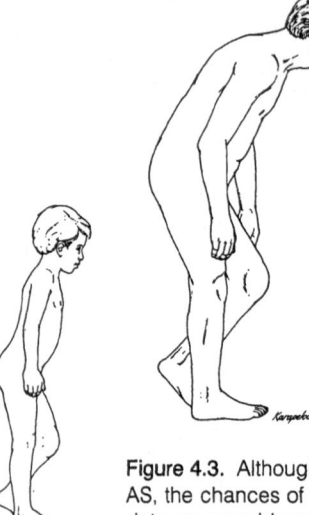

Figure 4.3. Although the boy with one swollen knee may end as the man with AS, the chances of this happening seem small. Based on currently available data, one would assume a risk of about 2%.

Table 4.2. Rome Criteria for Diagnosing Ankylosing Spondylitis

Clinical Criteria
1. Low back pain and stiffness for more than 3 months that is not relieved by rest
2. Pain and stiffness in the thoracic region
3. Limited motion in the lumbar spine
4. Limited chest expansion
5. History or evidence of iritis or its sequelae

Radiologic Criteria
6. X-ray showing bilateral sacroiliac changes characteristic of ankylosing spondylitis (this excludes bilateral osteoarthrosis of the sacroiliac joints)

From Moll, ref. 2.

diagnosis only after radiographic demonstration of sacroiliitis.[2] Although Scott had used sacroiliac x-ray changes as a means to early diagnosis but emphasized the importance of peripheral musculoskeletal pain, these criteria served to force some other (erroneous) diagnosis in essentially all children and most adults with spondyloarthritis. While these criteria may be used for classification, they are not useful for early diagnosis since they do not really identify a disease but rather a middle *stage* of a disease.[14,15] Their anomalous perpetuation is a result of (1) general agreement that the term *ankylosing spondylitis* is not an acceptable diagnostic term (it's too strong) for patients who have only peripheral arthritis and enthesopathy; (2) general willingness to accept the term ankylosing spondylitis for those with radiographic evidence of bilateral sacroiliitis (a 1961 effort at early identification of the

Table 4.3. New York Criteria for Ankylosing Spondylitis

A. Diagnosis
1. Limitation of motion of the lumbar spine in all three planes—anterior flexion, lateral flexion and extension
2. History or the presence of pain at the dorsolumbar junction or in the lumbar spine
3. Limitation of chest expansion to 1 inch (2.5 cm) or less, measured at the level of the fourth intercostal space

B. Grading
Definite Ankylosing Spondylitis
1. Grade 3–4 bilateral sacroiliitis with at least one clinical criterion *or*
2. Grade 3–4 unilateral or grade 2 bilateral sacroiliitis with clinical criterion 1 (limitation of back movement in all three planes) or with both clinical criteria 2 and 3 (back pain and limitation of chest expansion)*

Probable Ankylosing Spondylitis
Grade 3–4 bilateral sacroiliitis with no clinical criteria

---

*Radiographic grading of sacroiliitis: (2) marginal sclerosis; (3) erosions and sclerosis; (4) complete obliteration.
From Moll, ref. 2.

population susceptible to ankylosis of the spine); and (3) lack of recognition by pediatricians that this form of arthritis occurs in children and use of the criteria almost exclusively by physicians who do not see children.

Progress from this awkward state has been slow. While those who create classification criteria recognize that they are not useful for early diagnosis and must be subject to frequent revision as medical knowledge increases, there is nevertheless a tendency to perpetuate criteria as if they had been handed down on the tablets at Mount Sinai. However, in a disease in which the criteria being used for diagnosis require an average of 5 years in "limbo," modification would be an inevitable result of having a means of identifying especially susceptible individuals early in the course of their disease. The discovery by Brewerton, Schlosstein, et al. that HLA-B27 was associated with susceptibility to AS initiated another period of intensive study of this form of arthritis in children.[7-8]

Before detailing the clinical characteristics of spondyloarthritis in children, it would be appropriate to briefly review some relationships between HLA and disease.[16]

The Histocompatibility System and Disease

Definition of HLA

Grafts exchanged between major histocompatibility (MHC) identical donors survive significantly longer than grafts that are incompatible for this system.[17] Antigens present in the graft but absent from the host induce the primary immune response that leads to graft rejection. These antigens are called human leukocyte antigens (HLA). There are at least six HLA loci on the sixth chromosome; each locus has a substantial number of mutually exclusive alleles. The HLA system is complex, with a potential for over 355 million genotypes.

Methods of Study

Two different approaches may be used to determine whether a given HLA is related to a given disease. In *population studies*, the frequency of the HLA in unrelated patients can be compared with the frequency in a corresponding population of healthy controls. Since HLA occurs with different frequencies in different racial and ethnic groups, the study and control populations must be carefully matched to avoid erroneous conclusions. Many of these and other difficulties inherent in population studies can be overcome by *family studies*. This method, although difficult and expensive, has the additional capability of showing HLA linkage, if present, within an affected family, even in disorders in which no single HLA serves as a marker for the disease in all affected families.

Clinical Uses of HLA Typing

There are several different ways in which HLA typing may be useful in clinical practice (Table 4.4). When a heritable disorder first manifests itself late in life, effective genetic counseling is impossible. However, if the disorder is HLA-linked within a family (e.g., Marie's ataxia), early risk prediction and genetic counseling become possible.[18] In some other diseases (e.g., hemachromatosis) it may be possible to alter the environment of the identified susceptible individual so as to prevent or minimize the development of clinical manifestations of disease.[19] In yet other disorders (such as the 21-

Table 4.4. Uses of HLA Typing

1. Establishment of new classifications, definitions, and relationships between ill-defined syndromes
2. Elucidation of pathogenetic mechanisms
3. Identification of predisposed individuals and families
   a. Early diagnosis and treatment
   b. Avoidance of erroneous diagnosis and incorrect treatment
   c. Potential for altering environment to avoid disease-inducing factors
4. Identification of new precipitating environmental factors
5. Ensuring some uniformity in patients entered into clinical trials
6. Identification of some individuals at increased risk for certain drug reactions

hydroxylase-deficiency form of congenital adrenal hyperplasia), differentiation of heterozygote carriers from mildly affected individuals may be enhanced by HLA typing and then performing special provocative biochemical tests in those shown by HLA typing to have a high risk of having subclinical disease.[20] In these examples, it is clear that the genetic defects resulting in disease are HLA-linked and that HLA typing is clinically useful but that the HLA antigens themselves are not involved in the pathogenesis of disease. There is nothing to suggest that immunologic dysfunction is present.

The situation is considerably more complicated in the autoimmune disorders.[21,21a] It now appears likely that all immune responses are regulated both by a complex network of T-cell and B-cell interactions and by a linked set of genes that determine the structure of the HLA.[22-24] It is also likely that some anti-HLA antibodies have a direct pathogenic role in the creation or pattern of some diseases.[25] Some bacterial antigens, such as those of *Klebsiella pneumoniae*, for example, cross-react with HLA-B27.[26] The possible role of cross-reacting antibodies to bacteria in inducing spondyloarthritis requires further study.[27] Differing patterns of disease may result from HLA interactions: spondyloarthritic patients who carry DR4 are at higher risk of finger and toe arthritis.[28]

The major use of HLA typing in clinical work at present is to help in distinguishing between patients with similar clinical syndromes. Other benefits include the potential to assure some uniformity in clinical trials, enhanced diagnostic alertness, and the identification of individuals at increased risk for certain drug reactions (see Chapter 3 under Treatment with Gold and Penicillamine).

Immunoregulatory Functions of HLA Gene Products

In rats made transgenic by introduction of B27 and human β_2-microglobulin genes, spontaneous inflammatory disease resembling human B27-associated disease develops.[29] In at least some if not all species, HLA-A, -B, and -C gene products determine the number and specificity of cytotoxic killer T cells that can respond to viral and other foreign antigens. HLA-D-region gene products control the interactions of T and B cells and macrophages and thus determine whether an antibody response to a given antigen will develop.[30,31] While it is clear that susceptibility to autoimmune diseases is associated with the HLA system, the mechanisms for the actual production of disease remain speculative. As will be discussed in this chapter, HLA-B27–associated spondyloarthritis often begins as a response to specific infections. Some other attacks seem to result from skeletal trauma. Other precipitating factors remain unknown. Future study of the immunologic mechanisms that lead to the development of arthritis in B27-positive children may lead to preventive or curative maneuvers and may also answer many important questions relevant to the pathogenesis of a great variety of immunologic diseases.

HLA-B27 and Arthritis

Ankylosing Spondylitis

The strongest association of HLA with disease is that between B27 and AS.[8,17] Using radiographic evidence of significant sacroiliitis as the criteria for diagnosis of AS, the incidence of B27 in white AS patients is 90%, whereas the incidence of B27 in normal control populations is generally only about 8%. The frequency of AS in any population is correlated with the frequency of B27 in that population. In American blacks, where the frequency of B27 is 1–4%, the incidence of AS is much lower than in whites.[32] In Orientals, the frequency of HLA-B27 and AS is even lower. However, in British Columbian Haida Indians, where the incidence of B27-positive individuals is 50%, one-eighth of the entire male population develops radiographic evidence of AS in the sacroiliac joints.[33] In some Navajo Indian populations in eastern Arizona, the frequency of B27 is 36%, and as would be expected, AS is also unusually frequent.[34]

The risk of developing AS using SI calcification alone as a criteria for diagnosis is considerable for B27-positive individuals. Twenty to twenty-five percent of healthy B27-positive blood donors have AS by those criteria, and 40% of B27 relatives of an already-identified index case (a more susceptible group) have some spondyloarthritic symptoms.[8] The accurate prediction of lifetime risk would require prospective studies for a generation. Such studies have not yet been accomplished, so these risk estimates are underestimates. However, even with such underestimates, 2% of the white population can be expected to eventually develop radiographic changes in the SI joints that are characteristic of spondyloarthritis. Twenty-three percent of children of mothers diagnosed as AS will develop childhood arthritis.[35] Twenty-five percent of children diagnosed as AS have first-degree relatives who can be shown to have AS.[36] Other genetic material may greatly enhance the B27 risk.[37]

Other factors that affect the reported incidence of AS are age and sex. Females are usually affected more mildly than males, and the radiographic progression of disease is slower, causing delay in diagnosis. In published series, males outnumber females by eight to one, and diagnosis in males tends to be 5–10 years sooner than in females. It has long been recognized that because of the milder manifestations in women the disease often goes unrecognized, although spondyloarthritic manifestations are probably equally frequent in males and females.[38] Progression of disease is much slower in females, and calcification of ligaments is quite rare.

Ankylosing spondylitis with obvious involvement of the spine is rare in children, and there are relatively few reported cases.[39–46] While those cases of AS that do begin in childhood often present with peripheral spondyloarthritic symptoms rather than low back pain,[11,47] the frequency of progression from childhood spondyloarthritis to the stage of positive radiographic evidence of sacroiliitis, and the risk of subsequent progression to calcification of spinal ligaments, remain to be determined.[48] In a recent study, after 9 years, fewer than 6% of children with HLA-B27–associated arthritis had developed radiographic sacroiliitis.[49] The pattern within a family tends to remain constant; families with AS develop AS; those with spondyloarthritis without clear signs of AS tend to reproduce that pattern of disease.[50]

HLA-B27 is not the only marker that is associated with increased risk of developing AS; psoriasis, iritis, inflammatory bowel disease (IBD), or a family history of these disorders or spondyloarthritis also increases the risk of AS even in the absence of B27.[10] Some peculiar statistics emerge as a result of these associations. The frequency of B27 in patients with AS with psoriasis or IBD is lower than in AS without psoriasis or IBD. The presence of those diseases seems to make it less necessary for B27-associated gene material to be present to enhance development of AS.[10] On the other hand, the incidence of spondyloarthritis in B27 individuals who also have psoriasis or IBD is 50–100%.[10]

Testing for HLA-B27 is of little value in identifying cases of AS in unselected populations. In the absence of symptoms and effective measures to prevent disease, there even exits the potential disadvantage of creating anxiety and factitious or imagined illness. However, in patients in whom there is reason to believe that the diagnosis of spondyloarthritis is possible, the B27 test can be of help to the clinician. In those racial populations in which B27 is relatively rare (blacks and Orientals), a positive test in the presence of arthritis is of even more potential diagnostic importance, although a negative test is of relatively little importance.[32]

Reiter's Syndrome and "Reactive Arthritis"

Reactive arthritis is defined as a nonsuppurative process but there are increasing reports of localization and persistence of the inciting bacterial antigenic material in the synovial fluid and the synovium and the bowel wall of affected individuals.[51,51a] Reiter's syndrome (RS), initially described by Von Forest in 1507, and said to have affected Christopher Columbus,[52,53] defined as the classic triad of nongonococcal urethritis, arthritis, and ocular disturbances such as conjunctivitis, ketatitis, or iritis, is no longer an adequate name for a disease.[9,10,54] On the one hand, it is universally recognized that this disease process may be manifested by only one manifestation of the triad, resulting in the awkward phrase "incomplete Reiter's syndrome." On the other hand, the triad only represents a part of the disease, which may include severe mucocutaneous features and may also be indistinguishable in its course from AS.[9,10] It has recently been emphasized that RS is difficult to define because it is *always* incomplete.[10,11] One author stated that it was necessary to see 410 cases to appreciate the complete picture of the disease.[10] If RS and AS, as traditionally defined, are the only recognized and defined forms of spondyloarthropathy, no diagnostic terminology exists that applies to the majority of patients with reactive spondyloarthritis.[6] It is for this reason that we reserve the term Reiter's syndrome for the historically popularized triad, just as we reserve the term AS for patients with vertebral involvement.[55] In this schema, RS is merely one form of onset of spondyloarthritis and is not a separate disease, just as ankylosis of the spine is not a disease itself but rather the most severe end stage of spondyloarthritis.

The incidence of B27 in white individuals with RS is 80%; if the attack includes uveitis or keratoderma blennorrhagicum, features each individually associated with B27, the incidence of B27 is almost 100%.[9,10] When a patient presents merely with reactive arthritis without other features of RS after a known urethral or dysenteric infection, the incidence of B27 is only 65%.

The risk of developing reactive arthritis after certain infections is highly correlated with the presence of B27, however. In large *Salmonella typhimurium* epidemics, 7–27% of B27 individuals developed arthritis as opposed to only 1.35% of individuals without B27.[56,57] Other salmonella species may produce arthritis,[58] as may a reaction to salmonella vaccine.[59] In a study of nonspecific urethritis (36% were proved to be due to *Chlamydia trachomatis*), 20% of B27 individuals developed reactive arthritis as contrasted with only 2% of individuals without B27.[60] Thus, the risk of reactive arthritis in B27 individuals in a given infectious exposure may vary from 5 to 20 times that of other individuals. A child born with HLA-B27 is thought to be 300 times more likely to develop arthritis than one born without that antigen.[61] Other HLA antigens may determine which organisms set off the disease.[27]

Although the arthritis associated with RS is often pauciarticular and affects primarily large lower-extremity joints, the onset of this syndrome may be sudden acute, polyarticular, and accompanied by severe systemic manifestations simulating systemic JRA. While reactive arthritis has been generally thought of as a brief illness without long-term sequelae, there is considerable evidence that this presumption is not correct.[58–64] Of the 344 cases contained in Paronen's classic report, 42% of the 100 who could be located and examined 20 years later had some evidence of chronic arthritis,[65–67] 85% of these patients were B27-positive. While this is probably a selected sample (the sick were easier to find than the healthy) and so constitutes an overestimate, and while the majority of individuals with an attack of reactive spondyloarthritis make a complete recovery and are normal 20 years later, there is still considerable risk of chronicity. A 10-year follow-up of patients with *Yersinia* arthritis showed 46% with mild persistent peripheral symptoms; 40% of the B27 patients had radiographic sacroiliitis.[63]

JRA and HLA-B27

When typing sera for HLA-B27 became widely available, a number of children's arthritis clinics retrospectively typed the patients they were following who had fulfilled the established diagnostic criteria for JRA; 28–45% of these patients had HLA-B27. The majority of these were male children with "pauciarticular" JRA; however, there was an excess of B27 children in all subgroups of JRA. Many went on to fulfill the diagnostic criteria for AS, but the majority did not, at least within the period of these studies.[68,69] It is now apparent that most arthritic children with HLA-B27 have a disease pathogenetically and pathologically related to AS, a disease for which AS may be considered the prototype, which we term HLA-B27–associated spondyloarthritis.[5] HLA-B27 typing frequently permits a raised index of suspicion and is a means of achieving greater accuracy in differential diagnosis early in the course of arthritis in young people.[70–72] These children will continue to be at risk for arthritis throughout their lives, and their families are at greater risk for similar arthritis. Recent studies indicate that other different forms of heritable arthritis exist within the spectrum of what has been called JRA.[16] The B27 marker may be of use in differential diagnosis, in prospective study of arthritic children, in family counseling, and in therapy. It seems likely that it will be of further help in determining the pathogenesis of at least this form of arthritis and perhaps ultimately in developing methods of preventing these children from developing arthritis.

Limitations of HLA-B27 Testing

Laboratory tests should help to distinguish minimal disease from the normal state and from diseases with similar clinical manifestations.[15] HLA-B27 does not identify a disease; it is not a diagnostic test; its absence does not exclude any diagnosis. While it identifies a group of individuals with increased susceptibility to arthritis and may heighten the physician's sensitivity to previously ignored but significant symptoms, it also has the potentiality to encourage misdiagnosis of HLA-B27–associated arthritis in normals or in patients whose complaints are caused by other disorders. The physician who uses HLA typing as a clinical tool must recognize these limitations.[37]

HLA-B27-Associated Spondyloarthritis and Enthesopathy

For the purpose of this discussion, we have limited our analysis to children who are identified as having the HLA-B27 antigen.[73] We are aware that this is arbitrary and excludes patients with the identical syndrome who are not HLA-B27-positive. We have even excluded from our analyses a boy whose father and uncle have HLA-B27–associated arthritis and whose arthritis is obviously of this character but who is not HLA-B27-positive. We recognize that such a policy is illogical but believe it is temporarily appropriate. We have made the mistake of grouping all of these children under the heading "JRA" for many years; only this new marker has led to our ability to separate out this form of arthritis in childhood. For the moment, this method of defining the disorder, despite its shortcomings, seems most likely to lead to the most accurate collection of data and understanding of the disease process.

This is not to imply, however, that these manifestations are limited to patients with the B27 antigen; they do not seem to be so limited, and HLA-B27–associated spondyloarthritis itself appears to a prototype for spondyloarthritic disease not associated with HLA-B27.

The Clinical Presentation of Children with B27-Associated Arthritis

Epidemiology

Fifteen percent of children in our arthritis clinic have HLA-B27–associated spondyloarthritis.[4,5] Thirty percent of these B27 arthritic children are girls. The percentage of affected children increases with increasing age (Table 4.5). The male predominance is not apparent at 1–5 years of age and is most apparent between 6 and 9 years of age where newly recognized affected children are 90% males and in patients with the Reiter's triad, 80% of whom are males.

One-third of children with spondyloarthritis have a family history of arthritis, uveitis, sciatica, or inflammatory low back pain, which is acknowledged at the time of initial consulation. However, soon after the diagnosis was established in our patients, an additional 17% of the parents reported close relatives with similar arthritis. With the use of a mail questionnaire, we were able to document a significant arthritis history in 60% of the families of these children by the time the index cases had an average of 5 years of disease. Diagnosis of the child often leads to correction of misdiagnoses of disease in adult relatives.

More than one individual in a family may develop HLA-B27–associated spondyloarthritis at one time if B27 individuals acquire the same inciting infection at the same time or from each other.[74] Familial episodes of RS have been reported by others. Our experience suggests that most commonly this occurs without the complete triad: one individual may have iritis, another iritis with arthritis, etc. In our series in the two instances where more than

Table 4.5. Age at Onset of Arthritic Symptoms (58 Patients)

Age	Males	Females
1–2 years	3	3
3–5 years	3	3
6–9 years	10	2
10–15 years	24	10

From Jacobs, refs. 4 and 5.

one family member had a coincident onset of some manifestation of the triad, the relationships were father/son and brother/sister. In both families, the inciting illness was "traveler's diarrhea." HLA-B27+ relatives of B27+ arthritic probands are 16 times more likely to develop arthritis than B27+ individuals in the population as a whole.[75,76]

Epidemic RS has been associated with epidemics of specific types of *Shigella*,[77] *Campylobacter*,[78,79] *Salmonella*,[79] and *Yersinia enterocolitica*[80–81a] organisms. Sporotrichosis may also cause reactive arthritis.[82] Thus, susceptible individuals exposed to an environment where such infection is more likely are more likely to have an attack of RS. Similarly, males exposed to multiple sexual partners are more likely to develop nongonococcal urethritis with resultant RS. (Gonorrheal urethritis is not associated with this form of arthritis.) Male homosexuals have been shown to be at greater risk of acquiring dysenteric infection from oral-anal exposure and so may be expected to be more prone to RS. HIV infections may present with Reiter's syndrome.[83]

The Inciting Illness

In about 50% of cases, a history of antecedent illness or significant skeletal trauma can be elicited.[4,5] Most often, the illness is described as "flulike" with fever and vague musculoskeletal symptoms. A physician is often consulted because the fever is not accompanied by obvious signs of upper respiratory infection. Physical examination is usually normal, and in our series the children have not appeared ill enough to require laboratory study or medication. One to 3 weeks may elapse between the inciting illness and the onset of arthritis.

Significant skeletal trauma, defined as an injury that involves a documented bone fracture or a visit to the physician for evaluation within 24 h, occurred 1–3 weeks prior to the onset of this form of arthritis in 10% of our cases.

Diarrheal illness, while common in pediatrics in general, is not a frequent part of the prodromal illness. However, 7% of our patients had severe diarrhea as the inciting illness; usually, no effort had been made to ascertain that these illnesses were dysenteric, but we were able to document *Salmonella* and *Yersinia* in some cases. The children who had diarrheal illness as the inducer were most likely to have the RS triad of urethritis, arthritis, and conjunctivitis/keratitis/uveitis. Sexually acquired chlamydial urethritis as the inducer is uncommon in a pediatric series skewed to young children but is not so rare in teenagers.[84–86] As has been reported in all series of nongonococcal urethritis, patients usually developed urethritis following exposure to a new sexual partner. The interval between urethritis and arthritis may be as long as 8 weeks. Treatment for Chlamydral urethritis may reduce the risk of postvenereal arthritis.[86a] Occult gut inflammation is common in spondyloarthritis; up to 81% of patients with spondyloarthritis will have histologic signs of bowel inflammation on ileocolonoscopic biopsy.[87–88a]

Systemic Symptoms

Fever is not usually present when the arthritis appears except in those patients with RS following dysentery: half of those children have high spiking fever resembling that seen in systemic JRA and appear quite ill at the time the arthritis appears. Septic infection must be excluded; any child presenting with unilateral sacroiliac pain must be proven *not* to have pyogenic infection,[89] even though non-pyogenic inflammatory sacroiliitis does occur, even in infants and toddlers.[90]

Laboratory Studies

Most children have normal laboratory tests but some, as in other forms of arthritis, have elevated ESRs and positive tests for antinuclear antibodies.[5,91] Low-grade fever is noted by the parents in about 10% of the others. Most of the children do not appear systemically ill, but during the first month of illness, a few children have significant weight loss exceeding 10% of their onset weight.

Character of the Arthritis

The most common mode of onset is swelling of a single knee, and the arthritis is usually predominantly in the lower extremities (Table 4.6). Although occasional patients have more than four affected joints at onset, two is the average (Table 4.7); the ankle and wrist are commonly affected; and a single proximal interphalangeal joint (sausage finger) or the first metatarsophalangeal joint or the hip may also be involved.[92] Backache and sacroiliac pain are complaints in about 20% of patients. When associated with severe hip involvement these complaints identify a subset at increased risk for classical AS.[41,93,94] Severe destructive hip arthritis may antedate radiographic evidence of sacroiliitis in childhood AS. Severely affected individuals can usually be identified relatively early; mild disease tends to remain mild.[95]

The Evanescent Nature of the Symptoms

The fleeting symptoms, well described by Scott[13] and beautifully detailed by Hart,[47] tend to obscure the diagnosis. Since criteria for diagnosis of arthritis in childhood have required persistent arthritis in the same joint for 6 consecutive weeks, arthritis that comes and goes seems mysterious. The mother of one of our patients made a diary to convince the physician her child was ill since each time she went to the doctor, there were no findings (Fig. 4.4). This "mother's diary" is a good chronicle of a frequent pattern of disease in childhood spondyloarthritis.

Table 4.6. Joints and Entheses Affected in Childhood HLA-B27 Spondyloarthritis

	Number of Patients	
	At Onset	Sometime During Course
Knee	27	39
Ankle	16	29
Wrist	13	21
Finger (PIP) or toe (IP)	11 (3 sausage)	21
Metatarsal-tarsal*	9	10
Hip	7	21†
Heel pain*	6	16
First MTP	6	13
Sacroiliac	5	13
Achilles tendinitis*	5	12
Backache*	2	2
Elbow	2	12†
TMJ	0	4
Average number of swollen joints	2.5	4.5

* Enthesis.
† Disproportionate increase with time.
Key: PIP = Proximal interphalangeal joint; IP = interphalangeal joint;
TMJ = temporomandibular joint; MTP = metatarsophalangeal joint.
Modified from Jacobs, refs. 4 and 5.

Table 4.7. Number of Joints with Objective Evidence of Arthritis at Onset and During Course (Average 5 Years, 58 Patients)

Number of Joints Affected	At Onset	During Course
0	2	
1	27	12
2	14	7
3	4	11
4	5	10
5–8	4	9
9–11	2	8
14		1

Periarticular Inflammation

Enthesopathy. The enthesis is the site of attachment of ligaments and tendons to bone. This area is uniquely inflamed in spondyloarthritis, especially at the insertions of the Achilles tendon and plantar fascia into the calcaneus

8/13/73 Sat + Sun feet + knees swollen
little better today (Mon) but walking stiffly

8/27/73 Held up pretty well. Given aspirin while
they were away - today feet hurt

9/6/73 Went into swimming pool on Sunday
Mon: miserable
Tues: feels OK
Index finger since Monday badly swollen
+ painful

9/11/73 Fri + Sat night knees very painful
Crawled up stairs
Right area all swollen
Sat in eve - miserable again left knee
more painful.
Sun: all around hip area - very painful
had to carry him out of car van.
Mon: hardly any pain
Tues: not too painful

9-18-73 Past week - walking so-so. Stiff legged
Knees painful - can't sit any length of
time without becoming stiff and hurting
Rt thumb past 2 days very swollen
(difficulty in writing) Mon + Tues swollen (thumb)

9-26-73 Past week - R knee having mod severe
aching pain necessitating him pulling
himself up + down stairs, also swollen
need π ASA in am + covers him for daytime
Pain returns late afternoon + he needs
π ASA c̄ supper + π ā hs

Figure 4.4. Mother's diary brought to the physician in an effort to further diagnosis in an 8-year-old boy (facsimile).

and at synarthroses (articulations of joints without cavities) (Table 4.8). Orthopedists often do not realize spondyloarthritis/enthesopathy as the cause of painful heels.[96]

Bursitis and Tenosynovitis. Tenosynovitis around the joints, and bursitis, are often severe, and the clinical pattern may resemble that seen in osteomyelitis or in the gonococcal arthritis-tenosynovitis syndrome (Fig. 4.5).[47] Nuclear magnetic resonance imaging may show tendon thickening,

Table 4.8. Types of Synarthroses (Joints without Cavities)

Bony articulation (synostosis)
Bony articulation that is fibrous (syndesmosis)*
Bony articulation that is cartilaginous (synchondrosis)*
Bony articulation that is fibrocartilaginous (a symphysis)

* Ligaments are frequent articular components of syndesmoses and synchondroses.

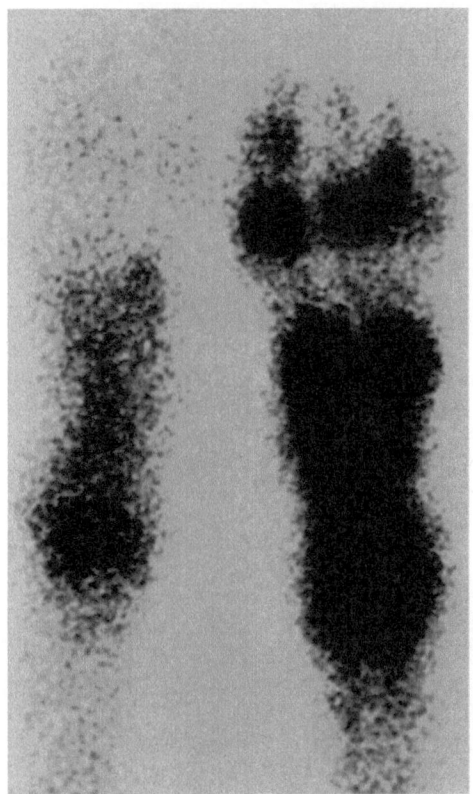

Figure 4.5. A typical bone scan shows diffuse uptake in the distal tibia, fibula, tarsal bones, and at the base of the metatarsals, consistent with diffuse hyperemia.

synovial-sheath swelting, particularly of the tibialis posterior and flexor digitorum longus tendons, and bursal swelling in those with tarsal involvement.[36] (Figs. 4.6 and 4.7)

Periostitis. Periosteal bone pain is a significant early manifestation in 20% of cases and may also resemble that seen in osteomyelitis (Figs. 4.8 and 4.9). When the articular and periarticular inflammation is generalized and very severe, as in some cases of acute RS, transverse metaphyseal lucent lines resembling those seen in acute leukemia may be seen, and the bones may have a patchy, moth-eaten appearance (Fig. 4.10). Disuse of an extremity as a result of pain may result in severe demineralization resembling that seen in reflex sympathetic dystrophy ("Sudeck's atrophy") (Fig. 4.11).

Eye Manifestations

Most children with HLA-B27–associated spondyloarthritis do not have eye manifestations. The most common eye manifestations, sometimes antedating

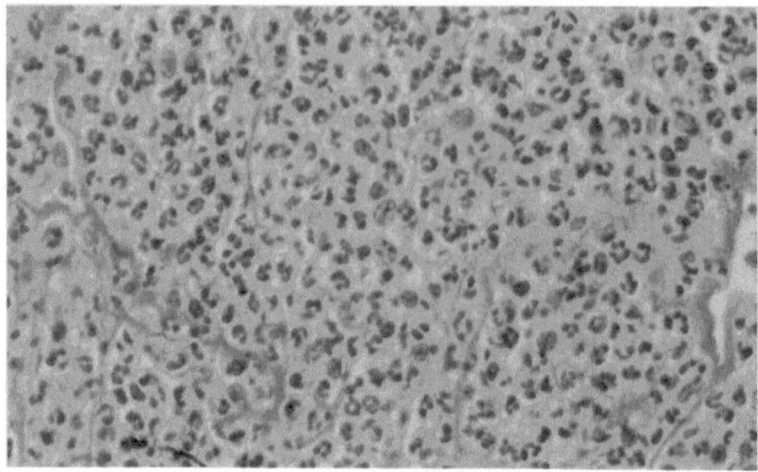

Figure 4.6. HLA-B27—associated arthritis may present with subacromial bursitis with persistent swelling and rice bodies; other joints may be affected later. The intensive inflammation is illustrated in a biopsy specimen from a 16-year-old girl (see also Thevenon A., Cocheteux P., Duquesnoy B., et al.: Subacromial bursitis with rice bodies as a presenting feature of seronegative rheumatoid arthritis. *Arthritis Rheum* 30:715–716, 1987).

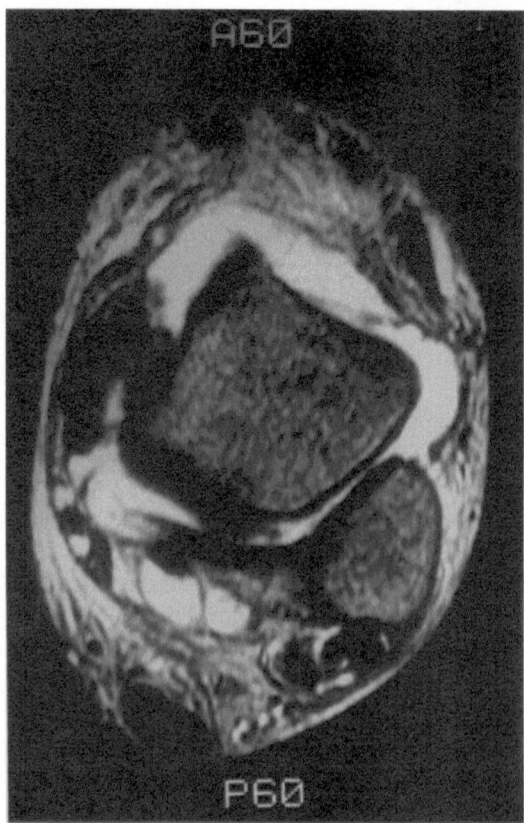

Figure 4.7. MRI of ankle in a 17-year-old boy with recent onset of HLA-B27—associated spondyloarthritis; white areas are large peritendinous effusions.

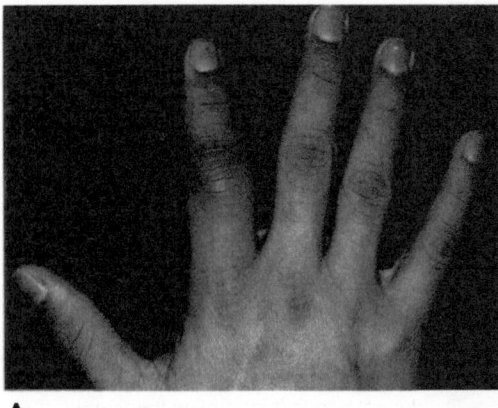

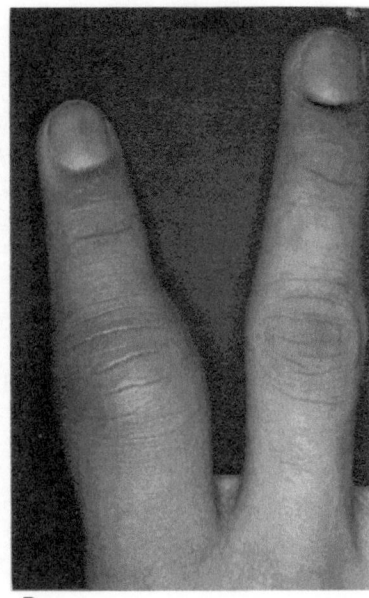

Figure 4.8. (**A**) "Sausage finger" simulating osteomyelitis in a 12-year-old boy. (**B**) Close-up view of a typical spondyloarthritic appearance.

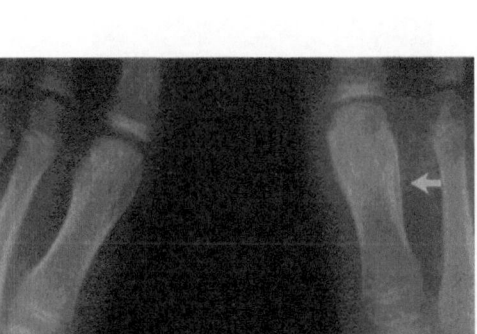

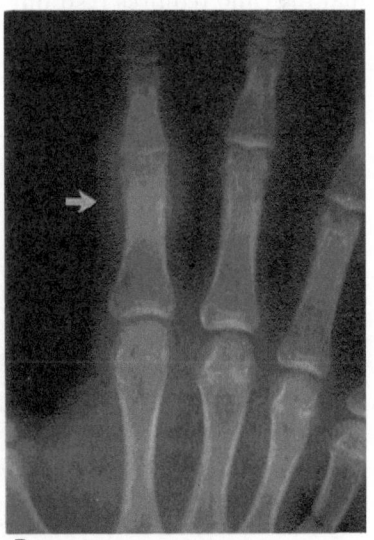

Figure 4.9. Two examples of periostitis. Note periosteal new bone with surrounding soft-tissue swelling. (**A**) On left, first metatarsal shows periosteal reaction and the first metatarsophalangeal joint is swollen. On right, sausage-shaped swollen index finger has periosteal reaction involving proximal phalanx (**B**) (same patient as in Fig. 4.8). (**A** Reprinted with permission from Jacobs et al., ref. 5.)

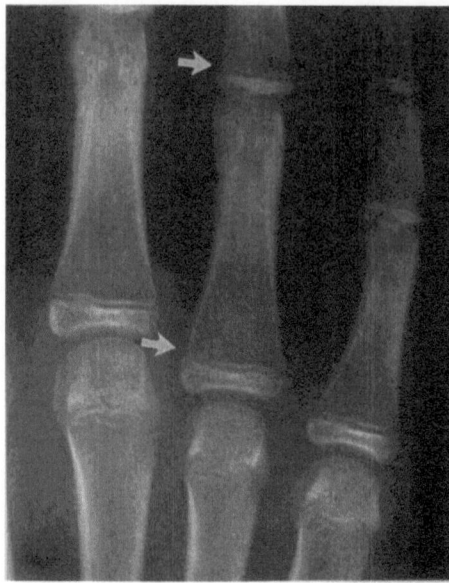

Figure 4.10. Transverse metaphyseal lucent bands (resembling the "lucent line of leukemia") are noted at the base of the proximal and middle phalanges above the dense epiphyseal lines. The bones also have a patchy, moth-eaten appearance similar to that seen in children with leukemia or other malignancy.

the arthritis by years, are chronic blepharitis or conjunctivitis[97] (Fig. 4.12). Reiter's syndrome may be accompanied by such severe keratoconjunctivitis that the child requires restraint to prevent self-injury from scratching.

Scars of prior attacks of iritis were noted in 3% of our spondyloarthritic

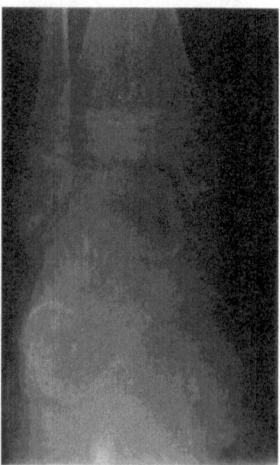
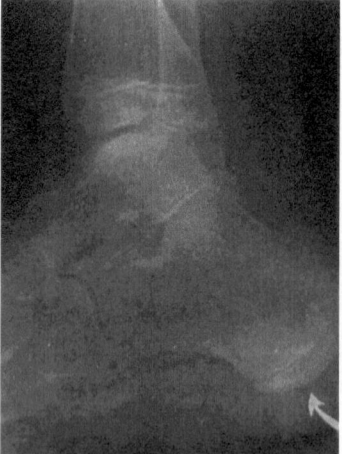

Figure 4.11. The normally sclerotic calcaneal apophysis (contrast Fig. 4.31) has become markedly osteopenic (*arrow*); similar severe density loss is apparent in the distal tibia/fibula with transverse metaphyseal lucent lines also noted; discrete lucent defects at tendinous insertions are not noted.

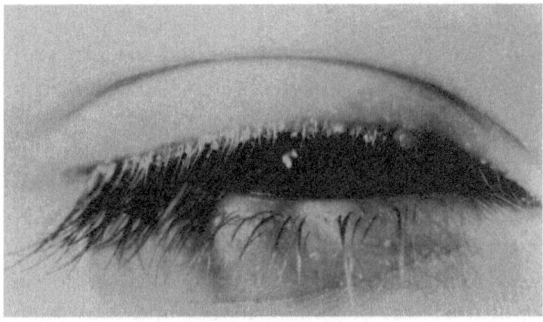

Figure 4.12. Crusty eyelashes are a manifestation of chronic blepharitis, the most common eye manifestation associated with spondyloarthritis.

children at the time of their initial eye examination. An additional 3% developed iritis within a month of onset of arthritis. An additional 2% developed iritis during an average follow-up period of 7 years; the total risk for life remains to be determined. Iritis was not always acute and symptomatic and so in some cases was indistinguishable from the subacute or chronic iritis that is associated with HLA-DR5–associated childhood arthritis. Intermediate uveitis ("pars planitis"[98]) may be associated with reactive arthritis[99] although this association has not previously been emphasized.

Case Report

A previously healthy 12-year-old girl and her family had a "viral" illness with mouth sores; the patient also had a red eye at that time, which subsided, but the eye became red again 3 weeks later in association with polyarthritis in the neck, temporomandibular joints, shoulders, hips, knees, and ankles. ESR was 25 but all other appropriate laboratory studies were normal or negative. Examination of the eyes revealed bilateral vitreous opacities with snowballing and banking at the ora, typical of pars planitis (intermediate uveitis).[98] The child was treated with naproxen and steroid eyedrops; arthritis persisted for 6 months and then remitted without recurrence over the past 2 years. The pars plantis was complicated by conjunctivitis after 1 month, and ±/+ cells were noted in the anterior chamber of each eye (anterior uveitis) after 2 months, in addition to the more posterior findings. Although vision remains normal mild evidence of pars planitis continues 2 years after onset. A recent report suggests that sulfasalazine might be tried in this patient.[100]

Genitourinary Manifestations

Occasional youngsters have dysuria, sometimes with considerable discomfort. Sterile pyuria can be demonstrated at the onset of the arthritis in 25% of children. Significant albuminuria and hematuria occur occasionally.

Skin Manifestations

The classic skin manifestations of RS—keratoderma blennorrhagicum and psoriasiform lesions of the penis—are rarely seen in children. Of 103 children with HLA-B27–associated spondyloarthritis followed prospectively, only 1 had skin lesions noted at onset. However, skin lesions have been reported in 25% of adult patients with RS following dysentery[65] and, if limited to small psoriasiform lesions at the tip of the penis (circinatic balanitis), may be easily overlooked (Fig. 4.13). In older teenagers and adults, the most striking skin changes are on the palms and soles and under the fingernails. The lesions on the palms and soles start as papulovesicles, become crusted, and may then develop into keratotic hornlike lesions (Fig. 4.14). The fingernails and toenails become uplifted by subungual hyperkeratosis (onycholysis), may be brittle, and may be associated with purulent paronychia (Fig. 4.15). In young children, lesions on the trunk, face, and extremities, which usually are mistaken for impetigo or psoriasis (Fig. 4.16), are more common.

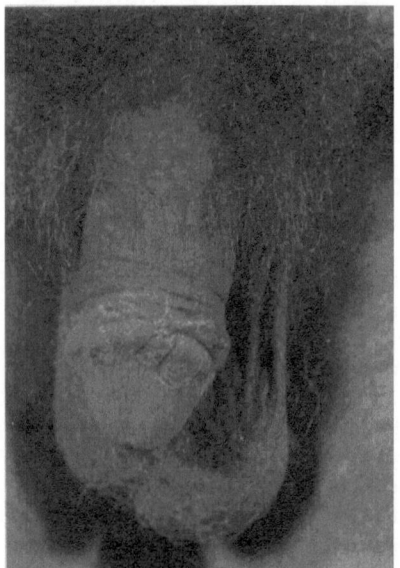

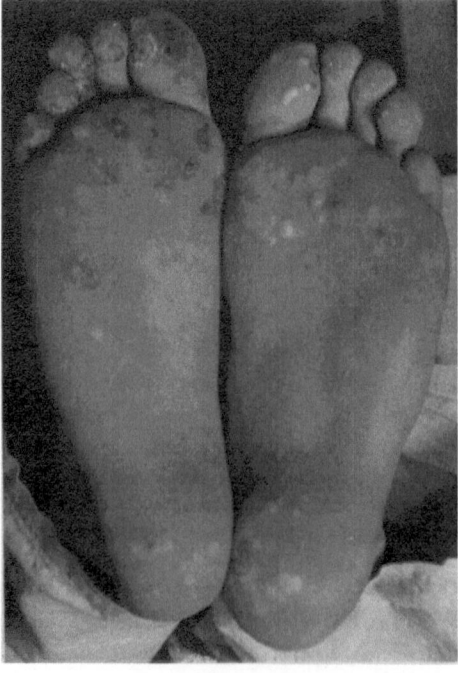

Figure 4.13. Penile balanitis typical of RS.

Figure 4.14. Classicial lesions of keratoderma blennorrhagicum on the soles of a teenage boy with RS.

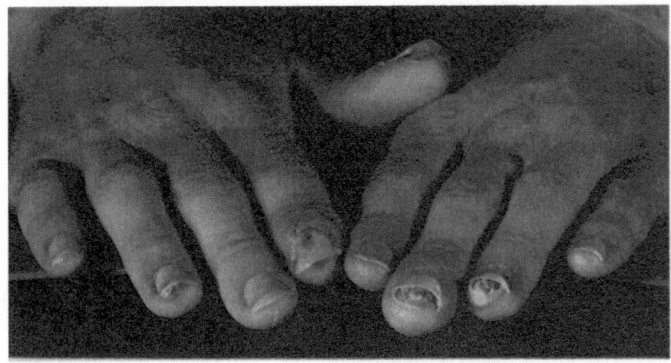

Figure 4.15. Subungual keratosis and onycholysis (RS). (Same patient as in Figs. 4.13, 4.14, and 4.17.)

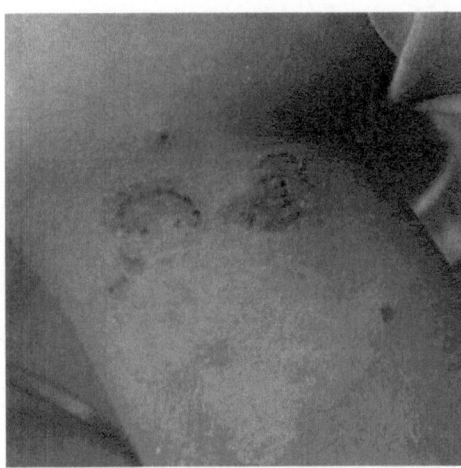

Figure 4.16. This keratoderma blennorrhagicum lesion was mistaken for impetigo in a 9-year-old boy with monarticular arthritis of this knee. This form of keratoderma (an infected psoriasiform eruption that appears at the time of an attack of arthritis) is seen in young children with RS (see Fig. 4.23).

Mucous Membrane Lesions

Lingual patches devoid of papillae may resemble geographic tongue (Fig. 4.17). Similar erosive lesions may occur on the mucous membranes of the lips, cheeks, and palate and at the urinary meatus. These lesions are usually painless and go unnoticed unless carefully and repetitively searched for during the early weeks of the acute attack.

Pleurisy

Mild complaints of pleuritic pain on respiration, occasionally accompanied by a pleural friction rub, are not uncommon in patients with RS.[65] Pleural effusion has rarely been reported.

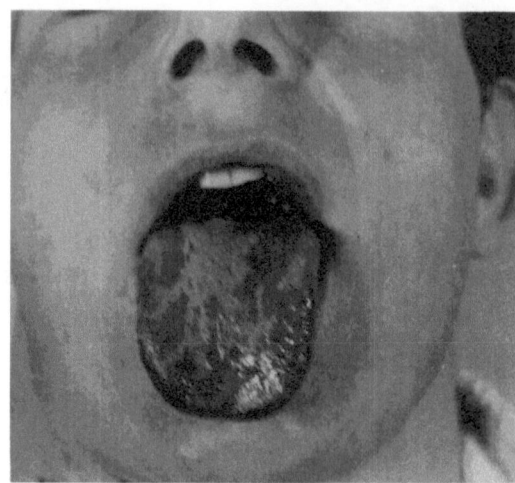

Figure 4.17. Lingual patches devoid of papillae on the tongue, RS.

Carditis

Two percent of patients with RS have pericarditis, sometimes during the acute attack but often months afterward.[65] Six percent of patients have associated myocarditis. Myocarditis and pericarditis are most often mild but may be associated with tamponade and cardiac failure. Occasional patients have aortic valvulitis with auscultatory evidence of aortic insufficiency at the onset of their illness.[100a] Atrioventricular conduction disturbances may cause confusion with rheumatic fever or Lyme disease.[101]

Gastrointestinal Manifestations

Some patients have the onset of diagnosable inflammatory bowel disease coincident with arthritis. Although diarrhea has been reported to be a frequent feature of RS, even in the absence of dysentery, this has not been our experience.

Renal Disease

Although hematuria and albuminuria may be associated with spondyloarthritis, there is no impairment of glomerular function.

Other Associated Manifestations

In our initial study of 58 cases, 8% of male patients with spondyloarthritis had unilateral nerve deafness with >50-dB loss.[4,5] Twenty percent of the 58 children had significant school-learning or behavioral problems, usually antedating the onset of arthritis. We do not know the significance of these observations, which require confirmation in larger series.

Muscular Pain

In addition to pain at the enthesis, especially at the heel, more diffuse muscle pain occurs in up to 30% of patients with RS and may be a prominent complaint in all forms of spondyloarthritis. In children, gastrocnemius pain seems most common. The onset of the spondyloarthritis syndrome may be insidious, with musculoskeletal pain and stiffness without arthritis.

Nervous-System Manifestations

Encephalitis has occasionally accompanied RS; a few adults have been reported with psychosis and seizures.[102] Polyneuritis, cranial nerve palsies, and peripheral neuropathy have also occasionally been reported. In nonepidemic situations such patients must be distinguished from those with Lyme disease (see Chapter 2).

Familial Hereditary Thrombocytopenia and Spondyloarthritis

Only a few families with hereditary thrombocytopenia have been reported and in the one reported family we have seen, severe HLA-B27–associated spondyloarthritis was seen in the thrombocytopenic father and one daughter (Fig. 4.18); another child has mild arthritis.[103] We have seen one other family with similar findings in father and daughter, albeit much milder than the original family.

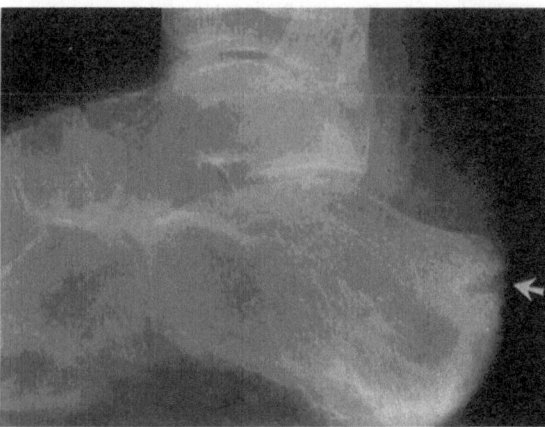

Figure 4.18. HLA-B27– associated spondyloarthritis with familial thrombocytopenia. Pain from the plantar and Achilles enthesopathy was so severe the 12-year-old patient crawled on her knees and developed giant knee calluses. Note lucencies in sclerotic calcaneal apophysis.

Pathology

Joints. The synovitis is nonspecific and seemingly identical with that of RA (see Chapter 3). The initial lesions may be mild with edema, vascular congestion, and a predominantly neutrophilic infiltrate. Later, the chronic manifestations associated with RA predominate with varying degrees of severity (Fig. 4.19).

Enthesopathy. This area is uniquely inflamed in spondyloarthritis; inflammation at the enthesis is the hallmark of the disease, which distinguishes it from RA.[2,104–106] To understand the pathology, it is necessary to review

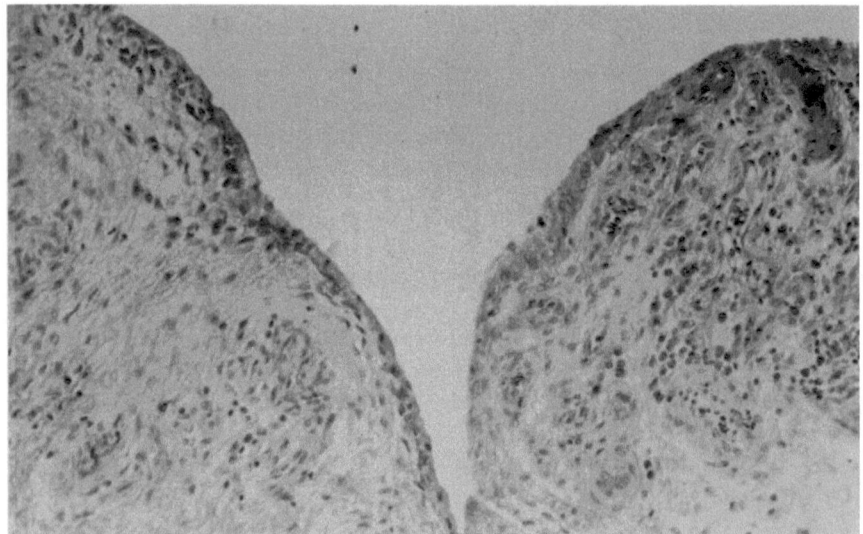

Figure 4.19. Chronic hypertrophic synovitis lined by enlarged histiocytes and populated by a mixed plasma-cell and lymphocytic exudate not morphologically differentiable from rheumatoid arthritis. ×120.

▷

Figure 4.20. (A) View of an enthesis (zone of tendinous insertion into cartilage (on right), which is suffused and partially destroyed by a "round-cell" inflammatory exudate that is almost entirely lymphocytic, in a 6-year-old boy who presented with monarticular arthritis of the first MTP joint with periostitis and was thought to have osteomyelitis (same patient as in Fig. 4.9A). **(B)** Central and upper-left zones represent the ligamentum teres. Its insertion into bone (an intraarticular enthesis), in lower- and middle-right sections, accommodates a chronic lymphocytic inflammatory exudate. This appears as irregularly outlined darker areas near the bone. The onset age was 10 years in this male. Specimen was obtained at the time of total hip replacement at age 20. **(C)** This is a higher magnification of the inflammatory exudate shown in **(B)**. The bone, on the right side of the field, is undergoing destruction, which was seen radiographically as bony erosions. **(A)** ×120; **(B)** ×30; **(C)** ×200.

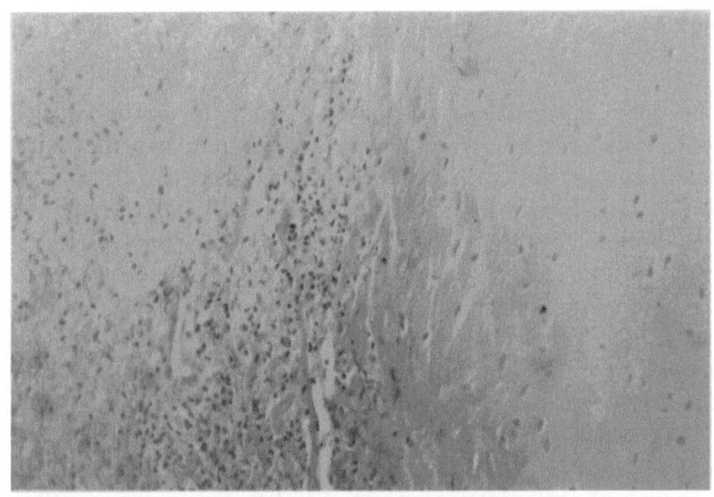

A

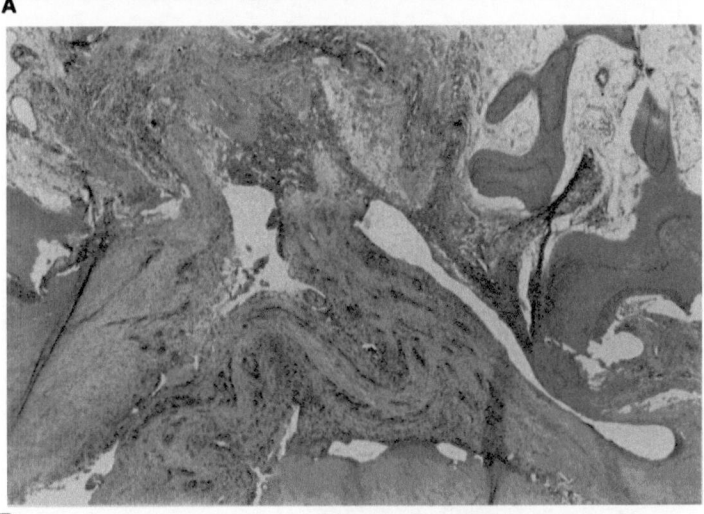

B

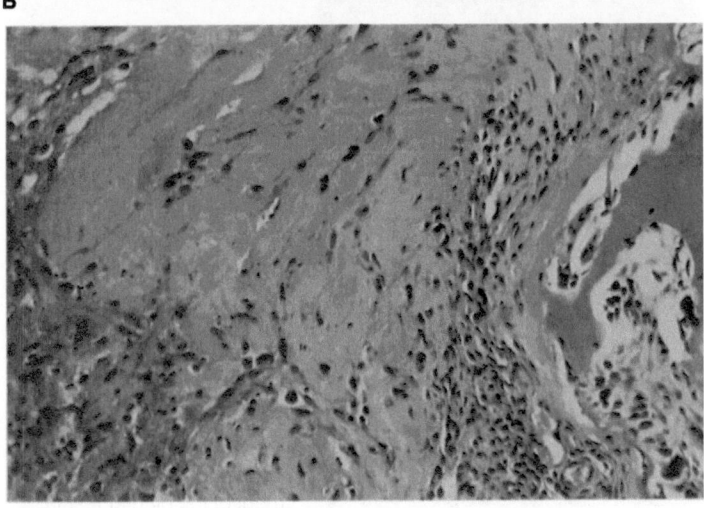

C

the anatomy of the site of ligamentous attachment to bone, the enthesis. Just before reaching the bone, the fiber bundles of the ligament become more compact, then cartilaginous, and then calcified. There is evidence that this area is quite vascular and, during growth, very active metabolically. When it becomes inflamed, lymphocytes, polymorphs, and plasma cells may be seen in the fibrous tissues. As the inflammation progresses, bony erosions become apparent at the attachment, and reactive new bone is seen in the inflamed fibrous tissue (Fig. 4.20). Eventually, the erosion is filled in with reactive new bone to which the ligaments become attached, forming a new enthesis. Plantar calcaneal spurs represent just such healed erosions with formation of a new enthesis at the insertion of the plantar fascia, which is commonly affected in spondyloarthritis (Fig. 4.21). Erosive lesions and spurs are also seen in the calcaneous at the insertion of the Achilles tendons and other ligaments.

The pathogenesis of the sacroiliac arthritis is similar. In addition to synovitis, there is endochondral ossification and replacement of the subchondral bone plate and cartilage with porous trabecular bone, producing the radiographically apparent bone sclerosis on the iliac side of the joint and eventual replacement of the joint with bone. The erosive lesions heal by deposition of reactive bone in connective tissue, without antecedent cartilage formation.

Apophyseal arthritis is probably the commonest cause of limited lumbar motion.[107] Inflammation of the spinal-disk ligament, the annulus fibrosis, at its site of insertion into the vertebra (its enthesis) results in the formation of bony spurs, which in this location are called syndesmophytes and are a hallmark of ankylosing spondylitis. Osteophytes, horizontal calcifications at the disk-bone border, together with syndesmophytes and osteitis causing des-

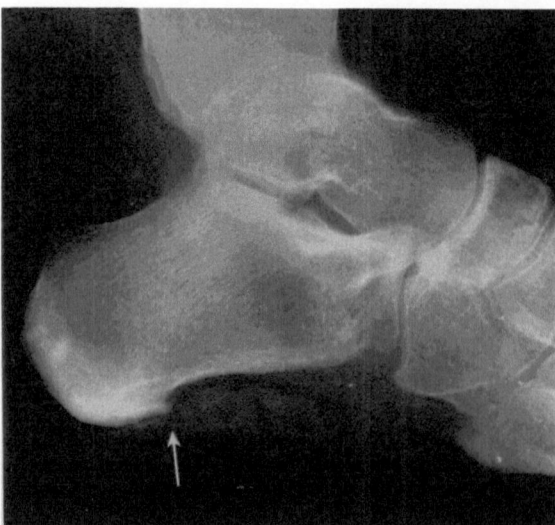

Figure 4.21. A well-defined spur has formed at the attachment of the plantar fascia.

truction, rebuilding, and squaring of the vertebral bodies[108] make up the bamboo spine of AS. These lesions are not generally seen in childhood, but signs of inflammation may be apparent at these sites even in young children.

Other fibrous attachments that are commonly inflamed in HLA-B27–associated spondyloarthritis are the ligamentum teres (producing tenderness of the greater trochanter), the anterior surface of the patella, the iliac crest, and the sternomanubrial joints.

Tendinitis and Fibrositis. Although inflammation at the enthesis is most common, there is evidence that inflammation of the fibrous tissues is not limited to the ligamentous attachments. Necrotizing vasculitis may rarely be seen in muscle[108a] (see Fig. 7.33). At other sites, in fibrous tissue, pathologic examination may show periarteriolar inflammation or focal areas of intense fibroblastic proliferation accompanied by reactive bone formation. Painful neuromas may be created within these fibrous scars as a result of nerve entrapment (Fig. 4.22).

Cardiovascular Lesions. The cardiovascular lesions are said to be morphologically unique.[108a,109] An inflammatory process with proliferation of small blood vessels, limited to the aortic wall behind and immediately above the sinuses of Valsalva, results in dense adventitial scar behind and adjacent to the commissures and extending below the base of the aortic valve to form a characteristic subvalvular ridge. The fibrous tissue may also extend into the base of the anterior mitral leaflet and into the most cephalad portion of the

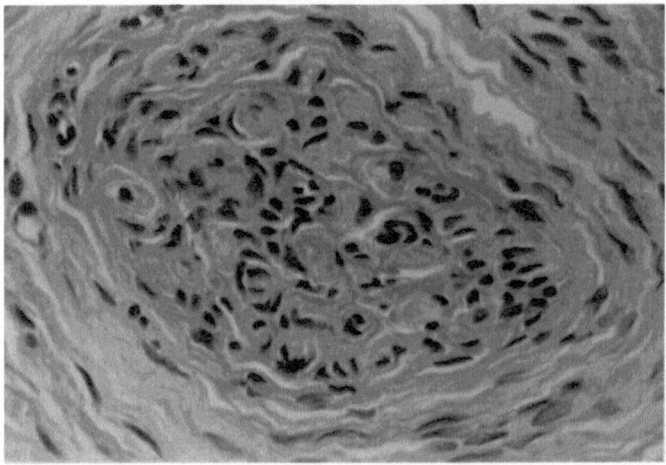

Figure 4.22. Plantar neuroma found on review of specimen removed from a boy with plantar fascial pain. The structures within this nerve are separated by scar tissue that is continuous with perineural scar, obliterating the perineurium and "tethering" the nerve to surrounding structures. Any motion that places tension on the nerve will cause lancinating pain. ×200.

muscular ventricular septum where it results in conduction defects.[110,111] Chronic panserositis may be seen in pericardium and pleura. Cardiovascular lesions are rare but commonly antedate or exceed the tempo of the arthritic process when they do occur.[108a] One case of giant-cell valvulitis has been reported.[112]

Renal Lesions. IgM and IgA nephropathy with vascular changes in small arteries and arterioles of the kidney may occur.[113–118] Segmental or circumferential subintimal deposits may extend throughout entire vessel walls. Deposits of immunoglobulin, complement, and fibrinogen in the glomerular and tubular basement membranes as well as in the vessel walls suggest that immunologic processes are associated with these renal lesions. Clinically significant amyloidosis occurs only occasionally, but with special study amyloid deposits may ultimately be demonstrated in 4% of severely affected patients.[119]

Keratoderma Blennorrhagicum. This classic skin manifestation of RS may be histologically indistinguishable from pustular psoriasis (Fig. 4.23).[120]

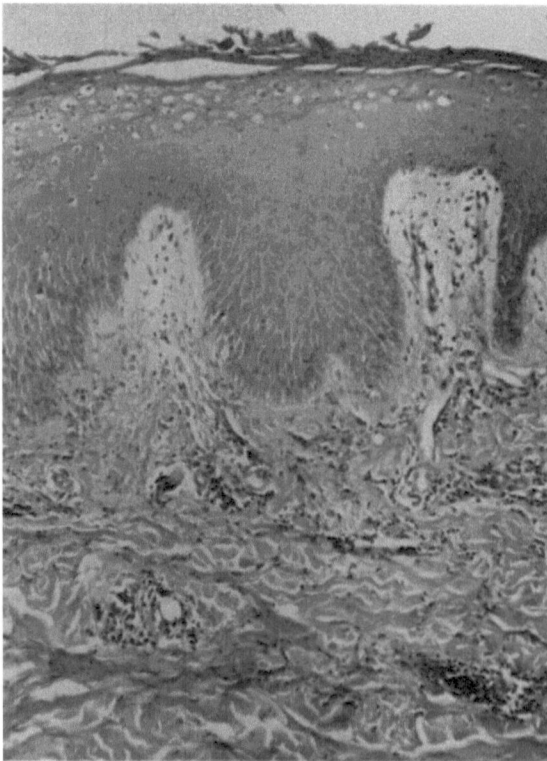

Figure 4.23. Punch-biopsy specimen of lesion pictured in Fig. 4.16, showing psoriasiform epidermal hyperplasia with vacuolated cells and collections of neutrophils in the stratum malpighii typical of keratoderma blennorrhagicum.

Tortuous capillaries spiral upward in the dermal papillae and are surrounded by inflammatory cells. There are parakeratotic mounds containing neutrophils on the surface. Neutrophils may accumulate in various layers of the epidermis, creating microabscesses resembling impetigo. Extremely keratotic horn formation may be seen under the fingernails. The moist penile and tongue lesions are similar but do not have the keratotic crusting seen elsewhere.

Course of the Disease

Pediatric series have not been followed long enough yet to provide good outcome data.[121] However, it seems likely from our series that the course of B27-positive spondyloarthritis will generally resemble that described for adult RS. Patients may be classified into three groups (Fig. 4.24).[122] The first group of patients remains well after a single attack (25%). The second group recovers from the initial attack, but months to years later has recurrent attacks involving one or more systems (50%). Some of these patients recover completely again, (two-thirds may be symptomless after 3 years)[123] but others go on to have mild chronic activity. A third group remains continuously active, usually with mild symptoms (25%).[124] However, some of these patients develop chronic polyarthritis with joint destruction, most often in the hips.[94] After years of chronic disease, a few patients go on to develop ankylosis of the spine.

Published series of symptomatic children who fulfill the current sacroiliac joint radiologic criteria for AS suggest that this group, as might be expected, constitutes a higher-risk subpopulation. Among these individuals, the risk of spinal disease would appear to be about 50% with 20-year follow-up.[44]

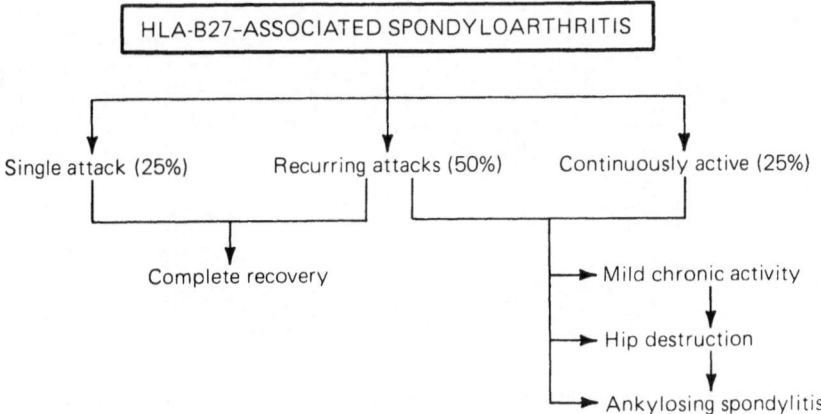

Figure 4.24. Varying course of patients with HLA-B27-associated spondyloarthritis.

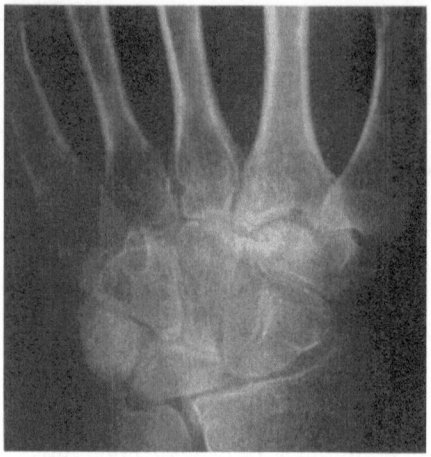 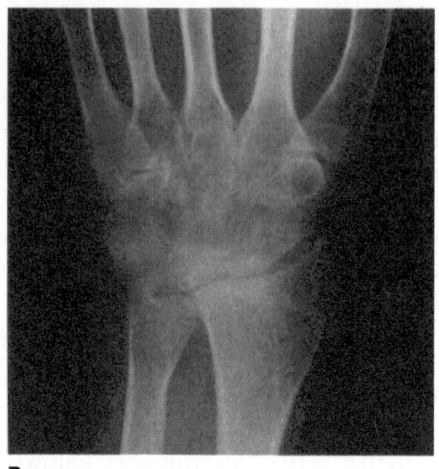

A   **B**

Figure 4.25. Rapidity of carpal destructive changes is revealed in films over 14 months of observation in a 12-year-old girl. (**A**) On left, initial film shows early joint-space narrowing, erosions, and osteopenia. (**B**) Follow-up study 14 months later shows "carpal crowding" due to diffuse destruction of joint spaces; reactive sclerosis is present adjacent to joint destruction against background of osteopenic bone. (Reprinted with permission from Jacobs et al., ref. 5.) Reactive arthritis may be rapidly destructive.[128]

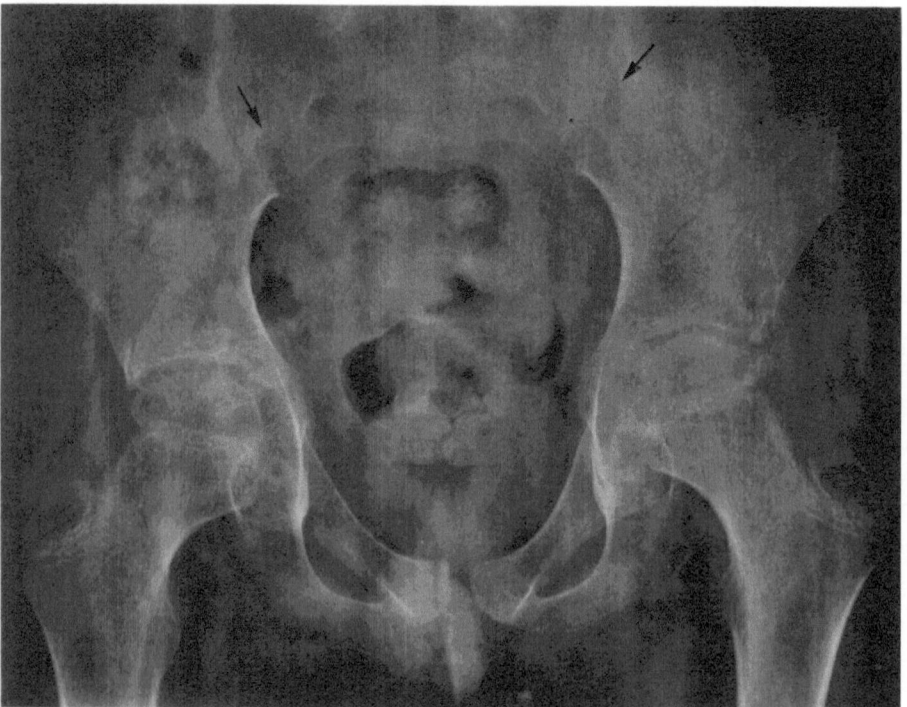

A

Figure 4.26. HLA-B27–associated spondyloarthritis; progressive destruction of the hips (1969–1977; age 9–17 years). Sacroiliac changes are apparent but were unrecognized in the earliest films. Despite these radiographic findings, this boy was an excellent basketball player (see Fig. 3.55; see also Fig. 4.28).

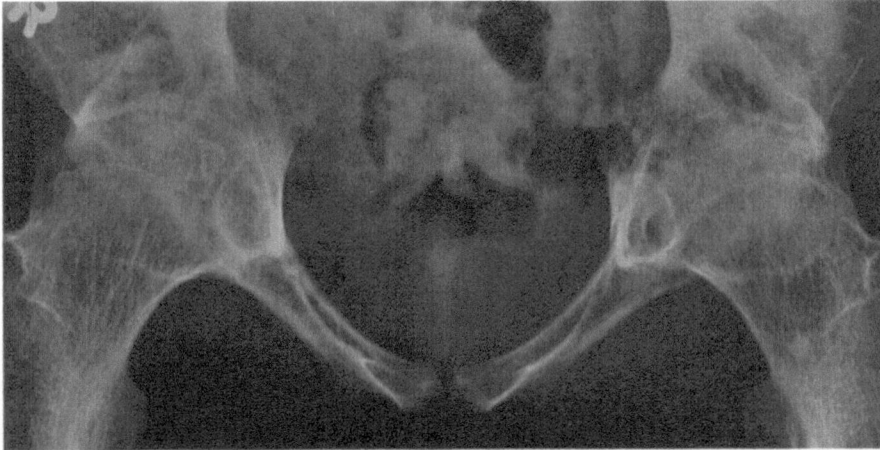

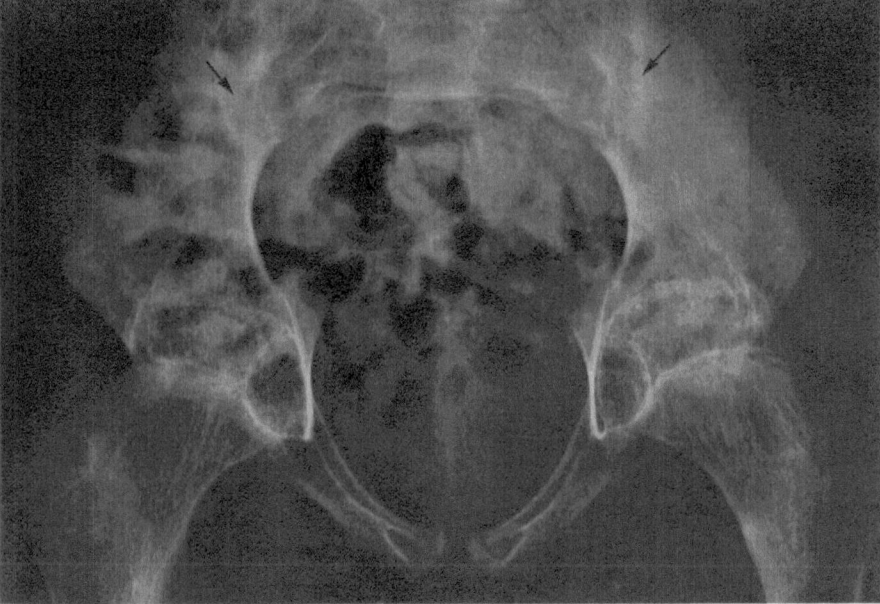

Figure 4.26. **B** and **C**.

Most patients with spondyloarthritis, with proper diagnosis and care, can be expected to lead normal lives. This is also true for the most seriously affected subpopulation, those with AS. While the disease is steadily progressive in some patients, exacerbations and remissions, sometime resembling attacks of RS, are a more common pattern.[8] Chronic otitis media may occur.[125]

Course of the Arthritis

Rapid joint destruction occurs in occasional patients (Fig. 4.25). Hips are the most frequent severely affected joint, although occasional patients may have destructive arthritis at the knees; wrists; shoulders; ankles; elbows; feet; hands; cricoarytenoid,[126] atlantoaxial,[127] and temporomandibular joints; in addition to progressive sclerosis, and ultimately fusion, of the sacroiliac joints. In the peripheral joints, demineralization, sometimes striking in nature, is the first radiologic manifestation and may be followed by joint-space narrowing, subchondral sclerosis, erosions of the articular surfaces, and proliferative changes at the joint margins. Bilateral hip destruction occurs in about 10% of boys who fulfill the diagnostic criteria for AS (Fig. 4.26).[94]

When temporomandibular joint disease occurs early in childhood, cosmetic and functional disability may result, requiring later surgical correction (see Fig. 3.28).

Sacroiliac arthritis is radiographically characterized by the appearance of indistinct joint margins and subchondral sclerosis, often asymmetric at first but becoming symmetric as the disease progresses. Initially, the joint space might appear widened due to erosions, but ultimately it is narrowed and finally ankylosed (Fig. 4.27). We find a 23° supine cephalad film of the pelvis the most satisfactory screening procedure. A complementary 15° prone caudad film may enhance accuracy to 85%.[129] MRI does not enable earlier radiographic diagnosis.[130]

In the spine, narrowing and ultimately fusion of the cervical apophyseal joints, previously thought typical of JRA, may be seen in these children (Fig. 4.28). Squaring of the lumbar vertebra may occur in the late teens, but cal-

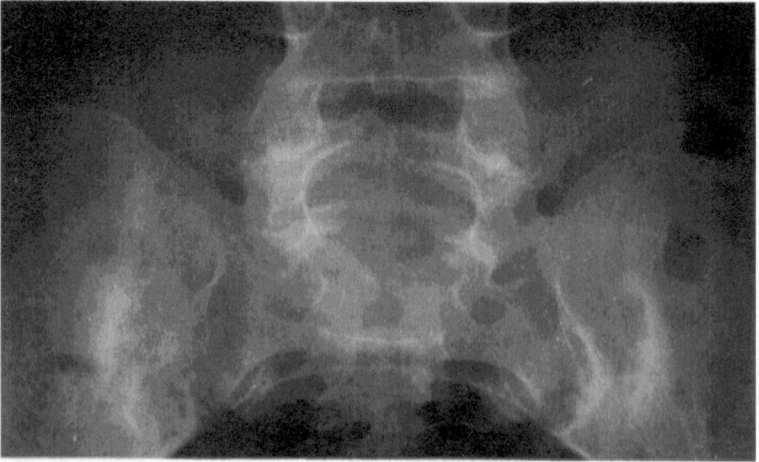

Figure 4.27. Asymmetric sacroiliac involvement typical of early childhood (age 10½ years) AS; right greater than the left.

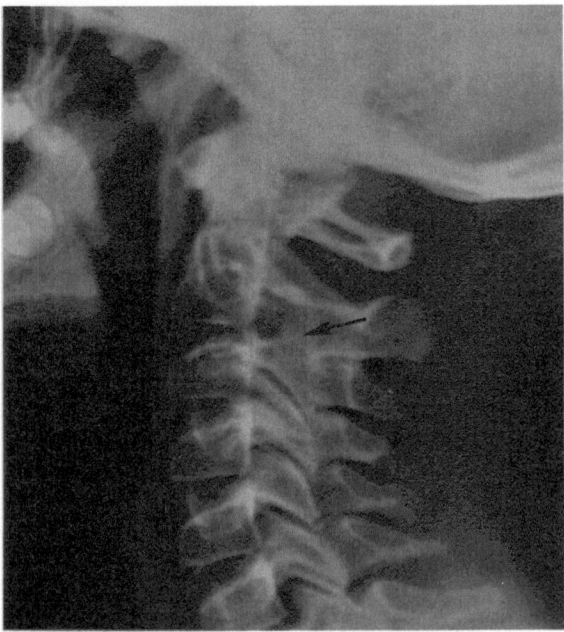

Figure 4.28. C-2-C-3 apophyseal joint fusion, previously thought to be specific for JRA, was also demonstrated in the boy whose hips are pictured in Fig. 4.26. We have observed this finding in a number of our spondyloarthritic children; it may occur in any form of arthritis that involves the neck during growth, and is not specific for JRA.

cification of the spinal ligaments and disks, spondylodiskitis, and formation of the bamboo spine are not radiologically apparent until later.

Pain in the heels and across the metatarsals is frequent and may make walking difficult.[131] Radiographic evidence of inflammation at the attachment of ligaments and tendons in the calcaneus may be manifest by demineralized lesions at various sites (Figs. 4.29–4.31).[132] These demineralized areas or erosions represent areas of osteitis and vascular proliferation extending from the inflammatory reaction in the fibrous tissues and retrocalcaneal bursa.[2] Spurs frequently form. At the site of the insertion of the plantar fascia, inflammation may also result in erosions, followed by calcification of the inflamed enthesis and formation of a bony spur, a new enthesis. The spur may fracture, resulting in more severe pain (Fig. 4.32). An additional cause of pain may be inflammation in the plantar fascia at a distance from the enthesis; if the inflammatory reaction and scarring bind down a nerve forming a neuroma, another source of pain may be established (Fig. 4.22). Similar signs and symptoms may be noted at the sites of attachment of ligaments to the iliac crest.

Low back pain is the most common manifestation of this enthesopathy in adults. While not common in children, it is a manifestation of all of those with AS. At first, the only symptom may be some paravertebral muscular spasm and tenderness and an inability to touch the toes with unbended knees. Flattening of the lumbar lordotic curve then becomes apparent, followed by limitation of lateral spine flexion and spinal extension. Limitation

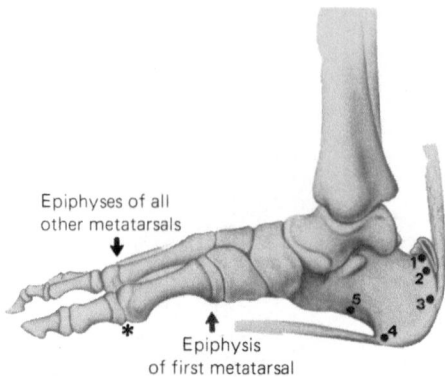

Epiphyses of all
other metatarsals

Epiphysis
of first metatarsal

Figure 4.29. Sites of inflammation in the heel in HLA-B27-associated spondyloarthritis. Characteristic target sites of calcaneal erosions are (1) superior surface, (2) above insertion of the Achilles tendon, (3) at the attachment of the Achilles tendon, (4) at the attachment of the plantar aponeurosis, and (5) anterior to attachment of the plantar aponeurosis. Inflammation results in thickening of the Achilles tendon and obliteration of the normal retrocalcaneal radiolucency due to inflammation of the retrocalcaneal bursa. The first MTP joint (*) is especially frequently affected. As shown, the first MTP anatomically resembles an IP joint and differs from the other MP Joints. (Modified with permission from Resnick et al., ref. 132.)

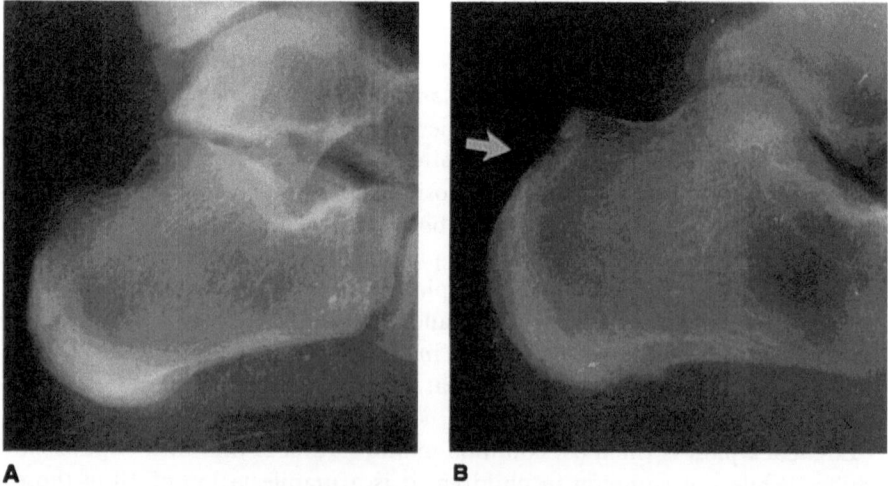

A

B

Figure 4.30. Rapid appearance/evolution of lucent defects at tendinous insertions. (**A**) Initial film fails to show definite abnormality at tendinous insertions. (**B**) Within 10 months, lytic defects have appeared (*arrow*), and a spur is beginning to form (sites 1, 2, 4 in Fig. 4.29).

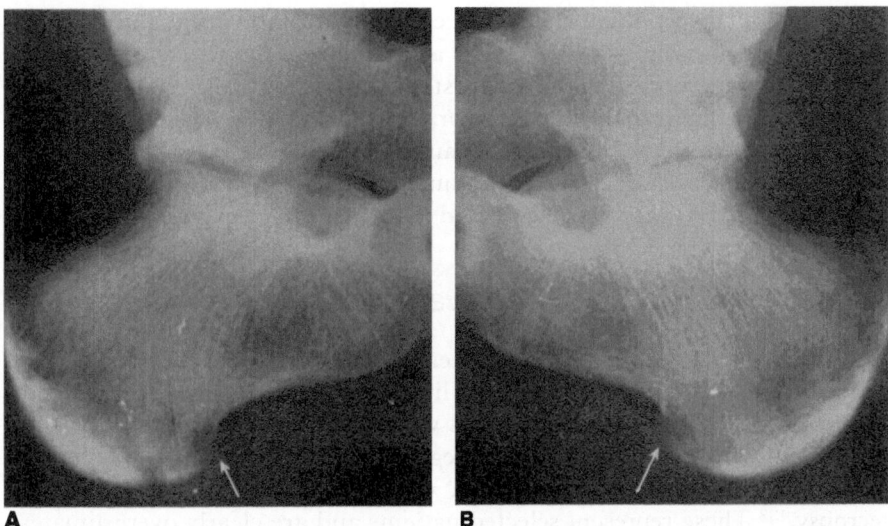

Figure 4.31. Discrete lucent defects at tendinous insertions of the left (**A**) and right (**B**) anterior and inferior calcaneus (site 4 in Fig. 4.29). The adjacent calcaneal apophysis retains some of its normal density, although there is a lucent line paralleling it. (Reprinted with permission from Jacobs et al., ref. 5.)

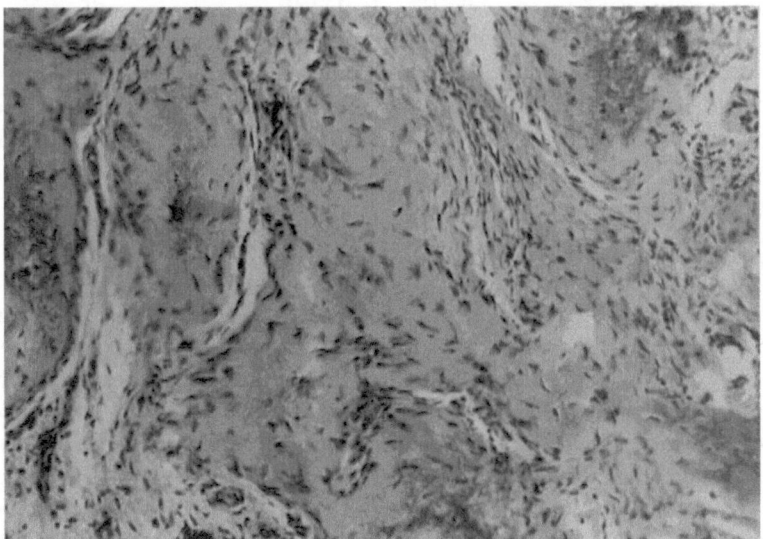

Figure 4.32. There are irregular microtrabeculae of essentially unmineralized osteoid, forming plastic shapes. Such patterns characterize fracture callus. This photomicrograph was taken from the vicinity of a ligamentous or tendinous insertion (enthesis) into the os calcis in a boy with heel pain due to unrecognized fracture of this heel spur. ×200.

of extension of the cervical spine may accompany the lumbar manifestations, resulting in the beginning of the classic appearance of the severe spondylitic patient with bent neck (Fig. 4.3). Chest expansion may also be decreased, secondary to arthritis of the costovertebral joints, and episodes of chest pain, localized to these joints, are not uncommon. Sleep may be disturbed, and morning stiffness is characteristic. Minimal exercise provides relief, although all of the symptoms may be exacerbated following severe exertion.

Extra-articular Disease: Cardiovascular Disease

The risk of development of clinical evidence of aortic insufficiency during the course of HLA-B27—associated spondylitis has not been completely defined but may be as high as 10% in patients with radiographically demonstrated sacroiliitis followed for 10 years after registry in an adult arthritis clinic.[132a] In one autopsy study, 20% of such patients had detectable lesions at necropsy.[133] These represent selected patients and are clearly overestimates of the incidence of this complication in patients with mild spondyloarthritis. However, aortic and mitral insufficiencies have been seen during childhood in these patients and may occur in the presence of even minimal arthritis.[108a–112,134–137] Cardiac manifestations are occasionally the presenting manifestations of spondyloarthritis.[100a] Atrioventricular conduction disturbances, pericarditis and myocarditis may be part of the initial attack or may occur as part of an exacerbation of the disease or as manifestations of RS within the context of AS.[43,132a,136] Spondyloarthritis should be considered in the differential diagnosis of unexplained pericarditis or aortic insufficiency in both children and adults.[136] In adults with aortic insufficiency and conduction disturbances requiring a pacemaker 88% are HLA-B27-positive.[138]

The Prognosis for Patients with Severe AS

Most patients with AS lead normal lives provided they receive appropriate medical care.[93] The mortality in women and in mild or moderately affected males is probably the same as that for the general population. Although different studies with different patient populations and data analysis offer conflicting conclusions, the mortality for severely affected men is probably considerably higher than that of the general male population.[139] In a study of severely affected individuals with a median age of entry of 41 years and an average follow-up period of 13 years mortality risk was fourfold for gastrointestinal disease; twofold for respiratory disease, accidents, suicide, and cerebrovascular diseases; and 40% in excess for circulatory disease, primarily cardiovascular diseases. Some of the latter may be reduced by modern surgical treatment. Secondary amyloidosis is the cause of death in a few severely affected patients (Fig. 4.33).[93]

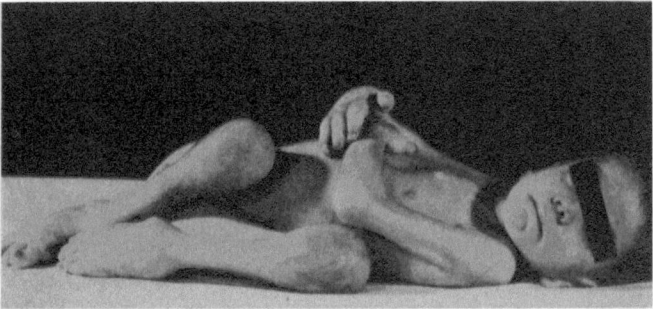

Figure 4.33. Cardiac and skeletal lesions characteristic of AS were found at autopsy in this 8-year-old youngster who was thought to have JRA. Many reports of JRA include data from patients who would now be recognized as having spondyloarthritis. Cauda equina syndrome with sensory impairment of the lower limbs and sphincter disturbances may occur in such severe cases.[144] (Reprinted with permission from Pirani C.L., Bennet G.A.: "Rheumatoid Arthritis: A Report of Three Cases Progressing from Childhood and Emphasizing Certain Systemic Manifestations. *Hospital for Joint Diseases Bulletin* 12:336–367, 1951. Copyright by the Hospital for Joint Diseases.)

Treatment

The management of children with HLA-B27 spondyloarthritis is not significantly different from that of children with JRA (see Chapter 3). Aspirin is sometimes the drug of choice; tolmetin or naproxen[8] frequently is most satisfactory in young children. However, older children often respond better to indomethacin. Naproxen has the advantage of twice-daily administration with better general compliance in teenagers. We have found the patient the best discriminator in selecting the optimal drug regimen. Our approach when initially offering drug therapy is to suggest brief trials of at least two agents, with the patient selecting the drug that provides the most relief of stiffness with the fewest side effects. Patients with sexually acquired disease induced by chlamydia may benefit from three months of antibiotic treatment (doxycycline, 200 mg. daily).[140]

Sulfasalazine is an extremely good agent for spondyloarthritis and may be used either alone or in combination with NSAIDs.[141–143] Benefit is commonly not noted for several weeks but then improvement may be expected to continue over a period of several months. Sulfasalazine may reduce the frequency of attacks of anterior uveitis.[100]

We have not found the slower-acting agents, gold and penicillamine, necessary or useful in these patients. While phenylbutazone might be of temporary use in severe exacerbations, we have avoided using it because of the life-threatening side effects. Corticosteroid regimens identical to those used for JRA (see Chapter 3) are reserved for acute iritis or carditis, for temporary use in severe attacks of RS that are incapacitating, and for peripheral arthritis that prevents walking.[145] We despair continuing reports of children allowed to become bedridden in one year.[146] Corticosteroids, azathioprine, and methotrexate are appropriate agents when necessary.[147] The aim of drug therapy is to suppress pain and inflammation so that normal activities may be maintained and the exercise program can be carried out. There is little evidence that the drugs affect the ultimate course of the disease.

Limitation of activities in these children is harmful, causing increasing stiffness and leading to depression and a constricted life-style. A vigorous exercise program including special exercises to encourage a straight back and neck is taught. Patients are instructed to stand erect and to stretch the back so as to "grow taller." Forward flexion is actively discouraged, and patients are encouraged to read and watch TV in the prone position, with the head held extended. If they cannot sleep in that position and must sleep supine, a firm mattress is prescribed, without a pillow. Deep-breathing exercises are provided. Smoking is discouraged. Severely affected youngsters should not choose an occupation that requires constant bending.

It is hard to say that the optimistic attitude of the physician is more important in the care of spondyloarthritis than in the other rheumatic diseases. However, there are some special features to be dealt with in these youngsters. The disorder is heritable, and some parents are guilty about this. Lay literature may be misleading, and parents may assume that their child will almost surely progress to AS, while just the opposite is true. We have found the most effective way to relieve the guilt and be optimistic is to indicate that the child can lead the same normal life as his parent. If the youngster is sports-oriented, we acknowledge the handicap of stiffness, try to adjust the medication schedule to provide optimum relief of symptoms at the time of meets and games, and capitalize on every opportunity to enhance body image. Teenagers (and their parents) can focus on a swollen knee as they do on a pimple, forgetting how beautiful or handsome they are, both physically and in their human values. Everybody has some problem in life; successful functioning despite a "handicap" can be ego-rewarding. Our positive attitudes provide defenses to be used by these patients when they face other attitudes in their peers or from uneducated and thoughtless adults with whom they have contact. We make the youngster the senior partner in our collaboration; we're there to back him up in the control of his disease and in his effort to prevent the disease from controlling him.

References

1. Moll JMH, Maslock I, Macrae I, et al.: Association between ankylosing spondylitis, psoriatic arthritis, Reiter's disease, the intestinal arthropathies, and Behcet's syndrome. Medicine 53:343–346, 1974.
2. Moll JMH: Ankylosing Spondylitis. Churchill Livingstone, Edinburgh, 1980.

3. Jacobs JC: HLA-B27 associated spondyloarthritis in children. Arthritis Rheum 23:695–696, 1980.

4. Jacobs JC: Arthritis as a manifestation of connective tissue disease. In Moore TD (ed.) Arthritis in Childhood. Report of the Eightieth Ross Conference on Pediatric Research. Ross Laboratories, Columbus, OH, 1981, pp. 18–23.

5. Jacobs JC, Johnston AD, Berdon WE: HLA-β27 associated spondyloarthritis and enthesopathy in childhood. J Pediatr 100:521–528, 1982.

6. Dougados M, van der Linden S, Juhlin R, et al.: The European spondyloarthropathy study group preliminary critieria for the classification of spondylarthropathy. Arthritis Rheum 34:1218–1227, 1991.

7. Wright V: Seronegative polyarthritis: A unified concept. Arthritis Rheum 21:619–633, 1978.

8. Calin A: Ankylosing spondylitis. In Kelley WN, Harris ED Jr, Ruddy S, Sledge CB (eds.) Textbook of Rheumatology, Vol. 2. Saunders, Philadelphia, 1989, pp. 1021–1037.

9. Calin A: Reiter's syndrome. In Kelley WN, Harris ED Jr, Ruddy S, Sledge CB (eds.) Textbook of Rheumatology, Vol. 2. Saunders, Philadelphia, 1989, pp. 1038–1052.

10. Brewerton DA. Many genes, many clinical features. Ann Rheum Dis 38(Suppl. 1):145–148, 1979.

11. Willkens RF, Arnett FC, Bitter T, et al.: Reiter's syndrome: evaluation of preliminary criteria for definite disease. Arthritis Rheum 24:844–848, 1981.

12. Gaucher A, Weryha G, Perrier P, et al.: Autosomal dominant arthropathy in a French family. Arthritis Rheum 34:737–743, 1991.

13. Scott SG: A Monograph on Adolescent Spondylitis or Ankylosing Spondylitis. Oxford University Press, London, 1942.

14. Ransohoff DF, Feinstein AR: Problem of spectrum and bias in evaluating the efficacy of diagnostic tests. N Engl J Med 299:926–930, 1978.

15. Conn RB, Brynes RK: Transfer of research technology to clinical practice— what are the criteria? Editorial. N Engl J Med 302:686–688, 1980.

16. Schaller JG, Hansen JA: HLA relationships to disease. Hosp Pract 16:41–49, 1981.

17. Suici-Foca N, King DW: The HLA system; structure and function. In Saunter M. Talmage DW, Frank MM, Austen FK, Claman HN (eds.) Immunological Diseases. Vol. 1, Chapter 17, pp. 385–410, 1988; Little Brown, Boston.

18. Jackson JF, Currier RD, Terasaki PI, et al.: Spinocerebellar ataxia and HLA linkage: Risk prediction by HLA typing. N Engl J Med 296:1138–1141, 1977.

19. Kidd KK: Genetic linkage and hemochromatosis. Editorial. N Engl J Med 301:209–210, 1979.

20. Mauseth RS, Hansen JA, Smith EK, et al.: Detection of heterozygotes for congenital adrenal hyperplasia: 21-hydroxylase deficiency—a comparison of HLA typing and 17-OH progesterone response to ACTH infusion. J Pediatr 97:749–753, 1980.

21. Winchester RJ: The HLA system and susceptibility to diseases: an interpretation. Clin Aspects Autoimmun 1:9–26, 1986.

21a. Dalton TA, Bennett JC: Autoimmune disease and the major histocompatibility complex: Therapeutic implications. Am J Med 92:183–188, 1992.

22. Segall M, Bach FH: HLA and disease. The perils of simplification. N Eng J Med 322:1879–1881, 1990.

23. Koivuranta-Vaara P, Repo H, Leirisalo M, et al.: Enhanced neutrophil migration in vivo HLA B27 positive subjects. Ann Rheum Dis 43:181–185, 1984.

24. Pease CT, Fordham JN, Currey HLF: Polymorphonuclear cell motility, ankylosing spondylitis, and HLA B27. Ann Rheum Dis 43:279–284, 1984.

25. Robinson WP, van der Linden SM, Khan MA, et al.: HLA-Bw60 increases susceptibility to ankylosing spondylitis in HLA-B27 + patients. Arthritis Rheum 32:1135–1141, 1989.

26. Ebringer R, Ebringer A: Ankylosing spondylitis: host-parasite interaction in the production of rheumatological disease. In Buchanan WW, Dick WC (eds.) Recent Advances in Rheumatology, Number two. Churchill Livingstone, Edinburgh, 1981, pp. 107–120.

27. Ford DK, da Roza DM, Ward RH: Arthritis confined to knee joints. Synovial lymphocyte responses to microbial antigens correlate with distribution of HLA. Arthritis Rheum 27:1157–1164, 1984.

28. Miehle W, Schattenkirchner M, Albert D, Bunge M: HLA-DR 4 in ankylosing spondylitis with different patterns of joint involvement. Ann Rheum Dis 44:39–44, 1985.

29. Hammer RE, Maka SD, Richardson JA, et al.: Spontaneous inflammatory disease in transgenic rats expressing HLA-B27 and Human B2m: An animal model of HLA-B27-associated human disorders. Cell 63:1099–1112, 1990.

30. McDevitt HO: Current concepts in immunology: Regulation of the immune response by the major histocompatibility system. N Engl J Med 303:1514–1517, 1980.

31. McGuigan LE, Geczy AF, Edmonds JP: The immunopathology of ankylosing spondylitis—A review. Semin Arthritis Rheum 15:81–105, 1985.

32. Hawkins BR, Dawkins RL, Christiansen FT, et al.: Use of the B27 test in diagnosis of ankylosing spondylitis: A statistical evaluation. Arthritis Rheum 24:743–744, 1981.

33. Cofton JP, Chalmers A, Price GE, et al.: HL-A 27 and ankylosing spondylitis in British Columbian Indians. J Rheumatol 2:314–318, 1975.

34. Rate RG, Morse HG, Bonnell MD, et al.: "Navajo arthritis" reconsidered. Relationship to HLA-B27. Arthritis Rheum 23:1299–1302, 1980.

35. Ostensen M, Romberg O, Husby G: Ankylosing spondylitis and motherhood. Arthritis Rheum 25:140–143, 1982.

36. Burgos-Vargas R, Petty RE: Juvenile ankylosing spondylitis. Rheum Dis Clin North Am 18:123–142, 1992.

37. McDaniel DO, Acton RT, Barger BO, et al.: Association of a 9.2-kilobase Pvu II Class I major histocompatibility complex restriction fragment length polymorphism with ankylosing spondylitis. Arthritis Rheum 30:894–900, 1987.

38. Kidd B, Mullee M, Frank A, Cawley M: Disease expression of ankylosing spondylitis in males and females. J Rheumatol 15:1407–1409, 1988.

39. Lynn TN: Rheumatoid spondylitis in a prepubertal female. Am J Dis Child 91:158–161, 1956.

40. Edstrom G, Thune S, Wittbom-Cigen G: Juvenile ankylosing spondylitis. Acta Rheum Scand 6:161–173, 1960.

41. Jacobs P: Ankylosing spondylitis in children and adolescents. Arch Dis Child 38:492–499, 1963.

42. Ellefsen F: Juvenile ankylosing spondylitis. Acta Rheum Scand 13:14-19, 1967.

43. Schaller JG, Bitnum S, Wedgwood RJ: Ankylosing spondylitis with childhood onset. J Pediatr 74:505–516, 1969.
44. Ladd JR, Cassidy JT, Martel W: Juvenile ankylosing spondylitis. Arthritis Rheum 14:579–590, 1971.
45. Bywaters EGL: Ankylosing spondylitis in childhood. In Ansell BD (ed.) Clinics in Rheumatic Diseases, Saunders, Philadelphia, 1976, pp. 387–396.
46. Kleinman P, Rivelis M, Schneider R, et al.: Juvenile ankylosing spondylitis. Radiology 125:775–780, 1977.
47. Hart FD: Ankylosing spondylitis. Lancet 2:1340–1344, 1968.
48. Bitter T, Jeannet M, deHaller E, et al.: Persistent yet reversible asymmetric pauciarthritis (PRAP): A B27-associated cluster. Ann Rheum Dis 38 (Suppl. 1):84–91, 1979.
49. Sheerin KA, Giannini EH, Brewer EJ, Barron KS: HLA-B27-associated arthropathy in childhood: long-term clinical and diagnostic outcome. Arthritis Rheum 31:1165–1170, 1988.
50. Calin A, Marder A, Marks S, et al.: Familial aggregation of Reiter's syndrome and ankylosing spondylitis: a comparative study. J Rheumatol 11:672–677, 1984.
51. Hammer M, Zeidler H, Klimsa S, Heesemann J: Yersinia enterocolitica in the synovial membrane of patients with Yersinia-induced arthritis. Arthritis Rheum 33:1795–1800, 1990.
51a. Arnett FC: Pathogenesis of the spondylarthropathies. Bull Rheum Dis (Arthritis Foundation) 40:(#6)1–3, 1991.
52. Hoenig LJ: The arthritis of Christopher Columbus. Arch Intern Med 152:274–277, 1992.
53. Keat A: Reiter's sydrome and reactive arthritis in perspective. N Eng J Med 309:1606–1615, 1983.
54. Shafer, N: Why Reiter's disease? NY State Med 77:1913–1918, 1977.
55. Rosenberg AM, Petty RE: Reiter's disease in children. Am J Dis Child 133:394–398, 1979.
56. Hakansson U, Low B, Eitrem R, et al.: HLA-B27 and reactive arthritis in an outbreak of salmonellosis. Tissue Antigens 6:366–367, 1975.
57. Inman RD, Johnston MEA, Hodge M, et al.: Postdysenteric reactive arthritis. A clinical and immunogenetic study following an outbreak of salmonellosis. Arthritis Rheum 31:1377–1383, 1988.
58. Hannu TJ, Leirisalo-Repo M: Clinical picture of reactive salmonella arthritis. J Rheumatol 15:1688–1671, 1988.
59. Calin A, Goulding N, Brewerton D: Reactive arthropathy following Salmonella vaccination. Arthritis Rheum 30:1197, 1987. (see also correspondence 31:1454–1455).
60. Keat, AC, Maini RN, Nkwazi GC, et al.: Role of *Chlamydia trachomatis* and HLA-B27 in sexually acquired reactive arthritis. Br Med J 1:605–607, 1978.
61. Editorial. Ankylosing spondylitis and its early diagnosis. Lancet 2:591–592, 1977.
62. Leirisalo M, Skylv G, Kouse M, et al.: Followup study on partients with Reiter's disease and reactive arthritis, with special reference to HLA-B27. Arthritis Rheum 25:249–259, 1982.
63. Leirisalo-Repo M, Suoranta H: Ten-year follow-up study of patients with Yersinia arthritis. Arthritis Rheum 31:533–537, 1988.

64. Mau W et al.: Clincal features and prognosis of patients with possible ankylosing spondylitis: Results of a 10-year follow-up. J Rheumatol 15:1109–1114, 1988.

65. Paronen I: Reiter's disease; a study of 344 cases observed in Finland. Acta Med Scand 131 [Suppl.] 212, 1948.

66. Sairanen E, Paronen I, Mahonen H: Reiter's syndrome: A follow-up study. Acta Med Scand 185:57–63, 1969.

67. Aho K, Ahvonen P, Alkio P, et al.: HL-A27 in reactive arthritis following infection. Ann Rheum Dis 34(Suppl.):29–30, 1975.

68. Rachelefsky GS, Stiehm ER: Histocompatibility locus antigen W27 and the rheumatic diseases. Pediatrics 56:498–500, 1975.

69. Schaller JG, Ochs HD, Thomas ED, et al.: Histocompatibility antigens in childhood-onset arthritis. J Pediatr 88:926–930, 1976.

70. Constantz R, Bluestone R: Diagnosis of the seronegative spondyloarthropathies: HLA-B27 testing as an aid to diagnosis. Contemp Orthop 2:141–147, 1980.

71. Nasrallah NS, Masi AT, Chandler RW, et al.: HLA-B27 antigen and rheumatoid factor negative (seronegative) peripheral arthritis. Studies in younger patients with early-diagnosed arthritis. Am J Med 63:379–386, 1977.

72. Khan MA: Editorial Comment. J Rheumatol 16:634–636, 1989.

73. Reynolds TL, Khan MA, van der Linden S, Cleveland RP: Differences in HLA-B27 positive and negative patients with ankylosing spondylitis: study of clinical disease activity and concentrations of serum IgA, C reactive protein, and haptoglobin. Ann Rheum Dis 50:154–157, 1991.

74. Calin A, Elswood J: Relative role of genetic and environmental factors in disease expression: Sib pair analysis in ankylosing spondylitis. Arthritis Rheum 32:77–81, 1989.

75. van der Linden SM, Valkenburg HA, de Jongh BM, Cats A: The risk of developing ankylosing spondylitis in HLA-B27 positive individuals. A comparison of relatives of spondylitis patients with the general population. Arthritis Rheum 27:241–249, 1984 (see also correspondence p. 1438).

76. Khan MA, van der Linden SM, Kushner I, et al.: Spondylitic disease without radiologic evidence of sacroilitis in relatives of HLA-B27 positive ankylosing spondylitis patients. Arthritis Rheum 28:40–43, 1985.

77. Lauhio A, Lahdevirta J, Janes R, et al.: Reactive arthritis associated with shigella sonnei infection. Arthritis Rheum 31:1190–1193, 1988.

78. Eastmond CJ, Norris Rennie JA, Reid TMS: An outbreak of campylobacter enteritis—A rheumatological followup survey. J Rheumatol 10:107–108, 1983.

79. Ebright JR, Ryan LM: Acute erosive reactive arthritis associated with campylobacter jejuni-induced colitis. Am J Med 76:321–322, 1984.

80. Ganfors K, Jalkanen S, VonEssen R, et al.: Yersenia antigens in synovial-fluid cells from patients with reactive arthritis. N Engl J Med 320:216–221, 1989.

81. Lahesmaa-Rantala R, Granfors K, Isomaki H, Toivanen A: Yersinia specific immune complexes in the synovial fluid of patients with yersinia triggered reactive arthritis. Ann Rheum Dis 46:510–514, 1987.

81a. Nikkari S, Merilathi-Palo R, Saario R, et al.: Yersinia-triggered reactive arthritis. Arthritis Rheum 35:682–687, 1992.

82. Shepherd RC, Smail PJ, Sinha GP: Reactive arthritis complicating cryptosporidial infection. Arch Dis Child 64:743–744, 1989.

83. Reveille JD, Conant MA, Duvic M: Human immunodeficiency virus-associated

psoriasis, psoriatic arthritis, and Reiter's syndrome: A disease continum? Arthritis Rheum 33:1574–1578, 1990.

84. Keat A, Dixey J, Thomas B, et al.: Chlamydia trachomatis and reactive arthritis: The missing link. Lancet 1:72–74, 1987.

85. Taylor-Robinson D, Thomas BJ, Dixey J, et al.: Evidence that Chlamydia tractomatis causes seronegative arthritis in women. Ann Rheum Dis 47:295–299, 1988.

85a. Rahman MU, Cheema MA, Schumacher HR, Hudson AP: Molecular evidence for the presence of clamydia in the synovium of patients with Reiter's syndrome. Arthritis Rheum 35:521–529, 1992.

86. Schumacher HR Jr, Magge S, Cherian PV, et al.: Light and electron microscopic studies on the synovial membrane in Reiter's syndrome. Immunocytochemical identification of chlamydial antigen in patients with early disease. Arthritis Rheum 31:937–946, 1988.

87. Mielants H, Veys EM, Joos R, et al.: Late onset pauciarticular juvenile chronic arthritis: relation to gut inflammation. J Rheumatol 14:459–465, 1987.

88. De Vos M, Cuvelier C, Mielants H, et al.: Ileocolonoscopy in seronegative spondylarthropathy. Gastroenterology 96:339–344, 1989.

88a. Bardin T, Enel C, Cornelius F, et al.: Antibiotic treatment of veneral disease and Reiter's syndrome in a Greenland population. Arthritis Rheum 35:190–194, 1992.

89. Reilly JP, Gross RH, Emans JB, et al.: Disorders of the sacro-iliac joint in children. J Bone Joint Surg 70-A:31–40, 1988.

90. Gedalia A, Watemberg N, Rotschild M, et al.: Inflammatory sacroiliitis in childhood. J Rheumatol 17:255–257, 1990.

91. Tomlinson IW, Jayson MIV: LE cells in Reiter's syndrome. Arthritis Rheum 25:239–240, 1982.

92. Siegel DM, Baum J: HLA-B27 associated dactylitis in children. J Rheumatol 15:976–977, 1988.

93. Calin A, Elswood J: The natural history of juvenile-onset ankylosing apondylitis: a 24-year retrospective case-control study. Br J Rheumatol 27:91–93, 1988.

94. Dwosh IL, Resnick D, Becker MA: Hip Involvement in ankylosing spondylitis. Arthritis Rheum 19:683–692, 1976.

95. Carette S, Graham D, Little H, et al.: The natural disease course of ankylosing spondylitis. Arthritis Rheum 26:186–190, 1983.

96. Schepsis AA, Leasch RE, Gorzyca J: Plantar Fasciitis. Etiology, treatment, surgical results, and review of the literature. Clin Orthop and Related Research 266:185–196, 1991.

97. Lee DA, Barker SM, Su WPD, et al.: The clinical diagnosis of Reiter's syndrome. Ophthalmology 93:350–356, 1986.

98. Eichenbaum JW, Friedman AH, Mamelok AE: A clinical and histopathological review of intermediate uveitis ("pars planitis"). Bull NY Acad Med 64:164–174, 1988.

99. Rosenbaum JT: Characterization of uveitis associated with spondyloarthritis. J Rheumatol 16:792–796, 1989.

100. Dougados M, Berenbaum F, Maetzel A, et al.: The use of sulfasalazine for the prevention of attacks of acute anterior uveitis associated with spondyloarthropathy. Arthritis Rheum 34:S195, 1991.

100a. Misukiewicz P, Carlson RW, Rowan L, et al.: Acute aortic insufficiency in a patient with presumed Reiter's syndrome. Ann Rheum Dis 51:686–687, 1992.

101. Haverman JF, Van Albada-Kuipers GA, Dohmen HJM, Dijmans BAC: Atrioventricular conduction disturbance as an early feature of Reiter's syndrome. Ann Rheum Dis 47:1017–1020, 1988.

102. Good AE: Reiter's disease: A review with special attention to cardiovascular and neurologic sequelae. Semin Arthritis Rheum 3:253–286, 1974.

103. Naparstek Y, Abrahamov A, Cohen T, Brautbar C: Familial hereditary thrombocytopenia and HLA. Am J Hematol 17:113–116, 1984.

104. Niepal GA, Kostka D, Kopecky S, et al.: Enthesopathy. Acta Rheum et Balneologica Pistiniana, No. 1., 1966.

105. Ball J: Enthesopathy of rheumatoid and ankylosing spondylitis. Ann Rheum Dis 30:213–223, 1971.

106. Resnick D, Niwayama G: Entheses and enthesopathy. Radiology 146:1–9, 1983.

107. Simkin PA, Downey DJ, Kilcoyne RF: Apophyseal arthritis limits lumbar motion in patients with ankylosing spondylitis. Arthritis Rheum 31:798–802, 1988.

108. Aufdermaur M: Pathogenesis of square bodies in ankylosing spondylitis. Ann Rheum Dis 48:628–631, 1989.

108a. Pile K, Kwong T, Fryer J, Laurent R: Polyarteritis associated with yersinia enterocolitica infection. Ann Rheum Dis 51:678–680, 1992.

109. Bulkley BH, Roberts WC: Ankylosing spondylitis and aortic regurgitation. Circulation 48:1014–1027, 1973.

110. Alexander B, Feiner H: Ankylosing spondylitis with cardiac dysrhythmia. Pathologic changes in cardiac conduction system. NY State J Med 79:1585–1588, 1979.

111. Shah A: Echocardiographic features of mitral regurgitation due to ankylosing spondylitis. Am J Med 82:353–356, 1987.

112. Podell TE, Wallace DJ, Fishbein MC, et al.: Severe giant cell valvulitis in a patient with Reiter's sydrome. Arthritis Rheum 25:232–234, 1982.

113. Linder E, Pasternack A: Immunofluorescence studies on kidney biopsies in ankylosing spondylitis. Acta Pathol Microbiol Scand [A] 78B:517–525, 1970.

114. Steinsson K, Hirszel P, Wiensten A: Mesangial IgM nephropathy in a patient with HLA-B27 spondylarthropathy. Arthritis Rheum 25:1056, 1982.

115. Jennette JC, Ferguson AL, Moore MA, Freeman DG: IgA nephropathy associated with seronegative spondyloarthropathies. Arthritis Rheum 25:144–149, 1982.

116. Neng Li K, Li PKT, Hawkins B, Mac-Moune Lai F: IgA nephropathy associated with ankylosing spondylitis: occurrence in women as well as in men. Ann Rheum Dis 48:435–437, 1989.

117. Collado A, Sanmarti R, Bielsa I, et al.: Immunoglobulin A in the skin of patients with ankylosing spondylitis. Ann Rheum Dis 47:1004–1007, 1988.

118. Shu KH, Lian JD, Yand YF, et al.: Glomerulonephritis in ankylosing spondylitis. Clin Nephrol 25:169–174, 1986.

119. Miller LD, Brown EC Jr, Arnett FC: Amyloidosis in Reiter's syndrome. J Rheum 6:225–231, 1979.

120. Weinberger HW, Ropes MW, Kulka JP, et al.: Reiter's syndrome, clinical and pathologic observations. A long-term study of 16 cases. Medicine 41:35–91, 1962.

121. Burgos-Vargas R, Clark P: Axial involvement in the seronegative entheso-

pathy and arthropathy syndrome and its progression to ankylosing spondylitis. J Rheumatol 16:192–197, 1989.

122. Calabro JJ, Grag SL, Khoury MI, et al.: Reiter's syndrome. Am Fam Physician 9:80–94, 1974.

123. Nissila M, Isomaki H, Kaarela K, et al.: Prognosis of inflammatory joint diseases. A three-year follow-up study. Scand J Rheumatol 12:33–38, 1983.

124. Sambrook P, McGuigan L, Champion D, et al.: Clinical features and followup study of HLA-B27 positive patients presenting with peripheral arthritis. J Rheumatol 12:526–528, 1985.

125. Camilleri AE, Swan IRC, Murphy E, Sturrock RD: Chronic otitis media: a new manifestation in ankylosing spondylitis? Ann Rheum Dis 51:655–657, 1992.

126. Helfgott SM, Treseler PA: Cricoarytenoid synovitis in ankylosing spondylitis. Arthritis Rheum 33:604–605, 1990.

127. Kernodle GW Jr, Allen NB, Kredich D: Atlantoaxial subluxation in juvenile ankylosing spondylitis. Arthritis Rheum 30:837–838, 1987.

128. Elbright JR, Ryan LM: Acute erosive reactive arthritis associated with campylobacter jejuni-induced colitis. Am J Med 76:321–323, 1984.

129. Brower AC: The sacroiliac joint. In: Arthritis in Black and White. p. 10, Philadelphia, WB Saunders, 1988.

130. Ahlstrom H, Feltelius N, Nyman R, Hallgren R: Magnetic resonance imaging of sacroiliac joint inflammation. Arthritis Rheum 33:1763–1769, 1990.

131. Gerster J-C, Piccinin P: Enthesopathy of the heels in juvenile onset seronegative B-27 positive spondyloarthropathy. J Rheumatol 12:310–314, 1985.

132. Resnick D, Feingold ML, Curd J, et al.: Calcaneal abnormalities in articular disorders. Radiology 125:355–366, 1977.

132a. O'Neill TW, King G, Gramham IM, et al.: Echocardiographic abnormalities in ankylosing spondylitis. Ann Rheum Dis 51:652–654, 1992.

133. Radford EP, Doll R, Smith PG: Mortality among patients with ankylosing spondylitis not given x-ray therapy. N Engl J Med 297:572–576, 1977.

134. Stewart SR, Robbins DL, Castles JJ: Acute fulminant aortic and mitral insufficiency in ankylosing spondylitis. N Engl J Med 299:1448–1449, 1978.

135. Reid GD, Patterson MWH, Patterson AC, et al.: Aortic insufficiency in association with juvenile ankylosing spondylitis. J Pediatr 95:78–80, 1979.

136. Gore JE, Vizcarrondo FE, Rieffel CN: Juvenile ankylosing spondylitis and aortic regurgitation: A case presentation. Pediatrics 68:423–426, 1981.

137. Pelkonen P, Byring R, Pesonen E, et al.: Rapidly progressive aortic incompetence in juvenile ankylosing spondylitis: a case report. Arthritis Rheum 27:698–700, 1984.

138. Bergfeldt L, Insulander R, Lindblom D, et al.: HLA-B27: An important genetic risk factor for lone aortic regurgitation and severe conduction system abnormalities. Am J Med 85:12–18, 1988.

139. Kaprove RE, Little AH, Graham DC, et al.: Ankylosing spondylitis: Survival in men with and without radiotherapy. Arthritis Rheum 23:57–61, 1980.

140. Zeidler H, Wollenhaupt J, Bialowons A: Chlamydia-induced arthritis: Antibiotic treatment and follow-up study. Arthritis Rheum 34:S61, 1991.

141. Bosi Ferraz M, Tugwell P, Goldsmith CH, Atra E: Meta-analysis of Sulfasalazine in Ankylosing Spondylitis. J Rheumatol 17:1482–1486, 1990.

142. Lehtinen MN, Leirisalo-Repo M, Luukkainen R, et al.: Sulfasalazine in the

treatment of ankylosing spondylitis. A twenty-six-week, placebo-controlled clinical trial. Arthritis Rheum 31:1111–1116, 1988.

143. Mielants H, Veys EM: HLA-B27 related arthritis and bowel inflammation. Part 1. Sulfasalazine (Salazopyrin) in HLA-B27 related reactive arthritis. J Rheumatol 12:287–293, 1985.

144. Mitchell MJ, Sartoris DJ, Moody D, Resnick D: Cauda equina syndrome complicating ankylosing spondylitis. Radiology 175:521–525, 1990.

145. Mintz G, Enriquez, RD, Mercado U, et al.: Intravenous methylprednisolone pulse therapy in severe ankylosing spondylitis. Arthritis Rheum 24:734–736, 1981.

146. Jay MS, Seymore C, Jay WM, Durant RH: Reiter's syndrome in an adolescent female with systemic sequelae. J Adolescent Health Care 8:280–285, 1987.

147. Calin A: A placebo controlled, crossover study of azathioprine in Reiter's syndrome. Ann Rheum Dis 45:653–655, 1986.

5

Systemic Lupus Erythematosus

Prologue

It was 1954. A 13-year-old girl became ill with fever, arthritis, a butterfly facial rash, diplopia, alopecia, and subcutaneous nodules (Fig. 5.1). Her urinalysis showed some protein and 20 red blood cells. A diagnosis of systemic lupus erythematosus (SLE) was made, and treatment was begun with 50 mg of prednisone daily. There was a dramatic response, and she began to feel well. Her chart was filled with notes of concern about the potential fearsome side effects of prednisone and its merely palliative benefits. As soon as she felt a little better, her doctors would reduce the prednisone; she would promptly become ill again. During the 21 months she survived, she was continuously ill and was hospitalized 10 times for a total 220 hospital days before she died of renal failure.

In May 1977, a 6-year-old girl became ill with fever, arthritis, extremity rashes, subcutaneous nodules, and pleuritic chest pains. Urinalysis was normal. She was treated with 40 mg of prednisone daily. There was a dramatic response. As soon as she felt well, her doctors began to reduce the prednisone and within 3 months had gotten it down to 15 mg daily. Five months later, she was found to have cotton-wool retinal exudates (cytoid bodies), hypertension (140/120), 2+ proteinuria, and a urine loaded with red blood cells; creatinine clearance was 53 mg/ml/m^3. When we first saw her in May 1978, renal biopsy showed severe active diffuse proliferative and necrotizing glomerulonephritis with involvement of 80% of the glomerular surface area (class IV). Urine protein was 2 grams daily. Serum total hemolytic complement was low, and anti-DNA binding (Farr test) was 95%. She was treated with prednisone 40 mg daily and antihypertensive agents (hydrochlorothiazide and propranolol). After a month, azathioprine 50 mg daily was added, and the prednisone was changed to 150 mg on alternate mornings.

All parameters gradually improved; after a year, it was possible to

409

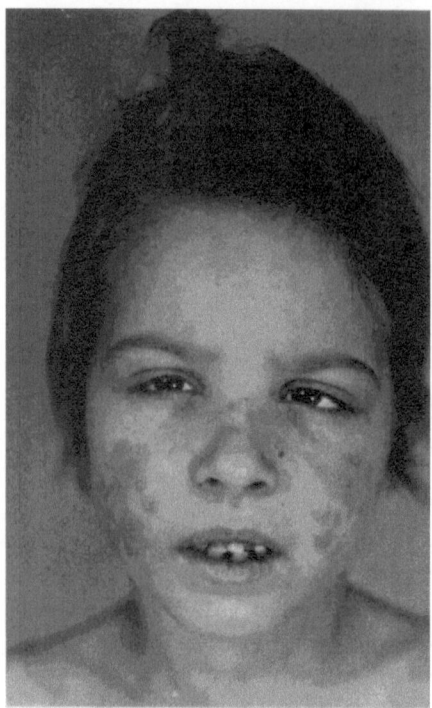

Figure 5.1. Typical rash of childhood systemic lupus; this child also has buccal and palatal ulcers and alopecia.

gradually reduce the prednisone to 100 mg on alternate mornings and to gradually withdraw the antihypertensive medications. After 2 years, the creatinine clearance was normal; the 24-h urine protein was 250 mg; the urinalysis was normal, except for a few white blood cells; the serum complement was normal; and the anti-DNA antibodies were only slightly elevated (37%) (Table 5.1). She had a brief hospitalization for cataract removal. She has attended school daily and led a normal life. Total hospitalization during the 39 months summarized here was 35 days. Since then she has been well.

Prior to 1955, 100% of children with SLE in one large pediatric center died within 1 year of apparent clinical onset of the disease.[1] In 1980, our clinic and others achieved 100% 5-year survival. Despite relatively little new understanding about pathogenesis and no "cure," there has been great progress in learning how to care for these children.

Epidemiology and Susceptibility

Systemic lupus erythematosus, the prototype of immunologically mediated disease in man, continues to excite substantial investigational interest in its etiology and pathogenesis.[2,3] It has become increasingly evident that im-

Table 5.1 Management Flowsheet for Systemic Lupus Erythematosus*

L.H. Onset, 6/77: Age, 6½; Arthritis, fever, adenopathy, rash, + LE Prep, ANA Rx. Prednisone 15–40 mg od

Date	Dose of Prednisone	Dose of Azathioprine	Complement (nl = > 160)	Farr Test (nl = < 20)	Cells	Urine Protein (mg)	Urine ClCr (ml/min/mm³)	Manifestations-Notations
4/78	40 od (2/kg)	37.5 od (1.5/kg)	75	95	Loaded	2100	53	Renal biopsy class IV BP 140/120; cytoid bodies Propranolol Hydrochlorothiazide Slow K
5/78	150 qod (6/kg)	50 od	84	74	Loaded			
8/78	150 qod (6/kg)	62.5 od	136	68	Loaded	800	81	
1/79	150 qod (6/kg)	75 od	85	69	6–8 RBCs	1600	90	
4/79	150 qod (6/kg)	75 od	123	63	Normal			
7/79	125 qod	75 od	164	31	Loaded	1200	90	Steroid cataract ʃ Propranolol
1/80	100 qod	75 od	202	53	Normal	300	120	ʃ Hydrochlorothiazide
8/80	75 qod	50 od	175	37	8–12 WBCs	250	121	Hepatitis A
7/81	75 qod	50 od	132	63	10–12 WBCs	440	120	Bilateral cataract removal

ʃ = discontinue.

*patient would probably be treated with IV pulse cyclophosphamide today but this patient is completely well in 1992 taking only azathioprine 25 mg daily (OD) plus prednisone 5 mg every second day (QOD).

Table 5.2. Factors Increasing Susceptibility to SLE

Age (early childhood and old age are protective; second decade highest susceptibility)
Sex (females most susceptible except under age 5 or over 65)
Family history:
   27% of affected children have an affected relative
   57% of monozygotic twins are concordant for SLE
Presence of HLA-DR3
Slow acetylator phenotypes
Chromosomal abnormalities
Presence of porphyria
Congenital deficiency of any component of complement or other immunologic
   deficiency
History of photosensitivity
Excessively proliferating B lymphocytes and B lymphocytes that hyperrespond to
   nuclear and lymphocyte antigens
Reduced numbers of T cells or impaired T-lymphocytes reactivity

---

mune reactions consist of an immensely complex, highly coordinated series of cell-to-cell effects involving macrophages and lymphocytes. Self-reactive clones are generally not permitted to develop or expand. Lupus seems to represent a breakdown of these regulatory mechanisms—an imbalance between what is beneficial to the organism and what is harmful. Current information suggests that lupus is a multifactorial disease requiring both genetic and environmental factors for disease expression (Table 5.2).[4,5] In individuals with a strong genetic predisposition, weak environmental factors may produce clinical disease, whereas in patients with a weak genetic predisposition, very strong environmental factors may be required to produce clinical symptoms. Experimental studies suggest that genetically determined predisposing factors differ in different individuals or families and that different environmental factors are operative in patients with differing genetic predispositions (Table 5.2).[6] "Lupus" may be a group of diseases rather than a single disease.[7,8]

Systemic lupus erythematosus is rare in young children; very few cases occur before age 5 and relatively few between 5 and 10 years of age.[9–17] Although females are more frequently affected at any age, the female preponderance of 90% in teenage and adult series is not seen during the first decade of life, when females exceed males only three to one in susceptibility. In a few families lupus is transmitted through the *male* line.[16,18] Black and Puerto Rican females seem to be considerably more susceptible than white females (Fig. 5.2).[17,19]

Lupus occurring in childhood often indicates strong familial susceptibility. Children are more frequently affected in multiple-case families; conversely, the incidence of affected close relatives is higher in childhood than in adult series.[1,12–12b] In one large pediatric series, 19 of 108 cases had affected first-

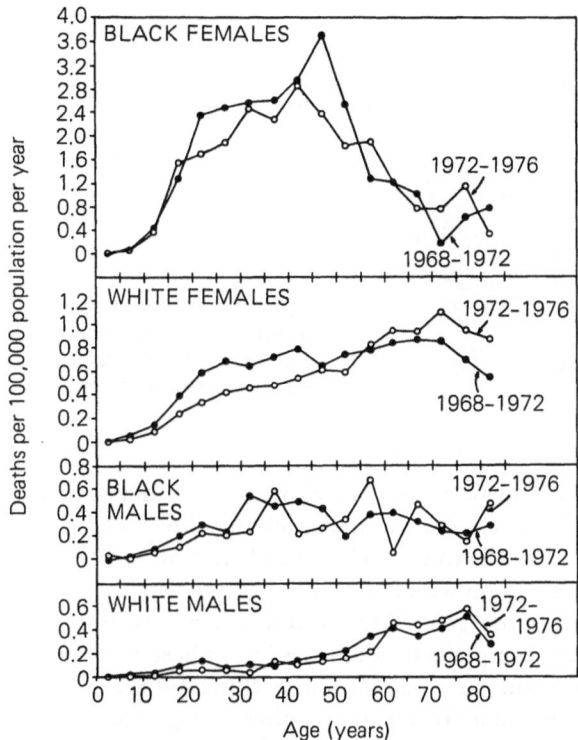

Figure 5.2. U.S. mortality rates for SLE (per 100,000 population per year) by 5-year age groups, sex, and race in 1968–1972 and 1972–1976. (Reprinted with permission from Gordon et al., ref. 608. Copyright by the American Rheumatism Association.)

degree relatives.[12] If aunts and uncles are included, 27% of childhood cases are familial in contrast to series using adults as the index case where only 5–10% are familial.[12,20] Furthermore, 57% of monozygotic twins are concordant for SLE, again indicating strong genetic predisposition.[21,21a] Monozygotic twins tend to develop SLE simultaneously (within 4 years) even if the children are reared apart.[10,22–23] Family studies suggest that coinheritance of two or more genes in linkage disequilibrium with a variety of HLA-D-region markers, especially DR3, is important in determining the full expression of disease in various families.[4] Additional genetic or environmental factors are required for full expression of the clinical illness in these families and in other patients.[4,24–27] There are certain other conditions associated with increased susceptibility to SLE (Table 5.2). All forms of drug-induced lupus have been shown to be correlated with the presence of the slow-acetylator phenotype; this phenotype probably is particularly associated with increased susceptibility to induction of SLE by aromatic or hydrazine chemical compounds.[28–29] Patients with various chromosomal abnormalities, including males with Klinefelter's syndrome (XXY), have an increased incidence of SLE and other autoimmune diseases.[30] All immunologic deficiency states predispose to SLE.[31] Patients with porphyria, especially porphyria cutanea tarda, also seem to be especially susceptible to SLE.[32]

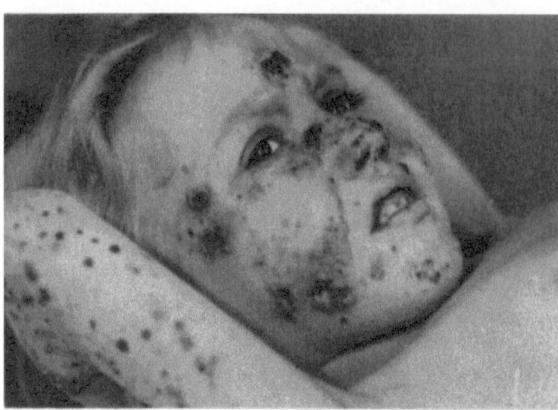

Figure 5.3. Photosensitive ulcerating rash in a child with SLE; 73% of lupus patients are photosensitive.[46]

Studies of immune regulation in patients with SLE suggest that genetic predisposition is related to (1) B-lymphocyte hyperactivity due either to a primary B-cell abnormality or ineffective T-cell control and/or to (2) unusually high response to immunization with lymphocyte antigens or modified lymphocyte antigens or nuclear antigens.[4,33,34] Macrophages are also intimately involved in all of these lymphocyte responses.[35,36] These variations from normal responses could result in precipitation of clinical disease after stimulation with a polyclonal B-cell activator, with either endogenous or exogenous nuclear antigens, or the disease could be a result of immunization with modified lymphocyte membranes (e.g., as a result of a viral infection). These immune functions are affected by hormones: male sex hormones suppress while female hormones increase humoral immune responses.[37] Estrogens in oral contraceptive pills may make lupus worse[38] and androgens may be protective.[39,40] In addition, females also have impaired cellular immunity relative to males, which may play a role in the increased female susceptibility to SLE.

Studies have suggested that in familial disease, in addition to transmission of genetic susceptibility factors, there is in some cases horizontal and in others vertical transmission of environmental factors (viruses?) which are required to precipitate disease, in addition to both random and nonrandom exposure to particular environmental inducers.[4,41–44]

One environmental factor that definitely can induce SLE in some individuals is ultraviolet light (Fig. 5.3). Recent evidence suggests that this may be from artificial as well as natural sunlight.[45] It may be wise to test children for the presence of congenital complement deficiencies and anti-Ro antibodies before beginning ultraviolet-light therapy for psoriasis.[46] We have seen a child develop a butterfly rash and arthralgia following ultraviolet-light therapy.[47] DNA may be denatured by ultraviolet light; it is not known whether some lupus exacerbations in sun-sensitive patients are a result of antibody formation to this denatured DNA.[48,49] Some patients with a congenital deficiency of one component of complement, C2, are especially prone to develop connective tissue diseases, including SLE, and are especially sun-sensitive.[50,50a] Sixty percent of homozygous C2-deficient individuals in families studied after an SLE-affected individual is identified ultimately develop SLE. In these C2-deficient individuals, exacerbations of lupuslike illness may occur after exposure to ultraviolet light and sometimes may remit spontaneously after discontinuing the exposure. There is also a high incidence of lupuslike disease in patients with hereditary angioneurotic edema associated with C1-inhibitor deficiency and in individuals with congenital deficiencies or dysfunction of other complement components (C1, C3, C4, C5, C6, C7, C8).[50-61] SLE in patients with C3 deficiency may be associated with lipodystrophy.[62] Combinations of defects also occur.[63] In a recent study of our pediatric lupus patients we found 42% to have congenital deficiencies of one or more complement components.[64]

Thus, susceptibility to SLE is affected by a multitude of genetic factors, including age, race, sex, and many different interrelated immunologic functions involving the handling of foreign or autologous proteins.[65] All of the potential mediators of the immune response—immunoglobulins, complement proteins, B and T lymphocytes, macrophages, and mast cells—seem to be involved.[35] A large number of environmental stimuli—some infectious, some not—may set off the disease in susceptible individuals. Some of the infectious environmental stimuli are transmitted from one parent to child at birth; others are acquired in the home, slightly increasing the risk for all household members. There has been considerable progress in recognizing and defining some of the at-risk population and some determinants of the disease, but much still remains to be done before we understand who will get SLE and why.

Immune Complexes and the Pathophysiology of SLE

Although SLE is characterized by the presence of many autoantibodies (antinuclear, gamma globulin [rheumatoid factors], white blood cell, red blood cell, platelet, coagulant, cytoplasmic and phospholipid [reagin] antibodies), the most troublesome and life-threatening immune reactions seem to be a result of the formation and defective clearing from the circulation of immune complexes of double-stranded (native) DNA with anti-DNA antibodies.[4,5] These DNA–anti-DNA complexes bind complement and can be important mediators of vascular and tissue injury, especially in the kidney.[66] Once the kidney is damaged by circulating complexes or by locally formed complexes of circulating antibody with antigenic glomerular constituents, it seems to be even more susceptible to binding such complexes, thereby sustaining more severe injury.[67] Although the evidence is less clear in other organs, it seems likely that DNA–anti-DNA complexes are responsible for much of the tissue damage in SLE. Experimental evidence suggests that damage in SLE is a result not only of unusual formation of these antibodies but is also fostered by local antibody production and fixation of antibodies by antigenic constituents of glomerular capillary walls.[67] To at least some extent, the size of the complexes is probably an important factor in their pathogenicity.[68]

In the healthy individual, DNA is not generally recognized as a foreign antigen, and the immune system seems to keep a close check on the formation and binding of the little anti-DNA that may occur normally.[5] Self-reactive clones are generally not permitted to develop or expand. In active SLE, those suppressor functions seem to be diminished, allowing for both excess production and binding of these antibodies. Although the study of immune complexes has provided some clarification of the mechanism of tissue injury in SLE, the factors that set off the formation of DNA-anti-DNA complexes remain obscure.[4,5] Viral antigens have repeatedly been implicated, but it is difficult to prove just what role, if any, they actually play in pathogenesis.[69,70] It is likely that the offending pathogens include a host of environmental substances and that the reactions involved in the production of SLE are a host of interdependent regulatory mechanisms that result in mishandling of foreign or autologous antigens so that an imbalance is created between what is beneficial to the organism and what is harmful. In most cases, this alteration of homeostatic control is self-sustaining and results in persistent immune-complex formation.

Clinical Measurement of Serum Immune Complexes, Complement, and Anti-DNA Antibodies

Immune Complexes

In recent years, many sensitive methods have been devised to directly demonstrate circulating immune complexes in serum. No one method identifies all forms of complexes, and none of the methods is without artifact and the potential for misinterpretation.[4] None of these assays are positive in all patients with SLE. Complexes are most commonly demonstrable in clinically active disease and, in general, correlate with high levels of anti-DNA antibody and low levels of total hemolytic complement. At present, the study of circulating immune complexes in SLE is of research interest, but these tests are not generally used in clinical decision-making.[2] With further study and refinement, they may turn out to be the most reliable laboratory indications of clinical activity in SLE.[71]

Cryoglobulins. Cryoglobulins, proteins that precipitate in the cold and redissolve on warming, are demonstrable in many patients with SLE, especially those with very active disease and with renal disease.[72] In lupus sera, these cryoprecipitates contain many different proteins (mixed cryoglobulinemia) and are thought to represent immune complexes. Demonstration of cryoprecipitates that redissolve on warming can be an easy and fast method of indirectly demonstrating the probable presence of immune complexes. Antibody tests performed on cold sera may be artifically negative if all the antibodies have settled on the bottom of the tube.

Complement

Antigen-antibody complexes bind complement that is either deposited in the tissues or cleared by the reticuloendothelial system. Serum total hemolytic complement may be conveniently measured and used as an indication of the activity of the disease.[5,73–75] Lowered levels of complement are not solely a reflection of tissue deposition since complement may be consumed as part of autoimmune hemolytic anemia, and in sick lupus patients complement synthesis may be decreased and catabolism may be increased.[76] Nevertheless, measurement of serum complement is an indirect but clinically useful technique for regulation of medications.[5,73–75] Complement levels fall before the appearance of increased proteinuria signals increasing renal damage. Therefore, a falling complement level is a predictor of renal insult at a time when therapeutic intervention may prevent immune-complex formation and deposition (Fig. 5.4).

In addition to measuring total hemolytic complement, it is possible to measure many of the specific components of complement. Some investigators prefer to use C3 or C4 determinations rather than total hemolytic complement.[76a] Determinations of total hemolytic complement require that blood be delivered promptly to the laboratory and the serum immediately separated and frozen at −70°C until the test can be performed. Improper handling or storage of specimens results in falsely low values.[77] Specimens cannot be easily transported to distant laboratories. When these handicaps are not insurmountable, total hemolytic complement, a reflection of the entire complement cascade, seems to us at this time to be the most useful complement determination for drug regulation.

Circulating split-products of complement may also cause tissue damage and split-product levels may also reflect disease activity and predict exacerbations.[78]

Anti-DNA Antibodies

Anti-DNA antibodies are the hallmark of SLE and are usually demonstrable in the presence of active disease.[79–83] Their presence is confirmatory of the diagnosis and, when present in association with low levels of complement, may have a specificity of 100%.[84] However, the absence of demonstrable anti-DNA antibodies may merely signify less activity of disease at a given time and must not be misinterpreted as meaning the child does not have SLE. A multitude of studies has confirmed the correlation of flare-ups of disease with preceding increasing levels of antibodies to both single-stranded

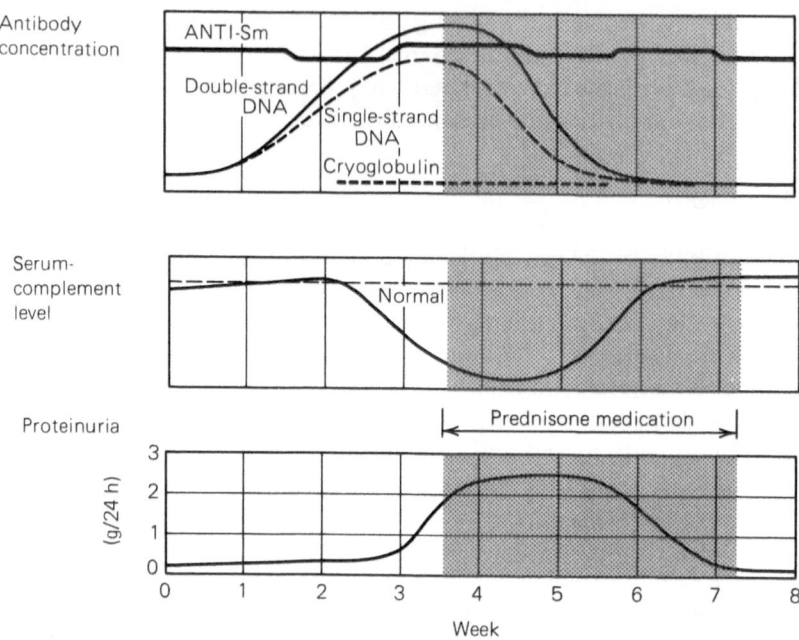

Figure 5.4. Flare-up of disease is traced for a typical SLE patient with limited kidney disease. The blood serum's content of antibodies against double- and single-strand DNA increases, and the complement level begins to decline, before the onset of proteinuria (increased urinary excretion of protein), a sign of kidney malfunction. Note the rapid increase in antibodies associated with extreme complement depression; the antibodies have combined with antigen to form immune complexes, which fix complement (and which may he observed in the serum as cryoglobulin, a gel-like precipitate formed at low temperature). Another antinuclear antibody, anti-Sm, does not increase during a flare-up; apparently only certain antibodies participate in forming immune complexes capable of inducing tissue damage. Prednisone, an anti-inflammatory steroid drug, is effective in treating an acute episode; its mechanism of action is not understood. (Reprinted with permission from Koffler, ref. 5.)

and double-stranded DNA (Fig. 5.4). Thus, demonstration of increasing and persistently very high levels of anti-native (double-stranded) DNA antibodies can be successfully used to predict exacerbations of disease and especially impending renal damage.[5,81–88] Therapeutic maneuvers can be instituted to prevent the formation of these antibodies and their deposition in blood vessels and tissues. Antibodies to DNA tend to appear before serum complement falls in lupus exacerbations, as one would expect if most of the reduction of complement is attributable to deposition of the immune complexes in tissue.[5] Measurement of both serum complement and anti-DNA antibodies is useful, as clinicians are more comfortable basing decisions on more than a single laboratory abnormality.

Autoantibody formation and immune-complex disease do not seem to be the only mechanisms of injury in SLE. Thus, in central-nervous-system disease, measurement of serum complement and anti-DNA antibodies may not be of as much help in predicting exacerbations as they are in renal disease.[89] This generally reported observation may, however, be a misinterpretation of the data: our experience suggests that in some instances very minor rises of anti-DNA antibodies and falls in serum complement may predict the onset of CNS symptoms. The problem, then, may be that these tests are not sensitive enough to distinguish CNS risk from no risk. In the CNS-susceptible patient, this may be primarily a reflection of increased sensitivity of the brain and of a smaller margin of residual safety in that organ as compared to the kidney.

Tests for Antinuclear Antibodies and the Diagnosis of SLE

The LE Cell

The presence of IgG antinuclear (anti-DNA-histone complex) factors in white blood cells subjected to specified laboratory trauma results in extrusion of the damaged nucleus, which is phagocytized by a healthy polymorph.[20] The phagocyte containing the engulfed homogeneous purple hematoxylin material is the LE cell. LE cells were demonstrable in 90% of the ARA series of patients with SLE and, when combined with three other criteria, achieved 99% specificity of diagnosis for SLE.[90] LE cells tend to disappear with treatment and with chronic renal failure.[20] They may be found in 9% of adults with RA, in lupoid hepatitis, and in some patients taking anticonvulsant drugs but are rarely seen in other childhood diseases, including other connective-tissue diseases. We have found LE cells in one child with acute lymphocytic leukemia,[91] and they have occasionally been seen in adults with lymphoma and other malignancies.

Buffy coat smears done as part of the LE cell preparation commonly show free *hematoxylin bodies* (awaiting phagocytosis) and *rosettes* of neutrophils surrounding a single purple nuclear mass.

LE cell preparations are time-consuming and require experienced technicians for accuracy. However, where they can be obtained promptly and are dependable, they are still very useful for diagnosis. Occasionally, LE cells may be demonstrated in the lupus patient whose ANA test is negative. In general, this is for technical reasons, i.e., lack of fixation of the antibody in preparation of the ANA test. Certain antibodies may be more likely to be "lost" in fixation. We find LE cell preparations still of significant-enough clinical value to warrant their being done.

Immunofluorescent Antinuclear Antibody Tests

Antinuclear antibody (ANA) tests demonstrate the presence of a variety of IgG and IgM antibodies to various nuclear antigens but are extremely poorly standardized. False positives range as high as 30%. Patients with other rheumatic diseases and relatives of lupus patients have a higher incidence of positive tests.[92-93]

Very few patients with active untreated lupus have a negative test for ANA, and 64% of these have antibody to Ro or anti-dsDNA antibodies which help to establish the diagnosis. In some instances the antibodies are present but lost to the test system.[94] Some, but not all, authors report that lupus patients with negative tests for both LE cells and ANA tend to have milder lupus with less renal disease.[94–96] Attempts to relate the titer of ANA to disease activity have not been altogether successful, although as a generality patients with lupus tend to have higher titers (at least 1:80 in most laboratories), and false-positive tests tend to be in the lower range.[97]

Different morphologic patterns of nuclear staining have been described:[98] (1) *Peripheral (shaggy or rim pattern):* antibodies to deoxyribonucleoprotein and native (double-stranded) DNA produce the peripheral pattern that is most specific for SLE, although not the most commonly demonstrated pattern in SLE. (2) *Homogeneous:* antibodies to deoxynucleoprotein or to histone produce the homogeneous pattern that is commonly seen in SLE. This pattern reflects the presence of many different antibodies. The other individually distinct patterns may be obscured into homogeneous staining. As the serum is diluted, the pattern may change, depending on the titers of the varying antibodies that are present. Antibody to histone is almost always present in drug-induced SLE. (3) *Nucleolar:* antibodies to ribosomal precursor ribonucleoproteins produce a nucleolar pattern that may be found in over 50% of patients with progressive systemic sclerosis and in many patients with dermatomyositis but is not typical of SLE. (4) *Speckled:* a variety of antibodies to nonhistone (acidic) nuclear proteins account for a speckled ANA pattern. These include antibodies to Sm, RNP, and SS-A (Ro) and SS-B (La) antigens. Antibodies to Sm and RNP together may be demonstrated by tests for extractable nuclear antibody (ENA). Antibodies to Sm are considered specific for SLE, while the presence of RNP antibody alone (without Sm) in high titer is a diagnostic criterion for the syndrome currently called mixed connective-tissue disease (MCTD). Antibodies to SS-A (Ro) and SS-B (La) are found in 15–20% of patients with SLE but also occur in 50% of patients with Sjögren's syndrome who do not have arthritis or SLE. Antibodies to topoisomerase (SCl-70) are thought to be specific for scleroderma, and antibodies to centromere are presumably specific for the CREST variety of scleroderma. The profile of these and other antinuclear antibodies may help in differentiating one rheumatic disease from another (Table 5.3).[98]

There antibody profiles are loosely related to disease heterogeneity.[99–101] However, they are not absolutely disease-specific, nor do they provide a simple guide to major subgroups of activity of disease.[97]

Children without identifiable rheumatic disease who present with musculoskeletal pain and positive ANA rarely if ever evolve into rheumatic disease.[102] We do not recommend repeat testing and arthritis-clinic follow-up for such children since such recommendations, so far as can be determined, provide no benefit and create unnecessary anxiety and expense.[102,103]

Table 5.3. Use of Antinuclear Antibodies in Diagnosis of Rheumatic Disease

Antibodies Specific for Disease		
Anti -	Sm	SLE
	SCl-70	Scleroderma
	Centromere	CREST scleroderma

Antibodies Used in Establishing ANA Profiles		
	Most frequent in	*Also Present in*
Antihistone	Drug-induced SLE (90%)	SLE, RA
Anti-RNP	MCTD (100%)	SLE, RA, Sjögren's syndrome
Ro, La (SS-A, SS-B)	Sjögren's syndrome without RA	SLE
Rheumatoid arthritis preciptin (RAP)	Sjögren's syndrome with RA	RA

Immunofluorescent Tests for Demonstrating Antinuclear Antibodies in Skin (the Lupus Band Test)

IgG or IgM antinuclear antibodies, with or without complement, can be demonstrated in *both* normal skin and lesional skin in patients with SLE and in patients with other connective-tissue diseases.[104] In patients with discoid lupus, the test is positive only in the lesional skin. Less intense reactions may be found in a variety of other disorders, including chronically sun-damaged skin, malignancy, infections, and certain endocrinologic disorders, so the test is not wholly specific for SLE. Although the deposition of immune complexes in the skin is of great interest, its relationship to the production of skin lesions is still unclear.

At times, the lupus band test, *performed on normal skin from an unexposed site*, helps to differentiate between cutaneous and systemic lupus or between lupus and other connective-tissue disorders. Its major (and rare) utility in our clinic, however, is for the occasional patient with equivocal signs and symptoms of lupus who has negative LE cell preparations and negative ANAs but a positive lupus band test, lending support to a presumed diagnosis of SLE. It may occasionally also be helpful in patients treated without a prior firm diagnosis, especially those with *membranous* nephritis who have a high incidence of negative ANA and LE preparations.[105,106] Lupus band test positivity correlates with disease activity, but studies trying to relate the test to renal disease have not been conclusive, and we do not find this test useful for regulating treatment.[107]

Anticardiolipin Antibodies

The presence of acquired antiphospholipid antibodies resulting in a biologic false-positive serologic test for syphilis, and of similar circulating anticoagulant antibodies which cause prolongation of the APTT, has been long known to be a feature of many patients with lupus. These antibodies are not specific for SLE and occur in other rheumatic and infectious diseases and occasionally in otherwise-normal children.[108,109] In recent years two additional tests to demonstrate anticardiolipin antibodies, an ELISA and a modified mixing PTT with kaolin, have come into common use. While the exact significance of the presence of each of these antibodies in SLE requires more study, they do seem to be generally associated with increased risk of thrombopenia, mitral- and aortic-valve disease with vegetations, pulmonary hypertension,[109a,110] thromboembolism,[110] adrenal insufficiency,[110a-110b] migraine, transient ischemic attacks, strokes, chorea, livedo reticularis[111] and recurrent fetal distress or death of the fetus with spontaneous abortion.[112-118] The presence of cofactor antibodies to β_2 glycoprotein I increases the risk of thrombosis.[118a] It is not yet certain whether any changes in therapy are indicated by the presence of these antibodies. However, in patients with these antibodies who have had *serious* thrombosis we maintain anticoagulation permanently.[119,120] Screening all patients with conditions for which ACA is a known risk factor leads to identification of a group of individuals who do not fulfill current diagnostic criteria for SLE; this has been called the "anticardiolipin syndrome."[113]

Occasional patients with anticardiolipin antibodies also have antibodies to other clotting factors resulting in increased risk of hemorrhage.[119,121,122] These patients may not be identifiable prior to surgery, leading some physicians to treat all such patients with steroids prior to surgery.[122,123]

The Pathology of SLE

Although it is sometimes referred to as a "collagen disease," there is no disorder of collagen in SLE.[20] The term *collagen disease* is a frequently used but inappropriate misnomer that often reflects sloppy diagnostic thinking. The two major unique pathologic findings in SLE are deposits of fibrinoid in blood-vessel walls and hematoxylin-staining degenerate nuclei (hematoxylin bodies) in affected tissues. Small arteries and arterioles of all organs may be affected, resulting in multisystem disease with manifestations in skin, subcutaneous tissue, fat, joints, muscles, tendons, kidney, heart, nervous system, lungs, and all gastrointestinal organs. Rheumatoid nodules (granulomas) are also seen in some patients.

Renal Pathology in SLE

The most extensive pathologic studies in SLE have been of the kidney since that organ's failure is the single most common cause of mortality. Renal biopsy provides a visual reflection of the microangiopathy of immune-complex disease.[5] In our experience, no SLE patient's kidney studied by light microscopy (LM), electron microscopes (EM), and immunofluorescent

(IF) techniques has been normal.[105] All have shown at least minimal abnormality with one or another of these methods. It is possible that if equally sophisticated pathologic studies were performed in other organs, similar pathologic changes could be demonstrated in every organ in all lupus patients.[124]

In our experience, renal biopsies of untreated patients with consistently normal urinalyses and creatinine clearance do not reveal lesions outside the mesangium, although others have reported occasional patients with generalized disease discovered solely as a result of renal biopsy despite normal renal function, urine sediment, and absence of proteinuria.[124–128] If every child with lupus has a renal biopsy at the time of diagnosis, only 7% will be normal.[129]

A system of classifying renal involvement was initially proposed by Baldwin[130] and has been continuously modified as a result of multi-institutional study under the auspices of the World Health Organization (WHO).[131] Determinations of morphologic patterns (histologic classes) of renal involvement in SLE is of general prognostic value since renal-biopsy findings defined in this fashion may be correlated statistically with prognosis (Fig. 5.5).[132,133] We use the WHO-proposed classification criteria as modified by Appel et al. in 1978.[105]

Mixed patterns are sometimes seen in the same biopsy, such as class III associated with class V. While these classes might be a reflection of different disorders or different host responses to different stimuli, little evidence has been accumulated to support such a hypothesis in humans. Transformation from one class to another is common, and the weight of evidence at present is

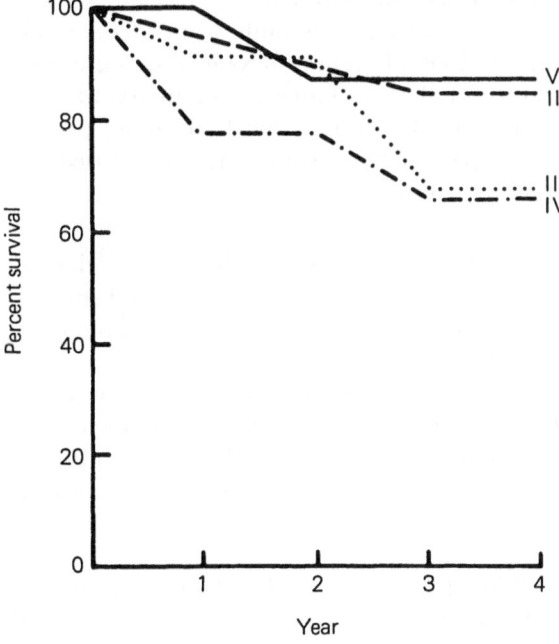

Figure 5.5. The predicted survival, in years, for SLE patients in each renal biopsy histologic class. (Reprinted with permission from Appel et al., ref. 105, copyright 1978, the Williams & Wilkins Co.)

that at least in the case of classes III and IV and probably in all classes, these divisions merely reflect severity of one disease process.[105]

Morphologic Classes or Patterns of Renal Involvement in SLE[105]

Class I: Normal Kidneys. No detectable changes by LM, EM, and IF.

Class II: Mesangial Changes

Class IIA: Minimal Alteration. No changes by light microscopy (Fig. 5.6A). By IF, deposits of immunoglobulin and complement in mesangial areas. Electron-dense deposits usually seen by EM in the mesangium (Fig. 5.6B). Experimental mesangial disease can be created by the injection of immune complexes into the circulation.[67]

Class IIB: Mesangial Glomerulitis. Segmental or global, focal or diffuse hypercellularity confined to the mesangium (more than three cells per mesangial area away from the vascular pole in 2- to 4-μm sections) and/or increased matrix with widening of the mesangial stalk (Fig. 5.7). No changes in the peripheral capillary wall. By EM and by IF, deposits of immunoglobulins and complement in the mesangial areas only. Tubular, vascular, and interstitial changes typically minimal or absent.

Class III: Focal and Segmental Proliferative Glomerulonephritis. In addition to mesangial changes as defined in class II, less than 50% of glomeruli involved with focal and segmental areas of intra- and often extracapillary cell proliferation, necrosis, karyorrhexis, and leukocytic infiltration affecting the capillary loops (Fig. 5.8). By EM and IF, abundant mesangial deposits and frequently subendothelial deposits. Tubular changes and interstitial inflammation (lymphocytes and plasma cells) usually focal and more prominent around glomeruli. A similar pattern may sometimes be created by injection of immune complexes into the circulation.

Class IV: Diffuse Proliferative Glomerulonephritis. Changes similar to those of class III but involving more glomerular surface area and greater than 50% of glomeruli (Fig. 5.9A). Subendothelial deposits often abundant and correspond to wire loops seen by LM (Fig. 5.9B).

The membranoproliferative variant of diffuse proliferative glomerulonephritis is characterized by prominent mesangial cell proliferation, circumferential mesangial extensions with reduplication of the basement membrane, lobular glomerular appearance, and either absent or minimal necrotizing changes.

Class V: Membranous Glomerulonephritis. Normal cellularity of glomeruli. Capillary walls diffusely and uniformly thickened (Fig. 5.10A). By IF

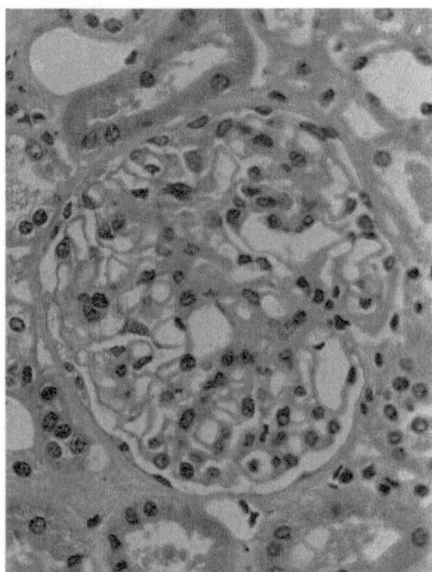

Figure 5.6. Class IIA. (**A**) Essentially normal glomerulus. H&E × 480. (**B**) Mesangial electron-dense deposits as seen in class IIA and IIB biopsies (*arrows*). (**A**: Reprinted with permission from Appel et al., ref. 64, copyright 1978, the Williams & Wilkins Co. **B**: Reprinted with permission from Pirani C.L., Silva F.G. In Churg J., et al. (eds.) *Kidney Disease: Present Status*. International Academy of Pathology Monograph Series No. 20. Williams & Wilkins Co., Baltimore, 1979.)

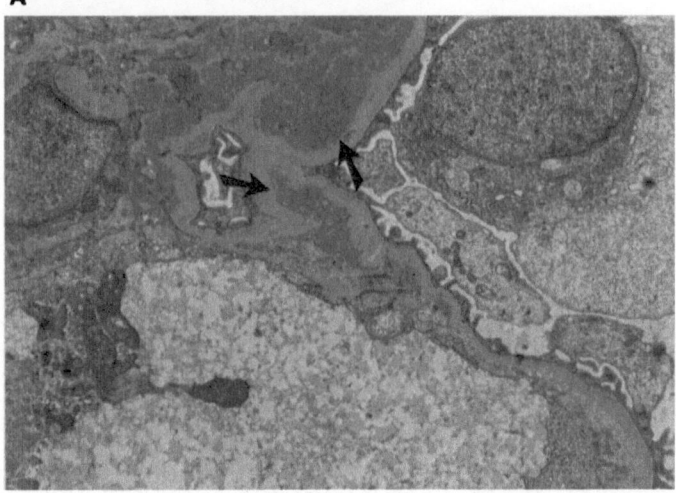

and EM, numerous subepithelial deposits along the GBM (Fig. 5.10B). Deposits also common within GBM and in mesangial areas. Protrusions of GBM-like material or "spikes" between subepithelial deposits. Subendothelial deposits absent or minimal and located near the mesangium. Tubular and interstitial changes less pronounced than in classes III and IV. This pattern cannot be experimentally created by circulating immune complexes that do not undergo intravascular dissociation.[67]

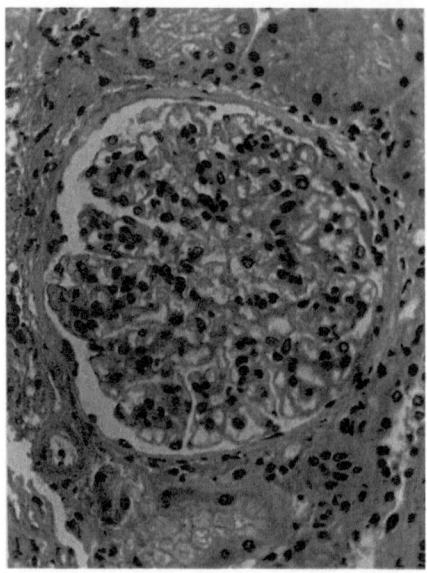

Figure 5.7. Class IIB. Mesangial glomerulitis. Representative glomerulus with mild diffuse mesangial hypercellularity. Tubules and interstitium are normal. H&E × 325. (Reprinted with permission from Appel et al., ref. 105.)

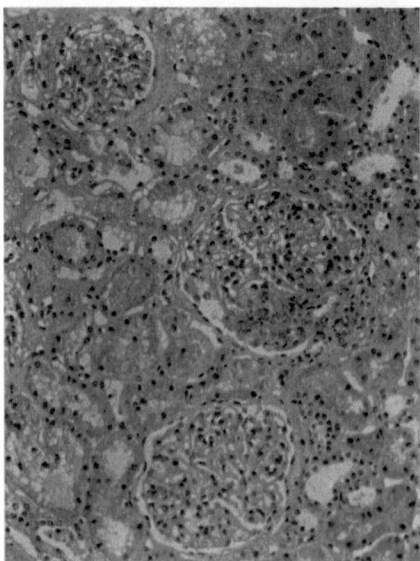

Figure 5.8. Class III. focal and segmental proliferative glomerulonephritis. Three glomeruli are seen. The one in the center exhibits segmental hypercellularity. A few inflammatory cells are present near this glomerulus. H&E × 176. (Reprinted with permission from Appel et al., ref. 105.)

Semiquantitative Scoring of Histologic Features

Activity and Chronicity Index Renal Pathology Scoring. To provide a more detailed description of the renal abnormalities of lupus nephritis for statistical analysis the N.I.H. group has used a semiquantitative scoring system which includes tubular, interstitial, and vascular changes as well as the severity of active and chronic lesions to enhance outcome predictions (Table

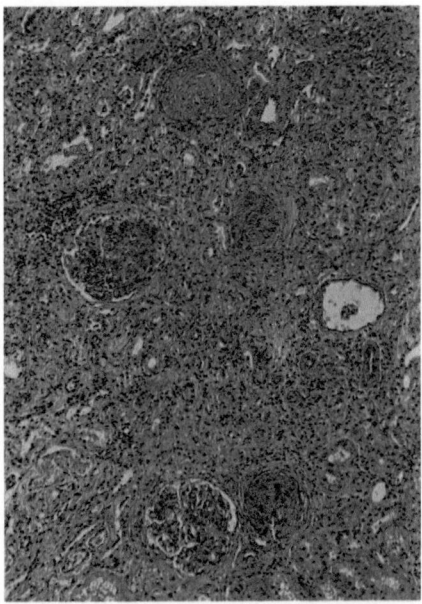

Figure 5.9. Class IV. (**A**) Diffuse proliferative glomerulonephritis. All glomeruli are involved either by proliferative or sclerotic changes. There is moderately severe tubular atrophy, interstitial inflammation, and fibrosis. H&E × 94. (**B**) Subendothelial electron-dense deposits as seen in class III and IV biopsies (*arrow*). Massive deposits indicate a poor prognosis.[134] (**A**: Reprinted with permission from Appel et al., ref. 105. **B**: Reprinted with permission from Pirani C.L., Silva F.G. In Churg J., et al. (eds.) *Kidney Disease: Present Status.* International Academy of Pathology Monograph Series No. 20. Williams & Wilkins, Baltimore, 1979.)

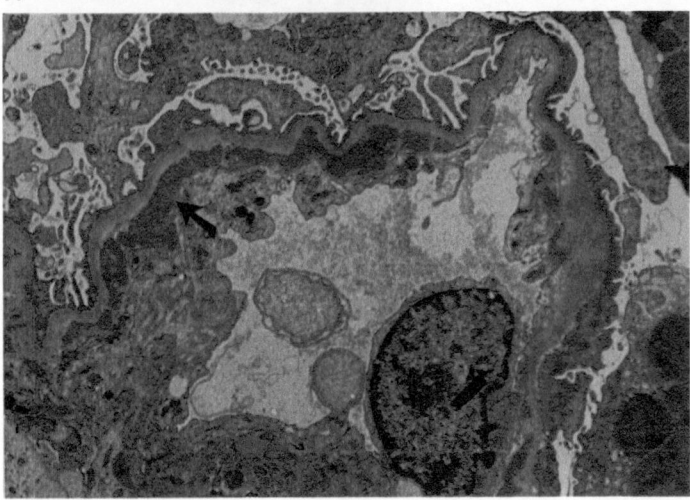

5.4).[135,136] The simultaneous occurrence of tubular atrophy, glomerular sclerosis, and cellular crescents identifies a very-high-risk subgroup among patients with diffuse proliferative disease.[136] A recent Dutch study confirmed that in young patients a chronicity index >3 was a poor prognostic sign for renal survival.[137] In a study of 20 children with class IV lupus nephritis seen between 1970 and 1984, 12/20 had a chronicity index >3 at the time of the initial biopsy; these children were at higher risk of a downward clinical course despite treatment with steroids and azathioprine.[138]

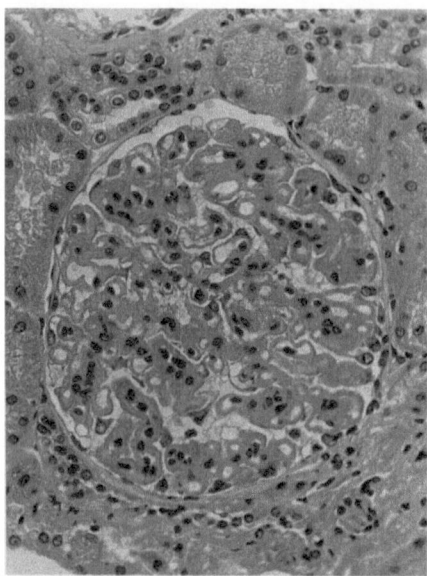

Figure 5.10. Class V. (**A**) Membranous glomerulonephropathy. Representative glomerulus with diffuse thickening of the capillary walls and mild segmental mesangial hypercellularity. H&E × 325. (**B**) Subepithelial electron-dense deposits as seen in class V biopsies (*arrows*). (**A**: Reprinted with permission from Appel et al., ref. 105. **B**: Reprinted with permission from Pirani C.L., Silva F.G. In Churg J., et al. (eds.) *Kidney Disease: Present Status*. International Academy of Pathology Monograph Series No. 20. Williams & Wilkins, Baltimore, 1979.)

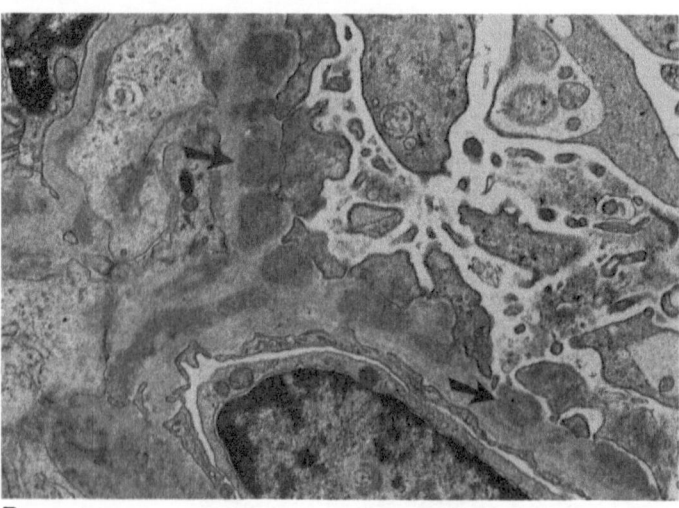

The Clinical Utilization of Information Obtained from Renal Biopsy

No pathologic parameters have so far been described that allow prediction of those at risk for transformation or progression, and even class IIA patients may progress rapidly to renal failure and death.[105,130,139] Thus, on the basis of presently available information, renal-biopsy findings alone cannot be suc-

Table 5.4 Inventory of Specific Renal Pathologic Lesions*

Activity Index (range 0 to 24)
Glomerular lesions
   Cellular proliferation
   Fibrinoid necrosis/karyorrhexis
   Hyaline thrombi
   Cellular crescents
   Leukocytic exudation
Tubulointerstitial lesions
   Mononuclear cell infiltration

Chronicity Index (range 0 to 12)
Glomerular lesions
   Sclerotic glomeruli
   Fibrous crescents
Tubulointerstitial lesions
   Tubular atrophy
   Interstitial fibrosis

* Individual lesions are scored 0 to 3+ (absent, mild, moderate, severe). Necrosis/karyorrhexis and cellular crescents are weighted by a factor of 2. Indexes are composite of scores for individual lesions in each category of activity or chronicity.
(Reprinted with permission from Balow I.E. ref. 136.)

cessfully used to determine treatment. If on the basis of a class IIA finding one offers less treatment, an individual may be allowed to progress unnecessarily to renal failure and death.[105,130,137,139]

However, severity of pathology shown on biopsy may be an aid to therapeutic decision-making. For example, when proliferative lesions are seen, there is less leeway for error in strategy. Progression from class III to class IV or V is associated with an almost certain expectation of renal failure.[105,130] Awareness of the risk of this progression may sharpen the clinician's intuition in class III patients and provide an incentive to both patient and physician for close monitoring and more aggressive (albeit hazardous) intervention if laboratory parameters suggest an increase in aggressiveness of the disease.

Conversely, class II patients have a relatively good prognosis in terms of potential for renal failure and so must be treated with a regimen that aims at prevention of progression of renal disease but takes no risk of causing death from complications of treatment. When this principle is not followed, deaths from treatment in this group may exceed deaths from disease.[105]

The clinician must be aware of two special problems that exist for patients demonstrated to be in class V. While overall such patients have a better prognosis after 4 years of disease, in the Columbia study 20% of class V patients had died within 8 years of the initial biopsy.[105] In these patients, autopsy showed this to be a result of transformation to more active forms of lupus nephritis. Baldwin has emphasized the improved prognosis for class V patients whose nephrotic syndrome can be brought into remission.[130] Thus, one challenge for therapy of class V patients is to promptly identify any tendency toward recrudescence of active disease that would require more aggressive therapeutic intervention to prevent progressive renal failure. Complacence based on class V biopsy findings can result in inadequate therapy; at the same time, the therapeutic regimen for class V patients must also carefully avoid unnecessary treatment that may cause deaths from complications of therapy.

The second special challenge of class V patients is their tendency to develop renal vein thrombosis, which puts them at considerable additional risk of pulmonary embolism.[140] Misinterpretation of proteinuria caused by renal vein thrombosis can result in inappropriate hazardous immunosuppressive therapy, whereas prompt diagnosis of renal-vein thrombosis and appropriate anticoagulation may prolong life in these patients.[141–144]

When data obtained from renal biopsy are used in this fashion to sharpen diagnostic and therapeutic decision-making, it may be helpful. Our experience suggests that if arbitrary regimens of therapy are prescribed solely on the basis of renal-biopsy findings, morbidity and mortality from the therapy in some patients may be sufficiently high to obscure the benefits obtained in others. This results in statistical data suggesting that no therapy equals any therapeutic regimen, a conclusion clearly outside the experience of anyone caring for children with this disease.

At present, no matter how mild the biopsy findings, no child with SLE should be considered safe from progression of renal disease. Moreover, no matter how "bad" the biopsy appears, there may still be room for improvement in renal function and morphology with therapy.[130,139] A biopsy obtained a few months previously is of limited value in making clinical decisions today; sampling errors and differing interpretations of the same slide by different observers further compromise the clinical utility of biopsies. In one clinic, when predictive information was studied by biopsy classification, by clinical classification, and by biopsy and clinical information combined, the total prognostic content was essentially that of the clinical information alone.[145] Knowledge of renal-biopsy results has generally failed to add important prognostic information about the future course of treated lupus nephritis to information already obtained from history, physical examination, and laboratory tests.[146] Thus, renal biopsy provides only a marginally useful increment in decision making at significant cost and hazard. However, in a disease requiring as complicated decision making as SLE, even marginal contributions may be valuable.

Estimating Prognosis in SLE

The importance of estimating the prognosis in determining the therapy for an individual patient in a disease of such variable severity and with such varied manifestations cannot be overestimated.[145-148] In a multicenter study of 1103 patients the presence of high serum creatinine and/or large amounts of urinary protein when first seen in 1965–1976 was associated with early death in large numbers of patients.[149] Patients with multisystem involvement at onset (seven or more ACR criteria) did poorly in the long run (63% were dead at 10 years). Patients with SS-B/La antibodies may have a better prognosis than others.[150]

The presence of low serum albumin, low hematocrit (<25), or low serum total hemolytic complement (<50) is also correlated with a poor prognosis in terms of renal function and survival.[145,147] Thrombocytopenia below 50,000/mm^3 in patients with severe disease is also extraordinarily dangerous, resulting in 100% death within 4 weeks in one series, indicating the need for aggressive intervention in that situation.[145,147] An elevated level of anti-DNA antibodies is less significant than low albumin, low hematocrit, or low complement in predicting deterioration. Other important observations of these studies were that progressive renal impairment was most likely in the first year and that new abnormalities were less likely to occur in the later years of disease.[145,147] These observations match our own: SLE in childhood tends to become a chronic disease of lower virulence provided the first few years are survived without severe permanent damage.[148,151]

Patients who are entered into a study with a longer average interval between onset of first symptom and entry have an overall better prognosis, since death is most common early in the course of disease.[9,20,147,148] Our own reported data in children are biased in this fashion. Also, studies such as our own, where no patients are lost to follow-up, achieve better survival since living patients are more likely to move away and be lost to the study than those who have died. All of these variables tend to be less significant when all of a large series of patients survive for 5–10 years after onset of symptoms. Survival data reported from a single institution become of general significance when survival is 100%. At that point, differences related to differing patient populations presenting to different institutions and varying points of entry into the study become less important. There is an increasing need for separate analysis of patients on dialysis or with "renal death."

Effects of Age, Sex, Race, and Socioeconomic Status on Prognosis. Although it used to be thought that lupus with early childhood onset tended to be more severe than lupus presenting after the 10th birthday, there is little evidence to support that belief.[152,153] Males are more severely affected.[154-156] Black and Hispanic patients do worse than whites[157] both in terms of frequency of renal disease and the outcome.[158] The prognosis for blacks with renal disease is not significantly different from whites if one controls for socioeconomic status, but the poor and poorly educated lupus patients with renal disease are at higher risk of renal failure than those with higher education and economic status.[158] They are also less likely to survive renal failure.[159,160]

Table 5.5. Causes of Death in Childhood SLE

First 5 Years of Disease	*Death in Adult Long-Term Survivors*
Infection	Pulmonary hypertension
Renal disease	Pulmonary embolism
Pulmonary hemorrhage	Infection
Management accidents in lupus crisis	Hypertension and stroke
	Myocardial infarction
	Suicide and Accident
	Renal disease

Causes of Death in SLE (Table 5.5)

The single most common cause of death is renal failure, but renal disease accounts for less than half of all deaths in SLE and did not account for most deaths even prior to dialysis and transplantation.[9–12,15,20,148,161–173] A major cause of death prior to the antibiotic era was infection, to which patients are more prone than normal. As deaths from renal disease have decreased, infection, enhanced by steroids and immunosuppressive drugs, has again become a major cause of fatality in some clinics where therapeutic regimens reduce renal death but at too high a risk for infection.[174] In some series CNS disease and bleeding from uncontrolled thrombocytopenia are frequent cause of death.[147] Many deaths in SLE occur from lack of control of complex disease manifestations.[147,175]

Recent deaths in adult long-term survivors of our earlier-reported children have been a result of pulmonary hypertension, late-diagnosed septic infection after tooth extraction, and pulmonary emboli and uncontrolled systemic hypertension following pregnancy. All were potentially preventable. In some other clinics, premature myocardial infarction and stroke are accounting for increased deaths in long-term childhood lupus survivors.[176] Suicide and accidents have also been important causes of loss in some clinics and may also be preventable.[20]

Lupus series often include large numbers of patients in whom the cause of death was not understood. Yet in therapeutic decision-making, it is most important for the physician to be aware of the various potential routes of demise. The large number of unexplained deaths may be interpreted as an indication of the need for safe control of the multisystem disease to avoid the physician being presented with mortal problems beyond clinical comprehension or control.

Spontaneous Remission in SLE

In a 1968 report, we described a 12-year-old child with SLE and renal disease who remitted without any treatment.[177] She remained well for 20 years before she needed treatment for SLE. At that time, we also reported on a 14-year-old girl with SLE whose aunt also had SLE. This girl had only a very brief course of low-dose prednisone following which she became well. She remained well, married, and had an uneventful pregnancy. A complete evaluation when she visited New York in 1978 showed that there was no longer any serologic evidence of SLE; the previously positive LE preparation, ANA, VDRL, and Coombs' test were all now negative. However, total hemolytic complement was low (105 CH50 units; nl = 155–210), although the determination of complement components did not demonstrate a deficiency of any presently identifiable component. Her first subsequent treatment for lupus was in 1983, 18 years after diagnosis. We have now seen three additional children with a family history of rheumatic disease who had brief self-limited lupuslike episodes after sun exposure. One is heterozygous C2-deficient. The other two have persistently low total hemolytic complements (as does one parent), although we are not yet able to document the presumed specific heritable complement deficiency.

Ropes[178] and Dubois[20] have emphasized the frequency of spontaneous remissions in adults with SLE. In their experience, 35–70% remit for from a few months to 10 or 20 years. Long remissions may also follow years of serious disease.[179] After 5 years without disease patients tend to remain well for many years.[180,181] Recent studies suggest that patients with quiescent lupus who are taking hydroxychloroquine are less likely to have a clinical flare.[182] The potential for spontaneous remission is important to understand for the care of patients, for interpretation of reports of therapeutic triumphs, and for its potential to teach us about the mechanisms involved in induction of SLE in susceptible individuals.

Several models for global assessment of disease activity are currently being developed.[182a]

The Clinical Picture of SLE in Childhood

Presenting Manifestations

Most children with SLE present with fever, arthralgia or arthritis, rashes, myalgia, malaise, fatigue, and weight loss. Abdominal pain, mouth sores, alopecia, and headache are also frequent.[9,12] A history of sun sensitivity is commonly elicited, as is a history of Raynaud's phenomenon. Lymphadenopathy and hepatosplenomegaly are commonly found on physical examination. Recurrent salivary gland swelling may occur, occasionally with dry eyes and dry mouth (Sjögren's syndrome). Laboratory evidence of renal and hematologic involvement is often demonstrable, and occasional children present solely with hematologic or renal manifestations.[183] Protein-losing enteropathy, acute or chronic constrictive pericarditis, interstitial pneumonia, and hyperlipidemia are occasionally the primary presenting manifestations.[184,185] Occasionally, neurologic or psychiatric symptoms predominate; chorea may antedate the onset of SLE by many years. SLE may mimic many other diseases and may present in many different ways.[9–13,15,20,145] In several of our patients the initial presentation was over-whelming sepsis.

Diagnosis

Initially, the diagnosis of SLE depended on the appearance of the classic butterfly rash. After Hargraves discovered the LE cell in 1948, diagnosis was based on the presence of such cells in a patient with multisystem disease; RA, lupoid hepatitis, and drug-induced disease had to be excluded.[20] These di-agnostic criteria have excellent specificity but do not allow for inclusion of patients with negative LE cell preparations. In 1971, a group of experienced rheumatologists under the auspices of the American Rheumatism Associa-tion (ARA) established a set of "classification" criteria that have 90% sensi-tivity and 98–99% specificity for SLE (Table 5.6).[90] The ARA (ACR) criteria have now been modified to include Sm antinuclear antibodies and anti-DNA antibodies, very specific laboratory determinations more exten-sively developed since the criteria were promulgated. A major criticism of the criteria has been that they do not identify patients early enough and that up

Table 5.6. Diagnostic Criteria of SLE (1982)[186,189]

Mucocutaneous Lesions
Butterfly rash
Discoid lupus
Photosensitivity
Oral or nasopharyngeal ulcers

Arthritis without deformity

Serositis
Pleurisy or pericarditis

Renal Disease
Proteinuria (>0.5 g daily) or cellular casts

Hematologic Abnormalities
Hemolytic anemia or leukopenia or lymphopenia or thrombocytopenia
LE cells or anti-DNA antibodies or Sm antigens or chronic false-positive test for
   syphilis
Positive fluorescence test for ANA

Neurologic Manifestations
Psychosis, convulsions, cerebral arteritis,* transverse myelitis,* peripheral
   neuropathy*

---

*Author's modifications from ACR criteria.
Note: Four of 11 items listed above are ultimately present in 96% of SLE patients; specificity is 96–99%.

to one-third of patients with SLE do not fulfill these criteria at the time of the first visit to the physician for the illness.[186-188]

As in all such proposed criteria, the physicians constructing the criteria sought an acceptable definition of patients for multi-institutional study of epidemiology, natural history, and efficacy of therapy rather than a set of diagnostic criteria. All experienced physicians make the diagnosis of SLE in patients who do not fulfill these criteria. Errors of diagnosis are more frequent in such "probable SLE" groups, and so they are generally omitted from multi-institutional studies to avoid differing investigator biases. The criteria serve an educational function; recognizing this, physicians tend to adopt them as diagnostic criteria. In inexperienced hands, such criteria lead to improved accuracy of positive diagnosis, but all large clinics include patients who are best considered to have SLE who do not fulfill these criteria, and not fulfilling these criteria does not exclude SLE as a diagnosis. Since patients are at greatly increased risk early in the course of the disease, there is no alternative to close monitoring and appropriate treatment of patients with SLE who do not fulfill these criteria for diagnosis.

One addendum to these criteria we would propose is the presumption that lupus is drug-induced in any child who develops the first sign of SLE while already receiving anticonvulsant medications or other drugs known to be capable of inducing lupus. This presumption may later be abandoned if not confirmed by the clinical course of the disease after the presumed offending agent is withdrawn. We have now seen two children whose DI-SLE remitted for years after withdrawal of anticonvulsant medication who then, years later, developed SLE. It seems likely that children with DI-SLE may be predisposed to develop SLE; however, only a few do so.

Clinical Manifestations[9-15,20,126,145,190]

Fever

In most children, the fever is low grade, reaching 102°F daily and returning toward normal. In occasional patients, there may be daily spikes to 104°F or more.

Weight Loss

Loss of weight is related to fever, anorexia, and mouth sores but seems more prominent in SLE than in other disorders. In some cases, great emaciation occurs (Fig. 5.11).

Rashes

Most children with SLE have a butterfly rash over the bridge of the nose and on the malar areas (see Figs. 5.1 and 5.3). Ro+ individuals are twice as likely

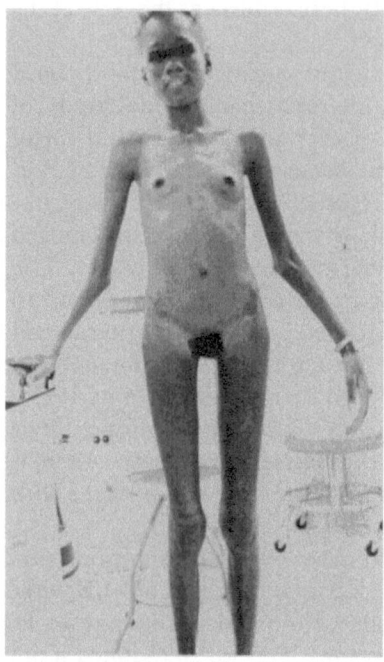

Figure 5.11. Girl, $15\frac{1}{2}$ years old, who had un-treated SLE for 8 months, with 30% weight loss (from 98 to 68 pounds). Psychotic behavior and other manifestations could be controlled with daily prednisone, but not with alternate-day prednisone (150 mg qod); psychosis was controlled by prednisone, 150 mg qod plus azathioprine, 75 mg daily.

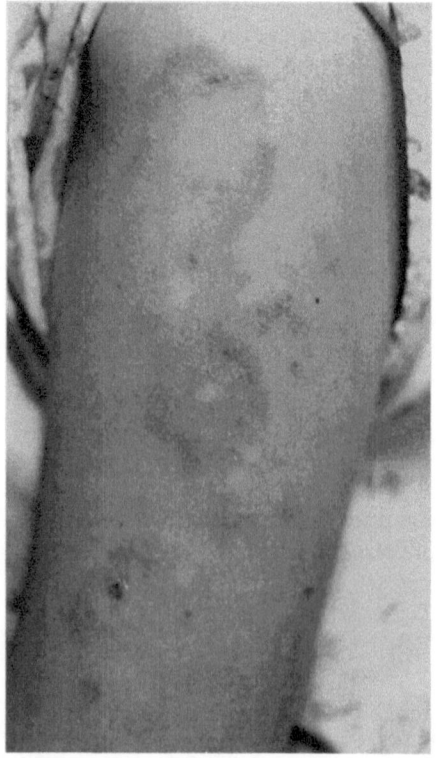

Figure 5.12. Discoid lupus lesions on arm of 11-year-old with SLE.

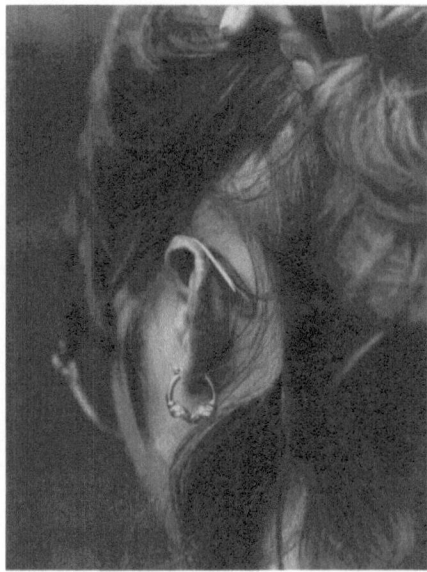

Figure 5.13. Discold lesions of ear pinna leading to diagnosis of SLE.

as other lupus patients to be photosensitive.[191] While in most cases the rash is maculopapular with fine scales, occasionally there are discoid lesions, and some children have only an erythematous blush. A similar rash in the V area of the anterior chest has been emphasized in adults but is rarely seen in children. Papules similar to those on the face may be seen on the extensor

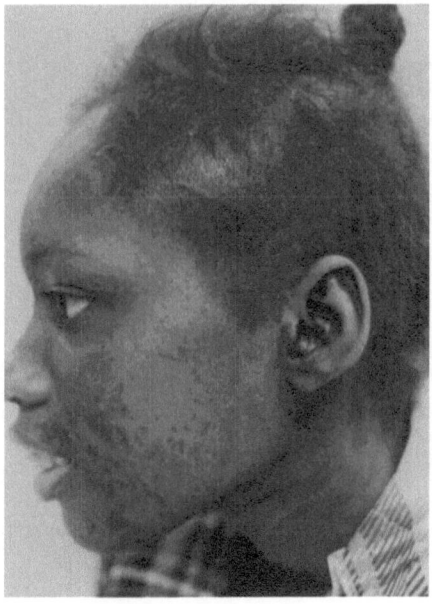

Figure 5.14 Facial and scalp hyperpigmentation seen in some black patients with SLE. Alopecia and frontal hair fracturing are apparent.

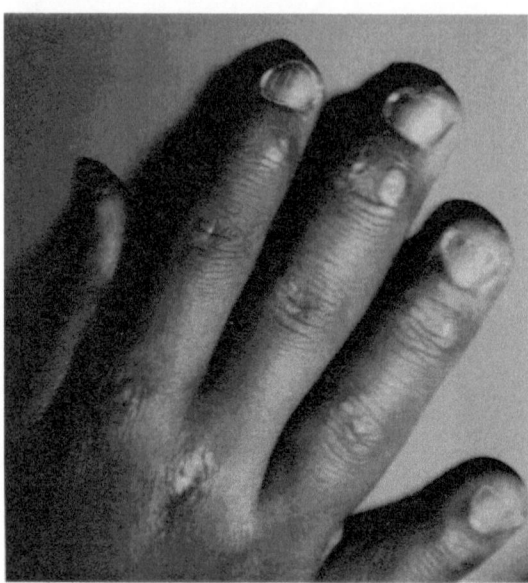

Figure 5.15. Blue discoloration of fingernails in a child with Ro + ANA – systemic lupus presenting with liver disease and discoid lesions of the ears similar to those in Fig. 5.13. Same patient as Fig. 5.19.

surfaces of the arms (Fig. 5.12) or solely on ear pinnae (Fig. 5.13). Diffuse hyperpigmentation may appear at sites of prior skin lesions, especially in blacks (Fig. 5.14); this may appear as a dark blue-black color to the fingernails (Fig. 5.15).[192] Sometimes the skin lesions ulcerate and crust (Fig. 5.3). Ulcerated infarcted lesions are frequent on the hands, especially on the

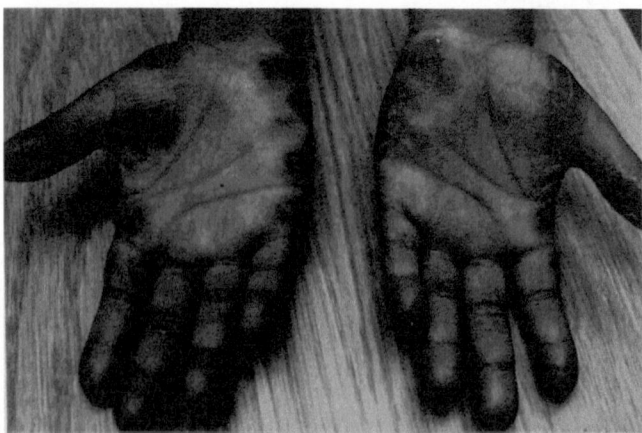

Figure 5.16. Digital and palmer necrotic vasculitic infarcts and ulcers are frequent in children with SLE.

palms (Fig. 5.16). Multiforme and purpuric lesions may also be seen. Subcutaneous nodules caused by panniculitis were common in our patients (see Prologue), and rheumatoid nodules may also occur.

Widespread photosensitive dermatophyte infections or pityriasis may mimic exacerbations of SLE.[193] Franks has recently published an extensive review of the dermatologic manifestations of SLE.[194]

Bullous SLE

Bullous (pemphigoidlike) lesions in SLE are rare but a disproportionate number of affected individuals are children.[195–199] Control may depend on the mechanisms involved in the pathogenesis of the bullae in the individual patient; where long-lived antibodies are responsible, pheresis may be required. Some patients respond to dapsone but our patient (Fig. 5.17) required plasmapheresis, intravenous cyclophosphamide, and intravenous prednisolone pulses for control.

Mucocutaneous Lesions

Shallow, painful ulcers of the lips (buccal mucosa), gums, and palate occur in 10–15% of patients, especially with exacerbations of disease (Fig. 5.18). Similar lesions are seen occasionally on the vulval surface.

Alopecia

A history of some increase in hair loss may be elicited from practically all patients with SLE and is a characteristic feature of the disease. Although generalized thinning or patches of hair loss may be disturbing to young girls, total alopecia does not occur. In addition to the hair falling out, the frontal hairs are brittle and prone to breaking off, leaving short lengths that stick out in unruly fashion (see Figs. 5.11 and 5.14).

The rash is photosensitive in about 40% of white females and less often in other groups. In some cases, systemic disease exacerbates or seems to have its onset with sun exposure. Contrary to the experience of Dubois, in our children this tends to occur most frequently in spring after the first day of considerable sun exposure. However, the majority of patients do not seem to be photosensitive. We do prohibit sunbathing in all our patients and urge caution about sun exposure. Broad-brim straw hats are in style and very attractive. Walking on the beach in late afternoon seems to do no harm. A reasonable attitude seems appropriate since social life at the beach is important for many of our teenage patients, and it would be wrong to prohibit this activity in its entirety, especially for those patients who are not known to be photosensitive.[20,145]

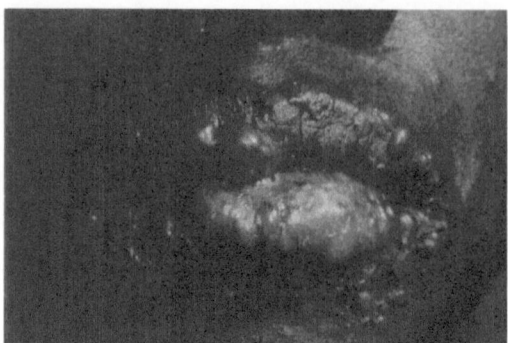

A

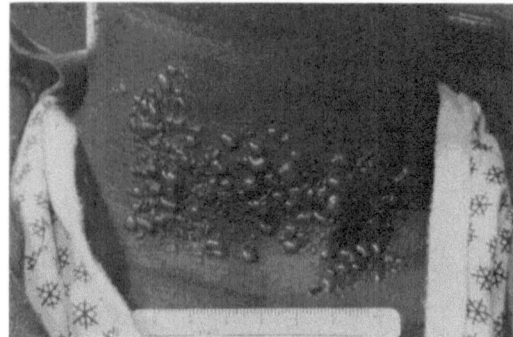

B

Figure 5.17. Bullous lupus. Immunofluorescence revealed thin linear deposits of IgG and C3 (but not IgM) at the dermal-epidermal junction deep down in the basement membrane; NaCl split-skin assay showed serum antiskin antibodies on the dermal side of the split as are seen in epidermolysis bullosa acquisiva and bullous lupus.[200]

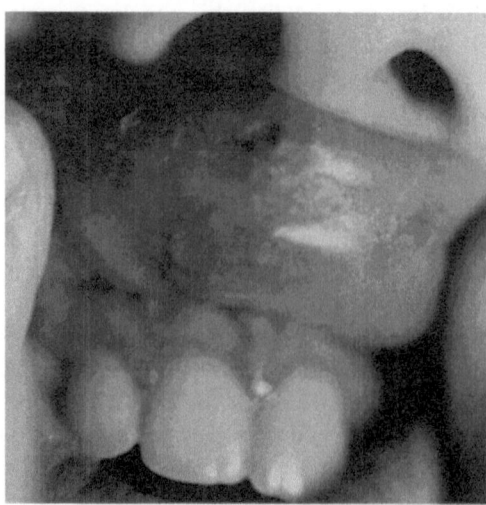

Figure 5.18. Ulcers of the lip and buccal mucosa are one of the diagnostic criteria of SLE.

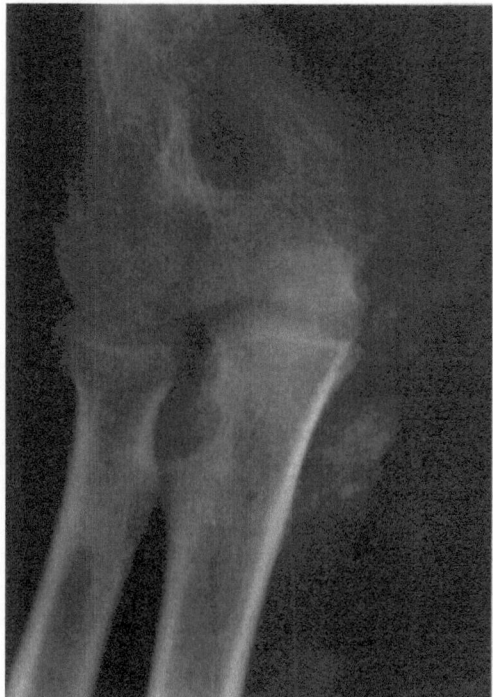

Figure 5.19. Diffuse calcinosis of the elbow with massive bony erosions in a 13-year-old girl with SLE which presented with severe polyarthritis. Same patient as Fig. 5.15.

Arthritis and Arthralgia

The most common arthritic manifestations are pain and transient joint swellings resembling mild RA, but without permanent deformity and scarring and with relatively little demonstrable arthritis at the time of examination. Morning stiffness and weather sensitivity are the same as in other forms of inflammatory arthritis. However, some of our patients have had flexion contractures and an arthritic picture indistinguishable from severe JRA at onset and for varying periods of time, even years, before other manifestations of SLE became apparent (Fig. 5.19). Similar cases have been reported by others;[201–203] hypertension and renal disease are less frequent in those with severe arthritis.[203a] Rheumatoid factor can be demonstrated in the serum of 25% of our childhood SLE patients.

A distinctive deformity of the hands has been reported in SLE (the "lupus hand").[203b,204] This is characterized by severe deformity of the fingers with subluxations that, at least initially, can be corrected by the patient unaided. Generally, there is little erosion or destruction. Ulnar deviation of the hand is typical. These hand deformities have been described under the eponym *Jaccoud's arthritis*, which was initially thought to represent chronic rheumatic fever but in most cases is a manifestation of SLE.[205,206] Patients with Jaccoud's arthropathy tend to have less renal disease.[203b]

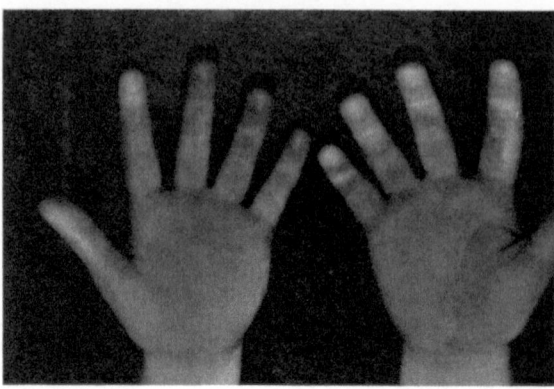

Figure 5.20. Raynaud's phenomenon with pallor and reactive hyperemia both visible at the same time in a 9-year-old boy with MCTD.

Myalgia

Inflammation of capillaries may sometimes be demonstrated in muscle, and myalgias are common. Occasional patients have inflammation and necrosis of muscle with elevation of muscle enzyme levels in blood. Most children seen in the past with severe myositis as part of SLE would probably be included in the subset now called mixed connective-tissue disease.

Raynaud's Phenomenon[207]

History of cold sensitivity with change in color to blue, then white, and then a red suffused dilation phase typical of Raynaud's syndrome may sometimes be elicited (Fig. 5.20). Raynaud's syndrome may precede the appearance of other signs of SLE by many years. Sometimes the fingers or toes are swollen and blue, and gangrene may occur with loss of a digit. In patients with severe peripheral ischemia treatment with prostaglandin E_1 infusions may save the digit.[207a–207b]

Case Report

A previously healthy 10-year-old black girl presented with 3 days of nighttime paresthesias in her left fourth and fifth fingers. Examination revealed sign of arterial insufficiency threatening loss of parts of the fourth and fifth fingers. Laboratory studies revealed the following abnormalities: CPK 911 (nl < 50 with proportionate increases in LDH, SGOT, SGPT), APTT 36.1 (nl < 35), ESR 30 mm/h, L.E. Prep. + ANA + 1:640 speckled, IgG anticardiolipin 1:322 (nl < 261), anti-DNA 350 (nl < 230), cryoglobulins + + + +, hemoglobin 11.1 grams, anti-Sm and RNP antibodies +. Further examination revealed mild swelling of PIP and MCP joints and of the knees, edema of the eyelids, generalized lymphadenopathy, a suggestion of a butterfly facial rash and muscle weakness. With treatment with IV solumedrol 1 gram daily plus nifedipine 20 mg qid, she improved daily but the tip of the fourth finger still remained

threatened after 72 h. Solumedrol was replaced after three daily "pulses" with prednisone 15mg q 6 h. At 96 h, when she developed increasing finger pain, an infusion of
PGE_1 was begun at a rate of 0.10 μg/kg/minute and the rate increased as needed to
maintain circulation (0.24 μg/kg/minute).

The dose could be titrated to maintain circulation. After 5 days the fourth distal
digit retained only minimal duskiness and the infusion of PGE_1 was discontinued.
Following discharge the patient moved to North Carolina where after 3 years
her disease continues to be adequately controlled with prednisone, nifedipine, and
hydroxychloroquine.

Gastrointestinal Manifestations

Episodes of abdominal pain ("gastrointestinal crises") are very frequent in
childhood lupus and may be confused with appendicitis or other acute abdominal problems (Table 5.7). Serositis accounts for some of these episodes,
but vasculitis of the mesentery and bowel wall is probably frequent, and
bowel hemorrhage, infarction, and perforation may occur.[20,178,209–211] Ischemic bowel may lead to overwhelming sepsis.[210]

Pancreatitis also occasionally occurs as a manifestation of SLE or may be
a complication of steroid therapy.[212–214] Acute pancreatitis in SLE has been
reported to be associated with an acute respiratory distress syndrome resembling hyaline membrane disease and requiring equally vigorous respiratory therapy.[215] In one child, SLE was reported to present with hyperlipoproteinemia resulting from pancreatitis.[216]

In addition to the acute abdominal crises of untreated or poorly controlled
SLE and those associated with pancreatitis, a third form of abdominal crisis

Table 5.7. Types of Abdominal Crisis in SLE

Serositis
Vasculitis of mesentery and bowel wall
   Hemorrhage
   Infarction
   Perforation (especially of colon)
Pancreatitis
   Related to uncontrolled SLE
   Related to steroid therapy
   Associated with acute respiratory distress
   syndrome
Sepsis with bacterial peritonitis
   Pneumococcal
   Group-A beta-hemolytic streptococcal
   Gram-negative
Intercurrent acute appendicitis, torsion of the
appendix epiploica,[208] etc.

is that associated with overwhelming sepsis, to which these patients are prone.[217] When a well-controlled patient with SLE taking the usual medications suddenly develops fever and abdominal pain, sepsis must be presumed and appropriate treatment instituted immediately. Sepsis associated with peritonitis in SLE may be gram-negative in origin but is also frequently pneumococcal or streptococcal. While acute appendicitis or other coincidental abdominal problems may rarely occur in a child with lupus, our experience is that abdominal problems are frequent in these children but usually are directly related in some fashion to the SLE. Surgery should only be performed when it is essential, as children ill with acute lupus and/or sepsis are not good surgical risks. However, early surgery may be lifesaving in cases of perforation.[209]

Gastrointestinal manifestations of SLE include malacoplakia,[218] hepatic infarctions, veno-occlusive disease, and retroperitoneal fibrosis[218–221a] (Fig. 5.21), ascites,[222,223] and protein-losing enteropathy.[210,224–226] Lupus may present in childhood with these manifestations. Diarrhea is not a common manifestation of childhood lupus, but occasionally a child presents in a fashion similar to ulcerative colitis or ileitis, so the diagnosis of SLE must also be considered in patients presenting with inflammatory bowel disease.

Decision-making in acute abdominal crises of childhood lupus is very difficult. Fortunately, modern management of childhood lupus has greatly reduced the frequency of abdominal crises requiring such decision-making. After careful study to rule out perforation and sepsis, abdominal pain in SLE is treated with prednisone.

Lymphadenopathy and Splenomegaly

Generalized significant lymphadenopathy occurs in 25–70% of children with SLE and may be a prominent presenting manifestation. Lymph nodes may become as large as several centimeters in diameter and suggest the possibility of lymphoma. Biopsied lymph nodes usually show edema and sinus hyperplasia similar to that seen in JRA, but sometimes areas of necrobiosis with masses of hematoxylin-stained material may be seen.[227]

Lymphoma may be associated with positive LE cells, and we have seen one case of acute lymphatic leukemia in which LE cells were demonstrated, raising diagnostic confusion. Lymph-node biopsies and bone-marrow aspirations may be necessary in patients with SLE with lymphadenopathy. Lymphoma and leukemia have not been reported to coexist with SLE in childhood, but they do occasionally coexist in adults. One youngster with both angioimmunoblastic lymphadenopathy and SLE has been described.[228,229]

Figure 5.21. (**A**) Retroperitoneal fibrosis causing renal obstruction in a 12-year-old girl with SLE. The IVP was obtained coincident with the renal biopsy and was noted to show medial deviation and partial obstruction of both ureters. (**B**) Follow-up films were normal after treatment with prednisone and azathioprine.

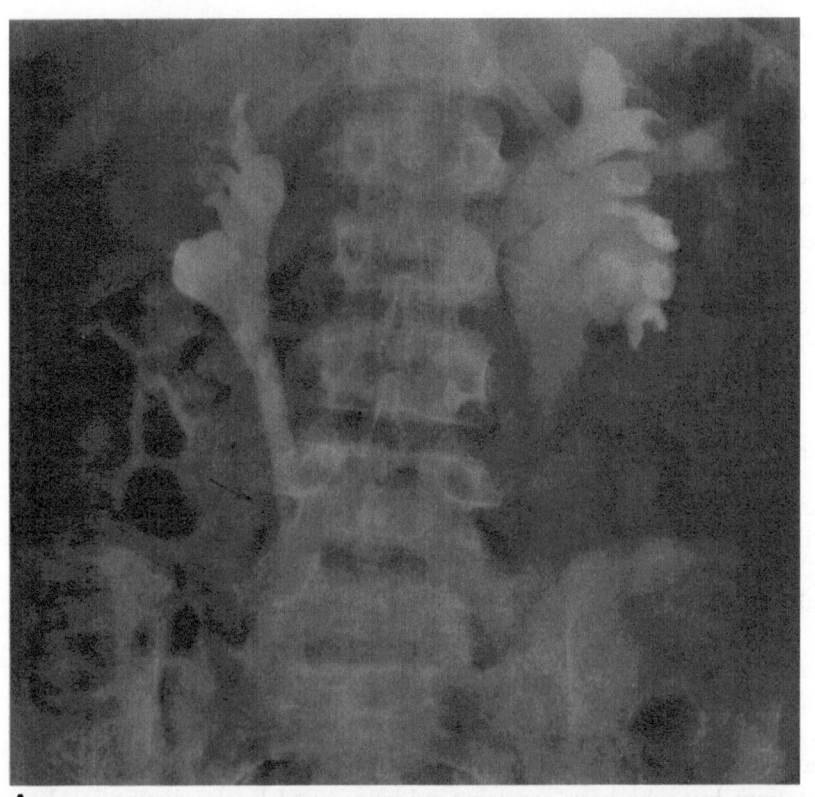

A

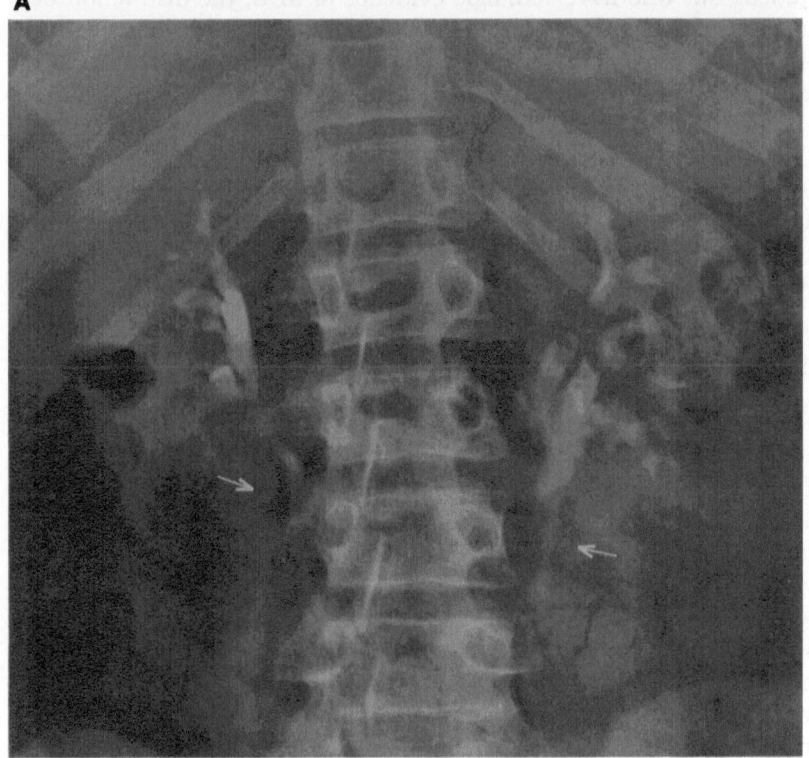

B

Splenomegaly is noted in about 25% of children with SLE. About 80% of spleens examined postmortem in SLE are said to show typical onionskin periarterial fibrosis, and in cases of SLE in which the spleen is removed for thrombocytopenic purpura, typical periarticular lesions often may be seen. In patients with SLE presenting solely with a clinical picture of idiopathic thrombocytopenic purpura (ITP) without other manifestations of SLE, serologic studies may be negative, and the diagnosis of SLE may first be established by demonstrating the lesions in the spleen after splenectomy is performed to control the purpura.

Hepatic Disease

Hepatomegaly occurs in about 15% of children with SLE, and abnormalities of the "liver enzymes" serum glutamic oxalacetic and pyruvic transaminases (SGOT and SGPT) are very common.[230] Jaundice, however, is rare in SLE. In the absence of severe hemolytic anemia, the presence of jaundice suggests that the patient does not have SLE but that the diagnosis is chronic active hepatitis ("lupoid hepatitis"), an illness that resembles SLE and may also be associated with antinuclear and anti-DNA antibodies and LE cells. This process may be very acute and require vigorous therapy.[231]

In patients in whom jaundice and liver disease are the most prominent manifestations but who have serologic evidence of SLE, the distinction between lupoid hepatitis and SLE has generally been made on the basis of liver biopsy. Piecemeal liver necrosis with plasma cell and lymphocyte infiltration have been considered pathognomonic of lupoid hepatitis. Patients with chronic active hepatitis rarely have significant renal disease or other significant organ involvement typical of SLE.

Occasionally, a patient with typical SLE also has chronic active hepatitis as one feature of her disease. Therapeutic regimens for such patients must take into account the degree of liver disease activity as well as the other manifestations of SLE.[230]

Hematologic Manifestations

Almost every patient with SLE has some manifestation of hematologic dysfunction.[20,232,233] *Anemia* (hemoglobin <10 grams) occurs in 50% of children with SLE and, when severe or accompanied by jaundice, is primarily due to autoimmune Coombs'-test-positive hemolytic anemia. SLE may begin in children with autoimmune hemolytic anemia, and years may elapse before other symptoms of lupus occur. However, other factors (e.g., iron deficiency, decreased life-span of red blood cells, and decreased bone-marrow activity) may also contribute to anemia, and most mild anemia in SLE is the "anemia of chronic disease" rather than autoimmune.[232] Occasionally, red cell or marrow hypoplasia or pancytopenia due to hemophagocytosis are seen in children with SLE.[234-235a]

Most forms of anemia in SLE respond to corticosteroid treatment. Anemia associated with renal failure may respond to treatment with recombinant erythropoietin.[236] Antibody-mediated manifestations may respond to intravenous gamma globulin,[237] cyclophosphamide,[238] and apheresis.[239,240] Aplastic anemia may respond to androgens.[241]

Leukopenia (<5000 WBCs/mm^3) is noted in 65% of children with SLE. The white blood cell counts are generally in the 2500–3500/mm^3 range. Although lymphopenia is apparent in the white blood count, the leukopenia is also a result of absolute granulocytopenia. The leukopenia is thought to be a result of antileukocyte antibodies and lymphocytotoxic antibodies and is very rarely due to marrow hypoplasia[242] or antibodies which prevent release from the marrow (myelokathexis).[243]

Case Report

A previously healthy 13-year-old girl developed fever, a malar rash, arthritis, anorexia, and weight loss; significant laboratory studies included ANA 1:1280 (homo), ESR 114, STS +, Coombs +, anti-DNA 358 (<160), C$_3$ 70 (83–177). Echocardiogram showed a small pericardial effusion. WBC was 4100 but fell to 2600. She was treated with prednisone 40 mg daily which was reduced quickly over 4 months to 5 mg daily, at which time (January 1985) she developed *Staphylococcus aureus* osteomyelitis of the right ankle which responded to antibiotic therapy. Prednisone was increased to 40 mg daily, weaned quickly to 25 mg daily, and reduced over the next 3 months to 17.5 mg daily. She transferred to our care in April 1985; laboratory studies revealed ESR 58; SGOT/PT 57/110; anti-DNA antibodies ++++; total hemolytic complement 90(160–210); anti-SM 1:40,960; WBC 3000 (P. 73); urine studies normal. Because the child was very Cushingoid, treatment was changed to prednisone 100 mg on alernate mornings at 7 A.M.; mouth sores and fever occurred in 3 weeks requiring increase to 125 mg qod; 4 weeks later she was noted to have an *E. coli* urinary tract infection, with plasma WBC only 800/mm^3. She was hospitalized and treated with antibiotics and prednisone was increased to 15 mg qid. She improved but WBC increased only to 1500. Bone-marrow aspirant showed maturational arrest at the myelocle stage with normal numbers of myelocytes but decreased erythroid precursors. Despite two plasmapheresis treatments, WBC fell to 900. Treatment with cyclophosphamide, 50 mg daily (1/kg), was then begun. A urinary infection recurred and was treated with trimethoprim-sulfa. Prednisone was changed to 150 mg qod, trimethoprin-sulfa 1 DS tablet continued daily and cyclophosphamide continued. WBC fell to 330 but bone-marrow aspirant was normal aside from slightly decreased polymorphonuclear cells. Prednisone was increased to 200 mg qod because of knee pains and nausea and then reduced again. After 3 months WBC was still only 600, after 6 months 1400, but after 1 year 2700. Prednisone was gradually reduced to 100 qod and after 14 months cyclophosphamide was discontinued. The patient remained well and 5$\frac{1}{2}$ years later is taking only 3 mg of prednisone qod. CBC, ESR, urinalysis, chemistries, and total hemolytic complement are normal and no anti-DNA antibodies are demonstrable.

Recombinant human granulocyte-macrophage colony-stimulating factor (GM-CSF) could now be tried in such a patient.[243a]

Autoimmune thrombocytopenia occurs in 10% of children with SLE and occasionally is the major presenting manifestation; (3–16% of patients with chronic ITP turn out to have SLE 1 to 10 years later).[244] Specific antiplatelet antibody studies may help to identify these individuals.[245] If the thrombopenia is sufficiently severe, petechia, purpura, hemorrhagic vesicles and bullae on the skin, bleeding from the gums, and GI bleeding may be noted.

Thrombopenia but not anticoagulant antibodies must be looked for prior to renal biopsy. Some patients with chronic thrombocytopenia can be managed with small doses of prednisone administered on alternate mornings. Patients unresponsive to this may occasionally be controlled with gamma globulin infusions[246] or with anti-D.[246a] For patients resistant to these regimens long-term danazol may be the the optimum agent.[247–251] Pulse cyclosphosphamide has been effective when other regimens, including splenectomy, have failed.[252] In the past, the indications for splenectomy in SLE were the same as those for other forms of thrombocytopenic purpura. Splenectomy should generally be avoided in SLE.[253,254] If splenectomy is performed, patients and their physicians must be aware of the increased risk of sepsis. Splenectomized children should be given pneumococcal vaccine and prophylactic penicillin therapy.

The circulating anticoagulant found in patients with SLE has no antithrombin activity and is not corrected by protamine; it interferes with prothrombin conversion to thrombin but does not cause bleeding. Rather, it induces a hypercoaguable state as does antithrombin III deficiency, another frequent abnormality in SLE.[255] There is considerable evidence that there is also true hypoprothrombinemia in some children with SLE. These defects often respond dramatically to prednisone treatment and may be corrected in a single day. Antibodies to clotting factors can be suppressed by gamma globulin.[256]

When the "lupus anticoagulant" is associated with clinically significant bleeding, it is because it is associated with hypoprothrombinemia and thrombopenia, which cause the hemorrhage. Deaths from pulmonary hemorrhage in children with lupus are common in some series.[12] These deaths are generally a result of pulmonary vasculitis and/or uncontrolled thrombocytopenia and can be prevented by vigorous treatment.

Thrombophlebitis is also unusually frequent in patients with SLE and, with improved survival, is becoming increasingly important as a cause of death.[257] A multitude of factors favors thrombophlebitis in SLE. Venulitis causes platelet activation, aggregation, and thrombus formation. Circulating anticoagulants cause a compensatory increase in thromboplastin generation and may be associated with very low levels of functional antithrombin III, also favoring thromboembolism.[255,258–260] Disseminated intravascular coagulation,[261] increased serum viscosity, and immobility of a sick patient may all contribute to the propensity to phlebitis. While prednisone has been said to also increase coagulability, our experience suggests that lack of control of the lupus activity is the primary cause of phlebitis in lupus.

Some patients with SLE present solely with the combination of auto-immune hemolytic anemia and thrombocytopenia (Evans syndrome).[262] In most of these children, anti-DNA antibodies and immune-complex formation can be demonstrated even though there are no other clinical manifestations of SLE; if renal biopsy is performed, mesangial deposits typical of SLE may be found even in the absence of abnormalities of the urine sediment.[263] With prompt treatment, most such patients have a more benign course than the usual group of patients with SLE. The potential does exist for the development of more generalized disease within this subset, and the hematologic manifestations may also be life-threatening. However, not all patients with Evans syndrome evolve into SLE[262,264] and, overall, patients with lupus presenting only with hematologic abnormalities have a milder course.[265,266]

Clinical symptoms suggesting arthritis are common in sickle hemoglobinopathies. In general, these are due to hemarthroses, dactylitis, bone infarcts, aseptic necrosis, osteomyelitis, septic arthritis, rheumatic fever, or JRA. Occasionally, a child with hemoglobinopathy also develops SLE, a possibility that must be considered when a child with known sickle-cell disease develops arthritis.[267]

Tests for infectious mononucleosis are commonly positive in SLE.[268,269]

Thrombotic thrombocytopenic purpura may occur as a life-threatening manifestation of SLE requiring daily plasmapheresis and fresh-frozen plasma in addition to other lupus medications.[270] Diagnosis depends on looking for and demonstrating red blood cell fragmentation on smear; failure to perform this simple examination and add the essential therapies will result in death of the patient.[271] (See p. 40.)

Renal Manifestations

Nephritis is clinically evident in 70% of children with SLE.[272]

Urinary Sediment. In our experience, leukocyturia is the most common single or early urinary manifestation of lupus nephritis; red cells and red cell casts tend to appear later and to reflect more aggressive disease than leukocytes alone. Urinary findings in mildly affected individuals vary from one urinalysis to the next; data collected on the basis of single determinations often do not accurately reflect the activity of the disease. Infection must be excluded in all patients with abnormal urinalyses, and obviously the possibility of menstrual red cells must also be excluded.

Hematuria alone has not been a useful prognostic factor in large series of patients with SLE, but it is generally found in patients whose renal biopsies will show *active* histologic lesions, while absence of hematuria is correlated with lack of presence of pathologic evidence of *active* renal lesions at the time of biopsy; however, the confidence limit of these statements is only about 82%.[145]

Proteinuria. Proteinuria is almost always present in patients with severe renal disease. While urinary protein determinations with dipsticks are easily performed, they are not wholly reliable in the low range. Orthostatic proteinuria is common in adolescents. Therefore, proteinuria is best expressed in terms of the more difficult to obtain, accurate 24-h collection.

Fries and Holman have emphasized the significance of the appearance of proteinuria in a lupus patient whose urine previously showed no protein; the likelihood of renal progression in this situation is more than doubled.[145] Increasing proteinuria correlates with decreasing renal function; 24-h quantitative determinations are necessary since 2+ qualitative values may be associated with normal 24-h excretion and 4+ values may represent values between 1 and 13 grams/24 h. The persistence of proteinuria is not a good guide to treatment since proteinuria may persist in patients with no pathologic evidence of active nephritis. Thus, although the advent of proteinuria or increases in the amount of proteinuria are cause for concern and reduction in the amount of protein in the urine is a good sign, persistence of proteinuria is of no necessary consequence.

Nephrotic Syndrome. Massive proteinuria and the nephrotic syndrome are correlated with an increased risk of renal-vein thrombosis. It is not certain that renal-vein thrombosis cannot cause the nephrotic syndrome, but the weight of evidence indicates that it is rather the nephrotic syndrome that predisposes the patient to renal-vein thrombosis. Patients with nephrotic syndrome and renal-vein thrombosis are prone to pulmonary emboli, an increasingly frequent cause of disability and ultimately death in SLE.[141]

Although the nephrotic syndrome occurs in patients with class III nephritis, it is more common in those whose biopsies show class IV and most common in patients with class V disease. Patients with purely membranous lesions on renal biopsy (class V) have an older average age of onset of SLE and a better prognosis than patients in class III or IV.[142] Aside from the lesser significance of proteinuria, however, the slightly improved prognosis for class V patients does not warrant any change in overall clinical management. It is common for patients with purely membranous disease to later develop diffuse proliferative (i.e., mixed) disease as time progresses.[105] In a recently reported series 36% of lupus patients with the nephrotic syndrome went on to renal failure as contrasted with 5% of lupus nephritis patients without the nephrotic syndrome.[273]

In patients with sudden massive increases in proteinuria, renal-vein thrombosis must be considered. Since proteinuria due to renal-vein thrombosis does not respond to prednisone or immunosuppressive therapy, a distinction should be made between increased proteinuria as a reflection of renal-vein thrombosis and increased proteinuria as a sign of more active nephritis. A duplex-Doppler ultrasound and/or a venogram should be done, and if a renal-vein thrombosis is demonstrated, anticoagulants should be given to prevent pulmonary embolism.[143,144]

Serum Creatinine and Creatinine Clearance. Renal function is better in children than in older individuals.[274] Elevation of serum creatinine is a relatively late manifestation of renal disease in SLE and so is not useful for early prediction of outcome. However, a rise in serum creatinine is a bad sign. Death within 2 years of demonstration of elevated serum creatinine (1.3 mg/100 ml) was seven times higher than in those with normal creatinine in Fries' and Holman's series.[145]

Creatinine clearance is a dynamic measurement of renal function. Unfortunately, accuracy of collection is difficult to achieve and a nuisance for the patient. Mobile teenagers resent the nuisance and when obtaining the urine tend to restrict their fluid intake to reduce the number of voidings to be collected. Such collections are inaccurate. Despite all of these problems, we find accurately determined creatinine clearance values a sensitive therapeutic indicator. Two days of cimetidine, 400 mg qid in fully grown individuals, may increase the accuracy of the clearance, which otherwise overestimates glomerular filtration rate by 48%.[275] Decreases in creatinine clearance suggest the need for more vigorous treatment when other parameters are equivocal.[276]

Renal Insufficiency. Patients with acute deterioration of renal function and anuria may respond to treatment and regain satisfactory renal function.[277–280] Acute deterioration of renal function is considered an indication for "pulse" steroid therapy in an effort to gain quick control of the process and cessation of immune-complex formation.[277,278] Pulse therapy has significant potential side effects, the most dangerous of which include life-threatening sepsis disseminating from an occult site of infection.[279] It is of little use in patients with chronic deterioration of renal function.[281]

Peritoneal and renal dialysis may be utilized as in other patients with renal insufficiency.[280] Patients with acute renal failure requiring dialysis may recover and be able to discontinue dialysis.[282] Renal transplantation has been successful in patients with SLE, and only a small number of patients have developed lupus in the transplanted kidney.[283] In part, this is because there is a tendency for the manifestations of active lupus to disappear in patients with chronic renal failure.[284] However, in part, this is also due to the use of immunosuppressive drugs as part of the posttransplantation regime.

Hyperkalemia. Even in the absence of oliguria, lupus patients may have persistent unexplained hyperkalemia, presumably due to immunologic injury to tubules and interstitial tissue. Impaired renin production and subsequently low aldosterone production are the most common causes of this hyperkalemia, which may be dangerously aggrevated by NSAIDs.[285]

Hypertension

Hypertension may be a prominent and life-threatening symptom of SLE and, if not controlled, induces more vasculitis and consequently more hypertension.[286] *If hypertension is not controlled, it tends to cause further deterioration in renal function and ultimately irreversible renal failure.*[286–288a] Children are especially susceptible to hypertensive encephalopathy, and death from stroke and premature coronary occlusion are increased if hypertension is not controlled.[289] Hypertension in SLE is often initially out of all proportion to other manifestations of renal disease and is often greatly aggravated by corticosteroid treatment. Urgent hypertensive crisis can usually be controlled with careful titration of oral doses of clonidine or nifedipine, producing a gradual safe reduction in mean arterial pressure.[290] Captopril and enalopril, inhibitors of angiotension-converting enzyme, are useful agents in these children but may themselves cause membranous nephropathy.[291]

Treatment of hypertension has been greatly improved in recent years. In general, we find the combination of hydrochlorothiazide and propranolol, a diuretic and a beta-blocker, an excellent and well tolerated regimen for these children. In addition to combating the salt- and water-retaining effects of prednisone, this regimen has the conceptual advantage of improving kidney blood flow while lowering blood pressure.[287] Verapramil, a calcium antagonist, has been effective in resistant cases and may become the first-line choice in black patients and patients taking cyclosporine.[292,292a] Potassium supplements are also routinely provided. Pediatricians are generally not the most experienced physicians in the use of antihypertensive drugs, and we have been fortunate in being able to secure advice for each patient from colleagues who devote their full time to the care of patients with hypertension. We are convinced that prompt effective blood-pressure control has significantly improved the prognosis for these children.

We also use hypertension as an indication for adding azathioprine to our therapeutic regimen to help assure control of the disease with alternate-day prednisone. The management of hypertension in these patients is greatly improved if it is possible to avoid daily prednisone administration.

In a few cases, hypertension may be a result of retroperitoneal fibrosis (Fig. 5.21).

The Ocular Fundus in SLE

The eye is a frequent "target organ" in SLE, and inflammation may be seen in optic nerve, conjunctiva, sclera, uveal tract, and retina.[293,294] Ocular pathology is generally associated with acute disease and, except for optic neuritis rarely causes visual impairment.[295] The most common eye findings in SLE are the fluffy white patches that may be seen in the retina in patients who are not hypertensive. These are called cytoid bodies and have been shown to represent foci of varicose hypertrophy, choroid inflammation, and gangliform degeneration of nerve fibers secondary to capillary endothelial damage.[20,296] Other funduscopic abnormalities described in SLE include small superficial retinal hemorrhages, very slight papilledema, and slight blurring of the choroidal reflex, thought to represent subretinal edema and central retinal-vein occlusion.[295] Hypertensive retinopathy may occur in children with uncontrolled hypertension; the cotton-wool exudates of hypertensive encephalopathy are hard to distinguish from the cytoid bodies of SLE.

Optic neuritis may be a presenting manifestations of SLE, and is often associated with transverse myelitis, a devastating neurologic complication.[297,298]

Neuropsychiatric Manifestations of SLE (Table 5.8)

Neuropsychiatric manifestations were recognized as a part of SLE in the original descriptions of the disease.[20] Major stroke, the most fearsome CNS manifestation,[162] is rare in childhood lupus and usually occurs as a result of uncontrolled hypertension rather than from cerebral vasculitis. Other neuropsychiatric manifestations have attracted greater interest in recent years, and with increasingly sophisticated observers and techniques for study, it may be possible to document some central or peripheral-nervous-system involvement at some time during the course of the disease in almost all patients.[299–302a] Neuropsychiatric symptoms may be the sole presenting manifestation of SLE[303] and may occur without the serologic abnormalities seen in lupus patients with active disease outside the nervous system.[304,305]

Pathophysiology of CNS Lupus. The increased number of deaths reported in patients with evident CNS lupus is due to severe vasculitis of the brain (Fig. 5.22). Johnson demonstrated that when the brains of all autopsied SLE

Table 5.8. Neuropsychiatric Manifestations of SLE

Headache
Seizures
Cerebral disorders of vision
Behavior disorders and psychosis
Cerebral infarcts[325a]
Chorea
Transverse myelitis
Pseudotumor cerebri and aseptic meningitis
Ascending polyneuritis (Guillain-Barré syndrome)
Peripheral neuropathy

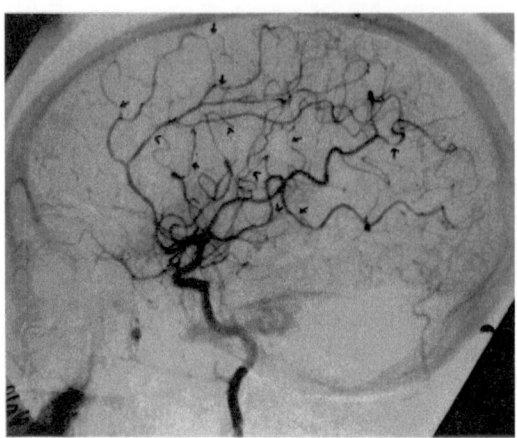

Figure 5.22. Angiogram showing diffuse vasculitis of the brain in childhood-onset SLE. Patient had deteriorating cerebral function.

patients were carefully examined, small hemorrhages, microinfarcts, and areas of perivascular gliosis were found in almost all patients whether they had recognized nervous-system manifestations or not.[306] The lesions are located in diverse areas of both cortex and brainstem and may be correlated with the diverse manifestations that may be seen clinically. Electron and fluorescent microscopy may reveal abnormalities in the brain when light microscopy is normal.[307] Immunoglobulins, complement, and anti-DNA antibodies may be deposited in the basement membrane of the choroid, a membrane biochemically similar to that of kidney.[307] Antineuronal and antiribosomal-P antibodies are associated with neuropsychiatric manifestations.[308–310] Most children with CNS manifestations of SLE have antiphospholipid antibodies.[311]

Electroencephalograms, brain scans, cerebrospinal fluid abnormalities, and angiograms may all reflect the CNS vasculitis in some patients.[312] Recently, elegant functional studies have also demonstrated abnormalities of blood flow and oxygen utilization in almost all patients with SLE, whether or not they have recognized neurologic abnormalities. The extent of the regionally diminished blood flow demonstrated with oxygen-15 or Xenon-133 brain scans correlates generally with the severity of the clinical neurologic manifestations. It is conceivable that the technique may someday be used to monitor the course and therapy of the disease.[313,314]

MRI and computed tomography have also documented evidence of CNS disease in many more patients with SLE than were previously recognized.[315,316] Cerebral infarcts and hematomas that went unrecognized in the past can be documented in patients with abnormal behavior or even in patients without any manifestation of CNS disease. The finding of perisulcal atrophy or basal-ganglion calcifications (Fig. 5.27) may help to differentiate organic from functional emotional disease.[317,318] In our experience, many patients previously considered to have emotional disturbances really had organic disease that might respond to treatment with corticosteroids or immunosuppressive agents. Very early in the course of CNS lupus, the CT scan may be normal. However, most patients with psychosis have perisulcal atrophy, and hemiparesis generally correlates with a finding of hematomas and infarcts on CT scan. It has even been reported that most young patients without a history of systemic disease who are found to have an atrophic pattern on CT scan of the brain have CNS lupus.

The recognition that most of what was previously called functional emotional disease in children with lupus is of organic origin and has a potential to respond to antilupus therapy has major therapeutic implications. If our patients are to live long and useful lives, our therapy will have to be aimed at preventing slow but progressive destruction of the central nervous system. Thus, long-term survival of children with lupus will require "prophylactic" protection of brain function just as it requires protection of renal, lung, and cardiac function.

Manifestations of CNS Lupus

Headache. Headache is a prominent symptom in children with active SLE and frequently is one of the presenting complaints.[20] The headaches usually subside as other manifestations of disease activity disappear. In some cases, the pattern of headache is identical to that of migraine with a visual aura, most commonly jagged lines resembling an aerial view of ancient fortifications (fortification specters).[319] When carefully sought, such complaints may be found in as many as 10% of patients with SLE. Half the patients with migrainous complaints have other evidence of CNS disease when the headache symptoms first occur. In general, the other CNS symptoms also tend to be transient and evanescent. Migrainous headaches generally occur in association with other signs of lupus activity and subside as those manifestations subside or are brought under control with drugs. In general, migrainous headache alone is not a cause for alarm in SLE, but on occasion this symptom may presage more significant CNS disease.

Headache may also be a manifestation of elevated blood pressure, intracranial hemorrhage, and meningitis (septic and aseptic) or may be a sign of increased intracranial pressure from pseudotumor cerebri due to SLE,[320] steroid withdrawal, or hypersensitivity to nonsteroidal anti-inflammatory drugs.[321]

Seizures. There are many potential causes of seizures in SLE (Table 5.9), and in the past convulsions occurred in about 17% of lupus patients.[20,162,322] Seizures directly related to lupus may be a manifestation of active vasculitis of the brain, injury caused by previously active vasculitis, hypertensive encephalopathy, or hemorrhage related to thrombocytopenia or coagulopathy.[20,322] In patients with renal failure, they may be related to azotemia

Table 5.9. Causes of Seizures in SLE

Directly Related to SLE
Active CNS vasculitis
Scars of prior CNS injury
Azotemia, fluid and electrolyte abnormalities
Hypertension
Hemorrhage due to thrombocytopenia, circulating anticoagulants, sepsis with
    disseminated intravascular coagulopathy
Bacterial meningitis (especially meningococcal and pneumococcal)
Shock, anoxia

Related to Therapy
Meningitis (tuberculous, bacterial, fungal)
Brain abscess
Sepsis with disseminated intravascular coagulopathy
Hyperosmolar diabetic coma (steroid-induced)
Postdialysis fluid and electrolyte shifts

Coincidental to SLE
Viral encephalitis/meningitis
Idiopathic epilepsy
Brain tumor

---

or fluid and electrolyte imbalances and postdialysis alterations. Viral CNS infection may occur in patients with SLE. Bacterial meningitis (especially with pneumococcal and meningococcal sepsis) is more frequent in children with SLE, and brain abscess may also be a complication of SLE and/or therapy. When a child with SLE has a seizure, bacterial meningitis must first be presumed to be present, and treatment for bacterial infection should be immediately instituted.[323] A presumptive diagnosis of CNS lupus may be made only after the possibility of infection is excluded.

It is difficult to interpret the prognostic implication of seizures in SLE since all studies include patients with seizures from a multitude of causes under one heading.[135] When seizures are really a manifestation of CNS lupus, they probably equal other severe neurologic manifestations in identifying a high-risk subset.[162]

Seizures may very rarely be one of the presenting manifestations of SLE, but most cases in the literature that were reported as SLE beginning with seizures long before any other manifestations represented cases of anticonvulsant drug-induced SLE.[4] Inclusion of such cases in statistical reviews resulted in the observation that seizures as a presenting manifestation in lupus are associated with a better prognosis than lupus without seizures.[162] It was this statistical peculiarity that first called our attention to the importance of anticonvulsant drugs as inducers of childhood lupus.[9]

Seizures caused by CNS vasculitis should be treated with anticonvulsant drugs as well as by achieving control of CNS lupus with prednisone and immunosuppressive drugs.

Cerebral Disorders of Vision. Involvement of visual pathways posterior to the optic chiasm may produce visual hallucinations and/or visual loss.[324] These sensorineural manifestations are a result of disease in the posterior cerebral artery circulation. At times, visual dysfunction is the most prominent symptom in SLE and may serve as an indication of impending CNS exacerbation. Rarely, sensory neuro-ophthalmologic complaints are the presenting manifestation of SLE, but complex formed visual hallucinations generally occur only after years of disease. In general, patients with involvement of visual pathways also have other manifestations of CNS lupus.

Hallucinations may be unformed (bright lights, straight lines, grids, or zigzag lines) or highly organized formed images (faces, hands, baseball bats, etc.) or both. Loss of vision may include multiple scotomata, homonymous visual-field defects, and transient (even momentary) blindness. These events characteristically last less than 30 min and often disappear in seconds or minutes. The tendency is for the physician to assume they are "psychological" in origin; those physicians who care for patients with lupus must discipline themselves to recognize this complaint as a sign of active lupus. At the same time, while they may presage more widespread and irreversible neurologic damage, they may also be a more benign manifestation of the disease and may subside without treatment or with little treatment.[320] When they occur in the presence of other evidences of deterioration, they call for vigorous action.

The absence of delirium, confusion, altered consciousness, or use of hallucinogenic drugs in these patients helps in distinguishing these lupus-induced cerebral disorders of vision from those of other etiologies. Seizures and signs of psychiatric abnormalities are generally absent in patients with these hallucinations. At times, patients with visual symptoms have other manifestations of diminished posterior cerebral circulation such as diminished gag reflex, tinnitus, diplopia, or vocal cord paralysis. Occasional patients have associated vascular headaches resembling migraine.

Behavioral Disorders and Psychosis. Numerous attempts have been made to separate organic mental changes caused by vasculitis of the brain from so-called functional behavioral disorders that may antedate the lupus or be precipitated by the additional stress caused by this severe and complicated illness in teenagers. Many years of experience with these patients have convinced me that it is impossible to exclude cerebral vasculitis as one cause of emotional disturbance and that better control of disease avoids most of the emotional manifestations. To some extent, of course, better control also makes it easier for the patient to adapt to having the disease. Insofar as emotional problems persist that can be benefited by psychotherapy, it is therapeutically irrelevant what proportion of their cause is organic since psychotherapy and psychotropic drugs have fewer adverse side effects than the drugs used for control of CNS lupus.

It is also apparent that emotional disorders are enhanced by steroids in some patients who require high doses for control of their SLE. Nervousness, tremors, and insomnia occur in almost all patients on high daily doses of steroids. When the emotional disorders induced or exaggerated by steroids warrant addition of immunosuppressive agents, there should be little hesitation about adding them. Many young patients who cannot tolerate daily prednisone because of the emotional side effects can tolerate alternate-day regimens.[325] Where either psychosis or other disease manifestations cannot be controlled with alternate-day prednisone, success may be achieved with an alternate-day regimen in association with azathioprine.

Case Report

A 15½-year-old girl was admitted with an 8-month history of facial rash, alopecia, arthritis, muscle weakness, anterior chest pain, amenorrhea, and cachexia (weight loss from 98 to 68 pounds) (Figs. 5.11 and 5.14). Laboratory studies reveal Hgb 6.0 grams; ESR 148 mm; 1 + urine protein with 5–8 RBC/hpf; ANA 1:160 speckled; elevated anti-DNA antibodies; lowered total hemolytic complement; and evidence of pericarditis on EKG. Percutaneous renal biopsy showed class 2-A lupus nephritis. At the time of examination, she reported "hearing voices" (auditory hallucinations). Treatment with prednisone 60 mg daily resulted in dramatic improvement but was associated with the development of significant hypertension and diabetes mellitus. When the prednisone was changed to 150 mg on alternate mornings, the hypertension and diabetes disappeared but on the "off" day she would hallucinate. With the addition of daily azathioprine to the alternate-day prednisone, all symptoms were controlled, and it was possible to discontinue insulin and antihypertensive medications. She made an excellent recovery and is currently maintained only on small doses of alternate-day prednisone (Fig. 5.23).

Cerebral Infarcts. With improved survival, it is becoming apparent that physicians will have to be more cognizant of the potential for gradual deterioration of cerebral function in lupus patients if they are permitted to have multiple small insults to the nervous system over a period of many years. Although major stroke is a relatively rare lupus manifestation in childhood, recurrent tiny ischemic cerebral insults may be more frequent than was previously recognized. This situation is analogous to the gradual destruction of lung function from interstitial scarring and recurrent tiny pulmonary emboli being seen as a new challenge in long-term childhood lupus survivors. While no single approach to this problem can be said to be of documented value, our present tendency is to prevent CNS exacerbations if we can even if some patients are overtreated in the effort. Special attention should be given to SLE patients with antiphospholipid antibodies who are at high risk.[325a–328]

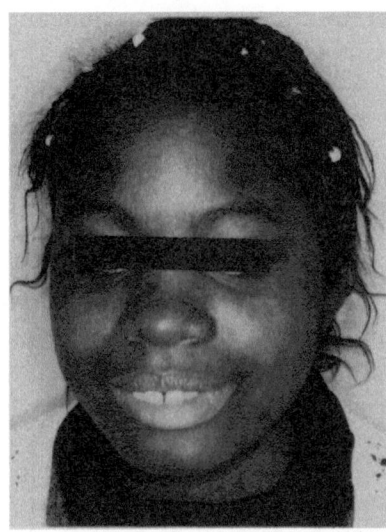

Figure 5.23. Patient shown in Figs. 5.11 and 5.14 after treatment. She completed high school and works full-time. She has taken full responsibility for her own medical care since recovery from the psychosis, which was a feature of her presentation at age $15\frac{1}{2}$.

Chorea. Chorea is not a common manifestation of SLE (only 70 cases have been reported) but, when present, tends to occur early in the disease, often before the diagnosis of SLE has been established.[289,329-332] Chorea is much more frequent in childhood than adult SLE: 53% of all reported cases of chorea due to SLE have been in children. In one series, 10% of all children with SLE had chorea.[289] Thus, pediatricians must be especially aware of chorea as a lupus manifestation, although most chorea is due to rheumatic fever and not to SLE.

Sometimes chorea is the sole presenting manifestation of lupus in childhood; 11 such cases have been reported. When SLE presents with chorea alone, many years (mean 3) may elapse between the onset of chorea and the next manifestation. Children whose SLE begins with chorea sometimes have a family history of SLE that alerts the physician to the potential diagnosis of SLE. We do all the appropriate serologic studies for SLE in all children with chorea, but even when the family history and serologic findings suggest that a brief episode of chorea was most likely a manifestation of SLE, no further manifestations of lupus may ever appear.

Pathologic studies of brains of patients with chorea have not revealed consistent basal-ganglia pathology. It is thought that multiple strategically placed vasculitic lesions result in dyskinesias by releasing motor activity from higher control. In some SLE patients, gamma-globulin deposits characteristic of immune-complex disease have been demonstrated in the choroid plexus, but this has not been a consistent finding in patients with chorea, and all patients with this finding do not have chorea. The explanations for the chorea in SLE stopping spontaneously or for the other manifestations of SLE not becoming apparent for many years are unresolved. Chorea in SLE may respond to haloperidol or to corticosteroid therapy. Some patients with anti-phospholipid antibodies and chorea without other signs of SLE have responded to anticoagulation alone.[329] The role of anticoagulants as therapy in lupus chorea remains to be determined.

Transverse Myelopathy in SLE. SLE may present with transverse myelitis, and in our experience this manifestation or presentation also seems more frequent in teenage than older patients. As with chorea, when transverse myelopathy is a feature of SLE, it is often part of the presenting syndrome; 40% of patients with this feature of SLE had not been known to have SLE prior to the onset of this neurologic manifestation. Thus, SLE is part of the differential diagnosis of unexplained transverse myelitis.[145,298,333–335]

The most common manifestations in these patients are numbness and weakness of the legs. Other clinical manifestations have included urinary retention, fecal incontinence, and paresthesias in the legs. Paraplegia occurs in most of these patients, although some have only paraparesis. Sensory loss is most common at the thoracic level but may be cervical or lumbar. A marked reduction in cerebrospinal fluid glucose is said to be a consistent early laboratory finding but may not be apparent until a week after onset. CSF protein is elevated on at least one determination in about 50% of patients with SLE myelopathy.

Autopsy studies reveal that the myelopathy is due to vasculitic ischemic necrosis of the spinal cord. Immunologic injury is believed to be responsible for the vascular lesions. Early vigorous corticosteroid therapy is probably effective in lupus myelopathy. Late treatment may also be of benefit but is less effective. In a study of 26 patients with this manifestation of SLE, 12 died, and only 4 recovered almost completely; 6 were wheelchair-bound.[145] We would advocate immediate treatment of transverse myelitis with prednisone before the etiology is established. Whether cyclophosphamide treatment and plasma exchange should also be used initially in this very threatening lupus manifestation remains to be determined, but I think most experts are now using pheresis and cyclophosphamide as soon as they see these patients.[336–339]

It has long been recognized that lupus may be mistaken for multiple sclerosis. Patients in whom multiple sclerosis is entertained as a diagnosis should have a complete laboratory evaluation for SLE since early drug intervention is crucial for patients whose neurologic symptoms are a manifestation of SLE. Both diseases may coexist in a single patient or family.[340]

Pseudotumor Cerebri and Aseptic Meningitis. Episodes of increased intracranial pressure (pseudotumor cerebri) may occur in SLE either as a manifestation of low-grade lupus vasculitis in the meninges (aseptic meningitis) or as a consequence of steroid withdrawal or from cerebral venous sinus thrombosis.[341,342] Pseudotumor has also been reported occasionally as a complication of nonsteroidal anti-inflammatory drug or azathioprine administration in SLE.[343] Increased intracranial pressure responds to prednisone treatment. We have found that many patients requiring steroid therapy for chronic meningitis and increased pressure can be maintained on alternate-day prednisone regimens. Rarely, chronic lupus inflammation may result in aqueductal stenosis requiring implantation of a shunt to relieve the pressure. *Inappropriate secretion of antidiuretic hormone* may be a manifestation of CNS lupus.[344]

Peripheral Neuropathy. Peripheral neuritis occurs in many vasculitic syndromes and has been reported to occur in 7% of patients with SLE.[20,155] In some instances, the peripheral neuritis is due to vasculitis in the nutrient blood vessels supplying the peripheral nerves; in other cases, the primary lesion seems to be degeneration of the posterior root spinal ganglia with secondary diffuse changes in the spinal nerves.[20] In one of our patients, the major finding at autopsy was infiltration of the endoneurium and perineurium by amorphous material that resembled hematoxylin bodies seen in other tissues. It was thought that this material compressed the nerve fibers, thus causing the polyneuritis.[345] These patients with Guillain-Barré–type syndromes may respond to intravenous immunoglobulin.[346]

In our experience, early treatment is associated with prompt improvement, but late treatment, while potentially beneficial, may not be associated with apparent benefit for many months or even more than a year.

Serologic Abnormalities in Patients with CNS Lupus. Abnormalities of serum complement and DNA binding (Farr test) are usually found in patients with CNS manifestations and in general can be used to predict CNS exacerbations in childhood lupus. However, studies in adults indicated a dissociation between the presence of these antibodies and decreases in complement when exacerbations included only CNS disease that was not associated with other system involvement.[347] Similar pediatric cases have not yet been reported but may occur. It is generally agreed that better serologic markers are needed for CNS lupus.[304,305]

Livedo reticularis and anticardiolipin antibodies predispose to cerebrovascular lupus.[348]

Cardiac Manifestations

Cardiovascular abnormalities have been reported in 50–80% of cases of SLE.[20,349-352] These range from nondiagnostic heart murmurs and electrocardiographic changes to pericarditis, myocarditis, Libman-Sachs endocarditis, subacute bacterial endocarditis,[353] arrhythmias, coronary arteritis, and complications of systemic and pulmonary hypertension. Long-term cardiac effects of corticosteroid therapy include deposits of myocardial and epicardial fat and accelerated coronary arteriosclerosis, which may result in early myocardial infarction.

Tachycardia and Heart Murmurs. Lupus cardiomyopathy associated with impaired left ventricular function is present in many young patients with SLE who have no clinical signs of cardiac dysfunction.[349,351,352] Uncharacteristic heart murmurs, heart-sound accentuation, and unexplained tachycardia are frequent findings. Strauer et al., in a small study of young women without clinically apparent cardiac involvement, found impaired function in all. Evidence of impaired pump function with reduced contractility and increased myocardial wall stiffness included increases of right and left ventricular end-diastolic pressure and decreases of cardiac output, stroke volume, ejection fraction, contractility indices, diastolic left ventricular volume inflow, and pharmacologically induced vasodilatation.

Pericarditis. Substernal or precordial pain typical of pericarditis occurs either as a presenting manifestation or during exacerbations of SLE in 30–45% of patients.[20] Friction rubs are heard relatively rarely. Occasionally, cardiac tamponade ensues;[354–356] there is suggestive evidence that this may be most frequent in patients with drug-induced disease.[357,358] Evidence of active or old pericarditis is found in 50–80% of autopsied patients.[350] Constrictive pericarditis also occurs in teenage lupus,[359] and may be the presenting manifestation. Bacterial or fungal pericarditis may be superimposed on lupus pericarditis.[360,361]

Myocarditis. The tachycardia often noted in afebrile lupus patients is thought to be a manifestation of subclinical myocarditis.[20] The myocarditis of SLE is frequently associated with generalized skeletal muscle myositis.[362] Cellular infiltrates, fibrinoid deposits, and interstitial connective tissue scars are found in 10–50% of autopsied patients.[350] Cardiac failure may occur, and at times myocarditis is the major manifestation of a lupus exacerbation. Evidence of active myocarditis is much less frequent in autopsies of steroid-treated patients.[350] Patients with anti-Ro antibodies are at higher risk for myocarditis and cardiac conduction defects.[363]

Endocarditis. Verrucae may occur on all four of the heart valves, but with steroid treatment they are essentially limited to the left side of the heart.[350,364] These vegetative valvular lesions (Libman-Sachs endocarditis) found at autopsy were the original pathognomonic diagnostic criterion for SLE and have been reported in a 1-year-old baby with SLE.[365] Although they are considered rarer now than was initially reported, they were noted in 50% of a recently reported autopsy series.[350] The lesions may heal, leaving scars that may ultimately calcify. Healing seems clearly to be fostered by corticosteroid therapy. Antiphospholipid antibodies are associated with increased risk of heart-valve lesions, intracardiac thrombus, and cerebral emboli.[366–370]

Cardiac Conduction Tissues. Arteries in the vicinity of the sinus and atrioventricular nodes and the atrioventricular bundle may be narrowed by

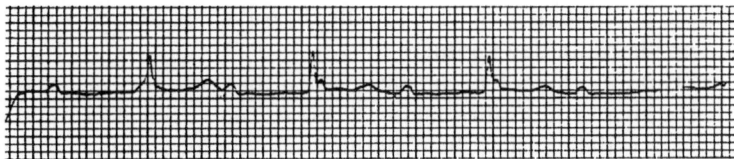

Figure 5.24. Complete heart block in course of childhood SLE; returned to normal with corticosteroid treatment (see Case Report).

intimal fibrosis and thickening of the media. Fibrous myocardial scars may occur in the bundle itself. While major arrhythmias or interference with atrioventricular conduction are rare,[350] lupus can present with complete heart block.[371]

Case Report

A 17-year-old boy developed fever, arthritis, abdominal pain, and a butterfly rash. He was started on aspirin and hydroxychloroquine; laboratory tests confirmed a diagnosis of SLE. Symptoms worsened and after 5 months he took prednisone 50 mg qod briefly but stopped as soon as he felt better. Within a week he was in complete heart block (Fig. 5.24). Ro and La antibodies were not present. The heart block responded promptly to conventional corticosteroid treatment but renal and psychiatric disease required the subsequent addition of azathioprine. His subsequent course over 4 years has been benign.

Coronary Arteries. Focal narrowing of intramural coronary arteries as a result of thromboembolism and vasculitis was noted in autopsied lupus patients prior to corticosteroid therapy. Naturally, as patients have lived longer, this has become a more significant problem. Even young children may die of myocardial infarction, and as other causes of death have been better controlled, myocardial infarction has become a more significant cause of mortality during the second decade of lupus disease and thereafter.[176,350,372–376]

Corticosteroids, while life-saving, induce a variety of increased coronary risk factors, including hyperlipidemia, hypertension, and diabetes mellitus. A number of studies show that steroids increase lipid and calcific deposits in vessel walls.[377]

Some children with lupus present with gigantic levels of triglycerides (2800–3800 mg) and dyslipoproteinemia may be a manifestation of SLE responsive to steroids, or may itself be a complication of steroid therapy.[378–381]

It is not yet known whether alternate-day steroid regimens reduce the increased coronary risk factors inherent in corticosteroid administration. However, such a presumption seems reasonable since clinical experience has shown that diabetes mellitus and hypertension induced by daily steroid administration to children with SLE usually disappear as soon as a patient is changed to an alternate-day regimen.

There are two ways to look at the observation that coronary artery disease is becoming a greater mortality factor in long-term survival of childhood-onset SLE. One is delight that the children are living long enough for this to happen. The other is to consider alternative forms of therapy that might have the potential to reduce the risk of early death from this cause. Ultimately, coronary arteriosclerosis avoidance may be a determining factor in deciding on alternate-day steroid regimens with immunosuppressive supplements if they are required. As always in SLE, net gain will have to be measured against the increased risks in terms of the potential for long-term induction of malignancy by the immunosuppressive agents.

Pulmonary Manifestations

Patients with SLE commonly have pleurisy and pleural effusion.[9,20,162,382–390] "Breathlessness" has long been recognized as a lupus manifestation. It may be a result of interstitial pneumonitis, pulmonary hypertension, pulmonary emboli, or pulmonary hemorrhage.[391] These are more common in childhood SLE than was previously appreciated and are becoming of increasing importance as patients are surviving for longer periods of time.

Pleurisy and Pleural Effusion. In our original series, 60% of children with SLE had pleuritic chest pain and/or effusion.[9] We see this manifestation less often now that patients are maintained on corticosteroids to avoid exacerbations of disease. Pleuritic chest pain often accompanied other signs of exacerbation but sometimes was the sole presenting manifestation or sign of exacerbation or the presenting manifestation of constrictive pericarditis.[392] Effusions are rarely large and usually do not interfere with aeration. Pleural-fluid protein in SLE is high (2.75–6.35 grams), and sugar ranges from 56 to 122 mg% in contradistinction to the low-pleural-fluid sugar that has been described in rheumatoid pleural effusions. Patients with pleural effusion often have streaky lesions at the base of the affected lung, presumably representing atelectasis from splinting and impaired cough. Chronic pleuritis is common in autopsy series of SLE.[20,162,387] Steroid-resistant pleural effusion may be treated with tetracycline pleurodesis.[389] Pneumothorax occurs rarely.[393]

Pneumonia. Patients with SLE are especially susceptible to pneumococcal infection and may develop lobar pneumonia with septicemia. Because of defective immunologic function both from the disease and its treatment, pneumonia of all sorts, lung abscess, and empyema are all seen in patients with SLE. Although parenchymal lung disease may be a manifestation of lupus exacerbation, one must initially presume that the patient has bacterial infection and obtain appropriate cultures and institute appropriate treatment based on that presumption.

Tuberculosis is also common in patients with SLE who are chronically ill and immunosuppressed and must be considered in the differential diagnosis of parenchymal lung disease. Patients with a known history of tuberculosis are given antituberculous therapy when corticosteroids or immunosuppressives are given.

Interstitial Lung Disease. The reported incidence of lupus pneumonitis without evidence of infection varies from 1% to 10%.[20] Pulmonary function studies are abnormal in most patients with SLE.[20] Acute lupus pneumonia with tachypnea, cyanosis, and respiratory distress may occur in children and may respond to corticosteroids and immunosuppression.[394] Chronic interstitial pneumonia has been found at autopsy in 98% of SLE patients; interstitial fibrosis, in 70%.[394] Individuals with anti-Ro antibodies may be at higher risk for severe lupus interstitial lung disease.[395] Diaphragmatic muscle fibrosis may contribute to "shrinking lung syndrome".[396] While in the past both acute and chronic interstitial lung disease seemed relatively minor problems in childhood SLE, our recent experience suggests that with improved survival from other lupus manifestations more attention will have to be paid to the pulmonary manifestations.[162]

As we have seen our patients survive into their twenties, we are becoming aware of an increased risk of slow but ultimately life-threatening progression of pulmonary fibrosis and pulmonary hypertension contributing significantly to ultimate lupus mortality. Recent studies suggest that lupus pneumonitis is merely one more manifestation of immune-complex disease with deposition of complexes in the interstitium of the alveolar walls and the alveolar capillary walls.[397] Theoretically, at least, better control of SLE should reduce the morbidity and mortality from this manifestation.

Pulmonary Hypertension and Pulmonary Emboli. Primary pulmonary hypertension, that is, pulmonary vascular hypertension without evidence of parenchymal disease clinically or at autopsy, also occurs in SLE.[398] Many such cases really represent the ultimate result of undiagnosed multiple pulmonary emboli.[109a,110,399] Thrombophlebitis is increased in SLE, and in recent years, as our patients have lived into their twenties, increasing morbidity and mortality have been observed from pulmonary emboli. Patients with antiphospholipid antibodies and/or membranous nephropathy are at greatest risk. In addition to diagnosable large emboli, we have recently become aware of patients developing pulmonary hypertension and breathlessness after clinical episodes of pain and acute respiratory distress suggesting pulmonary embolus but without sufficiently large areas of involvement to be confirmed on lung scan or electrocardiogram. Serial duplex-Doppler studies to exclude peripheral-vein thrombosis should be performed on all such patients and anticoagulation should be started promptly in those with peripheral- or renal-vein thrombosis.[400] If these studies and ventilation-perfusion lung scans[401] are negative, but there is a high index of suspicion for pulmonary embolus, pulmonary angiogram should be performed.[384,385] It may be advantageous in such patients to institute anticoagulation for the clinical signs of pulmonary embolism even when that diagnosis cannot be confirmed. Recent studies suggest that patients with pulmonary emboli should also be treated with thrombolytic agents.[402,403] New treatment modalities are not likely to have great impact on survival from pulmonary embolism. It is in the areas of more effective prevention, early diagnosis, and prompt treatment of deep-vein thrombosis and embolism that there is an opportunity for immediate improvement in survival. New, noninvasive, cost-effective techniques for documenting deep-vein thrombosis may help in achieving early accurate diagnosis.[401]

Acute Pulmonary Hemorrhage. Lupus may present with lung hemorrhage and is part of the differential diagnosis of all children with lung hemorrhage. A disproportionate number of deaths in childhood SLE may be caused by acute pulmonary hemorrhage related to pulmonary vasculitis and, in some cases, to thrombocytopenia and perhaps other coagulation defects.[12,382,383,404–411] When hemoptysis occurs in SLE, infection, emboli, and heart failure must all be considered, but hemoptysis must be thought to represent pulmonary hemorrhage in the absence of documentation of another explanation. However, most pulmonary bleeding in SLE occurs without hemoptysis[405] and is manifested solely by respiratory complaints and decreasing hematocrit.[406] Pulmonary bleeding in SLE is associated with a high immediate mortality and should be treated vigorously with IV pulse steroids;[412] transfusions (of fresh blood and of platelets if thrombocytopenia is present); tracheal lavage with epinephrine, saline, and bicarbonate; intubation; and oxygen and positive pressure. With improved diagnosis and institution of respiratory intensive care, previously hopeless cases may survive.

Pulmonary hemorrhage and acute renal failure (Goodpasture's syndrome) occur occasionally in SLE, as a manifestation of immune-complex disease. Plasmapheresis along with cyclophosphamide and pulse steroids is the favored therapy.[413]

Acute Laryngitis. Life-threatening respiratory distress caused by crio-arytenoid arthritis is rare and usually accompanies exacerbations of disease. Very high doses of intravenous steroid may be required for control.[414]

Infection in SLE

The disease may present with overwhelming pneumonoccal or meningococcal sepsis, or with staphylococcal osteomyelitis and septicemia. Infection is the commonest cause of death and is more frequent in patients with uncontrolled disease.[415,416] This is both because low levels of complement and other immunologic deficiencies are increased in patients with active disease and because the more active the disease the more likely the patient will require increased and more dangerous immunosuppression.[417] In addition, patients with congenital deficiencies of complement are more prone to both lupus and infection.

Urinary-tract infections are also common in patients with SLE and a surprising number are due to salmonella;[418] salmonella bacteremia may cause salmonella arthritis. Cystitis may be a primary lupus manifestation[418] susceptible to secondary bacterial infection. Salmonella is the most common serious gram-negative infecting organism in SLE,[419,420] but meningococcus[323] and gonococcus are also frequent.[360] Functional asplenia may be a feature of SLE; all patients should be immunized with pneumocccal vaccine.[421,421a]

Superinfection with fungus and pneumocystis carinii are related to daily prednisone treatment.[415] In coccidiodomycosis-endemic areas immunosuppressed patients are at risk of fatal coccidiodomycosis.[422] Overwhelming strongyloides infection may be interpreted as uncontrolled SLE.[423] Pericardial effusion may predispose to septic pericarditis.[360] In our experience the best protection against infection is a commitment to alternate-day prednisone at 7:30 A.M.; no matter how high the alternate-day dose (? 550 mg of prednisone qod), we rarely see infection in our patients.

Acquired hypogammaglobulinemia as a manifestation of active SLE has only recently come to our attention as a cause of potentially fatal infection.[424–430] Recognition of this previously unrecognized problem and treatment with intravenous gamma globulin has enabled us to provide significant improvement to three children with SLE in the past few years.[431] With more immunosuppression and better control of the lupus, the hypogammaglobulinemia disappears (see case report, p. 469).[430]

Sjögren's Syndrome

Sjögren's syndrome (SS), the combination of dry eyes (xerophthalmia) and dry mouth (xerostomia)—known together as the "sicca complex"—is rare in childhood.[432–434] Recently, on the basis of both immunologic and clinical differences, two forms of SS have been distinguished.[435] The secondary form occurs in older children and adults who have had RA or other connective-tissue disease, usually for many years.[434] Its sole importance is that recognition allows treatment-aimed symptomatic relief and limiting the damaging effects of chronic dry eyes and dry mouth and an awareness of increased susceptibility to lymphoma and other B-cell neoplasms.[436] Sjögren's syndrome patients commonly manifest considerable evidence of B-lymphocyte hyperreactivity with polyclonal hypergammaglobulinemia and circulating immune complexes. In some adults, this may evolve into a malignant lymphoma. Although this has not been noted in childhood, the potential obviously exists.

In our experience and in the literature, most children with SS have the primary form. Most of these children either have or will develop SLE or the subset mixed connective-tissue disease (MCTD).[437,438] Most recurrent parotitis under age 5 years is not SS. Recurrent salivary-gland swelling in children over age 5 years (Mikulicz's syndrome), without the sicca complex, may be the first manifestation of these connective-tissue diseases and may antedate the development of other symptoms for years.[426] AIDS may also present this way[439] suggesting that viruses contribute to the development of Sjögren's syndrome.[440]

The diagnosis of SS may be confirmed by the so-called Schirmer test (less than 5 mm of wetting of filter paper inserted in the conjunctival sac for 5 min without anesthesia), by diminution of stimulated parotid saliva flow, by abnormal salivary ultrasound or scintigraphy, and by demonstration of aggregates of lymphocytes on a labial salivary-gland biopsy. Typical positive biopsies can be demonstrated in 20–30% of asymptomatic patients with RA and SLE. Although these procedures do define the disorder for multi-institutional study, we find them of little practical significance in the care of patients. Cannulation of the salivary duct in a patient with SLE or MCTD may result in life-threatening infection since these patients are more prone to sepsis. We have barely survived this problem with a child and no longer do that procedure.

Autoantibodies are common in SS and usually include rheumatoid factor and antinuclear antibodies. Particular ANAs formerly called SS-A (now Ro) and SS-B (now La) are characteristic of primary SS and may delineate a particular subset of SLE or MCTD.[43,428,441,442] These may be the only antinuclear antibodies present in some children with lupus (ANA-negative lupus).[93] If the patient has other manifestations of SLE or MCTD, management is dependent on those primary diagnoses. Close monitoring of all patients is essential since rapidly progressive renal disease and other threatening lupus manifestations may occur.

Case Report

A 10-year-old black girl whose mother had died of SLE 4 years earlier was brought from Florida to New York for further evaluation of intermittent bilateral nontender parotid-gland swelling over a 2-year period. Over the 2 weeks prior to admission, she developed dry eyes, dry mouth, easy fatiguability, and joint pains. Physical examination revealed an obese girl with rock-hard swellings of both parotid glands; xerostomia; xerophthalmia (positive Schirmer test); and restriction of motion in an ankle, knee, and PIP joints due to pain. Significant laboratory abnormalities included ESR 86; ANA +++ (speckled); latex fixation 1:4000; total protein 9 5; IgG 3200 (IgA,M normal); creatinine clearance 79 cc/min/mm², with serum creatinine 0.8 and 24-h urine protein 115 mg; LE prep and Farr test were negative; CH50 complement was normal; and skin tests revealed normal delayed hypersensitivity with negative tuberculin. Minor salivary gland biopsy revealed a prominent chronic inflammatory infiltrate composed of lymphocytes and plasma cells. Pulmonary function tests were interpreted as showing restrictive lung disease.

The grandmother was told the child had SS, that this could evolve into SLE, and that she should report promptly to the medical center near her home in Florida. She was first seen there 3 months later. At that time she was acutely ill and was found on admission to have a serum creatinine of 9. Renal biopsy showed end-stage lupus renal disease. After several years of hemodialysis and one unsuccessful renal transplant, she received a transplant from a cadaver in 1979 (age 16 years); since that time she has had normal renal function, has no clinical evidence of SLE, and is a straight "A" student in high school.

Hypothyroidism

Nine percent of children with SLE are hypothyroid and 20–34% are reported to have antithyroid antibodies;[443] 6.6% of adults with lupus are hypothyroid and in some series hyperthyroidism is also more frequent in SLE.[444] Patients with thyroid disease may also have more Sjögren's syndrome than others and more pure red-cell aplasia.[445] We have also seen hyperthyroidism as the presenting manifestation of childhood SLE.[446]

Hypoadrenalism (Schmidt's Syndrome)

Lupus may present with polyserositis (pericarditis and pleurisy) with adrenal failure and hypothyroidism (autoimmune endocrinopathy; Schmidt's syndrome type II).[447] Although this is rare, prompt recognition of the Addisonian crisis is essential to save the life of the patient before cardiac arrest occurs.[448]

Case Report

Following an episode of pneumonia, a previously healthy 12-year-girl whose mother's first cousin has SLE developed recurrent respiratory illnesses and was noted to have excessive and persistent tanning. After 9 months she was admitted to a local hospital with fever and chest pain; before treatment could be begun she became hypotensive with ventricular tachycardia requiring cardiac resuscitation twice. Pericardial tamponade was recognized and a pericardial window was created. Over the next few days bilateral pleural effusions developed and enlarged and, despite tube drainage, pericardial tamponade recurred, so that pericardial stripping and placement of pleural drainage tubes was required. Laboratory studies performed on admission confirmed that she was hypothyroid and had Addison's disease; tests for antiadrenal antibodies were negative but antimicrosomal antibodies were present in very high titer, confirming the diagnosis of Schmidt's syndrome (type II autoimmune endocrinopathy). She was treated with antibiotics, thyroid hormone, and corticosteroids and progressively improved. As the steroid dose was lowered she became thrombopenic (96,000) and psychotic and developed hematuria, proteinuria, and granular casts. Renal biopsy showed lupus nephritis class IIB with some membranous features; immunofluorescent staining was positive for IgG, IgM, C_3, C_1, kappa, and lambda. Tests for antinuclear antibodies were negative but although C_3 and C_4 were normal, total hemolytic complement was low; further study revealed C_2 deficiency and hypogammaglobulinemia with IgA 24 (70–350), IgM 75 (50–300), IgG 367 (540–1250), APPT was 54 (C = 29); lupus anticoagulant: +;[448] IgG1:294 (280–1020); IgG2:64 (60–790); IgG3:29 (14–240); IgG4:3 (11–330). She was treated with prednisone and monthly infusions of gamma globulin. It was possible to change from 80 mg of prednisone daily to 150 mg every second morning at 7 A.M. within a month and to wean the prednisone to 20 mg one day, 2.5 the next (for adrenal support), and stop the gamma-globulin infusions after 18 months. IgG in 1992 ($1\frac{1}{2}$ years later) = 708.

Vascular occlusions associated with anti-phospholipid antibodies in SLE may also result in adrenal failure.[110a,b,448a]

Avascular Necrosis of Bone

Avascular necrosis (AVN) of bone is a troublesome complication of steroid administration and also of SLE (Fig. 5.25); Dubois initially and others subsequently noted the frequency of this problem in SLE even without steroid therapy.[20,449] There is some increased risk with increasing doses of oral steroids but intravenous bolus steroids may be associated with lower risk.[450] Some recent reports suggest that this particular complication of SLE and its treatment are much more frequent in childhood; up to 40% of some pediatric SLE series can be affected, in most cases solely with radiologic manifestations rather than with clinical symptoms.[15,451] However, when only symptomatic patients are reported, the incidence of the problem appears to be the same in children and adults (4.5% of SLE patients).[452] In one young woman, AVN was the presenting manifestation of SLE.[453]

Pathophysiology of AVN. Experimentally, AVN has been produced by interruption of the blood supply to the capital femoral epiphysis.[452] Other clinical situations in which AVN occurs suggest a similar mechanism: trauma, decompression sickness as a result of intravascular nitrogen embolism, blood slugging in hemoglobinopathies, fat embolism in alcoholics, and obstruction by Gaucher cells. Its occurrence in SLE without steroid treatment is presumably a result of vasculitis. Its occurrence in steroid-treated humans without vasculitis or any other known predisposing factor and in Cushing's syndrome is presumed to be a result of hyperlipemia and decreased lipolytic activity of the blood.[452]

Symptoms. Persistent disproportionate localization of pain that is relieved by rest in a single joint is suggestive of AVN of bone. Symptoms may ante-

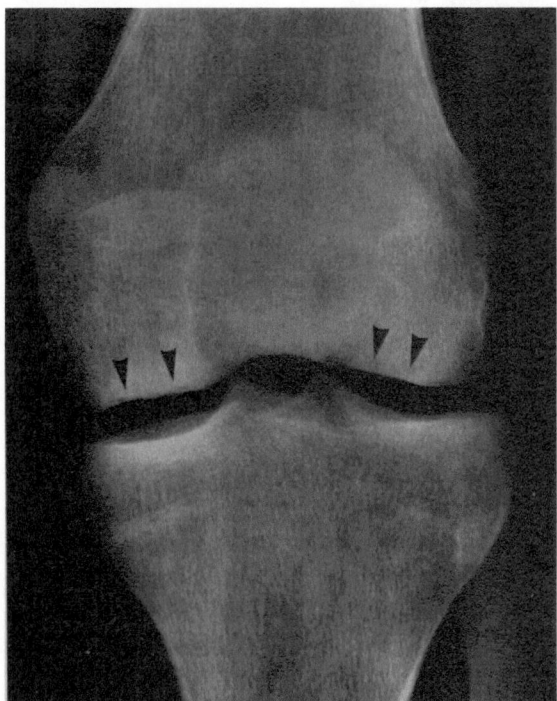

Figure 5.25. Avascular necrosis of the knee in a 15-year-old-girl with SLE who has received steroid treatment for 1 year. Surface of the distal femoral condyles shows a mixture of sclerosis, irregularities, and thin lucent line clefts (*arrows*).

date radiographic manifestations by many months; MRI enables earlier diagnosis. Hips and knees are most frequently affected, but multiple bone may be involved, and a mild reactive effusion may occur in adjacent joints. Loose bodies may break off and require removal to restore motion (Fig. 5.26). The hip is the clinically most significantly affected joint.

Treatment. The course of AVN of bone is variable. Most patients are asymptomatic, and the lesion is found only because of a radiologic survey. However, some patients progress rapidly to total joint destruction requiring joint replacement. Zizic has suggested that with early diagnosis and prompt surgical "core decompression" the prognosis for progression of symptomatic AVN can be greatly improved.[454] However, no randomized control study was presented, so most physicians have so far been reluctant to adopt this procedure.

We have not found the benefits of limitation of activities to equal the undesirable side effects of such limitation. Nonsteroidal anti-inflammatory agents are helpful to those patients with irritative synovitis and pain. Most patients with symptomatic AVN can manage without joint replacement, but there is no question that AVN remains one of the great clinical challenges now that children with lupus are surviving.

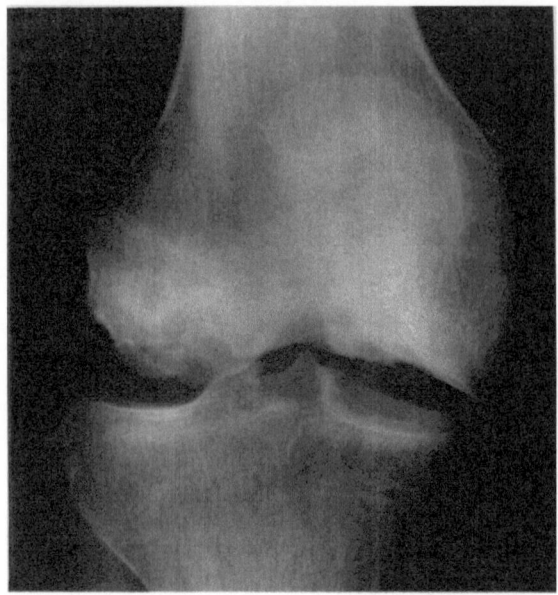

A

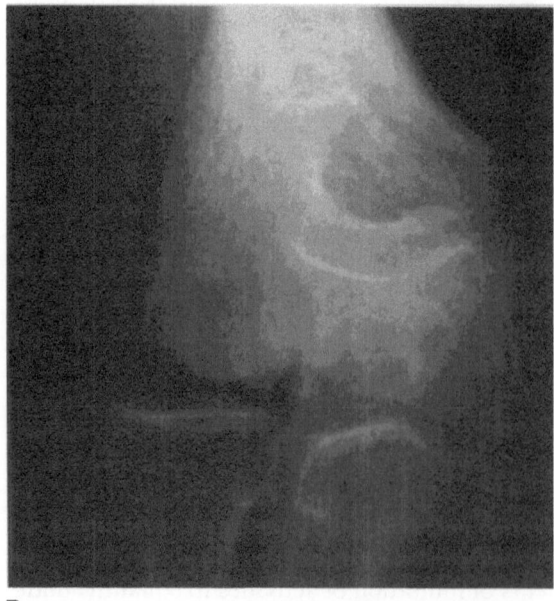

B

Figure 5.26. (**A**) AVN of knee with loose bodies causing locking in a 16-year-old girl with SLE. We have several similar patients who also required removal of such loose bodies from knees and elbows (**B**).

SLE and Pregnancy

Physicians for teenage girls must concern themselves with sexual intercourse, contraception, and pregnancy. These subjects should be discussed freely with all patients beginning at a young age.

Effects of SLE on Conception. Although it is probably hard for women to conceive when very ill, for a variety of reasons, conception does not seem adversely affected in mild lupus or by steroid therapy. Steroids may induce amenorrhea without interfering with ovulation. It is important that the girls understand that they must expect to become pregnant with unprotected intercourse.

Effects of SLE on the Outcome of Pregnancy. Placental size is reduced as a consequence of thrombosis, infarction, and immunologic injury.[455] Fetal wastage is increased in SLE, and the combination of spontaneous abortion and stillbirth may amount to 30%.[456–460] Those with hypocomplementemia or antiphospholipid antibodies are at highest risk[461,461a] but successful pregnancy often occurs without special treatment of even these high-risk women.[462] Some stillborn babies have fibrinous pericarditis and other signs of SLE. Premature delivery and small-for-dates babies are common, but with the exception of the small number of babies who develop neonatal SLE, most of the offspring are healthy, and we find it useful to reassure teenagers that they may expect to have normal children.[463]

Although no control studies have been performed it seems reasonable to treat women with a history of recurrent fetal loss associated with the presence of antiphopholipid antibodies with prednisone and one baby aspirin daily.[461a,464] While this does not always result in live birth it seems to be successful in some women.[465] There is no evidence that immunosuppressive drugs adversely affect pregnancy outcome in women with SLE.[466]

It is not known whether repetitive plasmapheresis and/or aggressive immunosuppression of a woman who has delivered a previous baby with congenital heart block will improve her chances of having a subsequent normal baby, or just how to time the treatment. Although myocarditis and heart failure (fetal hydrops) can be successfully treated in utero, congenital heart block, once established, persists.[467,468]

Effect of Pregnancy on SLE. Twenty-five to sixty percent of lupus patients worsen as a result of pregnancy.[469–470] It is not uncommon in these days of teenage pregnancy for lupus to present to the pediatrician in the first trimester, and it may be life-threatening, with sudden renal failure, hypertension, and thrombopenia. Low serum somplement values help to differentiate lupus from preeclampsia.[471] Some patients have some remission of symptoms during pregnancy similar to that seen in RA. The postpartum backlash that may occur is generally tolerable except for the problem of renal disease. Renal disease may first become apparent in patients during the pregnancy, may be associated with hypertension and toxemia, and may greatly worsen during the postpartum period. Three practical conclusions should be shared with patients: (1) Since pregnancy introduces an added risk, they should not get pregnant accidentally but reserve the added risk for a desired pregnancy. Undesired pregnancy could result in deterioration that prevents later desired pregnancy. (2) Pregnancy introduces a risk of increased renal disease, especially in the postpartum period or after abortion. There are problems about the use of medications.[471a] There is also increased risk of phlebitis and its complications. If renal disease is severe, with little reserve, pregnancy is undesirable and may result in death or renal death. (3) The postpartum and postabortion period will require close monitoring for hypertension, phlebitis, and pulmonary emboli and requires prompt care for even the slightest problem.

Contraception in SLE. Oral contraceptive agents are among the drugs that can worsen or induce SLE. However, the incidence of lupus induced by drugs is very small and certainly smaller than the risk of pregnancy. While the combination of condoms and foam provides good contraception (and protection from venereal disease), we are reluctant to have these patients dependent on male cooperation for contraception. If the girls will accept a diaphragm, that is our recommendation. Otherwise, we offer oral contraception as the initiating form of female birth control until they have become used to having sexual intercourse, replacing it with the diaphragm when that is acceptable to them. We discuss this with the girls and their parents, emphasizing that while we do not recommend sexual intercourse for young girls, we are prepared to provide the care they require in order not to become pregnant if they decide to become sexually active. We generally begin these discussions at about age 13.

Lupus in the Neonate

Ninety-percent of babies born to women with lupus are normal.[456,457] While the various manifestations of lupus that may be seen in the neonate presumably always reflect disease in the mother, the mother may be asymptomatic and not aware that she has any illness.[472,473] Thus, lupus in the infant may be a clue to diagnosis in the mother and may be used to provide lifesaving treatment to the mother during the postpartum period.

The risk of having an infant with neonatal lupus (categories 3–6 below) is greatly increased if the pregnant individual had a prior baby with neonatal lupus (25%) or has Ro antibodies (32%); La and RNP antibodies also increase risk but to a lesser extent.[474–476] The risk of having a baby with clinically evident heart disease is uncertain but much lower than 3% even in Ro + mothers with SLE.[474] However, a history of having had a baby with congenital heart block greatly increases the risk of having a second baby with congenital heart block. Most individuals who have babies with congenital heart block, however, are not known to have SLE.[475] Ro and La antibodies may be found in some normal individuals,[476,477] and the immunogenetics of congenital heart block is quite complex.[478–480a] Fraternal twins may be discordant for neonatal lupus![481] Lupus manifestations in the neonate can be divided into six categories.[482–486]

1. Babies with transplacental passage of antibodies resulting in serologic markers of lupus such as LE cells, ANA, Ro, La, anti-DNA antibodies, and even occasionally low serum complement reflecting immune-complex formation without symptoms. Tubuloreticular inclusions may be seen in cord blood lymphocytes or skin.[487,488] The exact frequency of these findings is unknown since they have not been systematically studied.
2. Babies with congenital cytomegalic infection (rare).[489]
3. Babies with Coombs-positive hemolytic anemia, thrombocytopenia, leukopenia, transient myesthenia gravis,[490] and/or neonatal hepatitis with cholestasis[491] with or without skin lesions.
4. Babies with discoid lupus skin lesions without other manifestations.
5. Babies with skin lesions and other symptoms, including heart disease.
6. Babies with complete congenital heart block without other signs of SLE.

This last category is the most frequent manifestation of neonatal lupus, and the mothers of all newborns with complete congenital heart block should be promptly evaluated for lupus. Most mothers of infants with complete congenital heart block do have connective-tissue disease or will develop it at some time in the future. Fetal bradycardia may alert the obstetrician to lupus in the pregnant woman and result in prompt diagnosis and therapy.[492]

Pathologic examination of a child with heart block revealed interruption of the conduction system by an unusually thick annulus fibrosis; there was also calcification and fibrosis along the ventricular portion of the conduction system and in the area of the sinoatrial node.[482] An AV node was not found either as a result of interference with cardiac organogenesis or, more likely, secondary to destruction of the node by inflammation during fetal life.[476,493] Occasionally, affected infants have other associated cardiac lesions.

Complete congenital heart block has long been known to have a high familial incidence. Mothers with infants having neonatal LE manifestation may deliver babies with the same or other manifestation in subsequent pregnancies.

Very few babies with neonatal lupus manifestations require therapy. However, a few who are sick with fever and systemic manifestations or thrombopenia, anemia, or renal disease require corticosteroid therapy. Almost all babies get well except for those with congenital heart block, some of whom require a pacemaker, and those with other cardiac lesions that require correction. It is rare for a baby with neonatal symptomatic SLE to get well and later again develop lupus. However, since susceptibility to lupus is increased in children of mothers with lupus, this does occasionally occur.[494,495]

Onset of Lupus in the First Year of Life

Increasing numbers of cases of lupus beginning in the first year of life are being reported.[95,365,496–498] As might be expected, progressive mental retardation might be a consequence.[497] Most of these babies probably had unrecognized neonatal lupus which evolved as a continuum into SLE. Here is an example of such a patient about whom we were consulted medicolegally:

Case Report

The infant was born with intrauterine growth retardation ($17\frac{1}{2}$ inches, 4 lb 3 oz) at 38 weeks gestation to a hypothyroid GIIABI 28-year-old woman. Physical exam revealed a heart murmur typical of a patent ductus arteriosus which was thought to close by age 2 months. There was a generalized "bruising" rash which lasted for 3 days. Platelet count was 53,000. The liver and spleen were enlarged; a liver biopsy at age $4\frac{1}{2}$ months showed the portal zones to be enlarged, fibrotic, and to contain small numbers of mononuclear inflammatory cells. She was noted to have hypertriglyceridemia (204 fasting). All developmental milestones were severely delayed with head lag still present at age 4 months. There was an episode of shock following liver biopsy. She remained profoundly retarded and microcephalic throughout her life. At age 15 months moderately severe diffuse calcifications were noted on CT scan of the brain; the calcifications in the white matter of the frontal and parietal lobes and in the basal ganglia and the thalami were typical of SLE[318] (Fig. 5.27). At age 4 she developed high fevers, a malar rash, arthritis, autoimmune hemolytic anemia, and thrombocytopenia. Laboratory studies revealed antinuclear and anti-DNA antibodies and low C3–C4 typical of SLE. Following institution of corticosteroid treatment she became hypertensive and after 1 year developed avascular necrosis of her hip. At age 6 years she had a midbrain infarct which progressed to include brainstem signs. A gastrostomy feeding tube was placed. At age $8\frac{1}{2}$ she died at home.

Special Lupus Erythematosus Syndromes

Drug-Induced Lupus

Systemic lupus erythematosus induced by anticonvulsant drugs (DI-SLE) constituted a significant segment of the childhood lupus population prior to 1963 when we first noted that of 35 children diagnosed as SLE, seven had drug-induced disease.[9] Several studies confirm the importance of this form of lupus in childhood.[9,499,500] Thorough reviews of drug-induced SLE were published by Rubin in 1988[501] and by Hess and Mongey in 1991.[502] We see fewer cases now, perhaps due to decreasing use of some of the drugs with a high risk of inducing SLE (Mesantoin and Tridione) and also perhaps because of prompt withdrawal of drug in seizure patients who develop even early or transient signs of SLE.

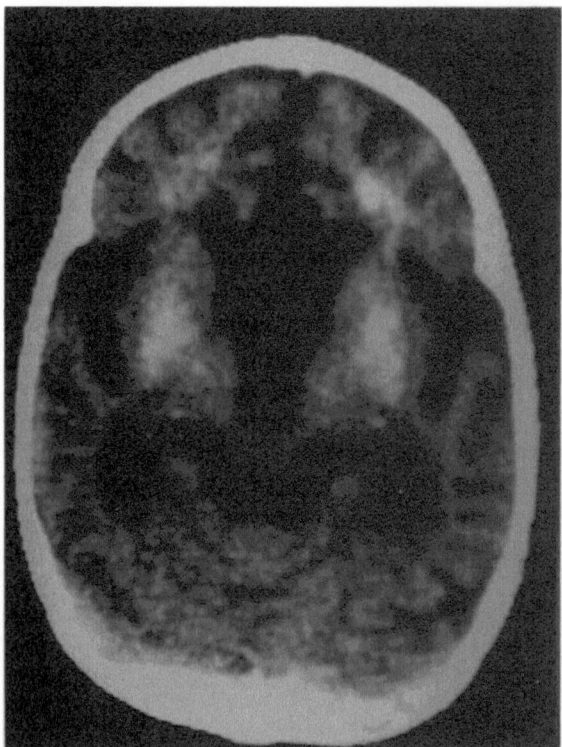

Figure 5.27. Congenital systemic lupus erythematosis. CT scan showing bilateral basal ganglia and thalamic calcification and bilateral frontal subcortical calcification with pronounced cerebral atrophy at age 18 months. Calcifications like these do not occur in congenital infection or following anoxia.

In addition to induction with anticonvulsant drugs, we have seen one child with lupus induced by hydralazine;[503] one with lupus induced by chlorpromazine[504] and/or an oral contraceptive agent; one with procainamide[505] and one with penicillamine.[506] The lupus disappeared with discontinuation of these drugs.[507] Sulfonamide-induced lupus, interferon-induced lupus[507a] and lupus induced by degraded tetracycline have also been reported in childhood. In addition to these drugs, methyldopa[508] and isoniazid induce lupus, but cases caused by these agents have not yet been reported in childhood. Other drugs can probably induce SLE in certain susceptible individuals (Table 5.10).

Susceptibility. Susceptibility studies suggest that DI-SLE is more frequent in individuals who are genetic slow acetylators[509] and that individuals who are both slow acetylators and positive for HLA-DR4 have a significant risk of developing hydralazine-induced SLE.[503] Similar studies need to be done with anticonvulsant drugs. Although females are more susceptible to DI-

Table 5.10. Drugs Capable of Inducing SLE and/or Positive ANA

Anticonvulsants
   Dilantin
   Mesantoin
   Tridione
   Zarontin
   Mysoline
   Phenobarbital
Antibacterials
   Sulfonamides
   Isoniazid
   Degraded tetracycline
Oral contraceptives
Antidepressants
   Chlorpromazine and other phenothiazides
   Nardil
Antithyroid drugs
   Propylthiouracil
Antihypertensive and cardiotonic agents
   Hydralazine
   Aldomet
   Procainamide
   Quinidine
Penicillamine
Vencuran and Practolol (Europe only)

Note: Single instances of drug-induced SLE have been reported from other drugs.

SLE than are males, DI-SLE is the most common form of lupus in adult males. Patients with a high family history of rheumatic disease also seem more susceptible to DI-SLE, as are individuals with the chromosomal abnormality that results in Klinefelter's syndrome.[501]

Mechanisms. The mechanisms by which drugs induce lupus in susceptible individuals are unknown and have only recently been subjected to intense study.[510,511] It is possible that rapid acetylation of hydrazine compounds is protective from DI-SLE as a result of the reduced quantity of the compound or a potentially toxic metabolite that is available. The observation that ANA develops more rapidly and with lower doses of drugs in slow acetylators would support such a hypothesis.[509] Other mechanisms may be involved with other compounds. The demonstrated ability of methyldopa and anticonvulsant drugs to depress T-cell functions, and especially the depression of T-suppressor cells, may be related to the induction of SLE by those agents.[512-514] Some cases of anticonvulsant DI-SLE appear to be dose-related. Other DI-SLE patients most resemble patients with hypersensitivity reactions. While the formation of DNA-drug complexes has been demonstrated and may be affected by various environmental stimuli, these complexes have not been pathogenic in humans or animals. Drug-induced disease can serve as an experimental model for studying the pathogenesis of SLE.

Antinuclear Antibodies. Drug-induced formation of antinuclear antibodies (DI-ANA) is much more frequent than symptomatic drug-induced lupus (DI-SLE). Approximately 20% of children receiving anticonvulsant drugs, including phenobarbital, have ANA.[499,500] Thus, the presence of ANA alone cannot be used as an indication for change of anticonvulsant medication.

Diagnosis of Drug-Induced SLE. Recent studies suggest that antihistone antibodies can be demonstrated in most or all patients with drug-induced SLE but are usually not found in patients with other forms of SLE or in asymptomatic individuals with ANA alone. The absence of antihistone antibodies in an individual with symptoms of SLE suggests that the disease is not drug-induced, while the presence of antihistone antibodies may be confirmative of the hypothesis that the disease manifestations are drug-induced.[515] Final diagnosis of DI-SLE is dependent on disappearance of symptoms. Prospective studies need to be done to see if patients with DI-ANA can be monitored with regular determination of antihistone antibodies in an effort to predict and avoid the subsequent appearance of DI-SLE.[516]

A special clinical syndrome of late-onset febrile hypersensitivity reactions to anticonvulsant drugs (and sulfonamides and propylthiouracil) has multisystem manifestations resembling SLE. Patients may continue to deteriorate weeks after the drug has been stopped.[517]

Manifestations. Pericardial tamponade is disproportionately frequent in DI-SLE and may be life-threatening.[9,357,358] On the whole, however, DI-SLE tends to be a milder form of lupus.[9,499–501] Renal disease is unusual, especially if the drug is withdrawn, but may occur and progress to renal failure if the drug is continued.[9] CNS disease has not been reported in DI-SLE. Immune complexes are rarely demonstrated in drug-induced disease, but they may occur, and while Farr test and complement are usually normal, they are occasionally abnormal.[518,519] Signs and symptoms of lupus usually begin to disappear promptly after the drug is withdrawn, but some symptoms may persist, and minor serologic abnormalities commonly persist for years.

Treatment. In addition to prompt drug withdrawal, patients should be treated in similar fashion to those with SLE, using the same observations and laboratory determinations as a guide to therapy. Steroid therapy is required by some patients, and prolonged immunosuppressive therapy is necessary in a few patients, especially those with immune complex nephropathy.

Mixed Connective Tissue Disease

In 1972, Sharp et al. described the clinical and serologic findings in 25 patients with what they proposed was an apparently distinct rheumatic disease syndrome, which they termed *mixed connective-tissue disease* (MCTD).[520] In addition to prominent arthritis, all the patients had features of scleroderma, dermatomyositis, and lupus erythematosus at some time during the course of their illness. The features that distinguished these patients from those with SLE were those of scleroderma (84% incidence of Raynaud's syndrome, 77% abnormal esophageal motility, and 88% swelling of the hands leading to a sausage appearance with tightening, thickening, and loss of elasticity) and myositis (present in 72%, who demonstrated muscle weakness and elevated muscle enzymes). Unlike scleroderma, the patients had an excellent response to corticosteroid therapy. There was a paucity of renal or CNS disease and of anti-DNA antibodies.

All the patients had a serologic marker, a hemagglutinating antibody to extractable nuclear protein (ENA), present in high titer, all of which was sensitive to ribonuclease (anti-RNP) and none of which contained the antibody to Sm (resistant to ribonuclease) considered specific for SLE.[521–523] A high-titer speckled pattern of ANA suggested the possibility of these antibodies being present. The major purpose of distinguishing this subset of patients from patients with SLE was their better prognosis and reduced steroid requirement.

Not all children with MCTD have a good prognosis.[438,524] About 47 children under age 16 have been reported or noted in the literature.[437,438,524–526a] In addition to the other features described by Sharp, Sjögren's syndrome or recurrent parotid swellings have been described in 30% of the children and were found at autopsy in children who had no salivary symptoms.[438] Severe thrombocytopenia resulted in two deaths, one from hemorrhage and one from sepsis following splenectomy.[438] There have been two other deaths from sepsis reported (pneumococcal and meningococcal),[438] and the largest reported series of pediatric cases reported a death rate of 4 of 15 after an average of only 5.4 years of disease.[438] Pulmonary abnormalities were frequent; 2 of 14 were already noted to have pulmonary hypertension. Myocarditis and pericarditis were frequent (9 of 14).[527] Neurologic abnormalities, rare in the original report, were noted in 3 of 14 children. Renal abnormalities were clinically apparent in 5 of 14 childhood patients in one series and 2 of 5 and 4 of 6 in two other series.[438,525,526] In reports of 14 renal pathologic examinations, there was total glomerular scarring in 1, membranoproliferative disease in 4, focal proliferative disease in 3, and mesangial lesions alone in 4.[524,525,528] Thus, the original report of absence of renal disease was not supported by cases reported in childhood.

Autopsy study of three children revealed striking proliferative vasculitis in both small and large vessels, including the aorta and larger coronary, pulmonary, and renal arteries. Inflammatory infiltrates, primarily with plasma cells, were prominent in many organs, including liver, intestine, and salivary glands; focal inflammatory lesions were present in the myocardium of all these children. There was a striking lack of cortical involution in the thymus with an unusual nodular hyperplasia of the medullary lymphocytes and plasma cells. In the esophagus, pylorus, and colon, there was alarming distinctive replacement of the inner, and occasionally the outer, muscle layers by an undefined hyaline-staining material.[438]

Nimelstein et al. reevaluated the 25 patients included in the original report of Sharp et al.[529] Of 22 patients who could be located, 8 had died—2 related to renal disease (1 scleroderma kidney and 1 membranous nephropathy), 2 of suicide, 3 of arteriosclerotic cardiovascular disease, and 1 of gastrointestinal hemorrhage. The age at onset of 2 of 8 dead patients was 12 years; 2 of 3 children or teenage patients in this series had died after an average of 12.5 years of disease. The prognosis for the older patients was better than for the children, although not as good as was originally suggested. Five patients had become virtually asymptomatic. With longer follow-up, the frequency and intensity of the arthritis and inflammatory muscle disease had decreased. However, features of scleroderma had assumed greater importance and cardiopulmonary deaths increased.[530,531]

Our own experience with nine children (seven girls, two boys) who fulfill the criteria for MCTD mirrors that of other authors. Two patients were receiving anticonvulsant drugs, one definitely prior to onset of the connective-tissue disease. The drug was discontinued in that boy with relief of most symptoms but without change in the serologic markers. One patient had manifestations of SLE and scleroderma with diffuse proliferative glomerulonephritis and severe swallowing difficulties requiring tube feeding. He was treated with prednisone and azathioprine but died following a pulmonary hemorrhage. Four patients have never received any treatment other than aspirin. This reflects the mildness of their disease in which the primary symptoms were arthritis, mild pericarditis, Raynaud's syndrome, and rash; one of these patients had mesangial nephritis on renal biopsy. One patient had psychotic behavior with a high titer of RNP antibody in the spinal fluid; she responded to steroid treatment, which was discontinued. Several years later we learned she had died unexpectedly. Two patients had severe myositis with CPK levels in the thousands that responded to steroids, which were then successfully discontinued (one began with parotid swelling). One patient has had a variety of lupus symptoms that were controlled with alternate-day prednisone treatment. Two patients had extraordinarily delayed puberty with menarche at age 18, different from our other girls with SLE.

In our experience, MCTD does seem to be a subset of connective-tissue disease, but the definition of the exact spectrum of disease in this subset requires a longer period of observation in both children and adults. Meanwhile, treatment must be individualized depending on the clinical situation and should be the same as would be given to a child with similar manifestations of dermatomyositis, scleroderma, or SLE. Thus, identification of patients with high titers of RNP and absence of Sm antibodies is of potential clinical and research importance but has only a little current practical utility,[529] as illustrated by this case report of a patient with MCTD whose disease and serologies changed to SLE, and, with treatment, changed back to MCTD.[532]

Case Report

A 10-year-old girl was seen in July 1981 with a history of months of fatigue, anorexia, and irritability followed by temperature of 105°F attributed to *E. coli* urine infection. At first she responded to appropriate antibiotic therapy but then fever recurred along with myalgia and arthritis. Laboratory studies were significant for ESR 89, hemoglobin 10.5; ANA 1:320 speckled; latex +; IgG 2440, IgM 355; direct Coombs test +; Sm −; RNP + 1:40,960. CH50 complement 230 (160–210), anti-DNA −; urine: nl. A growth chart showed progressive falloff from the 60th percentile to the 10th percentile beginning at age 7 years. She recovered without any treatment although the laboratory abnormalities persisted (ESR 119 in May 1982). When seen in 1983 she reported mild arthritic symptoms. In April 1984 she had grown 5 inches but gained only 3 lb since 1981. Puberty was progressing normally. There was obvious arthritis in one PIP joint and all DIP joints with nodules overlying the third metacarpals. No treatment was given; she did not return for 2 years but in April 1986 arrived complaining of a butterfly rash, mouth sores, and more arthritis, myalgias, abdominal pain, fatigue, and weakness. CH50 complement had fallen to 105 and anti-DNA antibodies had risen to 1143 (0–230). Sm antibodies were now demonstrated.[532,533] At first she responded to prednisone 125 mg qod, but by July 200 qod was insufficient. She became psychotic, did not respond to prednisone 15 mg qid, and was admitted. With azathioprine 50 mg od plus prednisone 15 mg qid plus stelazine she improved. By October she was well controlled with prednisone 150 qod plus the azathioprine; laboratory studies were normal. Prednisone was weaned over the next year to 50 mg qod and in 1988 to 25 mg qod; azathioprine was lowered to 25 mg od and prednisone was withdrawn over the next year. When seen in July 1989 she was taking 50 mg of azathioprine qod and had Raynaud's symptoms and Jaccoud's arthritic changes in her hands but felt well and had normal laboratory studies; Sm antibodies had disappeared. In 1990 she took azathioprine 50 mg every third day and attended college; routine laboratory studies were normal but APTT was elevated and IgM anticardiolipin antibodies were present. C2 was shown to be almost absent although CH50 was normal. During the past year she has remained well while taking azathioprine 25 mg every third day.

Other overlap syndromes occur without the specific serologic marker of MCTD.[534]

Discoid LE

Discoid LE is the mildest form of lupus, with the major manifestation limited to the skin.[20] It is not common in childhood. The dermal lesions are char-

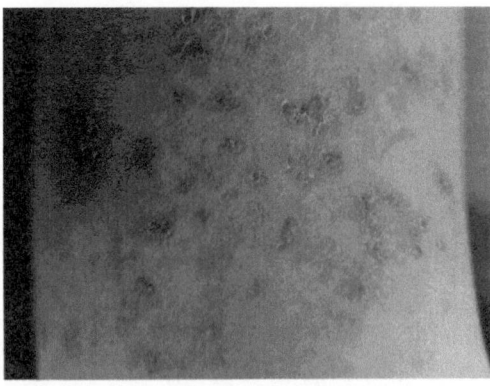

Figure 5.28. Discoid lupus lesions showing local erythema, adherent scales, follicular plugging, and atrophy. The acute lesions consist of ugly red edematous plaques (see also Figs. 5.12, 13).

acterized by persistent local erythema, adherent scales, follicular plugging, telangiectasia, and atrophy (Fig. 5.28). The face, ears, chest, arms, scalp, and mucous membranes are most frequently affected. Some patches resolve, but most leave flat white scars, and a few leave diffuse hyperpigmentation (Fig. 5.14). During the acute phase, the lesions are elevated and form ugly red edematous plaques that may enlarge peripherally and coalesce in bizarre patterns. Biopsy specimens of discoid lesions contain the membrane attack complex (C5b through C9) just as do dermal lesions of SLE patients.[535]

About one-quarter of patients with SLE are said to have had discoid lesions as their first manifestation (Fig. 5.13). Although no report analyzes children with discoid LE specifically to establish the risk of progression to SLE, in studies of all age groups, 7% of patients with discoid LE have progressed to SLE over an average period of about 5 years. Thus discoid lupus bears a significant but small risk of progression.[20] Patients with discoid lupus often have many of the laboratory determinants of SLE: positive LE preparation, ANA, elevated ESR, high gamma globulin, biologic false-positive serology, and mild leukopenia. In one series, 50% of discoid patients were reported to have mild proteinuria.

It is not to the patient's advantage to consider discoid lupus as SLE and offer treatment and prognosis appropriate to more severely ill patients. Nor is it appropriate to consider discoid LE as a wholly benign disease or one that is totally separate from SLE.[20] Patients with discoid lupus can be assured they have a small risk of progressing to a more threatening systemic illness and that once a year, or any time unusual symptoms appear, they should be evaluated in this regard. Hydroxychloroquine may reduce the frequency of progression. With the current success in management of children with SLE, we find it possible to avoid introducing a specter of frightening illness into the lives of these children and their families. An optimistic attitude prevents the creation of more iatrogenic disability than that created by the disorder.

A continuum of disease exists between discoid lupus with skin lesions only and severe SLE. Many dermal subdivisions have been proposed, but the distinctions between them are blurred, and the terminology tends to be ambiguous and confusing.[536-539] Isotretinoin[540] and interferon-alfa[541] have been reported to be helpful in a few patients with severe cutaneous disease which could not be controlled with hydroxychloroquine.

Treatment of SLE in Children

As emphasized by George Ehrlich, "SLE is no longer thought of as the dreaded killer of young women, the gory picture illustrated in older textbooks: disfiguring skin eruptions, depressed blood elements, polyserositis, and rapidly fatal proliferative glomerulonephritis."[542] With an empiric regimen determined by an experienced physician, the prognosis is relatively favorable for the majority of patients. The stage and severity of the disease dictate the therapy.[139,145,148]

Goals of Therapy

We have established the following current therapeutic goals:[543]

1. Control of the disease manifestations so the child may lead a normal life without major exacerbations
2. Prevention of scarring in any organ, which will adversely affect future life-span and function
3. Prevention of intolerable side effects of the therapeutic regimen

Principles of Therapy

Physicians tend to agree on the initial treatment of certain groups of patients, that is, those with mild arthritis as the major manifestation, those with active nephritis, and those with CNS disease.[544] Physicians also generally agree on steroid-tapering practices. Management of late-stage nephropathy is slightly more controversial. However, there is major disagreement among physicians regarding what is appropriate treatment of a "serologic flare," that is, the treatment of a patient who feels well despite deterioration of total hemolytic complement and anti-DNA antibody test values.[545] Our own approach to therapy is based on the following observations and principles:

1. Mild lupus in children is a rarity.[9-15] Most children with SLE develop nephritis.[272,546] Childhood lupus nephritis tends to be severe and carries a worse prognosis than adult lupus nephritis.[272,547]
2. Children with repeated exacerbations of nephritis tend to ultimately achieve a state of chronic renal failure.[548,549]
3. Children with exacerbations and complications of lupus and its therapy who become severely ill often present an insurmountable clinical chal-

lenge with a narrow therapeutic margin, and they may die as a result of reasonable but erroneous management decisions made in crisis situations. Treatment of exacerbations demands more dangerous drug regimens than are required for the prevention of exacerbations.[550]

4. Repeated exacerbations of serious disease, requiring repeated hospitalizations, are emotionally debilitating to the child and family and tend to result in poor compliance and a multitude of emotional problems that complicate therapy.

5. Decreases in serum total hemolytic complement and increases in anti-DNA antibodies (Farr test) predict impending exacerbation in most children with SLE. Decreasing creatinine clearance and increasing amounts of proteinuria demonstrated on 24-h urine collections also presage full-blown exacerbations. In other patients, minimal neurologic manifestations also signify impending exacerbation. Prompt institution of treatment can prevent exacerbations predicted by rising anti-DNA and decreasing serum complement levels.[5,73,75,80,83,86–88,139,550–559] Symptomatic treatment alone (i.e., late treatment of exacerbations) is associated with decreased survival, increased hospitalization, and increased total dose of medications.[560] In lupus nephritis, continuous normalization of C3 levels prevents histologic progression.[561]

6. Treatment of SLE with prednisone has been demonstrated to
   a. Control fever, arthritis, rash, mouth sores, myositis, anorexia, weight loss, lupus interstitial pneumonia, myocarditis, endocarditis, and pericarditis.[20,145]
   b. Reverse thrombocytopenia, hemolytic anemia, coagulopathy, and immune leukopenia.[20]
   c. Reduce production of anti-DNA antibodies and probably their deposition in the kidney.
   d. Result in improvement in renal biopsy findings, proteinuria, hematuria, and renal function.[73,277,562–567a]
   e. Prolong survival (Fig. 5.32).[10–15,73,87,139,148,277–280,553,562–565]

7. Treatment of SLE with azathioprine has been demonstrated to
   a. Improve survival of patients with a poor prognosis.[568–571]
   b. Reduce progression from a good-prognosis group to a poor-prognosis group.[569]
   c. Result in reduced need for hospitalization in patients with a good prognosis.[569]
   d. Suppress the nephrotic syndrome, and prevent its recurrence or later development if not present initially even in 92% of patients with diffuse or membranous renal lesions. Urinary protein excretion usually improves in azathioprine-treated patients and in many patients previously unresponsive to prednisone.[569,572–574]
   e. Cessation of azathioprine treatment in patients with severe SLE (defined as severe renal disease or CNS disease) was associated with exacerbation of disease in 85% of cases within 1 week to 15 months and

death in 30% within 10 months; 63% of those who survived found it necessary to reinstitute the drug within 15 months of stopping.[569]

f. Azathioprine could be discontinued in patients with a good prognosis without an absolute need to reintroduce it within 15 months but was associated with an exacerbation in an average of 3.6 months in 45% of patients.[569]

g. The risk of infection in patients being treated with prednisone has not been shown to be increased by the addition of azathioprine to their therapeutic regimen,[171,569] but the risks of azathioprine in terms of oncogenesis do not warrant its use where alternate-day prednisone alone provides adequate control of the disease.[575–580]

8. Treatment of class IV (diffuse proliferative) lupus nephritis with long-term[581] pulse IV cyclophosphamide has been demonstrated to

a. Improve probability of maintaining life-supporting renal function at 160 months more than 200% when compared with prednisone alone and 150% when compared with prednisone and azathioprine[567a] (Fig. 5.29). The difference was greater for those with chronicity index >1 (Fig. 5.30).[583] Probability of survival was also improved but only by about 10% (Fig. 5.31).[567,582]

b. Prevent progression of the chronicity index as contrasted with other agents.[138,567,583]

c. To have comparable safety and efficacy when administered to children compared with adults[584] with less risk of secondary amenorrhea.[567,582,584]

9. Treatment of severe CNS lupus with IV pulse cyclophosphamide may provide amelioration when steroids have failed.[585–587]

10. Alternate-morning prednisone regimens provide a satisfactory method of control of both symptoms and serologic parameters in most children with SLE with the only significant side effects being cataracts, slight shortness of stature, and aseptic necrosis of bone. This regimen allows growth and menarche, minimizes Cushingoid features, and is not associated with significant increased susceptibility to infection. It can be safely and successfully continued for many years. To achieve optimal results, alternate-day dosage must exceed twice the amount given daily. Many failures of alternate-day regimens result from giving the same dose every 2 days as was required daily,[73] rather than doubling the dose and adding 10%.[588–599] Large adults may tolerate and require doses as high as 500–600 mg; 350-mg dosing is frequent in adults treated in our clinic.[600]

11. When alternate-day prednisone does not seem to provide adequate control of other than class IV disease, supplementation with daily azathioprine usually suffices to achieve the goals of a normal life-style, no hospitalizations, no deterioration of renal function, and a minimum of side effects.[601] It is not known whether methotrexate could be used with comparable efficacy.[602] Restriction of the use of azathioprine to children whose disease is life- or function-threatening and not controlled with

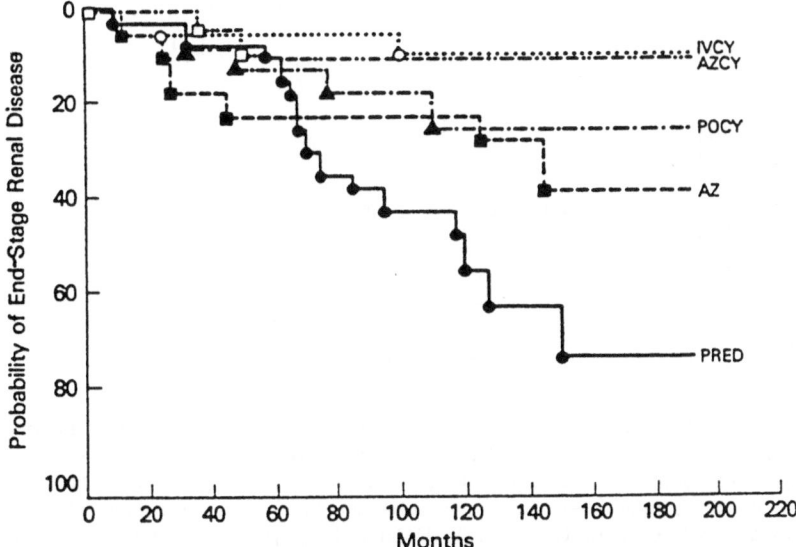

PRED	30	26	25	23	16	14	8	4	3	2	1
AZ	20	17	15	13	13	13	12	10	7	7	6
POCY	18	17	15	14	13	12	11	9	9	7	7
AZCY	23	23	21	19	18	17	12	11	4	2	0
IVCY	20	19	17	17	17	16	9	8	5	1	1

Figure 5.29. Probability of progression to end-stage renal disease in the study population by treatment group (prednisone only [PRED]: azathioprine [AZ]: oral cyclophosphamide [POCY]: oral azathioprine plus oral cyclophosphamide [AZCY]: and intravenous cyclophosphamide [IVCY]). Survival curves are shown, with end-stage renal disease as the outcome. The number of patients at risk in each group is shown for each 20-month time point. The curves for the AZCY, IVCY, and POCY groups were significantly different from that of the control (PRED) group ($P = 0.001$), $P = 0.0025$, and $P = 0.032$, respectively). The AZ group did not differ significantly from the PRED group ($P = 0.09$). The Mantel statistic from which the P values (versus PRED) were obtained were AZ 2.872, POCY 4.619. AZCY 10.571, and IVCY 9.169. The 95% confidence intervals at the 120-month (10-year) point were as follows: PRED 0.69–0.23, AZ 0.93–0.49, POCY 0.97–0.53, AZCY 1.00–0.78, and IVCY 1.00–0.74. (Reprinted with permission from: Steinberg and Steinberg, ref. 567a. Copyright by the American Rheumatism Associaton.)

    alternate-day prednisone alone makes concerns about future toxicity in terms of malignancy, sterility, and teratogenesis tolerable.

12. Current knowledge suggests that all children with class IV nephritis with chronicity scores >1 be treated with IV cytoxan pulses.

13. Since all patients with SLE appear to have mesangial changes prior to the development of other patterns of lupus nephritis and the more severe forms of lupus nephritis are more resistant to therapy and often have irreversible features, a "prophylactic" approach is warranted for all children with early SLE to prevent progression of renal disease.

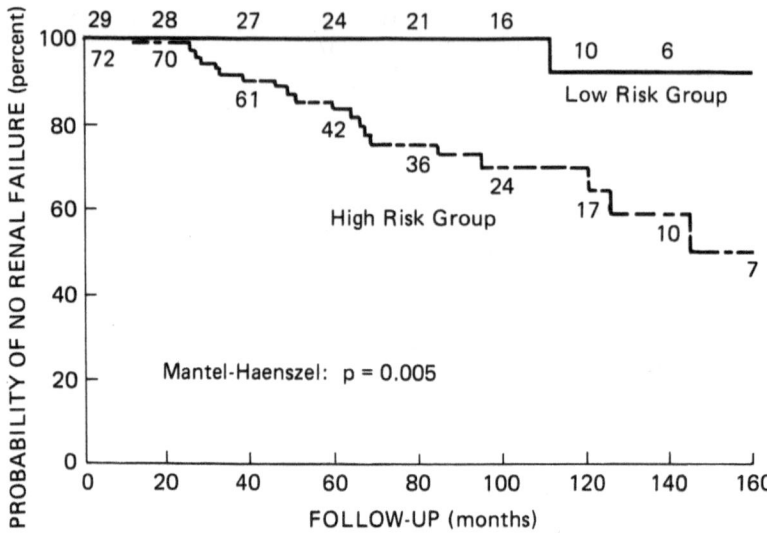

Figure 5.30. Probability of maintaining life-supporting renal function in patients with active lupus nephritis identified as being at high of low risk, according to the presence of chronic histologic changes. The high-risk group consisted of 72 patients whose renal biopsy specimens obtained before random assignment were graded with a chronicity index ≥ 1. (Reprinted with permission from Austin, Klippel, Balow et al. ref. 583.)

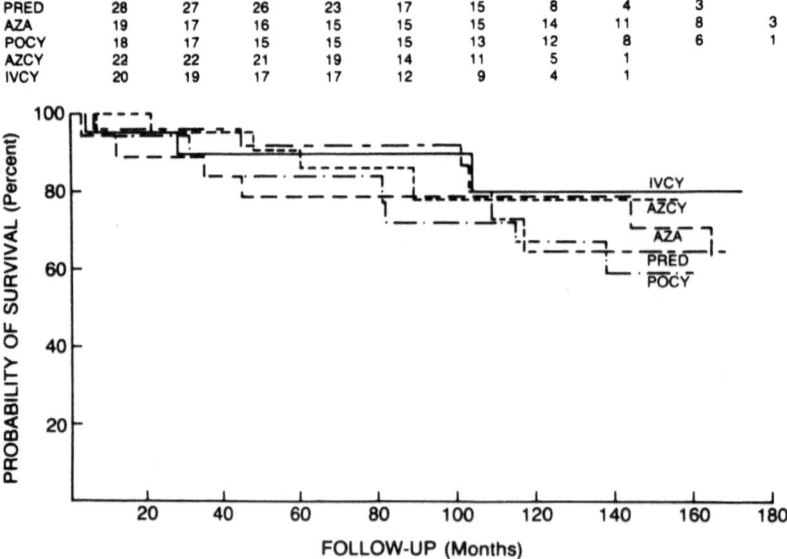

Figure 5.31. Probability of survival in patients with lupus nephritis by treatment group PRED denotes prednisone; AZA, azathioprine; POCY, oral cyclophosphamide; AZCY, combined oral azathioprine and cyclophosphamide; and IVCY, intravenous cyclophosphamide. (Reprinted with permission from Balow et al. ref. 567.)

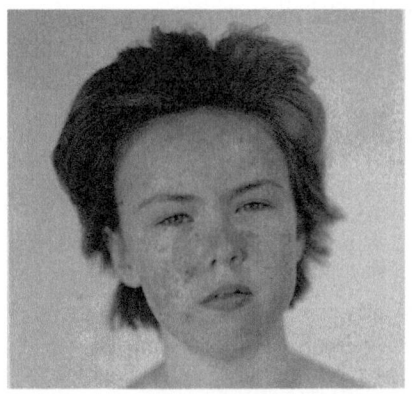

A

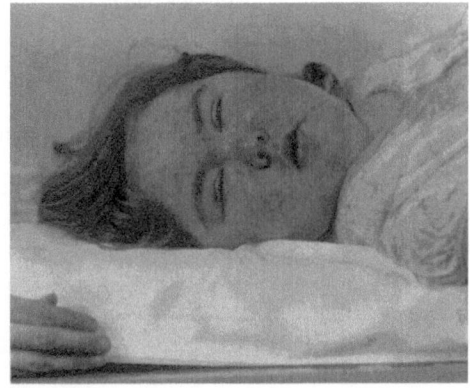

B

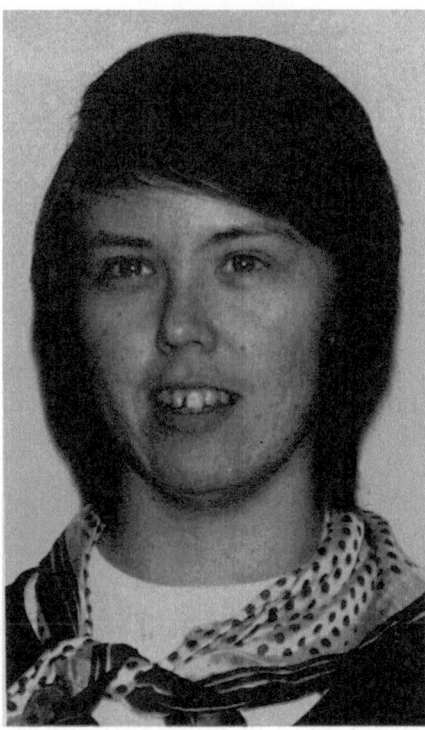

C

Figure 5.32. This 11-year-old girl (**A**) was the first patient with SLE accompanied by renal failure and hypertensive encephalo-pathy treated at this hospital with an arbit-rary regimen of high-dose (60 mg daily) prednisone (in 1962), following the pioneer-ing report of Pollak et al.,[562] indicating im-proved survival and improved renal-biopsy histology in patients managed with large doses of prednisone. All prior children with similar findings had died within a year. (**B**) Terrible Cushingoid complications that re-sulted from the lack of laboratory param-eters then available to guide reduction in steroid dosage, from failure to use an alternate-day regimen, and from a lack of understanding at that time of the need to keep the patient ambulatory to prevent demineralization and generalized vertebral collapse. (**C**) Patient in 1977 at time of adop-tion of a baby. She has since required renal transplant that has been successfully accomplished, and she is again doing well.

14. Optimal treatment of class V membranous lupus nephritis has not been determined. Cyclosporine may be the most effective agent.[603]
15. Treatment must be individually tailored for each patient based on the physician's up-to-the-minute knowledge of the current literature regard-ing SLE; understanding of the individual patient's prognosis, based on a

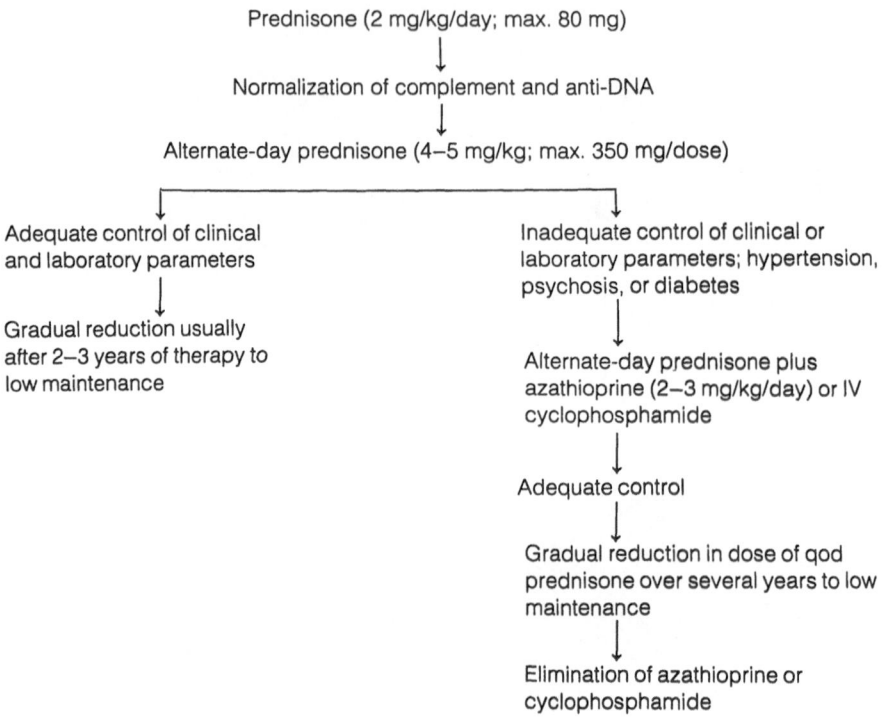

Prednisone (2 mg/kg/day; max. 80 mg)

↓

Normalization of complement and anti-DNA

↓

Alternate-day prednisone (4–5 mg/kg; max. 350 mg/dose)

Adequate control of clinical and laboratory parameters

↓

Gradual reduction usually after 2–3 years of therapy to low maintenance

Inadequate control of clinical or laboratory parameters; hypertension, psychosis, or diabetes

↓

Alternate-day prednisone plus azathioprine (2–3 mg/kg/day) or IV cyclophosphamide

↓

Adequate control

↓

Gradual reduction in dose of qod prednisone over several years to low maintenance

↓

Elimination of azathioprine or cyclophosphamide

Figure 5.33 Treatment plan for systemic lupus.

thorough synthesis of current data, physical findings, family history, and past history; and the physician's intuition resulting from broad experience in the care of other children with SLE.

Management Techniques

The following recommendations are proposed:

1. Newly diagnosed children with SLE who have no clinical evidence of renal disease, normal serum total hemolytic complement, and no demonstrable anti-DNA antibodies may be managed symptomatically provided they are closely monitored for signs of progressive disease. Arthritis alone or with rash and minor symptoms is treated with hydroxychloroquine and aspirin or nonsteroidal anti-inflammatory agents (See Chapter 3).

Patients with SLE may be especially susceptible to the hepatotoxic effects of salicylates[604] and nonsteroidal anti-inflammatory drugs.[605] Hypersensitivity reactions to nonsteroidal anti-inflammatory drugs in SLE patients have sometimes been characterized by aseptic meningitis. The evidence that this is an unusual and distinctive hypersensitivity reaction includes the immediate onset of symptoms following rechallenge and prompt resolution of symptoms following discontinuation of the drug.[605,606] The potential for these unusual reactions must be kept in mind when using aspirin and nonsteroidal anti-inflammatory drugs in patients with SLE.

2. In children who feel well but have abnormalities of total hemolytic complement and demonstrable anti-DNA antibodies, treatment may be begun with alternate-morning prednisone, 5 mg/kg/dose (150–250-mg maximum on alternate days [qod]—depending on the size of the patient).

3. In systemically ill patients and those with clinical evidence of renal, CNS, cardiac, pulmonary, or severe hematologic disease, treatment is begun with prednisone 2 mg/kg/day (maximum 80 mg daily), and this regimen is continued until the serum total hemolytic complement and anti-DNA antibody tests are normal (Table 5.1; Fig. 5.33). It is then changed abruptly to 250 mg on alternate mornings. If this change is not tolerated, the dose may be increased to 300 or 350 mg. If this still is not tolerated, a more gradual weaning process from daily therapy may be begun, increasing one day by 5 mg, while decreasing the next by 5 mg.

4. If clinical symptoms, urinary findings, renal function tests, or the presence of class IV nephritis warrants a more aggressive program, the alternate-day prednisone regimen is supplemented with azathioprine 2 mg/kg/day in a single dose or monthly IV cyclophosphamide, 500–1000 mg/mm^2 for 7 months followed by similar infusions every 3 months for maintenance, until remission occurs (minimum $2\frac{1}{2}$ years).[581,582,607] Recent studies favor cyclophosphamide for all class IV patients.[582] In our childhood series, blacks and males tend to have more severe disease and are more frequently treated with azathioprine or cyclophosphamide.[608] We are currently trying oral pulse cyclophosphamide, using the same dosage as IV, and successfully combatting nausea with oral ondansetron.[608a]

5. Severely ill, toxic, or moribund patients may require pulse steroid therapy (1 gram of methylprednisone daily for 3 days) or plasmapheresis three times weekly as initial therapy in addition to daily prednisone and IV cyclophosphamide. However, the exact roles of such regimens still remain to be determined.[609–617a]

6. All physicians who care for children with SLE must be prepared to offer intensive care for manifestations of the disease or catastrophic complications of therapy, especially during the first year of treatment.

7. Hypertension is recognized as begetting more hypertension and irreversible renal failure and is controlled with appropriate drugs.[290] Azathioprine is usually added to the regimen of children with significant hypertension for its steroid-sparing effect.

8. Patients are maintained on an alternate-day steroid regimen aimed at maintaining normal creatinine clearance, minimum achievable pro-

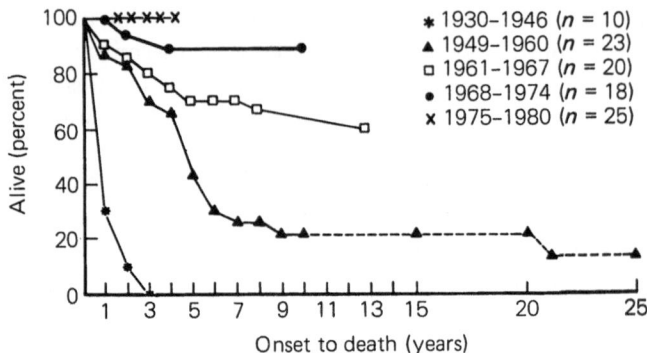

Figure 5.34. Cumulative survival rate of children with SLE at Columbia-Presbyterian Medical Center. No patients lost to follow-up. Curent 10-year survival without renal failure for white patients is 100%. For new black/Hispanic patients seen for at least one visit between 1985 and 1989 5-year survival without renal failure has fallen to 83%. Teenage pregnancy and lack of compliance have contributed to this discrepancy which, so far, persists despite our increasing support services to these patients.[623–627]

teinuria, and normal complement and anti-DNA binding. However, clinical judgment is used to weigh the need to increase the drug when complement and Farr test values are stable but not quite normal or when the opportunity exists to reduce the drug when the tests are "almost normal."

9. Stable patients are monitored at 3-month intervals, and the drug is increased for deteriorating laboratory values even in the absence of clinical symptoms.

10. Special attention is paid to any symptom of illness, and patients are promptly and carefully evaluated at any sign of illness. In addition to considering the possibility of exacerbation of the disease or its complications, we are constantly alert to the possibility of septic complications that demand immediate treatment and institute dynamic antibiotic therapy if there is any possibility that infection is present. Special care must be exercised during the postpartum period when hypertension or phlebitis/embolism may occur. "Stress" doses of steroids are administered for septic illness, trauma, or surgery.

11. At high doses of prednisone, the drug is weaned in 25-mg qod decrements at 3-month intervals if tolerated. Below 50 mg qod drug is weaned by 10-mg decrements with careful monitoring of all laboratory parameters and close attention to clinical detail (Table 5.1).

Any proposed therapeutic regimen in SLE represents a testimonial. As has been indicated, the most experienced physicians disagree frequently when presented with an individual case, especially when the patient is not critically ill.[544] Nevertheless, this is the regimen currently in use in our clinic, and it is more satisfactory than any of our other regimens that we have tried during 30 years of close monitoring of childhood lupus (Fig. 5.34), although it represents less than the optimal therapeutic goal—that is, cure of the disease without any side effects of the therapy.[618-622]

Obviously, by the time the reader sees this book, considering the pace of improvement in therapy for children with SLE, there will be new developments. Although plasmapheresis is not usually useful,[617a] in emergency situations, in addition to pulse steroids and IV cyclophosphamide, renal dialysis, plasma exchange and extracorporeal immunoadsorption may be lifesaving.[628-630] New regimens being developed for control of malignancy and renal allograft rejection will be tried in suitable high-risk patients with SLE.

Children with end stage renal failure requiring dialysis should receive transplants. After renal transplant, disease activity is sporadic and low and lupus nephritis recurs only rarely.[631]

Experience with childhood lupus over the past three decades indicates that when life or renal function is threatened, the patient is best off with aggressive management, provided it is delivered by experienced physicians alert to the potential hazards and ready to deal with them. Those who have continuously cared for these children from the time when SLE nephritis in childhood was considered 100% fatal within 1 year[1] cannot help but be pleased with the progress made during the past 30 years. It is hoped that improvement in the next 30 years will make this seem a small accomplishment.

References

1. Good RA, Venters H, Page AR, et al.: Diffuse connective tissue diseases in childhood. Lancet 81:192–204, 1961.
2. Morrow WJW, Youinou P, Isenberg DA, Snaith ML: Systemic lupus erythematosus: 25 years of treatment related to immunopathology. Lancet 2:206–210, 1983.
3. Steinberg AD, Raveche ES, Laskin CA, et al.: Systemic lupus erythematosus: Insights from animal model. Ann Intern Med 100:714–727, 1984.
4. Decker JL, Steinberg AD, Reinertsen JL, et al.: Systemic lupus erythematosus: Evolving concepts. Ann Intern Med 94:587–604, 1979.
5. Koffler D: Systemic lupus erythematosus. Scientific American, July 1980, pp. 52–61.
6. Reveille JD, Schrohenloher RE, Acton RT, Barger BO: DNA analysis of HLA-DR and DQ genes in American blacks with systemic lupus erythematosus. Arthritis Rheum 32:1243–1251, 1989.
7. Smolen JS, Chused TM, Leiserson WM, et al.: Heterogeneity of immunoregulatory T-cell subsets in systemic lupus erythematosus. Correlation with clinical features. Am J Med 72:783–790, 1982.
8. Stohl W, Crow MK, Kunkel HG: Systemic lupus erythematosus with deficiency of the T4 epitope on T helper/inducer cells. N Engl J Med 312:1671–1678, 1985.
9. Jacobs JC: Systemic lupus erythematosus in childhood. Pediatrics 32:257–264, 1963.

10. Meislin AG, Rothfield N: Systemic lupus erythematosus in childhood. Pediatrics 42:37–49, 1968.
11. Waldavens PA, Chase P: The prognosis of childhood systemic lupus erythematosus. Am J Dis Child 130:929–933, 1976.
12. King KK, Kornreich HK, Bernstein BH, et al.: The clinical spectrum of systemic lupus erythematosus in childhood. Arthritis Rheum 20:287–294, 1977.
12a. Winchester RJ, Nunez-Roldan A. Some genetic aspects of SLE. Arthritis Rheum 25:833–837, 1982.
12b. Shoenfeld Y, Slor H, Shafrir S, et al.: Diversity and pattern of inheritance of autoantibodies in families with multiple cases of systemic lupus erythematosus. Ann Rheum Dis 51:611–618, 1992.
13. Norris DG, Colon AR, Stickler GB: Systemic lupus erythematosus in children. Clin Pediatr 16:774–778, 1977.
14. Cassidy JT, Sullivan DB, Petty RE, et al.: Lupus nephritis and encephalopathy: Prognosis in 58 children. Arthritis Rheum 20:315–322, 1977.
15. Fish AJ, Blau EB, Westberg NG, et al.: Systemic lupus erythematosus within the first two decades of life. Am J Med 62:99–117, 1977.
16. Masi AT, Kaslow RA: Sex effects in systemic lupus erythematosus. Arthritis Rheum 21:480–484, 1978.
17. Siegel M, Lee SL: The epidemiology of systemic lupus erythematosus. Semin Arthritis Rheum 3:1–54, 1973.
18. Lahita RG, Chiorazzi N, Gibofsky A, et al.: Familial systemic lupus erythematosus in males. Arthritis Rheum 26:39–44, 1983.
19. Kaslow RA, Masi AT: Age, sex, and race effects on mortality from systemic lupus erythematosus in the United States. Arthritis Rheum 21:473–484, 1978.
20. Wallace DJ, Hahn BH (eds.): Dubois' Lupus Erythematous, 4th ed. Lee and Febiger, Philadelphia, 1993.
21. Deapen D, Escalante A, Weinrib L, et al.: A revised estimate of twin concordance in systemic lupus erythematosus. Arthritis Rheum 35:311–18, 1992
21a. Reichlin M, Harley JB, Lockshin MD: Serologic studies of monozygotic twins with systemic lupus erythematosus. Arthritis Rheum 35:457–64, 1992.
22. Arnett FC, Shulman LE: Studies in familial systemic lupus erythematosus. Medicine 55:313–322, 1976.
23. Kaplan D: The onset of disease in twins and siblings with systemic lupus erythematosus. J Rheumatol 11:648–652, 1984.
24. Scherak O, Smolen JS, Mayr WR: HLA-DRw3 and systemic lupus erythematosus. Arthritis Rheum 23:954–957, 1980.
25. Cleland LG: Familial lupus: Family studies of HLA and serologic findings. Arthritis Rheum 21:183–191, 1978.
26. Reville JO, Bias WB, Winkelstein JA, et al.: Familial systemic lupus erythematosus: Immunogenetic studies in eight families. Medicine 62:21–35, 1983.
27. Pronek Z, Timmerman LA, Alper CA, et al.: Major histocompatibility complex genes and susceptibility to systemic lupus erythematosus. Arthritis Rheum 33:1542–1553, 1990.
28. Morris RJ, Freed CR, Kohler PF: Drug acetylation phenotype unrelated to development of spontaneous systemic lupus erythematosus. Arthritis Rheum 22:777–780, 1979.
29. Reidenberg MM, Levy M, Drayer DE, et al.: Acetylator phenotype in idiopathic systemic lupus erythematosus. Arthritis Rheum 23:569–573, 1980.
30. Oritz Neu C, LeRoy EC: The coincidence of Klinefelter's syndrome and sys-

temic lupus erythematosus. Arthritis Rheum 12:241–246, 1969.
31. Schopper K, Feldges A, Baerlocher K, et al.: Systemic lupus erythematosus in Staphylococcus aureus hyperimmunoglobulinaemia E syndrome. Br Med J 287:524–526, 1983.
32. Rosemarin JI, Nigro EJ, Levere RD, Mascarenhas: Systemic lupus erythematosus and acute intermittent porphyria: Coincidence or association? Arthritis Rheum 25:1134–1137, 1982.
33. Sakane T, Steinberg AD, Green I: Studies of immune functions of patients with systemic lupus erythematosus. Arthritis Rheum 23:225–231, 1980.
34. Ruiz-Arguelles A, Alarcon-Segovia D, Llorenie L, et al.: Heterogeneity of the spontaneously expanded and mitogen-induced generation of suppressor cell function of T cells on B cells in systemic lupus erythematosus. Arthritis Rheum 23:1004–1009, 1980.
35. Unanue ER: Cooperation between mononuclear phagocytes and lymphocytes in immunity. N Engl J Med 303:977–985, 1980.
36. Frank MM, Hamburger MI, Lawley TJ, et al.: Defective reticuloendothelial system Fc-receptor function in systemic lupus erythematosus. N Engl J Med 300:518–523, 1979.
37. Inman RD: Immunologic sex differences and the female preponderance in systemic lupus erythematosus. Arthritis Rheum 21:849–852, 1978.
38. Jungers P, Dougados M, Pelissier C, et al.: Influence of oral contraceptive therapy on the activity of systemic lupus erythematosus. Arthritis Rheum 25:618–623, 1982.
39. Lahita RG, Bradlow HL, Ginzler E, et al.: Low plasma androgens in women with systemic lupus erythematosus. Arthritis Rheum 30:241–247, 1987.
40. Morley KD, Parke A, Hughes GRV: Systemic lupus erythematosus: Two patients treated with danazol. Br Med J 284:1431–1432, 1982.
41. DeHoratius RJ, Messner RP: Lymphocytotoxic antibodies in family members of patients with systemic lupus erythematosus. J Clin Invest 55:1254–1258, 1975.
42. Folomeeva O, Nassonova VA, Alekberova AS: Comparative studies of antilymphocyte, antipolynucleotide, and antiviral antibodies among families of patients with systemic lupus erythematosus. Arthritis Rheum 21:23–27, 1978.
43. Miller KB, Schwartz RA: Familial abnormalities of suppressor-cell function in systemic lupus erythematosus. N Engl J Med 301:803–809, 1979.
44. Messner RP, DeHoratius R, Ferrone S: Lymphocytotoxic antibodies in systemic lupus erythematosus patients and their relatives. Arthritis Rheum 23:265–270, 1980.
45. Seibold JR, Lynch CJ: Disco lupus, a new disease syndrome (letter). Arthritis Rheum 23:962–963, 1980.
46. Wysenbeek AJ, Block DA, Fries JF: Prevalence and expression of photosensitivity in systemic lupus erythematosus. Ann Rheum Dis 48:461–463, 1989.
47. Dowdy MJ, Nigra TP, Barth WF: Subacute cutaneous lupus erythematosus during Puva therapy for psoriasis: case report and review of the literature. Arthritis Rheum 32:343–346, 1989 (see also Correspondence 33:302–303, 1990).
48. Tan EM: Sunlight as a potential etiological factor in systemic lupus erythematosus. In Hughes GRV (ed.) Modern Topics in Rheumatology. Heinemann, London, 1976, pp. 99–106.
49. LeFeber WP, Norris DA, Ryan SR, et al.: Ultraviolet light induces binding of antibodies to selected nuclear antigens on cultured human keratinocytes. J Clin

Invest 74:1545–1551, 1984.

50. Agnello V: Complement deficiency states. Medicine 57:1–23, 1978.

50a. Johnson CA, Densen P, Wetsel RA et al Molecular heterogeneity of C2 deficiency. N Engl J Med 326:871–874, 1992.

50b. Nilsson UR, Nilsson B, Storm K-E, et al.: Hereditary dysfunction of the third component of complement associated with a systemic lupus erythematosus-like syndrome and meningococcal meningitis. Arthritis Rheum 35:580–586, 1992.

51. Zeitz HJ, Miller GW, Lint TF, et al.: Deficiency of C7 with systemic lupus erythematosus. Arthritis Rheum 24:87–93, 1981.

52. Colten HR, Alper CA, Rosen FS: Genetics and biosynthesis of complement proteins. N Engl J Med 304:653–656, 1981.

53. Fielder AHL, Walport MJ, Batchelor JR, et al.: Family study of the major histocompatibility complex in patients with systemic lupus erythematosus: Importance of null alleles of C4A and C4B in determining disease susceptibility. Br Med J 286:425–428, 1983.

54. Hannema AJ, Kluin-Nelemans JC, Hack CE, et al.: SLE like syndrome and functional deficiency of C1q in members of a large family. Clin Exp Immunol 55:106–114, 1984.

55. Wilson JG, Fearon DT: Altered expression of complement receptors as a pathogenetic factor in systemic lupus erythematosus. Arthritis Rheum 27:1321–1328, 1984.

56. Wisnieski JJ, Naff GB, Pensky J, Sorin SB: Terminal complement component deficiencies and rheumatic disease: development of a rheumatic syndrome and anticomplementary activity in a patient with complete C6 deficiency. Ann Rheum Dis 44:716–722, 1985.

57. Howard PF, Hochberg MC, Bias WB, et al.: Relationship between C4 Null genes. HLA-D region antigens, and genetic susceptibility to systemic lupus erythematosus in Caucasian and Black Americans. Am J Med 81:187–193, 1986.

57a. Suzuki Y, Ogura Y, Otsubo O, et al.: Selective deficiency of C1s associated with a systemic lupus erythematosus-like syndrome. Report of a case. Arthritis Rheum 35:576–579, 1992.

58. Lockshin MD, Qamar T, Redecha P, Harpel PC: Hypocomplementemia with C1s-C1 inhibitor complex in systemic lupus erythematosus. Arthritis Rheum 29:1467–1472, 1986.

59. Taieb A, Hehunstre J-P, Goetz J, et al.: Lupus erythematosus panniculitis with partial genetic deficiency of C2 and C4 in a child. Arch Dermatol 122:576–582, 1986.

60. Antes U, Heinz H-P, Loss M: Evidence for the presence of autoantibodies to the collagen-like portion of C1q in systemic lupus erythematosus. Arthritis Rheum 31:457–464, 1988.

61. Steinsson K, Erlendsson K, Valdimarsson H: Successful plasma infusion treatment of a patient with C2 deficiency and systemic lupus erythematosus: clinical experience over forty-five months. Arthritis Rheum 32:906–913, 1989.

62. Nusinow SR, Zuraw BL, Curd JG: The hereditary and acquired deficiencies of complement. Med Clin Nor Am 69:487–504, 1985.

63. Hauptmann G: Frequency of complement deficiencies in man; disease associations and chromosome assignment of complement genes and linkage groups. Complement Inflamm 6:74–80, 1989.

64. Foeldvari I, Kimura Y, Jacobs JC: Congenital complement deficiency in child-

hood lupus: 17% require little or no treatment. Arthritis Rheum 33S:144, 1990.

65. Kahl LE, Atkinson JP: Autoimmune aspects of complement deficiency. Clin Aspects Autoimmunity 2:8–20, 1988.

66. Wilson CB, Dixon FJ: Immunologic mechanisms in nephritogenesis. Hosp Pract 14:57–69, 1979.

67. Couser WG: What are circulating immune complexes doing in glomerulonephritis? N Engl J Med 304:1230–1232, 1981.

68. Waller SJ, Taylor RP, Wright EL, et al.: DNA/anti-DNA complexes. Arthritis Rheum 24:651–657, 1981.

69. Panem S, Ordonez NG, Kirstein WH, et al.: C-type virus expression in sytemic lupus erythematosus. N Engl J Med 295:470–475, 1976.

70. Phillips PE: Viruses and systemic lupus erythematosus. Bull Rheum Dis 28:954–958, 1978.

71. Abrass CK, Nies KM, Louie JS, et al.: Correlation and predictive accuracy of circulating immune complexes with disease activity in patients with systemic lupus erythematosus. Arthritis Rheum 23:273–282, 1980.

72. Yang LC, Norman ME, Doughty RA: A micromethod for the analysis of cryoglobulins via laser nephelometry: evaluation in comparison to Ciq binding activity in autoimmune diseases in pediatrics. Pediatr Res 14:858–862, 1980.

73. Lange K, Ores R, Strauss W, et al.: Steroid therapy of systemic lupus erythematosus based on immunologic considerations. Arthritis Rheum 8:244–259, 1965.

74. Gewurz H, et al.: The complement profile in acute glomerulonephritis, systemic lupus erythematosus and hypocomplementemic chronic glomerulonephritis. Contrasts and experimental correlations. Int Arch Allergy Appl Immunol 34:556–570, 1968.

75. Kohler PF, Ten Besel R: Serial complement component alterations in acute glomerulonephritis and systemic lupus erythematosus. Clin Exp Immunol 4:191–202, 1969.

76. Ruddy S, Carpenter CB, Chin KW, et al.: Human complement metabolism: an analysis of 144 studies. Medicine 54:165–178, 1975.

76a. Ricker DM, Hebert LA, Rohde, et al.: Serum C3 levels are diagnostically more sensitive and specific for systemic lupus erythematosus activity than are C4 levels. Am J Kid Dis 18:678–685, 1991. (See also: Editorial pp. 686–688.)

77. Takemura S, Hotta T, Matsumura N, et al.: Cold activation of complement. Arthritis Rheum 25:1138–1140, 1982.

78. Abramson SB, Weissmann G: Complement split products and the pathogenesis of SLE. Hosp Pract pp. 45–56, December 15, 1988.

79. Pisetsky DS: The role of anti-DNA antibodies in systemic lupus erythematosus. Clin Aspects of Autoimmunity 2:8–15, 1988.

80. Schur PH, Carr RI, Kunkel HG: Desoxyribonuclease acid (DNA) and antibodies to DNA in the serum of patients with systemic lupus erythematosus. J Clin Invest 45:1732–1740, 1966.

81. Pincus T, Schur PH, Rose JA, et al.: Measurement of serum DNA-binding activity in systemic lupus erythematosus. N Engl J Med 281:701–705, 1969.

82. Hughes GRV: Significance of anti-DNA antibodies in systemic lupus erythematosus. Lancet 2:861–863, 1971.

83. Pincus T, Hughes GRV, Pincus D, et al.: Antibodies to DNA in childhood systemic lupus erythematosus. J Pediatr 78:981–984, 1971.

84. Weinstein A, Bordwell B, Stone B, et al.: Antibodies to native DNA and serum complement (C3) levels. Application to diagnosis and classification of systemic

lupus erythematosus. Am J Med 74:206–216, 1983.

85. Koffler D, Agnello V, Winchester R, et al.: The occurrence of single-stranded DNA in the serum of patients with systemic lupus erythematosus and other diseases. J Clin Invest 52:198–204, 1973.

86. Lightfoot RW, Hughes GRV: Significance of persisting serologic abnormalities in systemic lupus erythematosus. Arthritis Rheum 19:837–843, 1976.

87. Appel AE, Sablay LB, Golden RA, et al.: The effect of normalization of serum complement and anti-DNA antibody on the course of lupus nephritis. Am J Med 64:274–283, 1978.

88. Adler MK, Baumgarten A, Hecht B, et al.: Prognostic significance of DNA-binding capacity patterns in patients with lupus nephritis. Ann Rheum Dis 34:444–450, 1975.

89. Winfield JB, Brunner CM, Koffler D: Serologic studies in patients with systemic lupus erythematosus and central nervous system dysfunction. Arthritis Rheum 21:289–294, 1978.

90. Cohen AS, Reynolds WE, Franklin EC, et al.: Preliminary criteria for the classification of systemic lupus erythematosus. Bull Rheum Dis 21:643–648, 1971.

91. Saulsbury FT, Sabio H, Conrad D, et al.: Acute leukemia with features of systems lupus erythematosus. J Pediatr 105:57–59, 1984.

92. Lehman TA, Hanson V, Singsen B, et al.: Serum complement abnormalities in the antinuclear antibody-positive relatives of children with systemic lupus erythematosus. Arthritis Rheum 22:954–958, 1979.

93. Tsokos GC, Pillemer SR, Klippel JH: Rheumatic disease syndrome associated with antibodies to the Ro (SS-A) ribonuclear protein. Semin Arthritis Rheum 16:237–244, 1987.

94. Gladman DD, Chalmers A, Urowitz MB: Systemic lupus erythematosus with negative lupus erythematosus cells and antinuclear factor. J Rheum 4:142–147, 1978.

95. Jordan SC, Lemire JM, Broder W, et al.: False-negative anti-DNA antibody activity in infantile systemic lupus erythematosus (SLE). J Clin Immunol 4:156–162, 1984.

96. Rothschild BM, Jones JV, Chesney C, et al.: Relationship of clinical findings in systemic lupus erythematosus to seroreactivity. Arthritis Rheum 26:45–51, 1983.

97. Sequi J, Leigh I, Isenberg DA: Relation between antinuclear antibodies and the autoimmune rheumatic diseases and disease type and activity in systemic lupus erythematosus using a variety of cultured cell lines. Ann Rheum Dis 50:167–172, 1991.

98. Fritzler MJ: Antinuclear antibodies in the investigation of rheumatic diseases. Bull Rheum Dis 35(6):1–10, 1985.

99. Harley JB, Sestak AL, Willis LG, et al.: A model for disease heterogeneity in systemic lupus erythematosus. Relationships between histocompatibility antigens, autoantibodies, and lymphopenia or renal disease. Arthritis Rheum 32:826–836, 1989.

100. Lehman TJA, Reichlin M, Santner TJ, et al.: Maternal antibodies to Ro (SSA) are associated with both early onset of disease and male sex among children with systemic lupus erythematosus. Arthritis Rhuem 32:1414–1420, 1989.

101. Reichlin M, Harley JB: Antibodies to Ro(SSA) and the heterogeneity of systemic lupus erythematosus. J Rheumatol 14:(Suppl)112–117, 1987.

102. Cabral DA, Petty RE, Fung M, Malleson PN: Persistent antinuclear antibodies

in children without identifiable inflammatory rheumatic or autoimmune disease. Pediatrics 89:441–444, 1992.

103. Chudwin DS, Ammann AJ, Cowan MJ, Wara DW: Significance of a positive antinuclear antibody test in a pediatric population. Am J Dis Child 137:1103–1106, 1983.

104. Velthuis PJ, Kater L, van der Tweel I, et al.: In vivo antinuclear antibody of the skin: diagnostic significance and association with selective antinuclear antibodies. Ann Rheum Dis 49:163–167, 1990.

105. Appel GB, Silva FG, Pirani CL, et al.: Renal involvement in systemic lupus erythematosus. Medicine 57:371–410, 1978.

106. Libit SA, Burke M, Michael A, et al.: Extramembranous glomerulonephritis in childhood: relationship to systemic lupus erythematosus. J Pediatr 88:394–402, 1976.

107. Morris RJ, Guggenheim SJ, McIntosh RM, et al.: Simultaneous immunologic studies of skin and kidney in systemic lupus erythematosus. Arthritis Rheum 22:864–870, 1979.

108. Singh AK, Rao KPP, Kizer J, Lazarchick J: Lupus anticoagulants in children. Ann Clin Lab Sci 18:384–387, 1988.

109. Myones BL, Anderson BD, Rivas-Chacon RF, Mercer WD: Anti-phospholipid antibodies in juvenile rheumatoid arthritis (JRA). Arthritis Rheum 33:S93, 1990.

109a. Luchi ME, Asherson RA, Lahita RG: Primary idiopathic pulmonary hypertension complicated by pulmonary arterial thrombosis. Arthritis Rheum 35:700–705, 1992.

110. Rider LG, Clarke WR, Rutledge J: Pulmonary hypertension in a seventeen-year-old boy. J Pediatr 120:149–159, 1992.

110a. Asherson RA, Hughes CRV: Recurrent deep vein thrombosis and Addison's disease in "primary" antiphospholipid syndrome. J Rheumatol 16:378–380, 1989.

110b. Carette S, Jobin F: Acute adrenal insufficiency as a manifestation of the anticardiolipin syndrome? Ann Rheum Dis 48:430–431, 1989.

111. Weinstein C, Miller MH, Axtens R, et al.: Livedo reticularis associated with increased titers of anticardiolipin antibodies in systemic lupus erythematosus. Arch Dermatol 123:596–600, 1987.

112. Kalunian KC, Peter JB, Middlekauff HR, et al.: Clinical significance of a single test for anti-cardiolipin antibodies in patients with systemic lupus erythematosus. Am J Med 85:602–608, 1988.

113. Harris EN, Phil M, Asherson RA, et al.: Antiphospholipid antibodies—autoantibodies with a difference. Ann Rev Med 39:261–271, 1988.

114. Love PE, Santoro SA: Antiphospholipid antibodies: anticardiolipin and the lupus anticoagulant in systemic lupus erythematosus (SLE) and in non-SLE disorders. Ann Intern Med 112:682–698, 1990.

115. Lockshin MD, Durzin ML, Goei S, et al.: Antibody to cardiolipin as a predictor of fetal distress or death in pregnant patients with systemic lupus erythematosus. N Engl J Med 313:152–156, 1985 (see also correspondence p. 1350–1351).

116. Branch DW, Scott JR, Kochenour NK, Hershoold E: Obstetric complications associated with the lupus anticoagulant. N Engl J Med 313:1322–1326, 1985 (see also Editorial p. 1348–1350).

117. Danao-Camara T, Clough JD: Anticardiolipin antibodies in systemic lupus erythematosus. Clev Clin J Med 56:525–528, 1989.

118. Pope JM, Canny CB, Bell DA: Cerebral ischemic events associated with endocarditis, retinal vascular disease, and lupus anticoagulant. Am J Med 90:299–309, 1991.

118a. Viard J-P, Amoura Z, Bach J-F: Association of anti-β_2 glycoprotein I antibodies with lupus-type circulating anticoagulant and thrombosis in systemic lupus erythematosus. Am J Med 93:181–186, 1992.

119. Bernstein ML, Salusinsky-Sternback M, Bellefleur M, et al.: Thrombotic and hemorrhagic complications in children with the lupus anticoagulant. Am J Dis Child 138:1132–1135, 1984 (see also Editorial p. 1098).

120. Case records of the Massachusetts General Hospital. Case 11-1990. N Engl J Med 322:754–769, 1990.

121. Ryan BR, Arkel Y, Walters TR, et al.: Acquired symptomatic inhibitors of plasma clotting factors in nonhemphilic children. Am J Ped Hematol/Oncol 8:144–148, 1986.

122. Simel DL, St. Clair EW, Adams J, Greenberg CS: Correction of hypoprothrombinemia by immunosuppressive treatment of the lupus anticoagulant-hypoprothrombinemia syndrome. Am J Med 83:563–566, 1987.

123. Ordi J, Vilardel M, Oristrell J, et al.: Bleeding in patients with lupus anticoagulant. Lancet 2:868–869, 1984.

124. Brentjens JR, Andres GA: The pathogenesis of extrarenal lesions in systemic lupus erythematosus. Arthritis Rheum 25:880–886, 1982.

125. Mahajan SK, Ordonez NG, Feitelson PJ, et al.: Lupus nephropathy without clinical renal involvement. Medicine 56:493–501, 1977.

126. Woolf A, Croker B, Osofsky SG, et al.: Nephritis in children and young adults with systemic lupus erythematosus and normal urinary sediment. Pediatrics 64:678–685, 1979.

127. Font J, Torras A, Cervera R, et al.: Silent renal disease in systemic lupus erythematosus. Clin Nephrol 27:283–288, 1987.

128. Stamenkovic I, Favre H, Donath A, et al.: Renal biopsy in SLE irrespective of clinical findings: Long-term follow-up. Clin Nephrol 26:109–115, 1986.

129. Baumal R, Farine M, Poucell S: Clinical significance of renal biopsies showing mixed mesengial and global proliferative lupus nephritis. Am J Kid Dis 10:236–240, 1987.

130. Baldwin DS, Gluck MC, Lowenstein J, et al.: Lupus nephritis. Clinical course as related to morphologic forms and their transition. Am J Med 62:12–30, 1977.

131. McCluskey RT: Lupus nephritis. In Sommers SC (ed.) Kidney Pathology Decennial 1966–1975. Appleton-Century-Crofts, New York, 1975, pp. 435–460.

132. McLaughlin J, Gladman DD, Urowitz MB, et al.: Kidney biopsy in systemic lupus erythematosus. II. Survival analyses according to biopsy results. Arthritis Rheum 34:1268–1273, 1991.

133. Dumas R: Lupus Nephritis. Collaborative study by the French Society of Paediatric Nephrology. Arch Dis Child 60:126–128, 1985.

134. Tateno S, Kobayashi Y, Hidekazu S, Hiki Y: Study of lupus nephritis: its classification and the significance of subendothelial deposits. Q J Med 207:311–331, 1983.

135. Austin HA III, Muenz LR, Joyce KM, et al.: Prognostic factors in lupus nephritis. Contribution of renal histologic data. Am J Med 75:382–391, 1983.

136. Balow JE: Lupus as a renal disease. Hosp Pract pp. 129–146, October 15, 1988.

137. Nossent HC, Henzen-Logmans SC, Vroom TM, et al.: Contribution of renal biopsy data in predicting outcome in lupus nephritis. Analysis of 116 patients.

Arthritis Rheum 33:970–977, 1990.

138. Rush PH, Baumal R, Shore A, et al.: Correlation of renal histology with outcome in children with lupus nephritis. Kidney Int 29:1066–1071, 1986.

139. Ginzler EM, Bollet AJ, Friedman EA: The natural history and response to therapy of lupus neph.itis. Ann Rev Med 31:463–487, 1980.

140. Hintz G, Acevedo-Vazquez E, Gutierrez-Espinosa G, Avelar-Garnica F: Renal vein thrombosis and inferior vena cava thrombosis in systemic lupus erythematosus. Frequency and risk factors. Arthritis Rheum 27:539–544, 1984.

141. Appel GB, Williams GS, Meltzer JI, et al.: Renal vein thrombosis, nephrotic syndrome, and systemic lupus erythematosus: An association in four cases. Ann Intern Med 85:310–317, 1976.

142. Donadio JV, Burgess JH, Holley KE: Membranous lupus nephropathy: A clinicopathologic study. Medicine 56:527–536, 1977.

143. Ross DI, Lubowitz R: Anticoagulation in renal vein thrombosis. Arch Intern Med 138:1349–1351, 1978.

144. Mailloux LU, Susin M, Stein HL, et al.: Nephrotic syndrome, membranous nephropathy, and renal vein thrombosis: Long-term follow-up. NY State J Med 78:1873–1879, 1978.

145. Fries JF, Holman HR: Systemic Lupus Erythematosus: A Clinical Analysis. Saunders, Philadelphia, 1975.

146. Whiting-O'Keefe Q, Riccardi PJ, Henke JE, et al.: Recognition of information in renal biopsies of patients with lupus nephritis. Ann Intern Med 96:723–727, 1982.

147. Fries JF, Weyl S, Holman HR: Estimating prognosis in systemic lupus erythematosus. Am J Med 57:561–565, 1974.

148. Jacobs JC: Childhood onset systemic lupus erythematosus. NY State J Med 77:2231–2233, 1977.

149. Ginzler EM, Diamond HS, Weiner M, et al.: A multicenter study of outcome in systemic lupus erythematosus. I. Entry variables as predictors of prognosis. Arthritis Rheum 25:601–611, 1982.

150. Reichlin M: Significance of the Ro antigen system. J Clin Immunol 6:339–348, 1986.

151. Rubin LA, Urowitz MB, Gladman DD: Mortality in systemic lupus erythematosus: the bimodal pattern revisited. Qtr J Med, New Series 55:87–98, 1985.

152. Lehman TJA, McCurdy DK, Bernstein BH, et al.: Systemic lupus erythematosus in the first decade of life. Pediatrics 83:235–239, 1989.

153. Hashimoto H, Tsuda H, Hirano T, et al.: Difference in clinical and immunological findings of systemic lupus erythematosus related to age. J Rheumatol 14:497–501, 1987.

154. Celermajer DS, Thorner PS, Baumal R, et al.: Sex differences in childhood lupus nephritis. Am J Dis Child 138:586–588, 1984.

155. Ward MM, Studenski S: Systemic lupus erythematosus in men: a multivariate analysis of gender differences in clinical manifestations. J Rheumatol 17:220–224, 1990.

156. Kaufman LD, Gomez-Reino JJ, Heinicke MH, Gorevic PD: Male lupus: analysis of the clinical and laboratory features of 52 patients, with a review of the literature. Semin Arthritis Rheum 18:189–197, 1989.

157. Tejani A, Nicastri AD, Chen C-K, et al.: Lupus nephritis in black and Hispanic children. Am J Dis Child 137:481–483, 1983.

158. Ward MM, Studenski S: Clinical manifestations of systemic lupus erythemato-

sus. Identification of racial and socioeconomic influences. Arch Intern Med 150:849–853, 1990.

159. Kasiske BL, Neylan III JF, Riggio RR, et al.: The effect of race on access and outcome in transplantation. N Engl J Med 324:302–307, 1991.

160. Callahan LF, Pincus T: Associations between clinical status questionnaire scores and formal education level in persons with systemic lupus erythematosus. Arthritis Rheum 33:407–411, 1990.

161. Urowitz MB, Bookman AAM, Koehler BE, et al.: The bimodal mortality pattern of systemic lupus erythematosus. Am J Med 60:221–225, 1976.

162. Estes D, Christian CL: The natural history of systemic lupus erythematosus by prospective analysis. Medicine 50:85–95, 1971.

163. Karsh J, Klippel JH, Barlow JE, et al.: Mortality in lupus nephritis. Arthritis Rheum 22:764–769, 1979.

164. Swaak AJG, Nossent JC, Bronsveld W, et al.: Systemic lupus erythematosus. I. Outcome and survival: Dutch experience with 110 patients studied prospectively. Ann Rheum Dis 48:447–454, 1989.

165. Ginzler EM, Schorn K: Outcome and prognosis in systemic lupus erythematosus. Rheum Dis Clin North Am 14:67–78, 1988.

166. Bresnihan B: Outcome and survival in systemic lupus erythematosus. Ann Rheum Dis 48:443–445, 1989.

167. Reveille JD, Bartolucci A, Alarcon GS: Prognosis in systemic lupus erythematosus. Negative impact of increasing age at onset, black race, and thrombocytopenia, as well as causes of death. Arthritis Rheum 33:37–48, 1990.

168. Helve T: Prevalence and mortality rates of systemic lupus erythematosus and causes of death in SLE patients in Finland. Scand J Rheum 14:43–46, 1985.

169. Jonsson H, Nived O, Sturfelt G: Outcome in systemic lupus erythematosus: a prospective study of patients from a defined population. Medicine 68:141–150, 1989.

170. Harisdangkul V, Nilganuwonge S, Rockhold L: Cause of death in systemic lupus erythematosus: a pattern based on age at onset. S Med J 80:1249–1253, 1987.

171. Rosner S, Ginzler EM, Diamond HS, et al.: A multicenter study of outcome in systemic lupus erythematosus. II. Causes of Death. Arthritis Rheum 25:612–617, 1982.

172. Caeiro F, Michielson FMC, Bernstein R, et al.: Systemic lupus erythematosus in childhood. Ann Rheum Dis 40:325–331, 1981.

173. Glidden RS, Mantzouranis EC, Borel Y: Systemic lupus erythematosus in childhood: clinical manifestations and improved survival in fifty-five patients. Clin Immun Immunopathol 29:196–210, 1983.

174. Rosner S, Ginzler E, Diamond H, et al.: Causes of death in systemic lupus erythematosus, abstracted. Arthritis Rheum 23:738, 1980.

175. Correria P, Cameron JS, Lian JD, et al.: Why do patients with lupus nephritis die? Br Med J 290:126–131, 1985.

176. Spiera H, Rothenberg RR: Myocardial infarction in four young patients with SLE. J Rheumatol 10:464–466, 1983.

177. Jacobs JC: Lupus erythematosus with nephritis. Pediatrics 41:369–370, 1968.

178. Ropes MW: Systemic Lupus Erythematosus. Harvard University Press, Cambridge, MA, 1976.

179. Heller CA, Schur PH: Serological and clinical remission in systemic lupus erythematosus. J Rheumatol 12:916–918, 1985.

180. Swaak AJG, Nossent JC, Bronsveld W, et al.: Systemic lupus erythematosus. II. Observations on the occurrence of exacerbations in the disease course: Dutch experience with 110 patients studied prospectively. Ann Rheum Dis 48:455–460, 1989.

181. Adelman DC, Wallace DJ, Klinenberg JR: Thirty-four-year delayed-onset lupus nephritis: a case report. Arthritis Rheum 30:479–480, 1987.

182. The Canadian Hydroxychloroquine Study Group: A randomized study of the effect of withdrawing hydroxychloroquine sulfate in systemic lupus erythematosus. N Engl J Med 324:150–154 (see also Editorial pp. 189–191), 1991.

182a. Bombardier C, Gladman DD, Urowitz MB, et al.: Derivation of the SLEDAI: A disease activity index for lupus patients. Arthritis Rheum 35:630–640, 1992.

183. Phadke K, Trachtman H, Nicastri A, et al.: Acute renal failure as the initial manifestation of systemic lupus erythematosus in children. J Pediatr 105:38, 1984.

184. Alverson DC, Chase HP: Systemic lupus erythematosus in childhood presenting as hyperlipoproteinemia. J Pediatr 91:72–75, 1977.

185. Falko JM, Williams JC, Harvey DG, et al.: Hyperlipoproteinemia and multifocal neurologic dysfunction in systemic lupus erythematosus. J Pediatr 95:523–529, 1979.

186. Tan EM, Cohen AS, Fries JF, et al.: The 1982 revised criteria for the classification of systemic lupus erythematosus. Arthritis Rheum 25:1271–1277, 1982 (see also Correspondence, 26:1055, 1983).

187. Ganczarczyk L, Urowitz MB, Gladman DD: Latent lupus. J Rheumatol 16:475–478, 1989.

188. Greer JM, Panush RS: Incomplete lupus erythematosus. Arch Intern Med 149:2473–2476, 1989.

189. Passas CM, Wong RL, Peterson M, et al.: A comparison of the specificity of the 1971 and 1982 American Rheumatism Association criteria for classification of systemic lupus erythematosus. Arthritis Rheum 28:620–623, 1985.

190. Szer IS, Jacobs JC: Systemic lupus erythematosus of childhood. In Lahita RG (ed.) Systemic Lupus Erythematosus. 2nd ed, 1992. Churchill Livingstone, New York, pp. 397–418.

191. Mond CB, Peterson MGE, Rothfield NF: Correlation of anti-Ro antibody with photosensitivity rash in systemic lupus erythematosus patients. Arthritis Rheum 32:202–204, 1989.

192. Vaughn RY, Bailey JP Jr, Field RS, et al.: Diffuse nail dyschromia in black patients with systemic lupus erythematosus. J Rheumatol 17:640–643, 1990.

193. Almeida L, Grossman M: Widespread dermatophyte infections that mimic collagen vascular disease. J Am Dermatol 23:855–857, 1990.

194. Franks AG Jr.: Identifying dermatologic manifestations of lupus erythematosus. J Musculoskel Med #4, pp. 59–75, #5 pp. 69–91, #7 pp. 39–57, 1988.

195. Kettler AH, Bean SF, Duffy JO, Gammon WR: Systemic lupus erythematosus presenting as a bullous eruption in a child. Arch Dermatol 124:1083–1087, 1988.

196. Olansky AJ, Briggaman RA, Gammon WR, et al.: Bullous systemic lupus erythematosus. J Am Acad Dermatol 7:511–520, 1982.

197. Hall RP, Lawlep TJ, Smith HR, et al.: Bullous eruption of systemic lupus erythematosus. Dramatic response to dapsone therapy. Ann Intern Med 97:165–170, 1982.

198. Dotson AD, Raimer SS, Pursley TV, Tschen J: Systemic lupus erythematosus

occurring in a patient with epidermolysis bullosa acquisita. Arch Dermatol 117:422–426, 1981.

199. Jacoby RA, Abraham AA: Bullous dermatosis and systemic lupus erythematosus in a 15-year-old boy. Arch Dermatol 115:1094–1097, 1979.

200. Helm KF, Peters MS: Immunodermatology update: The immunologically mediated vesiculobullous diseases. Mayo Clin Proc 66:187–202, 1991.

201. Ragsdale CG, Petty RE, Cassidy JT, et al.: The clinical progression of apparent juvenile rheumatoid arthritis to systemic lupus erythematosus. J Rheumatol 7:50–55, 1980.

202. Saulsbury FT, Kesler RW, Kennaugh JM, et al.: Overlap syndrome of juvenile rheumatoid arthritis and systemic lupus erythematosus. J Rheumatol 9:610–612, 1982.

203. Panush RS, Edwards L, Longley S, Webster E: 'Rhupus' syndrome. Arch Intern Med 148:1633–1636, 1988.

203a. Kaplan D, Ginzler EM, Feldman J: Arthritis and hypertension in patients with systemic lupus erythematosus. Arthritis Rheum 35:423–428, 1992.

203b. Spronk PE, ter Borg EJ, Kallenberg CGM: Patients with systemic lupus erythematosus and Jaccoud's arthropathy: a clinical subset with an increased C reactive protein response? Ann Rheum Dis 51:358–361, 1992.

204. Alarcon-Segovia D, Abud-Mendoza C, Diaz-Jouanen E: Deforming arthropathy of the hands in systemic lupus erythematosus. J Rheumatol 15:65–69, 1988.

205. Villiaumey J, Arlet J, Avouac B, et al.: Diagnostic criteria and new etiologic events in the arthropathy of Jaccoud: a report of ten cases. Clin Rheumatol Pract 7:156–174, 1986.

206. Martini A, Ravelli A, Viola S, Burgio RG: Systemic lupus erythematosus with Jaccoud's arthropathy mimicking juvenile rheumatoid arthritis. Arthritis Rheum 30:1062–1074, 1987.

207. Coffman JD: Raynaud's phenomenon. New York, Oxford University Press, 1989, pp. 1–186.

207a. Westphalen MA, McGrath MA, Kelly W, et al.: Kawasaki disease with severe peripheral ischemia: treatment with prostaglandin E_1 infusion. J Pediatr 112:431–433, 1988.

207b. Yoshikawa T, Suzuki H, Kato H, Yano S: Effects of prostaglandin E_1 on collagen diseases with high levels of circulating immune complexes. J Rheumatol 17:1513–1514, 1990.

208. Schikler KN, Nagaraj HS, Hodge KM: Torsion of appendix epiploica and acute abdominal pain in systemic lupus erythematosus. Am J Dis Child 136:748, 1982.

209. Zizic TM, Shulman LE, Stevens MB: Colonic perforations in systemic lupus erythematosus. Medicine 54:411–426, 1975.

210. Nadorra RL, Nakazato Y, Landing BH: Pathologic features of gastrointestinal tract lesions in childhood-onset systemic lupus erythematosus: study of 26 patients, with review of the literature. Ped Pathol 7:245–259, 1987.

211. Gladman DD, Ross T, Richardson B, Kulkarni S: Bowel involvement in systemic lupus erythematosus: Crohn's disease or lupus vasculitis? Arthritis Rheum 28:466–470, 1985.

212. Reynolds JC, Inman RD, Kimberly RP, et al.: Acute pancreatitis in SLE: report of twenty cases and a review of the literature. Medicine 61:25–32, 1982.

213. Marino C, Lipstein-Kresch E: Pancreatitis in systemic lupus erythematosus.

Arthritis Rheum 27:118–119, 1984.

214. Martini A, Notarangelo LD, Barberis L: Pancreatitis in systemic lupus. Arthritis Rheum 26:1173, 1983.

215. Goldberg BH, Bergstein JM: Acute respiratory distress in a child after steroid-induced pancreatitis. Pediatrics 61:317–318, 1978.

216. Alverson DC, Chase HP: Systemic lupus erythematosus in childhood presenting as hyperlipoproteinemia. J Pediatr 91:72–75, 1977.

217. Lipsky PE, Hardin JA, Schour L, et al.: Spontaneous peritonitis and systemic lupus erythematosus. JAMA 232:929–931, 1975.

218. Hamdan JA, Ahmad MS, Sa'adi AR: Malacoplakia of the retroperitoneum in a girl with systemic lupus erythematosus. Pediatrics 70:296–299, 1982.

219. Mor F, Beigel Y, Inbal A, et al.: Hepatic infarction in a patient with the lupus anticoagulant. Arthritis Rheum 32:491–495, 1989.

220. Averbuch M, Levo Y: Budd-Chiari syndrome as the major thrombotic complication of systemic lupus erythematosus with the lupus anticoagulant. Ann Rheum Dis 45:435–437, 1986.

221. Lloyd DD, Balfe JW, Barkin M, et al.: Systemic lupus erythematosus with signs of retroperitoneal fibrosis. J Pediatr 85:226–228, 1974.

221a. Buff DD: The etiology of retroperitoneal fibrosis. NYS J Med 91:336–338, 1991.

222. Bitran J, McShane D, Ellman MH: Ascites as the major manifestation of systemic lupus erythematosus. Arthritis Rheum 19:782–785, 1976.

223. Kaklamanis P, Vayopoulos G, Stamatelos G, et al.: Chronic lupus peritonitis with ascites. Ann Rheum Dis 50:176–177, 1991.

224. Tsutsumi A, Sugiyama T, Matsumura R, et al.: Protein losing enteropathy associated with collagen disease. Ann Rheum Dis 50:178–181, 1991.

225. Perednia DA, Curosh NA: Lupus-associated protein-losing enteropathy. Arch Intern Med 150:1806–1810, 1990.

226. Tsukahara M, Matsuo K, Kojima H: Protein-losing enteropathy in a boy with systemic lupus erythematosus. J Pediatr 97:778–780, 1980.

227. Case records of the Massachusetts General Hospital (case no. 42-1979). N Engl J Med 301:881–887, 1979.

228. Rosenstein ED, Wieczorek R, Raphael BG, Agus B: Systemic lupus erythematosus and angioimmunoblastic lymphadenopathy: case report and review of the literature. Semin Arthritis Rheum 16:146–151, 1986.

229. Steinberg AD, Seldin MF, Jaffe ES, et al.: Angioimmunoblastic lymphadenopathy with dysproteinemia. Ann Intern Med 108:575–584, 1988.

230. Runyon BA, Labrecque DR, Anuras S: The spectrum of liver disease in systemic lupus erythematosus. Am J Med 69:187–194, 1980.

231. Maggiore G, Porta G, Bernard O, et al.: Autoimmune hepatitis with initial presentation as acute hepatic failure in young children. J Pediatr 116:280–281, 1990.

232. Budman JR, Steinberg AD: Hematologic aspects of systemic lupus erythematosus. An Intern Med 86:220–229, 1977.

233. Schreiber AD: Immunohematology. JAMA 248:1380–1385, 1982.

234. Bailey FA, Lilly M, Bertoli LF, Ball GV: An antibody that inhibits in vitro bone marrow proliferation in a patient with systemic lupus erythematosus and aplastic anemia. Arthritis Rheum 32:901–905, 1989.

235. Heck LW, Alarcon GS, Ball GV, et al.: Pure red cell aplasia and protein-losing enteropathy in a patient with systemic lupus erythematosus. Arthritis Rheum 28:1059–1061, 1985.

235a. Wong K-F, Chan JKC: Reactive hemophagocytic syndrome-A clinicopathologic study of 40 patients in an oriental population. Am J Med 93:177–180, 1992.

236. Eschbach JW, Kelly MR, Haley NR, et al.: Treatment of the anemia of progressive renal failure with recombinant human erythropoietin. N Engl J Med 321:158–163, 1989.

237. McGuire WA, Yang HH, Bruno E, et al.: Treatment of antibody-mediated pure red-cell aplasia with high-dose intravenous gamma globulin. N Engl J Med 317:1004–1008, 1987.

238. Winkler A, Jackson RW, Kay DS, et al.: High-dose intravenous cyclophosphamide treatment of systemic lupus erythematosus-associated aplastic anemia. Arthritis Rheum 31:693–694, 1988.

239. Brooks Jr BJ, Broxmeyter HE, Bryan CF, Leech SH: Serum inhibitor in systemic lupus erythematosus associated with aplastic anemia. Arch Intern Med 144:1474–1477, 1984.

240. Fitchen JJ, Cline MJ, Saxon A, Golde DW: Serum inhibitors of hematopoiesis in a patient with aplastic anemia and systemic lupus erythematosus. Recovery after exchange plasmapheresis. Am J Med 66:537–542, 1979.

241. Stricker RB, Shuman MA: Aplastic anemia complicating systemic lupus erythematosus: response to androgens in two patients. Am J Hematol 17:193–201, 1984.

242. Cines DB, Passero F, Guerry IV D, et al.: Granulocyte-associated IgG in neutropenic disorders. Blood 59:124–132, 1982.

243. Wetzler M, Talpaz M, Kleinerman ES, et al.: A new familial immunodeficiency disorder characterized by severe neutropenia, a defective marrow release mechanism, and hypogammaglobulinemia. Am J Med 89:663–672, 1990.

243a. Wetzler M, Talpaz M, Kellagher MJ, et al.: Myelokathexis: Normalization of neutrophil counts and morphology by GM-CSF. JAMA 267:2179–80, 1992.

244. Karpatkin S: Autoimmune thrombocytopenic purpura. Clinical Aspects Autoimmunity, 2:21–37, 1988.

245. Imbach PI, Tani P, Berchtold W, et al.: Different forms of chronic childhood thrombocytopenic purpura defined by antiplatelet autoantibodies. J Pediatr 118:535–539, 1991.

246. Maier WP, Gordon DS, Howard RF, et al.: Intravenous immunoglobulin therapy in systemic lupus erythematosus-associated thrombocytopenia. Arthritis Rheum 33:1233–1239, 1990 (see also correspondence 34:787–789, 1991).

246a. Andrew M, Blanchette VS, Adams M, et al.: A multicenter study of the treatment of childhood chronic idiopathic thrombocytopenic purpura with anti-D. J Pediatr 120:522–527, 1992.

247. West SG, Johnson SC: Danazol for the treatment of refractory autoimmune thrombocytopenia in systemic lupus erythematosus. Ann Intern Med 108:703–706, 1988.

248. Ahn YS, Rocha R, Mylvaganam R, et al.: Long-term Danazol therapy in autoimmune thrombocytopenia: unmaintained remission and age-dependent response in women. Ann Intern Med 111:723–729, 1989.

249. Marino C, Cook P: Danazol for lupus thrombocytopenia. Arch Intern Med 145:2251–2252, 1985.

250. Ahn YS, Mylvaganam R, Garcia RO, et al.: Low-dose Danazol therapy in idiopathic thrombocytopenic purpura. Ann Intern Med 107:177–181, 1987.

251. Schreiber AD, Chien P, Tomaski A, Cines DB: Effect of Danazol in immune thrombocytopenic purpura. N Engl J Med 316:503–508, 1987.

252. Boumpas DT, Barez S, Klippel JH, Balow JE: Intermittent cyclophosphamide for the treatment of autoimmune thrombocytopenia in systemic lupus erythematosus. Ann Intern Med 112:674–677, 1990.

253. Rivero SJ, Alger M, Alarcon-Segovia D: Splenectomy for hemocytopenia in systemic lupus erythematosus. Arch Intern Med 139:773–776, 1979.

254. Gruenberg JC, VanSlyck EJ, Abraham JP: Splenectomy in systemic lupus erythematosis. Am Surgeon 52:336–370, 1986.

255. Gladman DD, Urowitz MB, Tozman EC, Glynn MFX: Haemostatic abnormalities in systemic lupus erythematosus. Q J Med 207:424–433, 1983.

256. Sultan Y, Kazatchkine MD, Maisonneuve P, Nydegger UE: Anti-idiotypic suppression of autoantibodies to factor VIII (antihaemophilic factor) by high-dose intravenous gammaglobulin. Lancet 2:765–768, 1984.

257. Peck B, Hoffman GS, Franck WA: Thrombophlebitis in systemic lupus erythematosus. JAMA 240:1728–1730, 1978.

258. Cosgriff TM, Martin BA: Low functional and high antigenic antithrombin III level in a patient with lupus anticoagulant and recurrent thrombosis. Arthritis Rheum 24:94–96, 1981.

259. St. Clair W, Jones B, Rogers JS, et al.: Deep venous thrombosis and a circulating anticoagulant in systemic lupus erythematosus. Am J Dis Child 135:230–232, 1981.

260. Boey ML, Loizou S, Colaco CB, et al.: Antithrombin III in systemic lupus erythematosus. Clin Exp Rheumatol 2:53–56, 1984.

261. Kerr LD, Spiera H, Aledort LN: Acute disseminated intravascular coagulation as a complication of systemic lupus erythematosus. NYS J Med 87:181–183, 1987.

262. Pui C-H, Wilimas J, Wang W: Evans syndrome in childhood. J Pediatr 97:754–758, 1980.

263. Favre H, Chatelanat F, Miescher P: Autoimmune hematologic diseases associated with infraclinical systemic lupus erythematosus in four patients: A human equivalent of the NZB mice. Am J Med 66:91–95, 1979.

264. Miller BA, Beardsley DS: Autoimmune pancytopenia of childhood associated with multisystem disease manifestations. J Pediatr 103:877–881, 1983.

265. Lavalle C, Hurtado R, Quezada JJ, et al.: Hemocytopenia as initial manifestation of systemic lupus erythematosus. Prognostic significance. Clin Rheumatol 2:227–232, 1983.

266. Miller MH, Urowitz MB, Gladman DD: The significance of thrombocytopenia in systemic lupus erythematosus. Arthritis Rheum 26:1181–1186, 1983.

267. White LE, Reeves JD: Polyarthritis and positive LE preparation in sickle hemoglobinopathies: A report of two cases. J Pediatr 95:1003–1004, 1979.

268. Young GAR, Vincent PC: Infectious mononucleosis and systemic lupus erythematosus. Lancet 1:971–972, 1982.

269. Hendry BM, Longmore JM: Systemic lupus erythematosus presenting as infectious mononucleosis with a false positive monospot test. Lancet 1:455, 1982.

270. Wu KK: Microvascular thrombosis: patholophysiology and new strategies. Hosp Pract 20:47–54, May 15, 1985.

271. Jain R, Chartash E, Furie R: Systemic lupus erythematosus complicated by thrombotic microangiopathy. Arthritis Rheum 34:S93, 1991.

272. Wallace DJ, Podell T, Weiner J, et al.: Systemic lupus erythematosus—survival patterns. Experience with 609 patients. JAMA 245:934–938, 1981.

273. Wallace DJ, Pistiner M, Klinenberg JR, et al.: 464 patients with idiopathic

SLE: natural course, treatment and causes of death. Arthritis Rheum 33S:130, 1990.

274. Elseviers MM, Verpooten GA, De Broe ME, DeBacker GG: Interpretation of creatinine clearance. Lancet 1:457, 1987.

275. Roubenoff R, Drew H, Moyer M, et al.: Oral cimetidine improves the accuracy and precision of creatinine clearance in lupus nephritis. Ann Intern Med 113:501, 1990.

276. Ratain JS, Petri M, Hochberg MC, Hellmann DB: Accuracy of creatinine clearance in measuring glomerular filtration rate in patients with systemic lupus erythematosus without clinical evidence of renal disease. Arthritis Rheum 33:277–280, 1990.

277. Cathcart ES, Scheinberg MA, Idelson BA: Beneficial effects of methylprednisone "pulse" therapy in diffuse proliferative lupus nephritis. Lancet 1:163–166, 1976.

278. Cole BR, Brocklebank JT, Kienstra RA, et al.: "Pulse" methylprednisolone therapy in the treatment of severe glomerulonephritis. J Pediatr 88:307–314, 1976.

279. Garrett R, Paulus H: Complications of intravenous methylprednisone pulse therapy, abstracted. Arthritis Rheum 23:677, 1980.

280. Moore WS, Guggenheim SJ, Anderson RJ: Diffuse proliferative lupus glomerulonephritis: Recovery from prolonged renal failure. JAMA 244:63–65, 1980.

281. Edworthy SM, Bloch DA, McShane DJ, et al.: A "state model" of renal function in systemic lupus erythematosus: its value in the prediction of outcome in 292 patients. J Rheumatol 16:29–35, 1989.

282. Kimberly RP, Lockshin MD, Sherman RL, et al.: Reversible "end-stage" lupus nephritis. Analysis of patients able to discontinue dialysis. Am J Med 74:361–368, 1983.

283. Nossent HC, Swaak TJG, Berden JHM, Dutch Working Party on SLE: Systemic lupus erythematosus after renal transplantation: patient and graft survival and disease activity. Ann Intern Med 114:183–188, 1991.

284. Nossent HC, Swaak TJG, Berden JHM, et al.: Systemic lupus erythematosus: analysis of disease activity in 55 patients with end-stage renal failure treated with hemodialysis or continuous ambulatory peritoneal dialysis. Am J Med 89:169–174, 1990.

285. Lee FO, Quismorio EP Jr. Troum OM, et al.: Mechanisms of hyperkalemia in systemic lupus erythematosus. Ann Intern Med 148:397–401, 1988.

286. Ostrov BE, Min W, Eichenfield AH, et al.: Hypertension in children with systemic lupus erythematosus. Semin Arthritis Rheum 19:90–98, 1989.

287. Laragh JH: Hypertension. Drug Therapy 10:71–88, January 1980.

288. McCurdy DK, Lehman TJA, Bernstein B et al.: Lupus nephritis: Prognostic factors in children. Pediatrics 89:240–249, 1992.

288a. Seleznick MJ, Fries JF: Variables associated with decreased survival in systemic lupus erythematosus. Semin Arthritis Rheum 21:73–80, 1991.

289. Dresner JG, Dysart NK, Michael AF, et al.: Central nervous system (CNS) lupus erythematosus (LE) in children, abstracted. Pediatr Res 12:551, 1978.

290. Weber MA: Editorials: Immediate treatment of severe hypertension. Widening the options. Arch Intern Med 149:2635–2636, 1989.

291. Sturgill BC, Shearlock KT: Membranous glomerulopathy and nephrotic syndrome after captopril therapy. JAMA 250:2343–2345, 1983.

292. Messerli FH (Editor): Calcium antagonists: current use and future implica-

tions: proceedings of a symposium. Am J Med 90(5A):1–53S, 1991.

292a. Epstein M: Calcium antagonists and renal protection. Arch Intern Med 152:1573–1584, 1992.

293. Klinkhoff AV, Beattie CW, Chalmers A: Retinopathy in systemic lupus erythematosus: relationship to disease activity. Arthritis Rheum 29:1152–1156, 1986.

294. Stafford-Brady FJ, Urowitz MB, Cladman DD, Easterbrook M: Lupus retinopathy. Patterns, associations, and prognosis. Arthritis Rheum 31:1105–1110, 1988.

295. Silverman M, Lubeck MJ, Briney EG: Central retinal vein occlusion complicating systemic lupus erythematosus. Arthritis Rheum 21:839–843, 1978.

296. Kraus A, Cervantes G, Barojas E, Alarcon Segovia D: Retinal vasculitis in mixed connective tissue disease: A fluorangiographic study. J Rheumatol 12:1122–1124, 1985.

297. Smith CA, Pinals RS: Optic neuritis in systemic lupus erythematosus. J Rheumatol 9:963–966, 1982.

298. Kenik JG, Krohn K, Kelly RB, et al.: Transverse myelitis and optic neuritis in systemic lupus erythematosus: a case report with magnetic resonance imaging findings. Arthritis Rheum 30:947–950, 1987.

299. Tsokos GC, Tsokos M, le Riche NGH, Klippel JH: A clinical and pathologic study of cerebrovascular disease in patients with systemic lupus erythematosus. Semin Arthritis Rheum 16:70–78, 1986.

300. Omdal R, Mellgren SI, Husby G: Clinical neuropsychiatric and neuromuscular manifestations in systemic lupus erythematosus. Scand J Rheumatol 17:113–117, 1988.

301. Yancey CL, Doughty RA, Athreya BH: Central nervous system involvement in childhood systemic lupus erythematosus. Arthritis Rheum 24:1389–1395, 1981.

302. Vermess M, Bernstein RM, Bydder GM, et al.: Nuclear magnetic resonance (NMR) imaging of the brain in systemic lupus erythematosus. J Comput Assist Tomogr 7:461–467, 1983.

302a. Hay EM, Black D, Huddy A, et al.: Psychiatric disorder and cognitive impairment in systemic lupus erythematosus. Arthritis Rheum 35:411–416, 1992.

303. King J, Aukett A, Smith MF, et al.: Cerebral systemic lupus erythematosus. Arch Dis Child 63:968–970, 1988.

304. Winfield JB, Brunner CM, Koffler D: Serologic studies in patients with systemic lupus erythematosus and central nervous system dysfunction. Arthritis Rheum 21:289–294, 1978.

305. Hopkins P, Belmont HM, Buyon J, et al.: Increased levels of plasma anaphylatoxins in systemic lupus erythematosus predict flares of the disease and may elicit vascular injury in lupus cerebritis. Arthritis Rheum 31:632–641, 1988.

306. Johnson RT, Richardson EP: The neurological manifestations of systemic lupus erythematosus. Medicine 47:337–369, 1968.

307. Gershwin ME, Hyman LR, Steinberg AD: The choroid plexus in CNS involvement of systemic lupus erythematosus. J Pediatr 87:588–590, 1975.

308. Zvaifler NJ, Bluestein HG: The pathogenesis of central nervous system manifestations of systemic lupus erytematosus. Arthritis Rheum 25:862–866, 1982.

309. Bonfa E, Golombek SJ, Kaufman LD, et al.: Association between lupus psychosis and anti-ribosomal P protein antibodies. N Engl J Med 317:265–311, 1987 (see also editorial p. 309–311).

310. Schneebaum AB, Singleton JD, West SG, et al.: Association of psychiatric manifestations with antibodies to ribosmal P proteins in systemic lupus erythemato-

sus. Am J Med 90:54–62, 1991.

311. Shergy WJ, Kredich DW, Pisetsky DS: The relationship of anticardiolipin anti-bodies to disease manifestations in pediatric systemic lupus erythematosus. J Rheumatol 15:1389–1394, 1988.

312. Nossent JC, Hovestadt A, Schonfeld DHW, et al.: Single-photon-emission computed tomography of the brain in the evaluation of cerebral lupus. Arthritis Rheum 34:1397–1403, 1991.

313. Pinching AJ, Travers RL, Hughes GRV: Oxygen-15 brain scanning for detection of cerebral involvement in systemic lupus erythematosus. Lancet 1:888–890, 1978.

314. Kushner MJ, Chawluk J, Fazekas F, et al.: Cerebral blood flow in systemic lupus erythematosus with or without cerebral complications. Neurology 37:1596–1598, 1987.

315. Bilaniuk LT, Patel S, Zimmerman RA: Computed tomography of systemic lupus erythematosus. Radiology 124:119–121, 1977.

316. Bell CL, Partington C, Robbins M, et al.: Magnetic resonance imaging of central nervous system lesions in patients with lupus erythematosus. Correlation with clinical remission and antineurofilament and anticardiolipin antibody titers. Arthritis Rheum 34:432–441, 1991.

317. Nordstrom DM, West SG, Andersen PA: Basal ganglia calcifications in central nervous system lupus erythematosus. Arthritis Rheum 28:1412–1416, 1985.

318. Yokota S, Mori T, Kosuge K, et al.: (Abstract) Basal ganglia calcification in two children with systemic lupus erythematosus and neuropsychiatric manifestations. Ryumachi 25:121–122, 1985.

319. Brandt KD, Lessell S: Migrainous phenomena in systemic lupus erythematosus. Arthritis Rheum 21:7–16, 1978.

320. Carlow TJ, Glaser JS: Pseudotumor cerebri in systemic lupus erythematosus. JAMA 228:197–200, 1974.

321. Shoenfeld Y, Livni E, Shaklai M, et al.: Sensitization to ibuprofen in systemic lupus erythematosus. JAMA 244:547–548, 1980.

322. Kassan SS, Lockshin MD: Central nervous system lupus erythematosus. Arthritis Rheum 22:1382–1385, 1979.

323. Lehman TJA, Bernstein B, Hanson V, et al.: Meningococcal infection complicating systemic lupus erythematosus. J Pediatr 99:94–96, 1981.

324. Jabs DA, Miller NR, Newman SA, et al.: Optic neuropathy in systemic lupus erythematosus. Arch Ophthalmol 104:564–568, 1986.

325. Sharfstein SS, Sack DS, Fauci AS: Relationship between alternate-day cortico-steroid therapy and behavioral abnormalities. JAMA 248:2987–2989, 1982.

325a. Dungan DD, Jay MS: Stroke in an early adolescent with systemic lupus erythematosus and coexistent antiphospholipid antibodies. Pediatrics 90:96–99, 1992.

326. Cronin ME, Biswas RM, Van der Straeton C, et al.: IgG and IgM anticardiolipin antibodies in patients with lupus with anticardiolipin antibody associated clinical syndromes. J Rheumatol 15:795–798, 1988.

327. Asherson RA, Lubbe WF: Editorial: Cerebral and valve lesions in SLE: association with antiphospholipid antibodies. J Rheumatol 15:539–543, 1988.

328. Harris EN, Gharvai AE, Asherson RA, et al.: Cerebral infarction in systemic lupus: association with anticardiolipin antibodies. Clin Exp Rheumatol 2:47–51, 1984.

329. Asherson RA, Derksen RHWM, Harris EN, et al.: Chorea in systemic lupus erythematosus and "lupus-like" disease: association with antiphospholipid anti-

bodies. Semin Arthritis Rheum 16:253–259, 1987.

330. Lusins JO, Szilagyi PA: Clinical features of chorea associated with systemic lupus erythematosus. Am J Med 58:857–861, 1975.

331. Groothius JR, Groothius DR, Mukhopadhyay D, et al.: Lupus-associated chorea in childhood. Am J Dis Child 131:1131–1134, 1977.

332. Herd JK, Medhi M, Uzendoski DM, et al.: Chorea associated with systemic lupus erythematosus: Report of two cases and review of the literature. Pediatrics 61:308–315, 1978.

333. Andrianakos AA, Duffy J, Suzuki M, et al.: Transverse myelopathy in systemic lupus erythematosus: Report of three cases and review of the literature. Ann Intern Med 83:616–624, 1975.

334. de Brum-Fernandes AJ, de F. Lucena-Fernandes M, Levy-Neto M, Cossermelli W: Myelitis in systemic lupus erythematosus. Arthritis Rheum 30:238–239, 1987.

335. Chang R, Quismorio FP Jr.: Transverse myelopathy in systemic lupus erythematosus (SLE). Arthritis Rheum 33S:102, 1990.

336. Guthrie JA, Turney JH: Plasma exchange for cerebral lupus erythematosus. Lancet 1:506–507, 1987.

337. Smith GM, Leyland MJ: Plasma exchange for cerebral lupus erythematosus. Lancet 1:103, 1987.

338. Warren RW, Kredich DW: Transverse myelitis and acute central nervous system manifestations of systemic lupus erythematosus. Arthritis Rheum 27:1058–1060, 1984.

339. Propper DJ, Bucknall RC: Acute transverse myelopathy complicating systemic lupus erythematosus. Ann Rheum Dis 48:512–515, 1989.

340. Sloan JB, Berk MA, Gebel HM, Fretzin DF: Multiple sclerosis and systemic lupus erythematosus. Arch Intern Med 147:1317–1320, 1987.

341. Kaplan RE, Springate JE, Feld LG, Cohen ME: Pseudotumor cerebri associated with cerebral venous sinus thrombosis, internal jugular vein thrombosis, and systemic lupus erythematosus. J Pediatr 107:266–268, 1985.

342. Li EK, Ho PCP: Pseudotumor cerebri in systemic lupus erythematosus. J Rheumatol 16:113–116, 1989.

343. Wasner CK: Ibuprofen, meningitis, and systemic lupus erythematosus. J Rheumatol 5:162–164, 1978.

344. Agus B, Nayar S, Patel DJ, McGrath M: Inappropriate secretion of ADH in a patient with systemic lupus erythematosus. Arthritis Rheum 26:237–238, 1983 (see also correspondence p. 1055).

345. Scheinberg L: Polyneuritis in systemic lupus erythematosus. Review of the literature and report of a case. N Engl J Med 255:416–421, 1956.

346. van Doorn PA, Vermeulen M, Brand A, et al.: Intravenous immunoglobulin treatment in patients with chronic inflammatory demyelinating polyneuropathy. Arch Neurol 48:217–220, 1991.

347. Winfield JB, Brunner CM, Koffler D: Serologic studies in patients with systemic lupus erythematosus and central nervous system dysfunction. Arthritis Rheum 21:289–294, 1978.

348. Englert HJ, Loizou S, Derue GGM, et al.: Clinical and immunologic features of livedo reticularis in lupus: a case-control study. Am J Med 87:408–410, 1989.

349. Strauer BE, Brune I, Schenk H, et al.: Lupus cardiomyopathy: Cardiac mechanics, hemodynamics, and coronary blood flow in uncomplicated systemic lupus erythematosus. Am Heart J 92:715–722, 1976.

350. Bulkley BH, Roberts EC: The heart in systemic lupus erythematosus and the changes induced in it by corticosteroid therapy. Am J Med 58:243–264, 1975.

351. Mandell BF: Cardiovascular involvement in systemic lupus erythematosus. Semin Arthritis Rheum 17:126–141, 1987.

352. Crozier IG, Li E, Milne MJ, Nicholls MG: Cardiac involvement in systemic lupus erythematosus detected by echocardiography. Am J Cardiol 65:1145–1148, 1990.

353. Lehman TJA, Palmeri ST, Hastings C, et al.: Bacterial endocarditis complicating systemic lupus erythematosus. J Rheumatol 10:655–658, 1983.

354. Averbuch M, Bojko A, Levo Y: Cardiac tamponade in the early postpartum period as the presenting and predominant manifestation of systemic lupus erythematosus. J Rheumatol 13:444–445, 1986.

355. Alpert MA, Goldberg SH, Singsen BH, et al.: Cardiovascular manifestations of mixed connective tissue disease in adults. Circulation 68:1182–1193, 1983.

356. Holloway JD, Garcia W, Espinoza LR: Cardiac tamponade in a healthy young woman. Hosp Pract 23:128–134, July 15, 1987.

357. Greenberg JH, Lutcher CL: Drug-induced systemic lupus erythematosus: a case with life-threatening pericardial tamponade. JAMA 222:191–193, 1972.

358. Carey RM, Coleman M, Feder A: Pericardial tamponade: a major presenting manifestation of hydralazine-induced lupus syndrome. Am J Med 54:84–87, 1973.

359. Jacobson EJ, Reza JJ: Constrictive pericarditis in systemic lupus erythematosus; demonstration of immunoglobulins in the pericardium. Arthritis Rheum 21:972–974, 1978.

360. Coe MD, Hamer DH, Levy CS, et al.: Gonococcal pericarditis with tamponade in a patient with systemic lupus erythematosus. Arthritis Rheum 33:1438–1441, 1990.

361. Kaufman LD, Seifert FC, Eilbott DJ, et al.: Candida pericarditis and tamponade in a patient with systemic lupus erythematosus. Arch Intern Med 148:715–717, 1988.

362. Borenstein DG, Fye WB, Arnett FC, et al.: The myocarditis of systemic lupus erythematosus: association with myositis. Ann Intern Med 89:619–624, 1978.

363. Logar D, et al.: Anti-Ro antibodies associated with cardiac manifestations of SLE. Ann Rheum Dis 49:627–629, 1990.

364. Galve E, Candell-Riera J, Pigrau C, et al.: Prevalence, morphologic types, and evolution of cardiac valvular disease in systemic lupus erythematosus. N Engl J Med 319:817–823, 1988 (see also correspondence 320–322, 1989).

365. Jordan JM, Valenstein P, Kredich DW: Systemic lupus erythematosus with Libman-Sachs endocarditis in a 9-month-old infant with neonatal lupus erythematosus and congenital heart block. Pediatrics 84:574–578, 1989.

366. Chartash EK, Lans DM, Paget SA, et al.: Aortic insufficiency and mitral regurgitation in patients with systemic lupus erythematosus and the antiphospholipid syndrome. Am J Med 86:407–412, 1989.

367. Asherson RA, Gibson DG, Evans DW, et al.: Diagnostic and therapeutic problems in two patients with antiphospholipid antibodies, heart valve lesions, and transient ischaemic attacks. Ann Rheum Dis 47:947–953, 1988.

368. Leung W-H, Wong K-L, Lau C-P, et al.: Association between antiphospholipid antibodies and cardiac abnormalities in patients with systemic lupus erythematosus. Am J Med 89:411–419, 1990.

369. Ford PM, Ford SE, Lillicrap DP: Association of lupus anticoagulant with severe

valvular heart disease in systemic lupus erythematosus. J Rheumatol 15:597–600, 1988.

370. Lubbe WF, Asherson RA: Intracardiac thrombus in systemic lupus erythematosus associated with lupus anticoagulant. Arthritis Rheum 31:1453–1454, 1988.

371. Maier WP, Ramirez HE, Miller SB: Complete heart block as the initial manifestation of systemic lupus erythematosus. Arch Intern Med 147:170–171, 1987.

372. Ishikawa S, Segar WE, Gilbert EF: Myocardial infarction in a child with systemic lupus erythematosus. Am J Dis Child 132:696–698, 1978.

373. Bonfiglio TA, Botti RE, Hagstrom JWC: Coronary arteritis, occlusion and myocardial infarction due to systemic lupus erythematosus. Am Heart J 83:153–158, 1972.

374. Englund JA, Lucas RV Jr: Cardiac complications in children with systemic lupus erythematosus. Pediatrics 72:724–730, 1983.

375. Friedman DM, Lazarus HM, Fierman AH: Acute myocardial infarction in pediatric systemic lupus erythematosus. J Pediatr 117:263–266, 1990.

376. Hosenpud JD, Montanaro A, Hart MV, et al.: Myocardial perfusion abnormalities in asymptomatic patients with systemic lupus erythematosus. Am J Med 77:286–292, 1984.

377. Etheridge EM, Hoch-Legeti C: Lipid deposition in aortas in younger age groups following cortisone and adrenocorticotropic hormone. Am J Pathol 28:315–332, 1952.

378. Alverson DC, Chase HP: Systemic lupus erythematosus in childhood presenting as hyperlipoproteinemia. J Pediatr 91:72–75, 1977.

379. Falko JM, Williams JC, Harvey DG, et al.: Hyperlipoproteinemia and multifocal neurologic dysfunction in systemic lupus erythematosus. 95:523–529, 1979.

380. Ettinger WH, Goldberg AP, Applebaum-Bowden D, Hazzard WR: Dyslipoproteinemia in systemic lupus erythematosus. Effect of corticosteroids. Am J Med 83:503–508, 1987.

381. Ilowite NT, Samuel P, Ginzler E, Jacobson MS: Dyslipoproteinemia in pediatric systemic lupus. Arthritis Rheum 31:859–863, 1988.

382. Haupt HM, Moore CW, Hutchins CM: The lung in systemic lupus erythematosus: analysis of the pathologic changes in 120 patients. Am J Med 71:791–798, 1981.

383. Pines A, Kaplinsky N, Olchovsky D, et al.: Pleuro-pulmonary manifestations of systemic lupus erythematosus: clinical features of its subgroups. Prognostic and therapeutic implications. Chest 88:129–135, 1985.

384. Saltzman HA, Alavi A, Greenspan RH, (PIOPED investigators), et al.: Value of the ventilation/perfusion scan in acute pulmonary embolism. Results of the prospective investigation of pulmonary embolism diagnosis (PIOPED). JAMA 263:2753–2759, 1990.

385. Gaither NS, Wortham D, Brinker JL: Current recommedations for use of pulmonary angiography. IM 12:19–34, August 1991.

386. De Jongste JC, Neijens HJ, Duiverman EJ, et al.: Respiratory tract disease in systemic lupus erythematosus. Arch Dis Child 61:478–483, 1986.

387. Nadorra RL, Landing BH: Pulmonary lesions in childhood onset systemic lupus erythematosus: analysis of 26 cases, and summary of literature. Ped Pathol 7:1–18, 1987.

388. Delgado EA, Malleson PN, Pirie GE, Petty RE: The pulmonary manifestations

of childhood onset systemic lupus erythematosus. Semin Arthritis Rheum 19:285–293, 1990.

389. Gilleece MH, Evans CC, Bucknall RC: Steroid resistant pleural effusion in systemic lupus erythematosus treated with tetracycline pleurodesis. Ann Rheum Dis 47:1031–1032, 1988.

390. Segel AM, Calabrese LH, Ahmad M, et al.: The pulmonary manifestations of systemic lupus erythematosus. Semin Arthritis Rheum 14:202–224, 1985.

391. Gross M, Esterly JR, Earle RH: Pulmonary alterations in systemic lupus erythematosus. Am Rev Resp Dis 105:572–577, 1972.

392. Tomaselli G, Gamsu G, Stulbary MS: Constrictive pericarditis presenting as pleural effusion of unknown origin. Arch Intern Med 149:201–203, 1989.

393. Jay MS, Jerath R, Van Derzalm T, et al.: Pneumothorax in an adolescent with fulminant systemic lupus erythematosus. J Adolescent Health Care 5:142–144, 1984.

394. Matthay RA, Schwartz MI, Petty TL, et al.: Pulmonary manifestations of systemic lupus erythematosus: review of twelve cases of acute lupus pneumonitis. Medicine 54:397–409, 1974.

395. Hedgpeth MT, Boulware DW: Interstitial pneumonitis in antinuclear antibody-negative systemic lupus erythematosus: a new clinical manifestation and possible association with Anti-Ro (SS-A) antibodies. Arthritis Rheum 31:545–548, 1988.

396. Rubin LA, Urowitz MB: Shrinking lung syndrome in SLE—a clinical pathologic study. J Rheumatol 10:973–976, 1983.

397. Inoue T, Kanayame Y, Ohe A, et al.: Immunopathologic studies of pneumonitis in systemic lupus erythematosus. Ann Intern Med 91:30–34, 1979.

398. Fayemi AO: Pulmonary vascular disease in systemic lupus erythematosus. Am J Clin Pathol 65:284–290, 1976.

399. Bjornsson J, Edwards WD: Primary pulmonary hypertension: a histopathologic study of 80 cases. Mayo Clin Proc 60:16–25, 1985.

400. White RH, McGahan JP, Daschbach MM, Hartling RP: Diagnosis of deep-vein thrombosis using duplex ultrasound. Ann Intern Med 111:297–304, 1989.

401. Hull RD, Raskob GE, Coates G, et al.: A new noninvasive management strategy for patients with suspected pulmonary embolism. Arch Intern Med 149:2549–2555, 1989.

402. Marder VJ, Sherry S: Thrombolytic therapy: current status, part II. N Engl J Med 318:1585–1593, 1988.

403. Mitchell JP, Trulock EP: Tissue-Plasminogen activator for pulmonary embolism resulting in shock: Two case reports and discussion of the literature. Am J Med 90:255–260, 1991.

404. Rajani KB, Ashbacher LV, Kinney TR: Pulmonary hemorrhage and systemic lupus erythematosus. J Pediatr 93:810–812, 1978.

405. Abud-Mendoza C, Diaz-Jouanen E, Alarcon-Segovia D: Fatal pulmonary hemorrhage in systemic lupus erythematosus. Occurrence without hemoptysis. J Rheumatol 12:558–561, 1985.

406. Miller RW, Salcedo JR, Fink RJ, et al.: Pulmonary hemorrhage in pediatric patients with systemic lupus erythematosus. J Pediatr 108:576–579, 1986.

407. Clinicopathologic Conference: anemia, abdominal pain, and death in a 19-year-old woman. Am J Med 83:93–100, 1987.

408. Castaneda S, Herrero-Beaumont G, Valenzuela A, et al.: Massive pulmonary hemorrhage: fatal complication of systemic lupus erythematosus. J Rheumatol

12:186–187, 1985.

409. Ramirez RE, Glasier C, Kirks D, et al.: Pulmonary hemorrhage associated with systemic lupus erythematosus in children. Radiology 152:409–412, 1984.

410. Howe HS, Boey ML, Fong KY, Feng PH: Pulmonary haemorrhage, pulmonary infarction, and the lupus anticoagulant. Ann Rheum Dis 47:869–872, 1988.

411. Leatherman JW, Davies SF, Hoidal JR: Alveolar hemorrhage syndromes: diffuse microvascular lung hemorrhage in immune and idiopathic disorders. Medicine 63:343–361, 1984.

412. Schwab EP, Freundlich B, Callegan PE: Prognosis and therapy of pulmonary alveolar hemorrhage in systemic lupus erythematosus. Arthritis Rheum 34: S188, 1991.

413. Simpson IJ, Doak PB, Williams LC, et al.: Plasma exchange in Goodpasture's syndrome. Am J Nephrol 2:301–311, 1982.

414. Raz E, Bursztyn M, Rosenthal T, Rubinow A: Severe recurrent lupus laryngitis. Am J Med 92:109–110, 1992.

415. Hellman DB, Petri M, Whiting-O'Keefe Q: Fatal infections in systemic lupus erythematosus: the role of opportunistic organisms. Medicine 66:341–348, 1987.

416. Nived O, Sturfelt G, Wollheim F: Systemic lupus erythematosus and infection: a controlled and prospective study including an epidemiological group. Q J Med 218:271–287, 1985.

417. Boghossian SH, Isenberg DA, Wright G, et al.: Effect of high-dose methylprednisolone therapy on phagocyte function in systemic lupus erythematosus. Ann Rheum Dis 43:541–550, 1984.

418. Orth RW, Weisman MH, Cohen AH, et al.: Lupus cystitis: primary bladder manifestations of systemic lupus erythematosus. Ann Intern Med 98:323–326, 1983.

419. Abramson S, Kramer S, Radin A, et al.: Salmonella bacteremia in systemic lupus erythematosus: eight-year experience at a municipal hospital. Arthritis Rheum 28:75–79, 1985.

420. Frayha RA, Jizi I, Saadeh G: Salmonella typhimurium bacteriuria. An increased infection rate in systemic lupus erythematosus. Arch Intern Med 145:645–647, 1985.

421. Malleson P, Petty RE, Nadel H, Dimmick JE: Functional asplenia in childhood onset systemic lupus erythematosus. J Rheumatol 15:1648–1652, 1988.

421a. Lipnick RN, Karsh J, Stahl NI, et al.: Pneumococcal immunization in patients with systemic lupus erythematosus treated with immunosuppressives. J Rheumatol 12:1118–1121, 1985.

422. Johnson WM, Gall EP: Fatal coccidiodomycosis in collagen vascular diseases. J Rheumatol 10:79–84, 1983.

423. Livneh A, Coman EA, Cho S, Lipstein-Kresch E: Strongyloides stercoralis hyperinfection mimicking systemic lupus erythematosus flare. Arthritis Rheum 31:930–931, 1988.

424. Ashman RF, White RH, Wiesenhutter C, et al.: Panhypogammaglobulinemia in systemic lupus erythematosus: in vitro demonstration of multiple cellular defects. J Allergy Clin Immunol 70:465, 1982.

425. Sussman GL, Rivera VJ, Kohler PF: Transition from systemic lupus erythematosus to common variable hypogammaglobulinemia. Ann Intern Med 99:32–35, 1983.

426. Goldstein R, Izaguirre C, Smith CD, et al.: Systemic lupus erythematosus and common variable panhypogammaglobulinemia: a patient with absence of circu-

lating B cells. Arthritis Rheum 28:100–103, 1985.

427. Stein A, Winkelstein A, Agarwal A: Concurrent systemic lupus erythematosus and common variable hypogammaglobulinemia. Arthritis Rheum 28:462–465, 1985.

428. Baum CG, Chiorazzi N, Frankel S, Shepherd GM: Conversion of systemic lupus erythematosus to common variable hypogammaglobulinemia. Am J Med 87:449–456, 1989.

429. Tsokos GC, Smith PL, Balow JE: Development of hypogammaglobulinemia in a patient with systemic lupus erythematosus. Am J Med 81:1081–1084, 1986.

430. Jacobs JC: Transient hypogammaglobulinemia (TH) with sepsis. A manifestation of childhood systemic lupus erythematosus (SLE) which improves with more immunosuppressive therapy. Pediatr Res 29(No. 4, Pt. 2):158A, 1991.

431. Akashi K, Nagasawa K, Mayumi T, et al.: Successful treatment of refractory systemic lupus erythematosus with intravenous immunoglobulins. J Rheumatol 17:375–379, 1990.

432. Bernstein B, Koster-King K, Singsen B, et al.: Sjögren's syndrome in childhood Arthritis Rheum 20:361–362, 1977.

433. Athreya B, Norman ME, Myers AR, et al.: Sjögren's syndrome in children. Pediatrics 59:931–938, 1977.

434. Jackson J, Anderson L, Schur P, et al.: Sjögren's syndrome in juvenile rheumatoid arthritis (JRA), abstracted. Arthritis Rheum 16:122, 1973.

435. Talal N, Moutsopoulos HM, Kassan S, (eds): Sjogren's Syndrome: Clinical and Immunological Aspects. Springer-Verlag: Heidelberg, 1987.

436. Kassan SS, Thomas TL, Moutsopoulos HM, et al.: Increased risk of lymphoma in sicca syndrome. Ann Intern Med 89:888–892, 1978.

437. Fraga A, Gudino J, Ramos-Niembro F, et al.: Mixed connective tissue disease in childhood: relationship with Sjögren's syndrome. Am J Dis Child 132:263–266, 1978.

438. Singsen BH, Swanson VL, Bernstein BH, et al.: A histologic evaluation of mixed connective tissue disease in childhood. Am J Med 68:710–717, 1980.

439. De Clerck LS, Coutteneye MM, de Broe ME, Stevens WJ: Acquired immunodeficiency syndrome mimicking Sjogren's Syndrome and systemic lupus erythematosus. Arthritis Rheum 31:272–275, 1988.

440. Flescher E, Talal N: Do viruses contribute to the development of Sjogren's Syndrome? Am J Med 90:283–294, 1991.

441. Harley JB: Autoantibodies in Sjogren's Syndrome. In Sjogren's Syndrome: Clinical and Immunological Aspects. Springer-Verlag, Berlin, New York, 1987, pp. 218–234.

442. Provost TT, Alexander EL, Reichlin M: The relationship between anti-Ro (SS-A) precipitin antibody positive Sjogren's syndrome and anti-Ro (SS-A) precipitin antibody positive lupus erythematosus. Ibid, pp. 247–257.

443. Eberhard BA, Laxer RM, Eddy AA, Silverman ED: Presence of thyroid abnormalities in children with systemic lupus erythematosus. J Pediatr 119:277–279, 1990.

444. Miller FW, Moore GF, Weintraub BD, Steinberg AD: Prevalence of thyroid disease and abnormal thyroid function test results in patients with systemic lupus erythematosus. Arthritis Rheum 30:1124–1131, 1987 (see also correspondence 31:1079–1080, 1980).

445. Franzen P, Friman C, Pettersson T, et al.: Combined pure red cell aplasia and primary autoimmune hypothyroidism in systemic lupus erythematosus. Arthitis

Rheum 30:839–840, 1987.

446. Utiger RD: The pathogenesis of autoimmune thyroid disease. N Engl J Med 325:278–279, 1991.

447. Tucker WS, Niblack GD, McLean RH, et al.: Serositis with autoimmune endocrinopathy: clinical and immunogenetic features. Medicine 66:138–146. 1987.

448. Case records of the Massachusetts General Hospital. Case 15-1985. N Engl J Med 312:976–983, 1985.

448a. Levy EN, Ramsey-Goldman R, Kahl LE: Adrenal insufficiency in two women with anticardiolipin antibodies. Cause and effect? Arthritis Rheum 33:1842–1846, 1990.

449. Klipper AR, Stevens MB, Zizic TM, et al.: Ischemic necrosis of bone in systemic lupus erythematosus. Medicine 55:251–257, 1976.

450. Felson DT, Anderson JJ: A cross-study evaluation of association between steroid dose and bolus steroids and avascular necrosis of bone. Lancet 1:902–905, 1987.

451. Bergstein JM, Wiens C, Fish AJ, et al.: Avascular necrosis of bone in systemic lupus erythematosus. J Pediatr 85:31–35, 1974.

452. Abeles M, Urman JD, Rothfield NF: Aseptic necrosis of bone in systemic lupus erythematosus: relationship to corticosteroid therapy. Arch Intern Med 138:750–754, 1978.

453. Crossman J, Koval NS, Condemi JJ: Systemic lupus erythematosus: Bilateral aseptic necrosis of hip. NY State J Med 75:1523–1526, 1975.

454. Zizic TM, Hungerford DS, Stevens MB: Ischemic bone necrosis in systemic lupus erythematosus. Medicine 59:134–148, 1980.

455. Hanly JG, Gladman DD, Rose TH, et al.: Lupus pregnancy. A prospective study of placental changes. Arthritis Rheum 31:358–366, 1988.

456. Wong K, Chan F, Lee C: SLE does not preclude normal pregnancy. Arch Intern Med 151:269–273, 1991.

457. Estes D, Larson DL: Systemic lupus erythematosus and pregnancy. Clin Obstet Gynecol 8:307–321, 1965.

458. McGee CD, Makowski EL: Systemic lupus erythematosus in pregnancy. Am J Obstet Gynecol 107:1008–1012, 1970.

459. Bear R: Pregnancy and lupus nephritis. Obstet Gynecol 47:715–718, 1975.

460. McCune AB, Weston WL, Lee LA: Maternal and fetal outcome in neonatal lupus erythematosus. Ann Intern Med 106:518–523, 1987.

461. Gatenby PA: Systemic lupus erythematosus and pregnancy. Aust NZ J Med 19:261–278, 1989.

461a. Shibata S, Sasaki T, Hirabayashi Y, et al.: Risk factors in the pregnancy of patients with systemic lupus erythematosus: association of hypocomplementemia with poor prognosis. Ann Rheum Dis 51:619–623, 1992.

462. Stafford-Brady FJ, Gladman DD, Urowitz MB: Successful pregnancy in systemic lupus erythematosus with an untreated lupus anticoagulant. Arch Intern Med 148:1647–1648, 1988.

463. Siamopoulou-Mavridou A, Manoussakis MN, Mavridis AK, Moutsopoulos HM: Outcome of pregnancy in patients with autoimmune rheumatic disease before the disease onset. Ann Rheum Dis 47:982–987, 1988.

464. Lubbe WF, Palmer SJ, Butler WS, Liggins GC: Fetal survival after prednisone suppression of maternal lupus-anticoagulant. Lancet 1:1361–1363, 1983.

465. Harris EN, Hughes GRV, Gharavi AE: Thrombosis, fetal loss and antiphospholipid antibodies. Clin Aspects Autoimmun 1:1–11, 1986.

466. Ramsey-Goldman R, Mientus JM, Medsger TA Jr.: Pregnancy outcome in women with systemic lupus erythematosus (SLE) treated with immunosuppressive drugs. Arthritis Rheum 33:S28, 1990.

467. Buyon JP, Swersky SH, Fox HE, et al.: Intrauterine therapy for presumptive fetal myocarditis with acquired heart block due to systemic lupus erythematosus. Experience with a mother with a predominance of SS-B (La) antibodies. Arthritis Rheum 30:44–49, 1987.

468. Bierman FZ, Baxi L, Jaffe I, Driscoll J: Fetal hydrops and congenital complete heart block: response to maternal steroid therapy. J Pediatr 112:646–648, 1988.

469. Lockshin MD: Pregnancy does not cause systemic lupus erythematosus to worsen. Arthritis Rheum 32:665–670, 1989 (see also correspondence 33:605–606, 1990).

469a. Buyon JP: Systemic Lupus Erythematosus and Pregnancy. Cliniguide to Rheumatology 1(#4):1–8, 1991.

470. Petri M, Perez-Gutthann S, Longenecker JC, Hochberg M: Morbidity of systemic lupus erythematosus: Role of race and socioeconomic status. Am J Med 91:345–353, 1991.

471. Buyon JP, Cronstein BN, Morris M, et al.: Serum complement values (C3 and C4) to differentiate between systemic lupus activity and pre-eclampsia. Am J Med 81:194–200, 1986.

471a. Soscia PN, Zurier RB. Drug therapy of rheumatic diseases during pregnancy. Bull Rheum Dis 41:#2:1–3, 1992.

472. Vonderheid EC, Koblenzer PJ, Ming PML, et al.: Neonatal lupus erythematosus. Arch Dermatol 112:698–705, 1976.

473. Crittenen IH: Rheumatoid arthritis in the mother of five siblings with congenital heart block. N Engl J Med 299:491–492, 1978.

474. Lockshin MD, Bonfa E, Elkon K, Druzin ML: Neonatal lupus risk to newborns of mothers with systemic lupus erythematosus. Arthritis Rheum 31:697–701, 1988.

475. Watson RM, Lane AT, Barnett NK, et al.: Neonatal lupus erythematosus. A clinical, serological and immunogenetic study with review of the literature. Medicine 63:362–378, 1984.

476. Buyon JP, Winchester R: Congenital complete heart block. A human model of passively acquired autoimmune injury. Arthritis Rheum 33:609–614, 1990.

477. Gaither KK, Fox OF, Yamagata H, et al.: Implications of anti-Ro/Sjogren's syndrome A antigen autoantibody in normal sera for autoimmunity. J Clin Invest 79:841–846, 1987.

478. Buyon JP, Ben-Chetrit E, Karp S, et al.: Acquired congenital heart block. Pattern of maternal antibody response to biochemically defined antigens of the SSA/Ro-SSB/La system in neonatal lupus. J Clin Invest 84:627–634, 1989.

479. Arnaiz-Villena A, Vaquez-Rodriguez JJ, Vicario JL, et al.: Congenital heart block immunogenetics. Evidence of an additional role of HLA Class III antigens and independence of Ro autoantibodies. Arthritis Rheum 32:1421–1426, 1989.

480. Provost TT, Watson R, Gammon WR, et al.: The neonatal lupus syndrome associated with U 1 RNP (nRNP) antibodies. N Engl J Med 316:1135–1138, 1987.

480a. Alexander E, Buyon JP, Provost TT, Guarnieri T: Anti-Ro/SS-A antibodies in the pathophysiology of congenital heart block in neonatal lupus syndrome, an experimental model. In vitro electrophysiologic and immunocytochemical studies. Arthritis Rheum 35:176–189, 1992.

481. Callen JP, Fowler JF, Kulick KB, et al.: Neonatal lupus erythematosus occuring in one fraternal twin. Serologic and immunogenetic studies. Arthritis Rheum 28:271–305, 1985.

482. Chameides L, Truex RC, Vetter V, et al.: Association of maternal systemic lupus erythematosus with congenital complete heart block. N Engl J Med 297:1204–1208, 1977.

483. Nolan RJ, Shulman ST, Victorica BE: Congenital complete heart block associated with maternal mixed connective tissue disease. J Pediatr 95:420–422, 1979.

484. Hardy JD, Banwell GS, Beach R, et al.: Congenital complete heart block in the newborn associated with maternal systemic lupus erythematosus and other connective tissue disorders. Arch Dis Child 54:7–13, 1979.

485. Editorial: Systemic lupus in the newborn. Lancet 1:859, 1979.

486. Doshi N, Smith B, Klionsky B: Congenital pericarditis due to maternal lupus erythematosus. J Pediatr 96:699–701, 1980.

487. Klippel JH, Grimley PM, Decker JL: Lymphocyte inclusions in newborns of mothers with systemic lupus erythematosus. N Engl J Med 290:97–98, 1974.

488. Levy SB, Goldsmith LA, Morohashi M, et al.: Tubuloreticular inclusions in neonatal lupus erythematosus. JAMA 235:2743–2744, 1976.

489. Jones MM, Lidsky MD, Brewer EJ, et al.: Congenital cytomegalovirus infection and maternal systemic lupus erythematosus: a case report. Arthritis Rheum 29:1402–1404, 1986.

490. Rider LG, Sherry DD, Glass ST: Neonatal lupus erythematosus simulating transient myasthenia gravis at presentation. J Pediatr 118:417–419, 1991.

491. Laxer RM, Roberts EA, Gross KR, et al.: Liver disease in neonatal lupus erythematosus. J Pediatr 116:238–242, 1990.

492. Ty A, Fine BP: Infantile systemic lupus erythematosus (SLE) associated with chromosomal abnormalities presenting as nephrotic syndrome, abstracted. Pediatr Res 12:548, 1978.

493. Taylor PV, Scott JS, Gerlis LM, et al.: Maternal antibodies against fetal cardiac antigens in congenital complete heart block. N Engl J Med 315:667–672, 1986.

494. Lanham JG, Walport MJ, Hughes GRV: Congenital heart block and familial connective tissue disease. J Rheumatol 10:823–825, 1983.

495. Reichlin M, Friday K, Harley JB: Complete congenital heart block followed by anti-Ro/SSA in adult life. Studies of an informative family. Am J Med 84:339–344, 1988.

496. Ty A, Fine B: Membranous nephritis in infantile systemic lupus erythematosus associated with chromosomal abnormalities. Clin Nephrol 12:137–141, 1979.

497. Cummings NP, Hansen J, Hollister JR: Systemic lupus erythematosus in a premature infant. Arthritis Rheum 28:573–575, 1985.

498. Anderson JR: Intracerebral calcification in a case of systemic lupus erythematosus with neurological manifestations. Neuropathol Appl Neurobiol 7:161–166, 1981.

499. Beernick DH, Miller JJ: Anticonvulsant-induced antinuclear antibodies and lupus-like disease in children. J Petiatr 82:113–117, 1973.

500. Singsen BH, Fishman L, Hanson V: Antinuclear antibodies and lupus-like syndromes in children receiving anticonvulsants. Pediatrics 57:529–534, 1976.

501. Rubin RL: Drug-induced lupus. Clin Aspects Autoimmun 2:16–29, 1988.

502. Hess EV, Mongey A-B: Drug-related Lupus. Bull Rheum Dis 40:#4, 1–8, 1991. Arthritis Foundation.

503. Litwin A, Adams LE, Zimmer H, et al.: Prospective study of immunologic effects of hydralazine in hypertensive patients. Clin Pharmacol Ther 29:447–456, 1981.

504. Steen VD, Ramsey-Goldman R: Phenothiazine-induced systemic lupus erythematosus with superior vena cava syndrome: case report and review of the literature. Arthritis Rheum 31:923–926, 1988.

505. Totoritis MC, Tan EM, McNally EM, Rubin RL: Association of antibody to histone complex H2A-H2B with symptomatic procainamide-induced lupus. N Engl J Med 318:1431–1436, 1988 (see also Editorial pp. 1460–1462).

506. Enzenauer RJ, West SG, Rubin RL: D-Penicillamine-induced lupus erythematosus. Arthritis Rheum 33:1582–1585, 1990.

507. Irias JJ: Hydralazine-induced lupus erythematosus-like syndrome. Am J Dis Child 129:862–864, 1975.

507a. Tolaymat A, Leventhal B, Sakarcan A, et al.: Systemic lupus erythematosus in a child receiving long-term interferon therapy. J Pediatr 120:429–432, 1992.

508. Nordstrom DM, West SG, Rubin RL: Methyldopa-induced systemic lupus erythematosus. Arthritis Rheum 32:205–208, 1989.

509. Woosley RL, Drayer DE, Reidenberg MM, et al.: Effect of acetylator phenotype on the rate at which procainamide induces antinuclear antibodies and the lupus syndrome. N Engl J Med 298:1157–1159, 1978.

510. Batchelor JR, Weish KI, Tinoco RM, et al.: Hydralazine-induced systemic lupus erythematosus: influence of HLA-DR and sex on susceptibility. Lancet 1:1107–1109, 1980.

511. Speirs C, Fielder AHL, Chapel H, et al.: Complement system protein C4 and susceptibility to hydralazine-induced systemic lupus erythematosus. Lancet 1:922–924, 1989.

512. Massimo L, Pasino M, Rosando-Vadala C, et al.: Immunological side-effects of anticonvulsants. Lancet 1:860, 1976.

513. Kirtland HH, Mohler DN, Horwitz DA: Methyldopa inhibition of suppressor-lymphocyte function. N Engl J Med 302:825–832, 1980.

514. Dosch H-M, Jason J, Gelfand EW: Transient antibody deficiency and abnormal T suppressor cells induced by phenytoin. N Engl J Med 306:406–409, 1982.

515. Craft JE, Radding JA, Harding MW, et al.: Autoantigenic histone epitopes: a comparison between procainamide- and hydralazine-induced lupus. Arthritis Rheum 30:689–694, 1987.

516. Epstein A, Barland P: The diagnostic value of antihistone antibodies in drug-induced lupus erythematosus. Arthritis Rheum 28:158–162, 1985 (see also correspondence p. 148, 1986).

517. Shear NH, Spielberg SP: Anticonvulsant hypersensitivity syndrome: in vitro assessment of risk. J Clin Invest 82:1826–1832, 1988.

518. Miller JJ III: Drug-induced lupus-like syndromes in children. Arthritis Rheum 20:308–311, 1977.

519. Weinstein J: Hypocomplementemia in hydralazine-associated systemic lupus erythematosus. Am J Med 65:553–556, 1978.

520. Sharp GC, Irvin WS, Tan EM, et al.: Mixed connective tissue disease—an apparently distinct rheumatic disease syndrome associated with a specific antibody to extractable nuclear antigen (ENA). Am J Med 52:148–159, 1972.

521. Sharp GC: Mixed connective tissue disease. Bull Rheum Dis 25:828–830, 1975.

522. Sharp GC, Irvin WS, May CM, et al.: Association of antibodies to ribonucleoprotein and Sm antigens with mixed connective-tissue disease, systemic

lupus erythematosus and other rheumatic disease. N Engl J Med 296:1149–1154, 1976.

523. Hamburger M, Hodes S, Barland P: The incidence and clinical significance of antibodies to extractable nuclear antigens. Am J Med Sci 273:21–28, 1977.

524. Singsen BH, Bernstein BH, Kornreich HK, et al.: Mixed connective tissue disease in childhood: a clinical and serologic survey. J Pediatr 90:893–900, 1977.

525. Baldassare A, Weiss T, Auclair R, et al.: Mixed connective tissue disease (MCTD) in children, abstracted. Arthritis Rheum 19:788, 1976.

526. Hutto JH, Ayoub EM: Mixed connective tissue disease in children, abstracted. Pediatr Res 11:488, 1977.

526a. Oetgen WJ, Boice JA, Lawless OJ: Mixed connective tissue disease in children and adolescents. Pediatrics 67:333–337, 1981.

527. Alpert MA, Goldberg SH, Singsen BH, et al.: Cardiovascular manifestations of mixed connective tissue disease in adults. Circulation 68:1182–1193, 1983.

528. Savouret J-F, Chudwin DS, Wara DW, et al.: Clinical and laboratory findings in childhood mixed connective tissue disease: presence of antibody to ribonucleoprotein containing the small nuclear ribonucleic acid U1. J Pediatr 102:841, 1983.

529. Nimelstein SH, Brody S, McShane D, et al.: Mixed connective tissue disease: a subsequent evaluation of the orginal 25 patients. Medicine 59:239–248, 1980.

530. Prakash UBS, Luthra HS, Divertie MB: Intrathoracic manifestations in mixed connective tissue disease. Mayo Clin Proc 60:813–821, 1985.

531. Lemmer JP, Curry NH, Mallory JH, Waller MV: Clinical characteristics and course in patients with high titer anti-RNP antibodies. J Rheumatol 9:536–542, 1982.

532. Fisher DE, Reeves WH, Wisniewolski R, et al.: Temporal shifts from Sm to ribonucleoprotein reactivity in systemic lupus erythematosus. Arthritis Rheum 28:1348–1355, 1985.

533. ter Borg EJ, Horst G, Hummel E, et al.: Sequential development of antibodies to specific Sm polypeptides in a patient with systemic lupus erythematosus: evidence for independent regulation of anti-double-stranded DNA and Anti-Sm antibody production. Arthritis Rheum 31:1563–1567, 1988.

534. Asherson RA, Angus H, Matthews JA, et al.: The progressive systemic sclerosis/systemic lupus overlap: an unusual clinical progression. Ann Rheum Dis 50:323–327, 1991.

535. Biesecker G, Lavin L, Zisking H, Koeffler D: Cutaneous localization of the membrane attack complex in discoid and systemic lupus erythematosus. N Engl J Med 306:264–270, 1982.

536. Sontheimer RD, Maddison PJ, Reichlin M, et al.: Serologic and HLA associations in subacute cutaneous lupus erythematosus, a clinical subset of lupus erythematosus. Ann Intern Med 97:664–671, 1982.

537. Callen JP, Klein J: Subacute cutaneous lupus erythematosus. Clinical, serologic, immunogenetic, and therapeutic considerations in seventy-two patients. Arthritis Rheum 31:1007–1013, 1988.

538. Weinstein C, Miller MH, Axtens R, et al.: Lupus and lupus-cutaneous manifestations in systemic lupus erythematosus. Aust NZ J Med 17:501–506, 1987.

539. Weinstein CL, Littlejohn GO, Thomson NM, et al.: Severe visceral disease in subacute cutaneous lupus erythematosus. Arch Dermatol 123:638–640, 1987.

540. Newton RC, Jorizzo JL, Solomon AR Jr, et al.: Mechanism-oriented assessment of isotretinoin in chronic or subacute cutaneous lupus erythematosus. Arch Der-

matol 122:170–176, 1986.

541. Nichalas J-F, Thivolet J: Interferon alfa therapy in severe unresponsive subacute cutaneous lupus erythematosus. N Engl J Med 321:1550–1551, 1989.

542. Ehrlich GE: Systemic lupus erythematosus. JAMA 232:1361–1365, 1975.

543. Jacobs JC: Treatment of systemic lupus erythematosus in childhood. Arthritis Rheum 20:304–307, 1977.

544. Wasner CK, Fries JF: Treatment decisions in systemic lupus erythematosus. Arthritis Rheum 23:283–286, 1980.

545. Gladman DD, Urowitz MD, Keystone EC: Serologically active clinically quiescent systemic lupus erythematosus: a discordance between clinical and serologic features. Am J Med 111:210–216, 1979.

546. Wallace DJ, Podell TE, Weiner JM, et al.: Lupus nephritis. Experience with 230 patients in a private practice from 1950 to 1980. Am J Med 72:209–220, 1982.

547. Donadio JV Jr: Cytotoxic-drug treatment of lupus nephritis. N Engl J Med 311:528–529, 1984.

548. Donadio JV Jr, Holley KE, Ferguson RH, et al.: Treatment of diffuse proliferative lupus nephritis with prednisone and combined prednisone and cyclophosphamide. N Engl J Med 299:1151–1155, 1978.

549. Ibid: Letter to the Editor. N Engl J Med 300:564–565, 1979.

550. Schur PH, Sandson J: Immunological factors and clinical activity in systemic lupus erythematosus. N Engl J Med 278:533–538, 1968.

551. Bardana EJ, Harbeck RJ, Hoffman AA, et al.: The prognostic and therapeutic implications of DNA: anti-DNA immune complexes in systemic lupus erythematosus (SLE). Am J Med 59:515–522, 1975.

552. Hecht B, Siegel N, Adler M, et al.: Prognostic indices in lupus nephritis. Medicine 55:163–181, 1976.

553. Urman JD, Rothfield NF: Corticosteroid treatment in systemic lupus erythematosus: Survival studies. JAMA 238:2270–2276, 1977.

554. Swaak AJG, Aarden LA, Van Exps LWS, et al.: Anti-dsDNA and complement profiles as prognostic guides in systemic lupus erythematosus. Arthritis Rheum 22:226–235, 1979.

555. Helve T, Kurki P, Teppo A-M, Wegelius O: DNA antibodies and complement in SLE patients. A follow-up study. Rheumatol Int 3:129–132, 1983.

556. Laitman RS, Glicklich D, Sablay LB, et al.: Effect of long-term normalization of serum complement levels on the course of lupus nephritis. Am J Med 87:132–138, 1989.

557. ter Borg EJ, Horst G, Hummel EJ, et al.: Measurement of increases in antidouble-stranded DNA antibody levels as a predictor of disease exacerbation in systemic lupus erythematosus. A long-term, prospective study. Arthritis Rheum 33:634–643, 1990.

558. Nossent JC, Huysen V, Smeenk RJT, Swaak AJG: Low avidity antibodies to double stranded DNA in systemic lupus erythematosus: a longitudinal study of their clinical significance. Ann Rheum Dis 48:677–682, 1989.

559. Swaak AJG, Groenwold J, Bronsveld W: Predictive value of complement profiles and anti-dsDNA in systemic lupus erythematosus. Ann Rheum Dis 45:359–366, 1986.

560. Jarrett MP, Walter L, Barland P, et al.: The effect of continuous normalization of serum complement (CH50) on the course of lupus nephritis. A five year prospective study, abstracted. Arthritis Rheum 23:697, 1980.

561. Garin EH, Donnelly WH, Shulman ST, et al.: The significance of serial measurements of serum complement C3 and C4 components and DNA binding capacity in patients with lupus nephritis. Clin Nephrol 12:148–155, 1979.

562. Pollak VE, Pirani CL, Kark RM: Effect of large doses of prednisone on the renal lesions and life span of patients with lupus glomerulonephritis. J Lab Clin Med 57:495–511, 1961.

563. Rothfield NF, McCluskey R, Baldwin DS: Renal disease in systemic lupus erythematosus. N Engl J Med 269:537–544, 1963.

564. Hagge WW, Burke EC, Stickler GB: Treatment of systemic lupus erythematosus complicated by nephritis in children. Rediatrics 40:822–827, 1967.

565. Ackerman GL: Alternate-day steroid therapy in lupus nephritis. Ann Intern Med 72:511–519, 1970.

566. Donadio JV Jr, Holley KE, Wagoner RD, et al.: Treatment of lupus nephritis with prednisone and combined prednisone and azathioprine. Ann Intern Med 77:829–835, 1972.

567. Balow JE, Austin HA III, Tsokos GC, et al.: Lupus nephritis. Ann Intern Med 106:79–84, 1987.

567a. Steinberg AD, Steinberg SC: Long-term preservation of renal function in patients with lupus nephritis receiving treatment that includes cyclophosphamide versus those treated with prednisone only. Arthritis Rheum 34:945–950, 1991. (See also: Correspondence, 35:605–607, 1992.)

568. Sztejnbok M, Stewart A, Diamond H, et al.: Azathioprine in the treatment of systemic lupus erythematosus: a controlled study. Arthritis Rheum 14:639–645, 1971.

569. Ginzler E, Sharon E, Diamond H, et al.: Long-term maintenance therapy with azathioprine in systemic lupus erythematosus. Arthritis Rheum 18:27–35, 1975.

570. Barnett EV, Dornfeld L, Lee DB, et al.: Long-term survival of lupus nephritis patients treated with azathioprine and prednisone. J Rheum 5:275–287, 1978.

571. Felson DT, Anderson J: Evidence for the superiority of immunosuppressive drugs and prednisone over prednisone alone in lupus nephritis. Results of a pooled analysis. N Engl J Med 311:1528–1533, 1984.

572. Drinkard JP, Stanley TM, Dornfeld L, et al.: Azathioprine and prednisone in the treatment of adults with lupus nephritis. Medicine 49:411–432, 1970.

573. Shelp WD, Bloodworth JMB Jr, Riselbach RE: Effect of azathioprine on renal histology and function in lupus nephritis. Arch Intern Med 128:566–573, 1971.

574. Hayslett JP, Kashgarian M, Cook CD, et al.: The effect of azathioprine on lupus glomerulonephritis. Medicine 51:393–412, 1972.

575. Hahn B, Kantor O, Osterland K: Azathioprine plus prednisone compared with prednisone alone in the treatment of systemic lupus erythematosus. Ann Intern Med 83:592–605, 1975.

576. Donadio JV, Holley KE, Wagoner RD, et al.: Further observations in the treatment of lupus nephritis with prednisone and combined prednisone and azathioprine. Arthritis Rheum 17:573–581, 1974.

577. Steinberg AD, Plotz PH, Wolf SM, et al.: Cytotoxic drugs in treatment of nonmalignant diseases. Ann Intern Med 76:619–642, 1972.

578. Schneck SA, Penn I: De-novo brain tumors in renal transplant recipients. Lancet 1:983–986, 1971.

579. Tallent MB, Simmons RL, Najarian JS: Birth defects in child of male recipient of kidney transplant. JAMA 211:1854–1855, 1970.

580. Malkzedah MH, Grushkin CM, Wright HT Jr. et al.: Hepatic dysfunction after

renal transplantation in children. J Pediatr 81:279–285, 1972.

581. Balow JE, Boumpas DT, Vaughan EM, et al.: Lupus nephritis (LN): Controlled trial of pulse methylprednisolone (MP) versus pulse cyclosphosphamide (CY). J Amer Soc Neph 2:263, 1991.

582. Wagner-Weiner L, Emery H, Spencer C, et al.: Intravenous pulse cyclophosphamide therapy (IVCY) for childhood lupus nephritis; Variable renal outcomes at 3 to 7 year follow-up. Arthritis Rheum 34:S58, 1991.

583. Austin HA III, Klippel JH, Balow JE, et al.: Therapy of lupus nephritis. Controlled trial of prednisone and cytotoxic drugs. N Engl J Med 314:614–619, 1986.

584. Lehman TJA, Sherry DD, Wagner-Weiner L, et al.: Intermittent intravenous cyclophosphamide therapy for lupus nephritis. J Pediatr 114:1055–1060, 1989.

585. McCune WJ, Golbus J, Zeldes W, et al.: Clinical and immunologic effects of monthly administration of intravenous cyclophosphamide in severe systemic lupus erythematosus. N Engl J Med 318:1423–1431, 1988.

586. McCune WJ, Fox D: Intravenous cyclophosphamide therapy of severe SLE. Rheum Dis Clin NA 15:455–477, 1989.

587. Boumpas DT, Yamada H, Patronas NJ, et al.: Intermittent pulse cyclophosphamide for the treatment of severe neuropsychiatric lupus. Arthritis Rheum 33S:130, 1990.

588. Reed WP, Lucas ZJ, Cohn R: Alternate-day prednisone therapy after renal transplantation. Lancet 1:747–749, 1970.

589. Walron J, Watson BS, Ney RL: Alternate-day vs. shorter-interval steroid administration. Arch Intern Med 126:601–607, 1970.

590. Jacobson ME: The rationale of alternate-day corticosteroid therapy. Postgrad Med 49:181–187, 1971.

591. McAdams AJ, McEnery PT, West CD: Mesangiocapillary glomerulonephritis: changes in glomerular morphology with long-term alternate-day prednisone therapy. J Pediatr 86:23–31, 1975.

592. Bolton WK, Atuk NO, Sturgill BC, et al.: Therapy of the idiopathic nephrotic syndrome with alternate-day steroids. Am J Med 62:60–70, 1977.

593. Fauci AS: Alternate-day corticosteroid therapy. Am J Med 64:729–731, 1978.

594. Coggins CH (ed.) A controlled study of short-term prednisone treatment in adults with membranous nephropathy: collaborative study of the adult idiopathic nephrotic syndrome. N Engl J Med 301:1301–1306, 1979.

595. Breitenfeld RV, Hebert LA, Lemann J, et al.: Stability of renal transplant function with alternate-day corticosteroid therapy. JAMA 244:151–156, 1980.

596. Macgregor RR, Sheagren JN, Lipsett MB, et al.: Alternate-day prednisone therapy: evaluation of delayed hypersensitivity responses, control of disease and steroid side effects. N Engl J Med 280:1427–1431, 1969.

597. McEnery PT, Gonzzlez LL, Martin LW, et al.: Growth and development of children with renal transplants. Use of alternate-day steroid therapy. J Pediatr 83:806–814, 1973.

598. Dale DC, Fauci AS, Wolff SM: Alternate-day prednisone: leucocyte kinetics and susceptibility to infections. N Engl J Med 291:1154–1158, 1974.

599. Shaprio GG, Tuttoni DS, Kelley VC, et al.: Growth, pulmonary, and endocrine function in chronic asthma patients on daily and alternate day adrenocorticoid therapy. J. Allergy Clin Immunol 57:430–439, 1976.

600. Bass AR, Kopelman R, McMahon D, et al.: High dose alternate-day steroid

(HDADS) therapy in lupus nephritis. Arthritis Rheum 33S:164, 1990.

601. Kimura Y, Foeldvari I, Jacobs JC. Azathioprine is a valuable agent in the treatment of pediatric lupus nephritis. Pediatr Res 29 (#4, pt 2):345A, 1991.

602. Rothenberg RJ, Graziano FM, Grandone JT, et al.: The use of methotrexate in steroid-resistant systemic lupus erythematosus. Arthritis Rheum 31:612–615, 1988.

603. Lemoine R, Favre H, Miescher P, et al.: Morphological evolution of membranous lupus glomerulonephritis on combined treatment of cyclosporine and steroids. Kidney Int 37:442, 1990.

604. Seaman WE, Ishak KG, Plotz PH: Aspirin-induced hepatotoxicity in patients with systemic lupus erythematosus. Ann Intern Med 80:1–8, 1974.

605. Ruppert GB, Barth WF: Tolmetin-induced aseptic meningitis. JAMA 245:67–68, 1981.

606. Codding C, Targoff IN, McCarty GA: Aseptic meningitis in association with diclofenac treatment in a patient with systemic lupus erythematosus. Arthritis Rheum 34:1340–1341, 1991.

607. Lehman TJA: Current concepts in immunosuppressive drug therapy of systemic lupus erythematosus. J Rheumatol 19:20–22, 1992.

608. Gordon MF, Stolley PD, Schinnar R: Trends in recent systemic lupus erythematosus mortality rates. Arthritis Rheum 24:762–765, 1981.

608a. Oster MW: Oral Ondansetron. Ann intern Med 115:233, 1991.

609. Orta-Sibu N, Chantler C, Bewick M, Haycock G: Comparison of high-dose intravenous methylprednisolone with low-dose oral prednisolone in acute renal allograft rejection in children. Br Med J 285:258–260, 1982.

610. Liebling MR, McLaughlin K, Boonsue S, et al.: Monthly pulses of methylprednisolone in SLE nephritis. J Rheumatol 9:543–548, 1982.

611. Barron KS, Person DA, Brewer EJ Jr, et al.: Pulse methylprednisolone therapy in diffuse proliferative lupus nephritis. J Pediatr 101:137–141, 1982.

612. Hoch S, Schur PH: Methylprednisolone pulse therapy for lupus nephritis: a follow-up study. Clin Exp Rheumatol 2:313–320, 1984.

613. Edwards JCW, Snaith ML, Isenberg DA: A double blind controlled trial of methylprednisolone infusions in systemic lupus erythematosus using individualised outcome assessment. Ann Rheum Dis 46:773–776, 1987.

614. Singer DRJ, Roberts B, Cohen J: Infective complications of plasma exchange: a prospective study: Arthritis Rheum 30:443–447, 1987.

615. Schroeder JO, Euler HH, Loffler H, Synchronization of plasmapheresis and pulse cyclophosphamide in severe systemic lupus erythematosus. Ann Intern Med 107:344–346, 1987.

616. Mackworth-Young CG, Morgan DSH, Hughes GRV: A double blind, placebo controlled trial of intravenous methylprednisolone in systemic lupus erythematosus. Ann Rheum Dis 47:496–502, 1988.

617. Balow JE: Lupus nephritis: pathogenesis, course and management. Adv Exp Med Biol 252:3–15, 1989.

617a. Lewis EJ, Hunsicker LG, Lan S-P, et al.: A controlled trial of plasmapheresis therapy in severe lupus nephritis. N Eng J Med 326:1373–9, 1992. (See also Editorial, pp 1425–1427).

618. Aptekar RG, Atkinson JP, Decker JL, et al.: Bladder toxicity with chronic oral cyclophosphamide therapy in non-malignant disease. Arthritis Rheum 16:461–467, 1973.

619. Warne GL, Fairley KF, Hobbs JB, et al.: Cyclophosphamide-induced ovarian failure. N Engl J Med 289:1159–1162, 1973.
620. Tannenbaum H, Schur PH: Development of reticulum cell sarcoma during cyclophosphamide therapy. Arthritis Rheum 17:15–18, 1974.
621. Pollock BH, Barr JH Jr, Stolzer BL, et al.: Neoplasia and cyclophosphamide. Arthritis Rheum 16:524–526, 1973.
622. Walker SE, Anver MR: Accelerated appearance of neoplasia in female NZB/NZW mice treated with high-dose cyclophosphamide. Arthritis Rheum 22:1338–1343, 1979.
623. Petri M, Perez-Gutthann S, Longenecker C, Hochberg MC: The association of black race with morbidity in patients with systemic lupus erythematosus (SLE) is explained by socioeconomic status (SES) and compliance. Arthritis Rheum 33S:83, 1990.
624. Petri M, Perez-Gutthann S, Longenecker JC, Hochberg M: Morbidity of systemic lupus erythematosus: Role of race and socioeconomic status. Am J Med 91:345–353, 1991.
625. Liang MH, Partridge AJ, Daltroy LH, et al.: Strategies for reducing excess morbidity and mortality in blacks with systemic lupus erythematosus. Arthritis Rheum 34:1187–1196, 1991.
626. Samanta A, Feehally J, Roy S, et al.: High prevalence of systemic disease and mortality in Asian subjects with systemic lupus erythematosus. Ann Rheum Dis 50:490–492, 1991.
627. Sidel VW: Nephrology in the inner city. NYS J Med 9:179–182, 1991.
628. Verrier Jones J, Fraser ID, Bothamley J, et al.: A therapeutic role for plasmapheresis in the management of acute systemic lupus erythematosus. Plasma Ther 1:33–41, 1979.
629. Lockwood CM, Worlledge S, Nicholas A, et al.: Reversal of impaired splenic function in patients with nephritis or vasculitis (or both) by plasma exchange. N Engl J Med 300:524–530, 1979.
630. Terman DS, Buffaloe G, Mattioli C, et al.: Extracorporeal immunoadsorption: initial experience in human systemic lupus erythematosus. Lancet 2:824–827, 1979.
631. Nossent JC, Swaack TJG, Berden JHM, et al.: Systemic lupus erythematosus after renal transplantation: Patient and graft survival and disease activity. Ann Intern Med 114:183–188, 1991.

6

Dermatomyositis

Dermatomyositis is a disease of the connective tissues that is characterized primarily by inflammation of skin and muscles. It is uncommon but not rare. Despite its initial description in 1887, the disease went virtually unnoticed in children until Wedgwood et al. (1953)[1] and Banker and Victor (1966)[2] kindled new interest with their pioneering clinical and pathologic studies. Since that time, there have been an increasing number of clinical reports and a few efforts at etiologic definition.

Clinical Presentation

There are two quite distinct patterns of presentation (Table 6.1): (1) an *acute onset* with high fever, prostration, rash, and profound muscle weakness seen in one-quarter of cases, and (2) the more common *insidious onset* in which sometimes only rash alone is apparent for months prior to obvious muscle weakness. In those with insidious onset, diagnosis is frequently delayed. These children are often thought to have eye or skin allergies, may be mis-

Table 6.1. Dermatomyositis—Patterns of Presentation

Acute	*Insidious*
High fever	Periorbital and skin rashes thought to be
Prostration	allergy
Profound muscle weakness	Arthralgia
Rash	Frequent falling or stumbling
	Inability to take the big step into the
	school bus or to turn a doorknob
	Frustration and irritablity

Table 6.2. Skin Manifestations of Dermatomyositis

Edema of the eyelids and supraorbital area
Heliotrope hue to the eyelids
Rashes over the knuckles, elbows, and knees (Gottron's sign)
Generalized rashes, sometimes most pronounced in the "V" area of the chest
Vertical ungual telangiectasias

taken for JRA if there is sufficient accompanying arthritis, or may be thought to merely have behavioral problems as they become more and more irritable as a result of pain and an increasing, unrecognized, frustrating inability to do what is required of them. Inability to take the big step onto the school bus, or to open the refrigerator door, and stumbling with a tendency to fall have been some of the complaints that have first brought these children to our attention.

Immunopathology

Skin[3]

The characteristic telangiectasias, edema and heliotrope hue to the eyelids, and rashes overlying joints (Gottron's sign) (Table 6.2) are due to superficial perivascular infiltration of lymphocytes and histiocytes with wide dilatation of blood vessels, vacuolar alteration at the dermoepidermal interface, and thinning of the epidermis. Considerable dermal edema accounts for the supraorbital swelling seen in most early cases (Fig. 6.1). Morphologic changes may best be viewed in the nailfold capillary bed and correlate with the clinical course.[4]

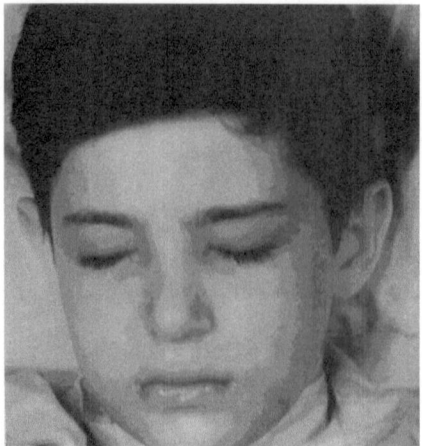

Figure 6.1. Supraorbital edema is the most common dermal manifestation in childhood dermatomyositis; at times, it is the sole dermal clue to diagnosis.

Muscle[5]

The primary lesion is active capillary necrosis although there may be destruction of arterioles in some cases. Most patients have foci of lymphocytic inflammation in the septa separating muscle fascicles. The predominant cells are usually CD8+ T cells. There may be necrosis and infarctlike lesions resulting from ischemia. Atrophy may be prominent. Electron microscopy shows tubuloreticular structures typical of connective-tissue disease. In histologically abnormal blood vessel walls, immunofluorescent staining reveals granular deposits of IgG, IgM, and C3, alone or in various combinations.[6] These studies suggest that childhood dermatomyositis is an immune-mediated vasculopathy in which the complement-membrane attack complex is the primary mediator of vessel injury.[7,8] The histologic and immunopathologic abnormalities are not diagnostic of this syndrome, may also be seen in other connective tissue disorders, and do not correlate well with prognosis.[5]

Other Organs[2]

Similar vasculitis has been demonstrated in the heart, GI tract, GU organs, and nervous system. It probably can occur in all organs.

Peripheral Blood Mononuclear Cytotoxicity to Muscle Cells[9,10]

Peripheral blood mononuclear cells from patients with dermatomyositis have been shown to be cytotoxic to muscle cells in tissue culture. The cytotoxicity, at least to some extent, correlates with the clinical activity of the disease. Numerous autoantibodies of uncertain significance have been identified in patients with dermatomyositis but cellular immune mechanisms seem most important.[11,12] CD8+ cytotoxic T cells are generally the hallmark of this disease but one case mediated by gamma/delta T cells has been reported.[13,14]

Epidemiology[15–17]

Epidemiologic studies suggest predisposition determined by age, sex, and genetic factors. Boys are less often affected than girls, but account for 35% of cases. Infants may be affected, but onset prior to age 2 is very rare. There are four reports of families with two affected siblings. We have cared for affected cousins and there is one other report of first cousins.[18] A common HLA antigen, B8, present in 21% of white controls, has been found in up to 72% of children with dermatomyositis; this was associated with the supratype A1,

Table 6.3. Diagnostic Criteria for Dermatomyositis

1. Symmetrical proximal muscle weakness
2. Elevation of skeletal muscle enzymes in serum
3. Electromyographic findings typical of myositis[27]
4. Classical dermatomyositis rash
5. Muscle-biopsy findings typical of dermatomyositis*

*Only performed in absence of 1, 2, or 3.
Note: A definite diagnosis requires rash plus any other three criteria.
From Bohan et al., ref. 28, with permission.

Cw7, B8, DR3. The antigens HLA-B8, DR3, and DQA1 are also associated with a wide variety of other "immunopathic" disorders, including myasthenia gravis, Sjögren's syndrome, dermatitis herpetiformis, celiac disease,
and endocrinopathies.[19] Homozygote C2 deficiency has been reported in an
adult with dermatomyositis.[17] Myopathy with and without skin lesions has
been reported in children with IgA deficiency.[16,19a]

Family members have developed the disease within 2 weeks of each other,
suggesting that an infectious exogenous factor sets off an autoimmune
reaction in a genetically susceptible host.[20-22] Coxsackie virus does it in some
mice and in adults[23,24]; it may be the exogenous factor for some cases in
childhood.[25,26]

Clinical Features

Diagnosis

The diagnosis of dermatomyositis is based on the presence of the characteristic dermal manifestations and myositis in the absence of laboratory evidence
of SLE or MCTD (Table 6.3). Other disorders to be considered in the differential diagnosis are discussed at the end of this chapter and listed in Table
6.6. Experienced observers can often make the diagnosis promptly by inspection. There are five skin signs to be looked for (Table 6.2).

Characteristics of the Rash. Swelling of the eyelids and supraorbital areas
is the most common dermal manifestation and can usually be seen even if
there are no other dermal manifestations (Fig. 6.1). There is often a characteristic heliotrope hue to the upper eyelids (a dusky lilac discoloration with
telangiectasias) (Fig. 6.2). An erythematous/violaceous maculopapular
eruption appears over the extensor surfaces, especially of the interphalangeal
joints, the elbows, and knees (Gottron's sign) (Figs. 6.3–6.6). In some cases,
there is an extensive rash in the V area of the chest (Fig. 6.7). Periungual
vasculitis is visible in the form of vertical telangiectasia in the cuticles (Figs.

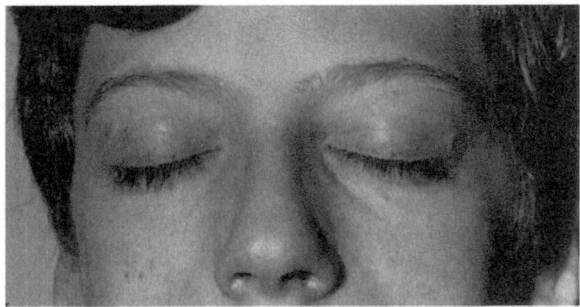

Figure 6.2. Heliotrope hue to eyelids with telangiectasias, a classic dermal manifestation of dermatomyositis.

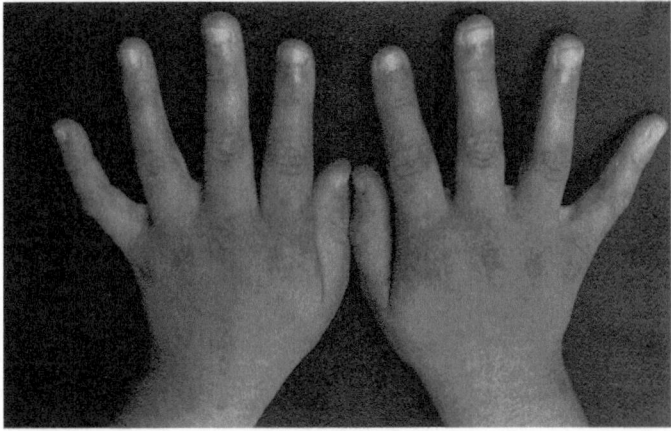

Figure 6.3. Gottron's sign—an erythematous rash over the extensor surfaces, especially over the knuckles. Vertical telangiectasia typical of dermatomyositis are seen in cuticles of the second and third fingers.[29]

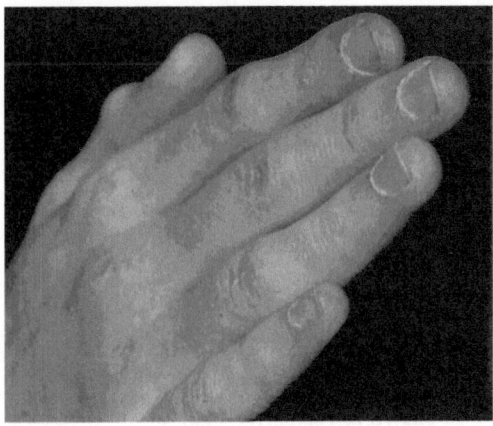

Figure 6.4. Gottron's sign and vertical telangiectasia of the cuticles in another boy with dermatomyositis.

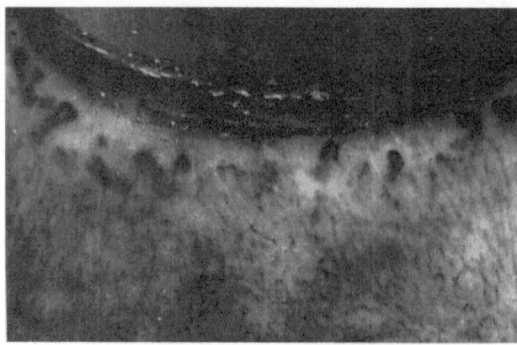

Figure 6.5. Ungual telangiectactic vessels viewed with the scanning microscope, a useful way of demonstrating these lesions. (Reprinted with permission from Maricq H: *Arthritis Rheum* 16:619–628, 1981.) (See patient 2, ref. 29.)

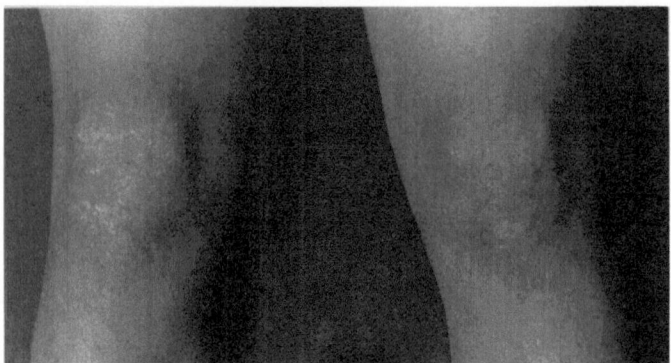

Figure 6.6. Erythematous lesions overlying the extensor surfaces of the knees.

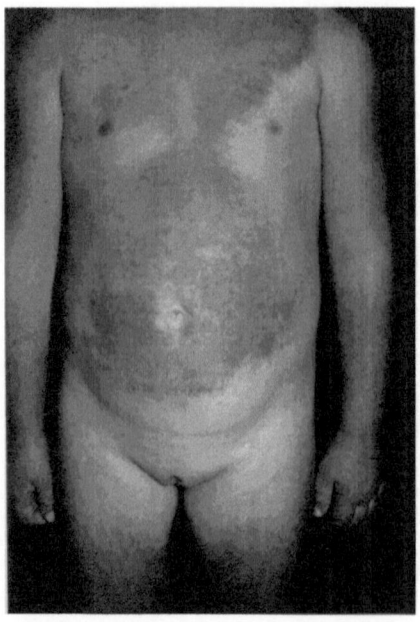

Figure 6.7. Diffuse red rash of dermatomyositis.

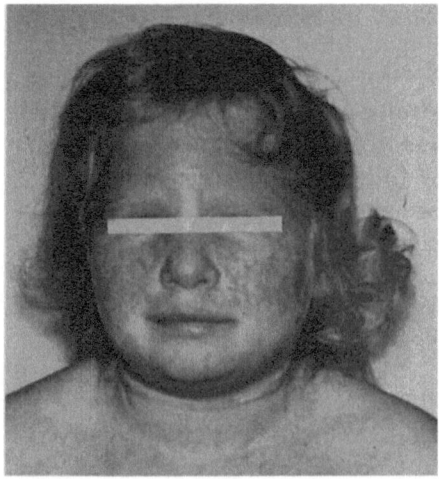

Figure 6.8. Facial butterfly and diffuse rash.

6.3–6.5); these sensitive areas may become infected, creating paronychia and a portal of entry for staphylococcal sepsis.

A mild butterfly eruption on the face is not uncommon in childhood dermatomyositis (Fig. 6.8) and does not, by itself, indicate the illness is a feature of SLE.

Muscle Weakness. Early in the disease, there may be considerable pain in the proximal muscles. The myopathy is clearly proximal with greater strength in distal muscle groups and may be most clearly demonstrated by the pediatrician as difficulty holding up the flexed thing or the laterally outstretched arms. Truncal weakness produces Gower's sign, an inability to rise from the supine position without turning over and "climbing up" with elbows and knees (see Fig. 1.1). Performing these simple maneuvers in children with swelling or rash about the eyes or on the extensor surfaces becomes routine. A simple grading system may be used to quantify the degree of muscle weakness (Table 1.3).

Inflammation in the muscles is confirmed with needle electromyography (EMG), which primarily reflects the state of the muscle membrane inflammation.[27] Abnormal spontaneous activity includes increased spontaneous and insertional activity, fibrillation potentials, positive sharp waves, bizarre high-frequency discharges, fasciculation potentials, and "coupled" discharges. Nerve conduction is demonstrated to be normal. Although typical of myositis, none of the findings are specific for this particular connective-tissue syndrome. The correlation of these findings with the other clinical manifestations, rash, weakness, and elevation of "muscle enzymes" in the serum (CPK, aldolase, GOT, GPT, and LDH) and the absence of laboratory determinants and other diagnostic features of SLE (Chapter 5), enable diagnosis.[28] A negative biopsy does not exclude the diagnosis; selection artifact results in at least 10% of biopsies in well-documented cases being normal.[30]

Diagnosis is usually established, therefore, without the need for muscle biopsy (Table 6.3).[28] The bad habit of subjecting children to unnecessary muscle biopsy to "confirm" what is already known is deplored, especially when the same diagnosis must be made in the presence of a normal biopsy. Muscle biopsies have a number of disadvantages: delay prior to institution of effective therapy (or failure to do so because the biopsy is artifactually normal); unnecessary hospitalization and risks of heavy sedation; expense of operating room and neurosurgeon to obtain adequate specimens; unpleasant scars; possibility of poor healing if it is necessary to institute therapy concomitantly; and creation of a portal for entry of infection. All of this morbidity is acceptable *when the diagnosis is uncertain* (i.e., does not fulfill these diagnostic criteria; Table 6.3) or if an established research protocol approved by the human experimentation committee seeks to establish the cause of this syndrome. The mere freezing away of specimens for further confirmation of knowledge already garnered from prior studies does not warrant the morbidity. Improved techniques for obtaining specimens with the Bergstrom percutaneous muscle-biopsy needle may resolve these problems.[31] MRI may also make biopsy a procedure of the past.[32]

Arthritis. Arthritis, manifested by joint effusion or pain and limitation of motion apart from that which may be a result of soft-tissue contractures in old chronic cases, occurs in about 25% of the children, and sometimes requires nonsteroidal anti-inflammatory drugs in addition to the medications being used for the control of muscle weakness. Two of our patients have developed arthritis following complete recovery from dermatomyositis, one spondyloarthritis and one severe psoriatic. Both had previously been treated with methotrexate.

Gastrointestinal Problems. Swallowing difficulty (dysphagia), as a result of myopathy of palatal muscles, is common;[33] fluids may emerge from the nose when the child drinks. In such severe cases, aspiration is the greatest risk to life, and hospitalization in an intensive-care unit is necessary. Severely ill children may have atony of gastrointestinal smooth muscle as a result of impaired vascular supply. One of our patients had the superior mesenteric artery syndrome with duodenal obstruction (Fig. 6.9). Gastrointestinal perforation from bowel-wall infarction and ulceration is now extremely rare but remains an important cause of death; the presumption that this was common in childhood dermatomyositis came from autopsy studies, a highly selected population of a small percentage of the most severely affected individuals. Pneumotosis intestinalis may occur, presumably as a result of impaired bowel circulation allowing gas-forming bacteria in the bowel wall. This may be asymptomatic (even with pneumoperitoneum) or may indicate sepsis and be a grave prognostic sign. The available data suggest that pneumotosis may

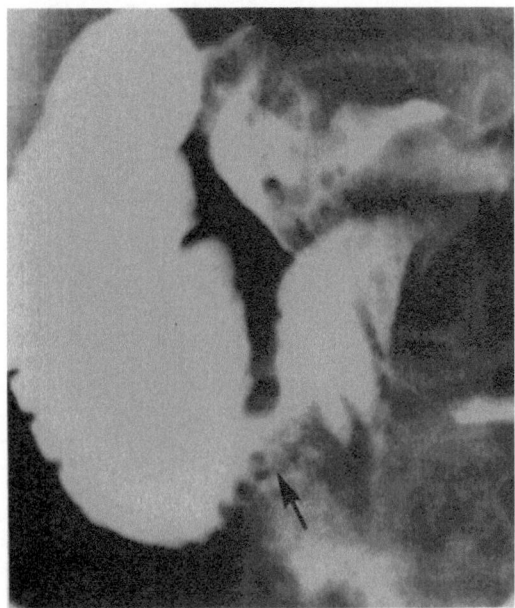

Figure 6.9. Superior mesenteric artery (SMA) syndrome in a 10-year-old girl with severe dermatomyositis. Obstructive symptoms were relieved by having the child sleep prone instead of supine. Note dilated duodenum with sharp cutoff *(arrow)*, findings typical for this syndrome.

be ignored if the patient has no abdominal symptoms and is having a steady rather than downhill course of his disease.[34] However, visceral perforation requires prompt diagnosis and surgery. With modern pediatric anesthesia, surgery, and intensive care, previously hopeless catastrophies can be overcome.[35,36]

Lung Disease. Weakness of the primary and accessory respiratory muscles may interfere with respiration and cough, fostering aspiration and hypostatic pneumonia, formerly a common cause of death in severely affected children. Interstitial pneumonia/fibrosis (fibrosing alveolitis) is probably more common than has been recognized.[37] In occasional patients, this inflammation in the interstitium and alveolar spaces of the lung may become the predominant manifestation of the disease and may be complicated further by pneumothorax.[38]

Interstitial lung disease in adult polymyositis occurs primarily in older patients, and it has been suggested that there may be an adjuvant effect from tuberculosis as in Caplan's syndrome.[39] Two of the four reported children with severe interstitial pneumonia as a feature of dermatomyositis have had a history of tuberculosis; in one of these patients, treatment for tuberculosis was begun just prior to the onset of obvious dermatomyositis. We have seen one child with dermatomyositis where interstitial pneumonia was the predominant manifestation (Fig. 6.10); there was no history or evidence of tuberculosis, however.

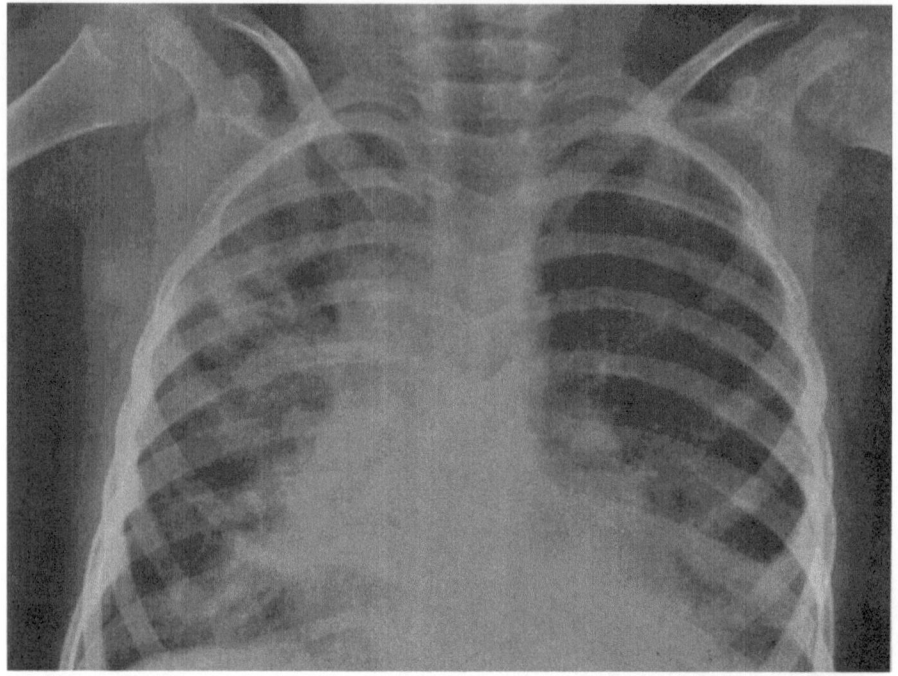

A

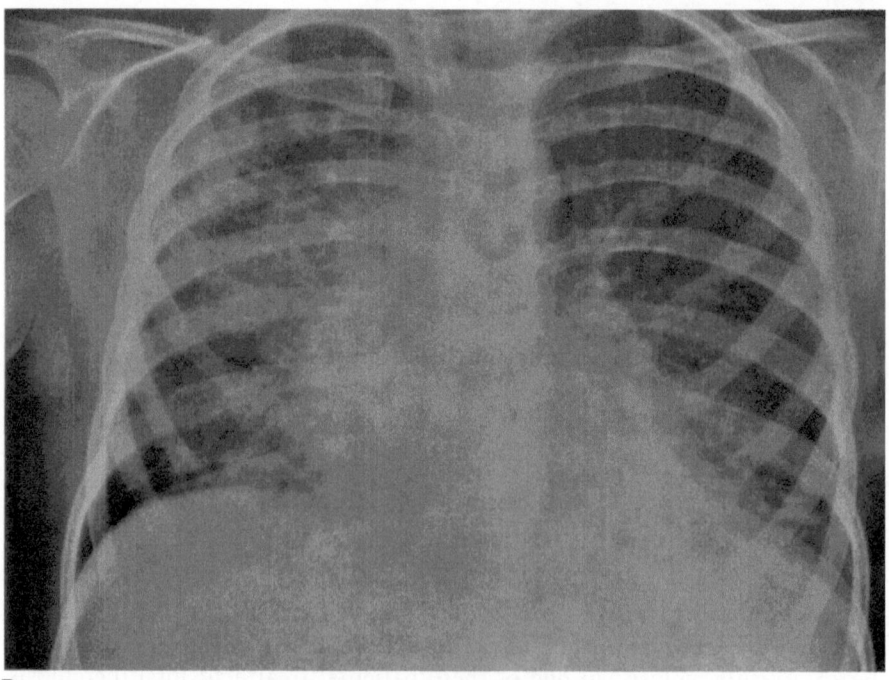

B

Figure 6.10. Recurrent episodes of interstitial pneumonia were the most prominent manifestation of dermatomyositis in this 5-year-old boy. Each episode responded to corticosteroid therapy, and the boy ultimately recovered completely and is receiving no medications.
(Courtesy of Dr. Martin Meltzer.)

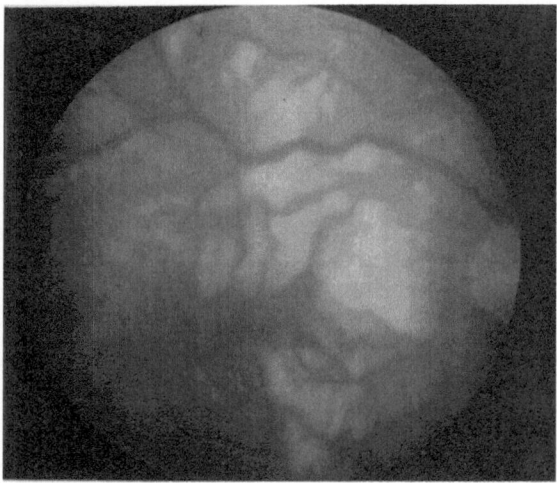

Figure 6.11. Acute retinitis seen in a boy with severe dermatomyositis. Retinopathy disappeared promptly with steroid therapy, and the patient made a complete recovery a few months later.

Anti-Jo antibodies are associated with increased risk of lung disease in adults but this association has not been established in children.[37] Methotrexate may cause interstitial pneumonia; drug-induced pulmonary disease would have to be distinguished from that associated with dermatomyositis.[37]

Cardiac Manifestations. Despite the presence of cardiac-muscle vasculitis in autopsied patients, there have been only three reports of clinical cardiac manifestations in children with dermatomyositis[40,40a]—one of cardiac conduction defects and two of pericarditis. Pericarditis, myocarditis, and arrhythmias have been reported in adults.[41]

Retinitis. Cytoid bodies, microscopic foci of degenerated retinal nerve fibers, result from capillary damage in the retina analogous to that elsewhere and are seen as fluffy cotton-wool exudates (Fig. 6.11). Although rarely reported in adults, retinitis is not uncommon in children; we have reported three cases from the Babies Hospital; subsequently, others have made similar observations.[17,42,43] The children were not visually symptomatic, but they were all very ill at the time of discovery of the eye lesions during daily examinations of the fundi. The retinopathy subsides with steroid treatment, leaving no residua.

Renal Biopsy Findings. There sometimes is proteinuria, but there are no significant clinical renal manifestations. Bitnum reported hypercellularity of the glomerular tufts, hyperplastic changes in small blood vessels, and thickening of the basement membranes.[44] Shortly after that report appeared, we biopsied a patient, although, in retrospect, there is no indication for renal biopsy in childhood dermatomyositis. Our findings—mild focal segmental

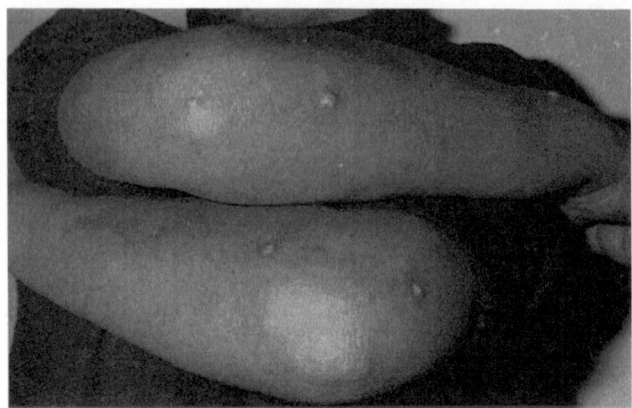

Figure 6.12. Isolated small calcium nodules in a patient who has recovered from dermatomyositis.

and global mesangial proliferation and glomerulosclerosis—were similar to those reported by Bitnum. Similar renal-biopsy findings have been documented in a young woman with dermatomyositis with acute renal failure due to myoglobinuria.[45] Kagen has demonstrated that most patients with dermatomyositis have myoglobinemia and myoglobinuria.[46] We suspect that the renal-biopsy findings are best interpreted as evidence for subclinical renal injury from myoglobin. While acute renal failure from myoglobinuria in dermatomyositis is so far unreported in children, the potential for this complication certainly exists; its prompt recognition would allow appropriate therapeutic, possibly lifesaving, maneuvers.

Renal stones with obstructive uropathy and sepsis may be a complication of osteoporosis resulting from weakness and lack of mobility complicated by prednisone administration.

The Nervous System. Anoxic encephalopathy may occur if adequate blood oxygen saturation is not maintained.[2] Despite the presence of pathologic evidence of vasculitis in the nervous system in autopsy studies (and in the retina), central- or peripheral-nervous-system manifestations have not been reported in children. However, detailed modern studies aimed at trying to document unnoticed abnormalities have not been performed. Miller has suggested that more than an expected number of these children have residual psychological and learning disabilities,[47] possibly residua from unrecognized cerebral vasculitis.

Calcinosis. Children with dermatomyositis are prone to calcify skin, fascia, subcutaneous tissue, and fat (but not muscle) during the healing phase (Fig. 6.12). The extremities and trunk, pelvis, and neck may all be affected. Most

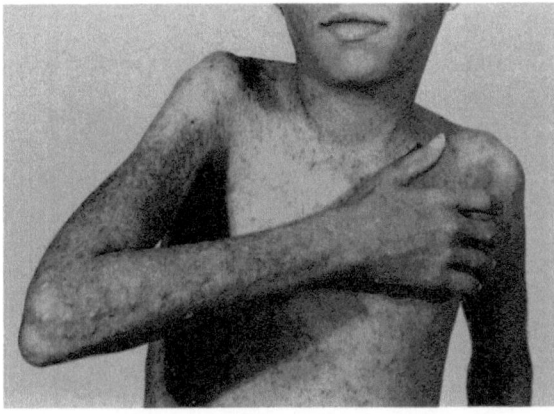

Figure 6.13. Calcium exoskeleton with multiple calcium nodules.

of the calcium deposits are small punctate or clumpy-popcorn-like and, when they are superficial, may become painful and then open, discharging calcium with relief of pain (Figs. 6.13 and 6.14). Sheets of calcium are occasionally laid down, forming an exoskeleton that prevents adequate mobility of the joints (Figs. 6.15–6.18). Probenecid and warfarin have been reported to help a few patients.[48,49] Improvement may take place during the late teens in these patients, with almost total disappearance of the sheets of calcium and improvement in function as a result.[50] In one reported case this was associated with life-threatening hypercalcemia[51] and we have seen one such patient who, following cyclosporine treatment, developed hypercalcemia and

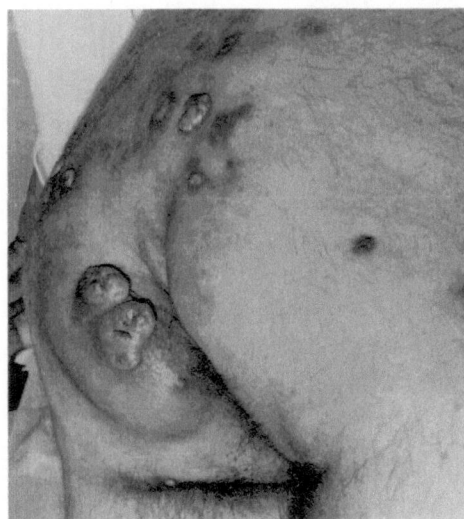

Figure 6.14. Large calcium nodules in the buttock that make sitting painful.

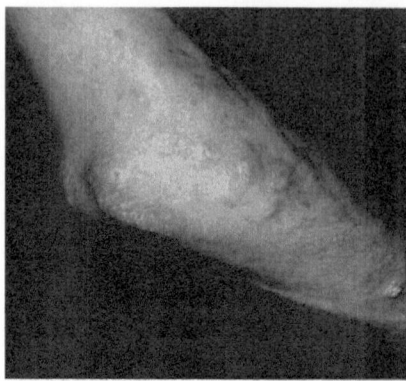

Figure 6.15. Limited movement of the elbow results from calcium exoskeleton.

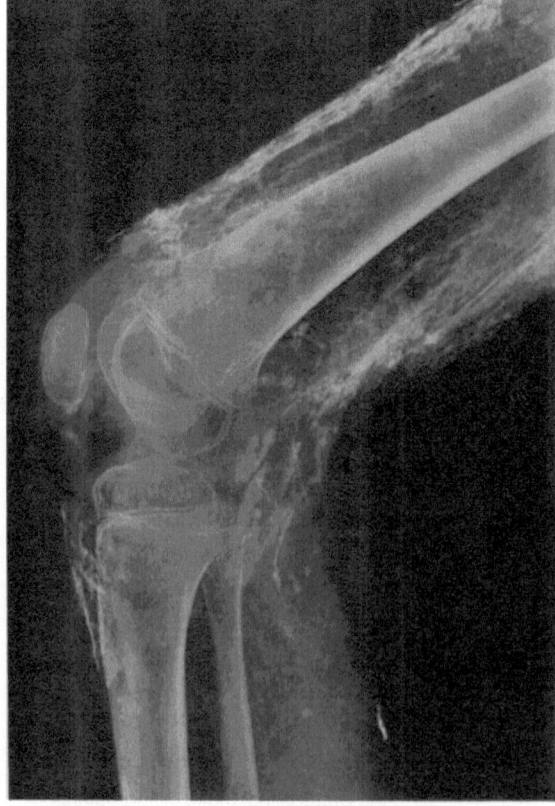

Figure 6.16. Radiograph showing ectopic calcification forming sheets in the subcutaneous tissues.

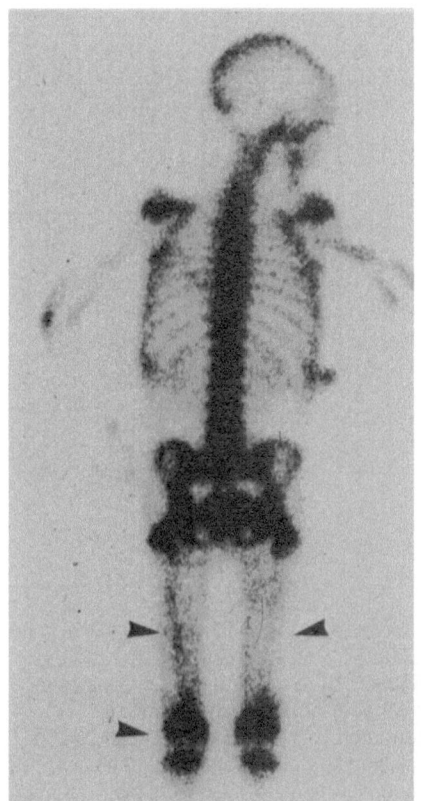

Figure 6.17. Technetium bone scan in same patient at age 10 showing extensive calcinosis in soft tissues.

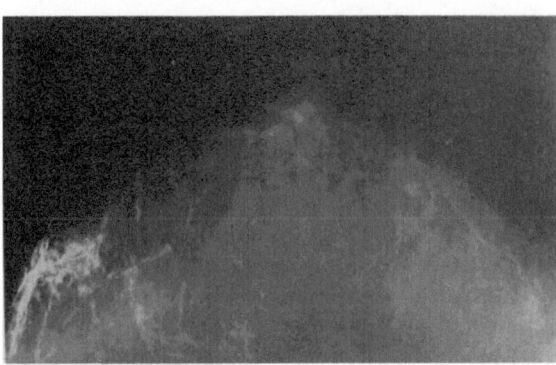

Figure 6.18. Mammogram showing calcinosis of breast following childhood dermatomyositis. (Courtesy of Dr. Thane Asch.)

hypercalcuria. Tumorous calcinosis occurs occasionally and in rare cases requires surgical removal to improve local function (Fig. 6.19).

Children with calcinosis are prone to staphylococcal infections and may have a granulocyte chemotactic defect with raised IgE concentratons.[51a]

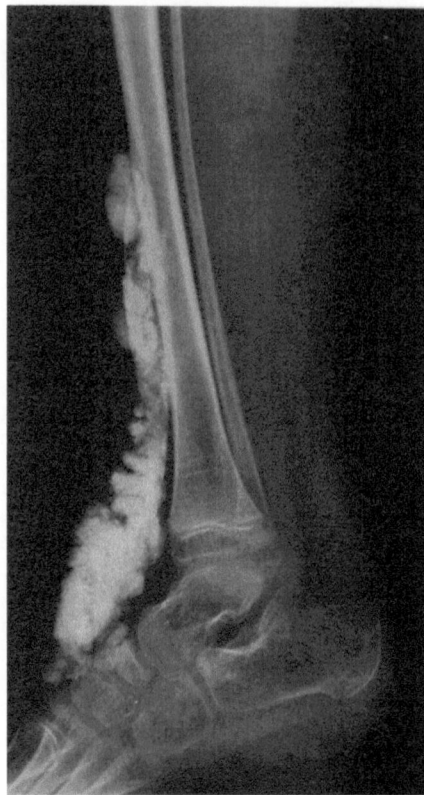

Figure 6.19. Severe tumorous calcinosis in a 4-year-old boy with very mild dermatomyositis. Removal of calcium and calcified tendon sheaths is sometimes necessary to restore function; the underlying tendons are normal.[53]

Course of the Disease

Two courses of illness are apparent. A small group of patients recovers within about 1 year. They are often the most systemically ill at onset and may constitute a separate disease.

Most of the children are ill for a number of years.[52] The disease is almost always uniphasic, although there may be relative exacerbations and remissions while it is active or a polyphasic course may be created by premature withdrawal of medications. Occasional patients are reported in whom the disease remains active for many years. In our clinic, one girl was continously ill for 15 years (Fig. 6.20). However, the disease becomes inactive in almost all children, and medication can usually be discontinued within 5 years. In one series, all patients who survived (90%) tolerated withdrawal of medication after 2 years, although this has not been the experience of most physicians.[30,40,50,52,52a]

Sixty percent or more of children make a complete recovery without any

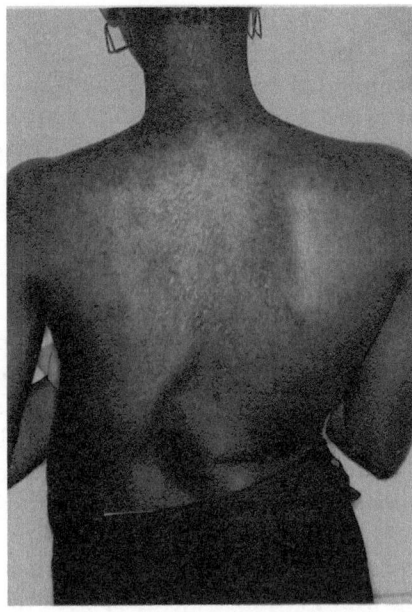

Figure 6.20. Twenty-three-year-old girl who had active dermatomyositis for 15 years. Muscle weakness and marked elevations of muscle enzymes (CPK, 1000) persisted, with progressive scoliosis and appearance of sclerodermatous pigmentation and scarring of the skin. There are no serologic markers of MCTD; she has graduated from college and is employed full-time.

residua.[52] All of our patients are functioning relatively normally despite, in the most severe chronic cases, disfigurement from skin and muscle atrophy and scarring, growth retardation, calcinosis, limitation of motion of some joints, and CPK elevations and persistent abnormalities in muscle histology.[47] In our experience, these muscle-biopsy findings are of no clinical significance and are not associated with progression of muscle weakness or decrease in physical function.[30,54,55]

It is not known whether calcinosis and scarring could be further reduced by more aggressive early use of prednisone, of gamma globulin, or of the newer immunosuppressive agents. The relatively small number of patients seen even in the largest centers, together with the relatively good prognosis for most children with dermatomyositis, has made it impossible to study this poignant question. However, even without the development of new and better agents for the treatment of childhood dermatomyositis, the physician faced with a new patient has every reason to be optimistic.

One clinic has observed an increased risk of autoimmune hypothyroidism after recovery from dermatomyositis.[56] Lipodystrophy may also be a sequelae.[57] In our experience these patients with lipodystrophy may have insulin resistance, hyperinsulinemia, hypertriglyceridemia, hypertension, diabetes, and liver disease in addition to short stature. This problem is just beginning to be studied.[58,59]

One of our patients has had a full-blown recurrence after being completely well for 6 years, without medication.

Management and Prognosis

Despite repeated laments about the lack of blinded randomized control studies of the efficacy of corticosteroid therapy, the response of most patients is dramatic, with relief of pain and gradual increase in muscle strength.[28] Within a week, myoglobinemia and myoglobinuria may be shown to disappear, followed by more gradual improvement in the muscle enzyme determination.[46] Lymphocyte cytotoxicity to muscle cells in vitro may also be shown to normalize with treatment. All of these laboratory parameters exacerbate if treatment is prematurely withdrawn.[9]

Treatment regimens must be individualized, and no single regimen is applicable to all patients (Fig. 6.21).[40,52,52a,59a] We start with prednisone, presumably the safest drug. Most patients receive 2 mg/kg/day in divided doses. If at the end of several months they seem completely well, we try to gradually reduce the medicine over a period of many months. This can be accomplished without exacerbation in approximately 10% of patients, often those who were most ill at onset.

In patients who continue to require prednisone treatment, we change to an alternate-day regimen, usually beginning with 2½ times the daily dose that was required. This is given as a single bolus on arising. We have also used this regimen as the initial treatment in a few patients whose disease was quite mild. After control is achieved, we seek the lowest alternate-day dose. Some patients have exacerbations and remissions requiring dosage adjustments. In our series, medication could be discontinued in most patients after a period of a few years. In one recent report, the average length of active disease in the group who did not recover during the first year of disease was just under 5 years.[52]

We have used weekly oral doses (2–3 mg/kg)[60] or biweekly intravenous injections of methotrexate (2–3 mg/kg/dose, or 7–10 mg/kg/dose with leukovorin rescue in 2 resistant cases) or oral daily azathioprine (50–125 mg daily) or cyclophosphamide (2 mg/kg/day) when the disease was either life-threatening or, on clinical criteria, could not be adequately managed over the long-term with alternate-day prednisone alone. We have supplemented alternate-day prednisone with pulse IV prednisolone as frequently as every eighth morning on arising, in selected patients, with success.[61,62] Plasmapheresis does not seem to be effective.[63] The only two patients we have treated with cyclophosphamide have had gastrointestinal perforations soon after its introduction; this may have been merely a reflection of the severity of their illness, or may have been related to antecedent azathioprine treatment. All of our previously reported patients have recovered and have been receiving no medicines for 10–8 years.[40,59a] We and others have begun to use cyclosporine in refractory cases;[61,64] higher than usual adult doses may be required.[65–65b] Although patients with autoimmune disease are at higher risk of cyclosporine renal toxicity than others, children are at much lower risk than adults.[65c] Gamma globulin is sometimes also effective;[66–67c] an NIH

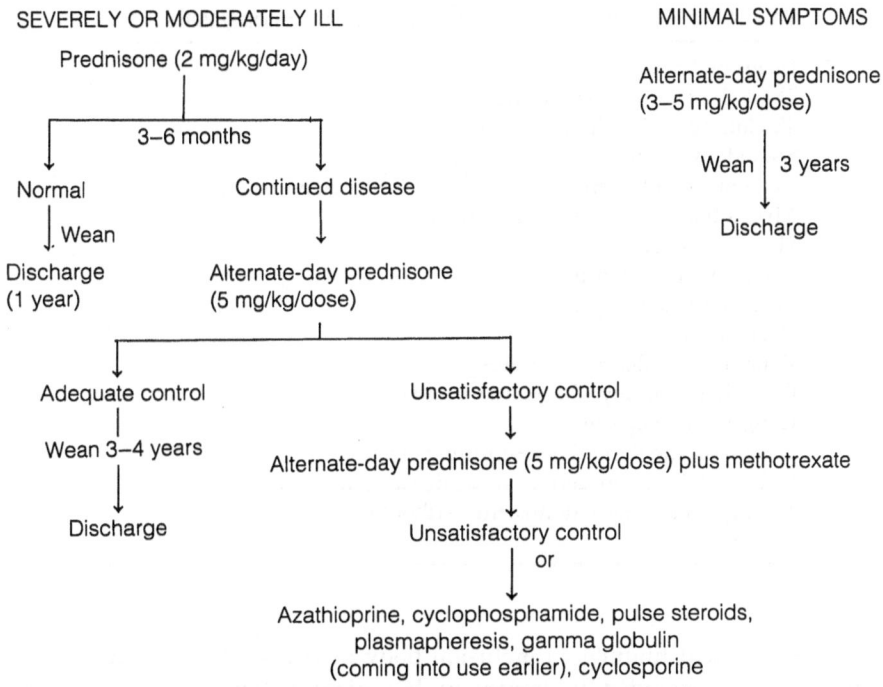

SEVERELY OR MODERATELY ILL

Prednisone (2 mg/kg/day)

3–6 months

Normal   Continued disease

Wean

Discharge   Alternate-day prednisone
(1 year)   (5 mg/kg/dose)

Adequate control   Unsatisfactory control

Wean 3–4 years   Alternate-day prednisone (5 mg/kg/dose) plus methotrexate

Discharge   Unsatisfactory control

or

Azathioprine, cyclophosphamide, pulse steroids,
plasmapheresis, gamma globulin
(coming into use earlier), cyclosporine

MINIMAL SYMPTOMS

Alternate-day prednisone
(3–5 mg/kg/dose)

Wean | 3 years

Discharge

Figure 6.21. Treatment plans for childhood dermatomyositis.

trial is currently in progress. (Caution must be taken in IgA-deficient patients.) Any patient whose disease is not controlled with one drug should have a trial of another agent or a combination of agents,[68] with aggressive management.

Very few children with dermatomyositis now die of the disease. Recent reports continue to indicate a mortality rate of 10%, but half of the deaths, on review, seem avoidable. Even this greatly reduced mortality rate may be expected to be improved upon in the future.

Disorders Resembling Dermatomyositis (Table 6.4)

Inclusion Body Myositis[69]

Although most often seen in elderly men, this subset of dermato/polymyositis, characterized by electron-microscopy demonstration of intracytoplasmic or intranuclear tubular or filamentous inclusions which resemble paramyxovirus nucleocapsid, has a bimodal age of onset with one peak in teenagers. Some patients have skin features indistinguishable from dermatomyositis; all fulfill diagnostic criteria for polymyositis, but asymmetry and distal (as well as proximal) muscle weakness, rare in dermatomy-

Table 6.4. Conditions that May Resemble Dermatomyositis

Inclusion body myositis
Transient acute viral myositis
Trichinosis and eosinophilic myositis[81]
Steroid myopathy
Agammaglobulinemia with persistent CNS echovirus infection
Myoglobinuria and rhabdomyolysis
Hypothyroidism
Leukemia with myositis
Muscular dystrophy
Toxoplasmosis
Drug-induced dermatomyositis
Granulomatous myositis (sarcoid and Crohn's disease)
Congenital myopathies
Calcinosis and dermal bone-forming disorders
SLE, MCTD, scleroderma, systemic vasculitis
Polymyositis (? dermatomyositis without rash)
AIDS[82,83]

ositis, are frequent findings in inclusion body myositis. Only about 20% of patients have responded to treatment but gammaglobulin has not been tried.[70] A major reason for reviewing all muscle-biopsy specimens (some cases can be diagnosed with light-microscopy findings of vacuoles rimmed with basophilic granular material) or rebiopsying treatment-resistant patients for election microscopy not obtained at the first biopsy is the frequency of these findings not being appreciated by those not looking specifically to exclude this diagnosis. When a new therapeutic approach is discovered this will be of greater significance.

Transient Acute Viral Myositis[71–73]

Arthralgia and myalgia are common in viral illnesses. Myositis, verified by elevation of CPK, has been documented with influenza A and B, coxsackie A9 and B5, herpesvirus hominus, Epstein-Barr, adenovirus 21, and hepatitis B infections. A 17-year-old girl with hepatitis B infection had a rash suggestive of dermatomyositis. The other viremias were not associated with a dermatomyositislike rash.

A number of epidemics of influenza-virus infection have been associated with severe myositis in children. The illnesses were similar in each child: following an initial flulike illness and a day or 2 of recovery, the child awakens with severe, excruciating pain and tenderness in the calves and thighs. The pain is so severe that the children cannot walk. The syndrome is dramatic; as a result, these children are frequently hospitalized and subjected to unnecessary intensive study. Diagnosis is easily established by a simple determination of CPK. Elevations range from 10 to 60 times normal. The children recover completely within 72 h. Once the physician is aware of this syndrome, it is easily recognized, and the family is quickly reassured. These children do not manifest the prostration and electrolyte abnormalities occasionally seen following viral illness in children with unrecognized lipid storage myopathy, a condition which may be fatal.[74]

A one-family epidemic of myositis lasting 1–4 weeks was associated with anti-Jo antibodies in the patients and in rodents infesting their home.[22] We have seen one case after insecticide spray.

Trichinosis and Hypereosinophilic Syndromes[75,76]

In typical cases, trichinosis starts with gastrointestinal symptoms followed by fever, urticaria, orbital edema, subungual petechiae, myalgia, and muscle weakness. Eosinophilia is a constant finding, may rise to 70%, and persists for months. Diagnosis is by serologic test. Myositis may also be seen in the hypereosinophilic syndrome as one feature of a systemic illness.

Steroid Myopathy[77]

Myopathy is a well-known complication of treatment with corticosteroids and presents a special problem when it occurs during the course of dermatomyositis. Onset usually is insidious but may be quite acute over a period of only a few days. Weakness is most severe in the hip flexors. Symptomatic improvement may take place with reduction in dose, but recovery may take months. Differentiation of steroid myopathy from exacerbation of dermatomyositis depends on demonstration of worsening weakness and increasing urinary creatine with normal serum muscle enzymes. Usually, if progressive weakness is caused by dermatomyositis itself, the enzymes will be increasing at the same time. Reduction in urine creatine with reduction in dose of prednisone confirms the diagnosis.

Persistent and Fatal Central Nervous System Echovirus Infections in Patients with Agammaglobulinemia[78–80]

This syndrome was first reported in 1956 when it was recognized that some patients with agammaglobulinemia developed a dermatomyositislike syndrome (Fig. 6.22). Arthritis often precedes skin and muscle involvement, and it remains to be determined whether echovirus can be cultured from the spinal fluid at that stage. Later, erythema, edema, and induration of the skin, together with muscle weakness and flexion contractures of the extremity joints, signal the onset of this syndrome. Neurologic symptoms may become prominent. Cultures of spinal fluid reveal echovirus. Intravenous or intraventricular gamma globulin may control the disease.

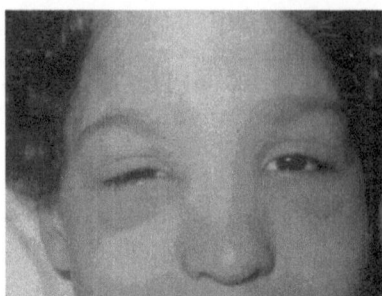

Figure 6.22. Periorbital edema and erythema typical of the dermatomyositislike syndrome that occurs in agammaglobulinemic boys as a manifestation of chronic echovirus meningitis.

Pitfalls in Interpreting Serum CPK Activity[84]

Assay for CPK is commonly used in diagnosing disorders of skeletal or cardiac muscle but may be elevated in a variety of circumstances: exercise, even as mild as repetitive pumping of the hand during blood donation; insertion of needles into muscle, as in EMG; head injury or cerebral insult; psychoses; amyotrophic lateral sclerosis; hypokalemia; alcohol ingestion; hypothyroidism, even without symptoms of myopathy; McLeod syndrome; pulmonary disease; and a variety of other pathophysiologic states. The CPK value must be interpreted along with other clinical data.

Hypothyroidism[85,86]

Muscle weakness, sometimes associated with cramps, pain, stiffness, and myotonia, may be the presenting manifestations of hypothyroidism. This is almost always associated with elevation of muscle enzymes and sometimes with abnormalities on EMG. A similar syndrome has recently been reported in association with adult celiac disease. Muscular symptoms disappeared with treatment of the basic disease. Muscle weakness may be a manifestation of many endocrine disorders.[87]

Rhabdomyolysis and Lipid Storage Myopathy[87-91]

Recurrent rhabdomyolysis may occur in children whose skeletal muscle metabolism of carbohydrates is deficient, as in deficiency of muscle phosphorylase, phosphofructokinase, or carnitine palmityltransferase. These patients usually have diminished ketone production and high levels of plasma free fatty acids and triglycerides during fasting, suggesting a deficiency in the liver as well as the muscle. Some of these disorders are treatable with diet. Diagnosis is important since recurrent rhabdomyolysis may be associated with severe electrolyte imbalance, cardiac arrhythmias, renal failure, and respiratory failure.

Rhabdomyolysis may occur in seemingly normal individuals with infection,[92] trauma, exercise, and cold exposure. Children may have severe symmetrical pain and swelling in specific leg muscles and may appear very ill. If sufficient myoglobin is in the urine, it will appear pink/brown; positive hematest with negative microscopic examination for red blood cells together with the child's symptoms helps to differentiate this from acute nephritis.

One instance of rhabdomyolysis after injection of iron-dextran has been reported.[93]

Dermatomyositis and Malignancy[94,95]

There is a significantly increased incidence of cancer in adults with dermatomyositis; recognition of that association may lead to early cancer diagnosis and treatment. This association has not been present in children, although occasionally leukemia may present with symptoms suggestive of dermatomyositis.

Muscular Dystrophy[96]

Children with muscular dystrophy present with a selective pattern of progressive weakness without inflammatory disease and so are easily distinguished from children with dermatomyositis. Diagnosis is confirmed by family history, muscle enzyme abnormalities in other family members, and muscle biopsy.

Toxoplasmosis[97]

Acute toxoplasmosis can be accompanied by myositis; rarely, the organism can be isolated from affected muscle tissue. Serologic evidence of recent toxoplasma infection can be demonstrated in some adults with polymyositis but not in children and not in patients with dermatomyositis.

Drug-Induced Dermatomyositis[98,99]

Two cases of dermatomyositis appeared coincident with *BCG vaccination*. Typical skin rash, myositic symptoms, characteristic findings on muscle biopsy, EMG abnormalities, and elevations of muscle enzymes may result from treatment with *penicillamine* in 1.4% of patients, especially individuals with HLA-DR2/DQw1,[100] and disappear on withdrawal of the drug. Drug-induced muscle disease has been reported with carbimazole, lovastatin, hydroxychloroquine, colchicine, clofibrate, emetine, corticosteroids,[87,101,102] and zidovudine (AZT).[83]

Granulomatous Myositis[103]

Muscle pain and granulomata on biopsy may be found in Crohn's disease and in sarcoidosis.

Chronic Congenital Myopathy Associated with Coxsackie Virus A9[104]

Two infants with congenital Coxsackie virus A9 disease with myopathy continued to shed virus in stool throughout their lives, and in one the virus could be grown from muscle tissue obtained postmortem at age 11 years.

Calcinosis and Dermal Bone-Forming Disorders

Tumeral calcinosis may occur as a manifestation of a heritable disorder causing increased renal phosphate absorption and resultant hyperphosphatemia.[105] Dermal ossification is a feature of Albright hereditary osteodystrophy, fibrodysplasia ossificans progressiva, and a newly described disorder of mesenchymal differentiation which begins soon after birth.[106]

References

1. Wedgwood RJP, Cook CD, Cohen J: Dermatomyositis: report of 26 cases, in children with a discussion of endocrine therapy in 13. Pediatrics 12:447–466, 1953.
2. Banker BQ, Victor M: Dermatomyositis (systemic angiopathy) of childhood. Medicine 45:261–289, 1966.
3. Ackerman AB: Histologic Diagnosis of Inflammatory Skin Diseases. Lea and Febiger, Philadelphia, 1978.
4. Silver RM, Maricq HR: Childhood dermatomyositis: serial microvascular studies. Pediatrics 83:278–283, 1989.
5. Crowe WE, Bove KE, Levinson JE, et al.: Clinical and pathogenetic implications of histopathology in childhood polydermatomyositis. Arthritis Rheum 25:126–139, 1982.
6. Whitaker JN, Engel WK: Vascular deposits of immunoglobulin and complement in idiopathic inflammatory myopathy. N Engl J Med 286:333–338, 1972.
7. Kissel JT, Mendrell JR, Rammonohan KW: Microvascular deposition of complement membrane attack complex in dermatomyositis. N Engl J Med 314:329–334, 1986.
8. Miller FW: Humoral immunity and immunogenetics in the idiopathic inflammatory myopathies. Curr Opin Rheumatol 3:902–910, 1991.
9. Dawkins RL, Mastaglis FL: Cell-mediated cytotoxicity to muscle in polymyositis. N Engl J Med 288:434–438, 1973.
10. Kalovidouris AE, Pourmand R, Passo MH, Plotkin Z: Proliferative response of peripheral blood mononuclear cells to autologous and allogenetic muscle in patients with polymyositis/dermatomyositis. Arthritis Rheum 32:446–453, 1989.
11. Fudman EJ, Schnitzer TJ: Clinical and biochemical characteristics of autoanti-

body system in polymyositis and dermatomyositis. Semin Arthritis Rheum 15:255–260, 1986.

12. Saito E, Murabayashi K, Ogawa T, et al.: Etiological difference between dermatomyositis and polymyositis. Jap J Rheumatol 3:85–93, 1991.

13. Kalovidouris AE: The role of cell-mediated immunity in polymyositis. Curr Opin Rheumatol 3:911–918, 1991.

14. Hohlfeld R, Engel AG, Li K, Harper MC: Polymyositis mediated by T lymphocytes that express the gamma/delta receptor. N Engl J Med 324:877–881, 1991.

15. Friedmen JN, Pachman LM, Mary jowski KL, et al.: Immunogenetic studies of juvenile dermatomyositis: HLA-DR antigen frequencies. Arthritis Rheum 26:214–216, 1983.

16. Carroll JE, Silverman A, Isobe Y, et al.: Inflammatory myopathy, IgA deficiency, and intestinal malabsorption. J Pediatr 89:216–219, 1976.

17. Leddy JP, Griggs RC, Klemperer MR, et al.: Hereditary complement (C2) deficiency with dermatomyositis. Am J Med 58:83–91, 1975.

18. Hennekam RCM, Hiemstra I, Jennekens FGI, Kuis W: Juvenile dermatomyositis in first cousins. N Engl J Med 323:199, 1990.

19. Reed AM, Ober C, Pachman LM: Increased risk for juvenile dermatomyositis (JDMS) is associated with HLA-DQA1. Arthritis Rheum 33:S15, 1990.

19a. Liblau R, Morel E, Bach J-F: Autoimmune diseases, IgA deficiency, and intravenous immunoglobulin treatment. Am J Med 93:114–115, 1992.

20. Harati Y, Niakan E, Bergman EW: Childhood dermatomyositis in monozygotic twins. Neurology 36:721–723, 1986.

21. Walker EJ, Jeffrey PD: Polymyositis and molecular mimicry, a mechanism of autoimmunity. Lancet 2:605–608, 1986.

22. Garcia-de-la-Torre I, Ramirez-Casillas A, Hernandez-Vazques L: Acute familial myositis with a common autoimmune response. Arthritis Rheum 34:744–750, 1991.

23. Ytterberg SR, Mahowald ML, Messner RP: Coxsackie virus B1-induced polymyositis. Lack of disease expression in nu/nu Mice. J Clin Invest 80:499–506, 1987.

24. Yousef GE, Isenberg DA, Mowbray JF: Detection of enterovirus specific RNA sequences in muscle biopsy specimens from patients with adult onset myositis. Ann Rheum Dis 49:310–315, 1990.

25. Christensen ML, Pachman LM, Schneiderman R, et al.: Prevalence of Coxsackie-B virus antibodies in patients with juvenile dermatomyositis. Arthritis Rheum 29:1365–1370, 1986.

26. Bowles NE, et al.: Dermatomyositis, polymyositis, and Coxsackie-B virus infection. Lancet 1:1004, 1987.

27. Liveson JA, Spielholz NI: Peripheral Neurology; Case Studies in Electrodiagnosis. Davis, Philadelphia, 1979.

28. Bohan A, Peter JB, Bowman RL, et al.: A computer-assisted analysis of 153 patients with polymyositis and dermatomyositis. Medicine 56:255–286, 1977.

29. Spencer-Green G, Schlesinger M, Bove KE, et al.: Nailfold capillary abnormalities in childhood rheumatic disease. J Pediatr 102:341–346, 1983.

30. Bowyer SL, Blane CE, Sullivan DB, Cassidy JT: Childhood dermatomyositis: factors predicting functional outcome and development of dystrophic calcification. J Pediatr 103:882–888, 1983.

31. DiLiberti JH, D'Agostino AN, Cole G: Needle muscle biopsy in infants and children. J Pediatr 103:566–570, 1983.

32. Hernandez RJ, Keim DR, Sullivan DB, et al.: Magnetic resonance imaging appearance of the muscles in childhood dermatomyositis. J Pediatr 117:546–550, 1990.

33. de Merieux P, Verity A, Clements PJ, Paulus HE: Esophageal abnormalities and dysphagia in polymyositis and dermatomyositis. Arthritis Rheum 26:961–968, 1983.

34. Fischer TJ, Cipel L, Stiehm ER. Pneumotosis intestinalis associated with fatal childhood dermatomyositis. Pediatrics 61:127–130, 1978.

35. Schullinger JN, Jacobs JC, Berdon WE: Diagnosis and management of gastrointestinal perforations in childhood dermatomyositis with particular reference to perforations of the duodenum. J Pediatr Surg 123:1117–1119, 1988.

36. Downey EC, Woolley MM, Hanson V: Required surgical therapy in the pediatric patient with dermatomyositis. Arch Surg 123:1117–1120, 1988.

37. Dickey BF, Myers AR: Pulmonary disease in polymyositis/dermatomyositis. Semin Arthritis Rheum 14:60–76, 1984.

38. Singsen BH, Tedford JC, Platzker ACG, et al.: Spontaneous pneumothorax: a complication of juvenile dermatomyositis. J Pediatr 92:771–774, 1978.

39. Schwartz MI, Matthay RA, Sahn SA, et al.: Interstitial lung disease in polymyositis and dermatomyositis: analysis of six cases and review of the literature. Medicine 55:89–104, 1976.

40. Jacobs JC: Methotrexate and azathioprine treatment of childhood dermatomyositis. Pediatrics 59:212–218, 1977.

40a.Pereira RM, Lerner S, Maeda WT et al.: Pericardial tamponade in juvenile dermatomyositis. Clin Cardiol 15:301–303, 1992.

41. Gottdiener JS, Sherber HS, Hawley RJ, et al.: Cardiac manifestations in polymyositis. Am J Cardiol 41:1141–1144, 1978.

42. Bruce GM: Retinitis in dermatomyositis. Trans Am Ophthalmol Soc 32:282–295, 1938.

43. Fruman LS, Ragsdale CG, Sullivan DB, et al.: Retinopathy in juvenile dermatomyositis. J Pediatr 88:267–269, 1976.

44. Bitnum S, Daeschner CW, Travis LB, et al.: Dermatomyositis. J Pediatr 64:101–131, 1964.

45. Pirovino M, Neff MS, Sharon E: Myoglobinuria and acute renal failure with acute polymyositis. NY State J Med 79:764–767, 1979.

46. Kagen LJ: Myoglobinemia in inflammatory myopathies. JAMA 237:1448–1452, 1977.

47. Miller JJ: Late progression in dermatomyositis in childhood. J Pediatr 83:543–548, 1973.

48. Skuterud E, Sydnes OA, Haavik TK: Calcinosis in dermatomyositis treated with probenecid. Scand J Rheum 10:92–94, 1981.

49. Burger RG, Featherstone GL, Raasch RHE, et al.: Treatment of calcinosis universalis with low-dose warfarin. Am J Med 83:72–75, 1987 (see also correspondence 84:795–796, 1988).

50. Steiner RM, Glassman L, Schwartz MW, et al.: The radiologic findings in dermatomyositis of childhood. Radiology 111:385–393, 1974.

51. Wilscher ML, Holdawat IM, North JDK: Hypercalcaemia during resolution of calcinosis in juvenile dermatomyositis. Br Med J 288:1345, 1984.

51a.Moore EC, Cohen F, Douglas SD, Gutta V: Staphylococcal infections in childhood dermatomyositis—association with the development of calcinosis, raised

IgE concentrations and granulocyte chemotactic defect. Ann Rheum Dis 51:378–383, 1992.

52. Spencer CH, Hanson V, Singsen BH, et al.: Course of treated juvenile dermatomyositis. J Pediatr 105:399–408, 1984.

52a. Oddis CV: Therapy for myositis. Curr Opin Rheumatol 3:919–924, 1991.

53. Ames EL, Posch JL: Calcinosis of the flexor and extensor tendons in dermatomyositis. Case Report. J Hand Surg 9A:876–879, 1984.

54. Chalmers A, Sayson R, Walters K: Juvenile dermatomyosisits: medical, social, and economic status in adulthood. Can Med Assoc J Med 314:329–334, 1986.

55. Miller LC, Michael AF, Kim Y: Childhood dermatomyositis. Clin Pediatr 26: 561–566, 1987.

56. Wexter ID, Newman AJ, Dhams WT: Hypothyroidism occurring in patients with childhood dermatomyositis. Pediatr Res 255:170A, 1989.

57. Tucker LB, Sadeghi-Nejad A, Schaller JG: The association of acquired lipodystrophy with juvenile dermatomyositis. Arthritis Rheum 33:S146, 1990.

58. Sissons JG, West RJ, Fallows J, et al.: The complement abnormalities of lipodystrophy. N Engl J Med 294:461–465, 1976.

59. Reaven GM: Insulin resistance, hyperinsulinemia, and hypertriglyceridemia in the etiology and clinical course of hypertension. Am J Med 90(Suppl A):7S–12S, 1991.

59a. Jacobs JC: Treatment of dermatomyositis. Arthritis Rheum 20:338–341, 1977.

60. Teresi ME, Crom WR, Choi KE, et al.: Methotrexate bioavailability after oral and intramuscular administration in children. J Pediatr 110:788–792, 1987.

61. Kula RW: In Delakas MC (ed.) Polymyositis and dermatomyositis. Butterworths, Boston, pp. 255–279, 1988.

62. Laxer RM, Stein LD, Petty RE: Intravenous pulse methylprednisolone treatment of juvenile dermatomyositis. Arthritis Rheum 30:328–334, 1987.

63. Miller FW, Leitman SF, Cronin ME et al.: Controlled trial of plasma exchange in polymyositis and dermatomyositis. N Engl J Med 326:1380–1384, 1992.

64. Heckmatt J, Saunders C, Peters AM, et al.: Cyclosporin in juvenile dermatomyositis. Lancet 1063–1066, 1989.

65. Kahan BD, Conley S, Portman R, et al.: Parent-to-child transplantation with cyclosporine immunosuppression. J Pediatr 111(6, pt. 2):1012–1016, 1987.

65a. Whang R, Whang DD, Ryan MP: Refractory potassium repletion. A consequence of magnesium deficiency. Arch Intern Med 152:40–45, 1992.

65b. Burack DA, Griffith BP, Thompson ME, Kahl LE: Hyperuricemia and gout among heart transplant recipients receiving cyclosporine. Am J Med 92:141–146, 1992.

65c. Feutren G, Mihatsch MJ et al.: Risk factors for cyclosporine-induced nephropathy in patients with autoimmune diseases. N Engl J Med 326:1654–1660, 1992.

66. Lang BA, Laxer RM, Murphy G, et al.: Treatment of juvenile dermatomyositis with intravenous gammaglobulin. Am J Med 91:169–172, 1991.

67. Di Nicolo R, Hutto J, Jyonouchi H, et al.: Intravenous gammaglobulin (IVGG) improves treatment of dermatomyositis. Pediatr Res 27:155A, 1990.

67a. Cherin P, Herson S, Wechsler B, et al.: Efficacy of Intravenous Gammaglobulin Therapy in Chronic Refractory Polymyositis and Dermatomyositis: An Open Study with 20 Adult Patients. Am J Med 91:162–168, 1991.

67b. Dwyer JM: Manipulating the immune system with immune globulin. N Eng

Med 326:107–116, 1992.

67c. Viard J-P, Vittecoq D, Lacroix C, Bach J-F: Response of HIV-1-associated polymyositis to intravenous immunoglobulin. Am J Med 92:580–581, 1992.

68. So SKS, Najarian JS, Nevins TE, et al.: Low-dose cyclosporine therapy combined with standard immunosuppression in pediatric renal transplantation. J Pediatr 11:1017–1021, 1987.

69. Cohen MR, Sulaiman AR, Garancis JC, Wortmann RL: Clinical heterogeneity and treatment response to inclusion body myositis. Arthritis Rheum 32:734–740, 1989.

70. Case Records of the Massachusetts General Hospital. Case 40-1991 N Engl J Med 325:1026–1035, 1991.

71. Pittsley RA, Shearn MA, Kaufmam L: Acute hepatitis B simulating dermatomyositis. JAMA 239:959, 1978.

72. Dietzman DE, Schaller JG, Ray G, et al.: Acute myositis with influenza B infection. Pediatrics 57:255–258, 1976.

73. Grunwald Z, Ashkenazi S, Peterbourg I, et al.: Acute transient myositis secondary to viral infection in childhood. A report of two patients and review of the literature. Intl Pediatr 6:301–303, 1991.

74. Kelly KJ, Garland JS, Tang TT, et al.: Fatal rhabdomyolysis following influenza infection in a girl with familial carnitine palmityl transferase deficiency. Pediatrics 84:312–316, 1989.

75. Drachman DA, Tuncbay TO: The remote myopathy of trichinosis. Neurology 15:1127–1135, 1965.

76. Layzer RB, Shearn MA, Satya-Murti S: Eosinophilic polymyositis. Ann Neurol 1:65–71, 1977.

77. Askari A, Vignos PJ, Moskowitz RW: Steroid myopathy in connective tissue disease. Am J Med 61:485–492, 1976.

78. Bardelas JA, Winkelstein JA, Seto DSY, et al.: Fatal echo 24 infection in a patient with hypogammaglobulinemia: Relationship to dermatomyositis-like syndrome. J Pediatr 90:396–399, 1977.

79. Crennan JM, Van Scoy RE, McKenna CH, Smith TF: Echovirus polymyositis in patients with hypogammaglobulinemia. Am J Med 81:35–42, 1986.

80. Mease PJ, Ochs HD, Wedgwood PJ: Successful treatment of echovirus meningoencephalitis and myositis-fasciitis with intravenous immune globulin therapy in a patient with X-linked aggammaglobulinemia. N Engl J Med 304:1278–1281, 1981. (see also: N Engl J Med 313:758, 1985)

81. Herrera R, Varela E, Morales G, et al.: Dermatomyositis-like syndrome caused by Trichinae. Report of two cases. J Rheumatol 12:782–784, 1985.

82. Nordstrom M, Petropolis AA, Giorno R, et al.: Inflammatory myopathy and acquired immunodeficiency syndrome. Arthritis Rheum 32:475–479, 1989.

83. Walter EB, Drucker RP, McKinney RE, Wilfert CM: Myopathy in human immunodeficiency virus-infected children receiving long-term Zidovudine therapy. J Pediatr 119:152–155, 1991.

84. Nevins MA, Saran M, Bright, M, et al.: Pitfalls in interpreting serum creatine phosphokinase activity. JAMA 224:1382–1387, 1973.

85. Hochberg MC, Koppes GM, Edwards CQ, et al.: Hypothyroidism presenting as a polymyositis-like syndrome. Arthritis Rheum 19:1363–1366, 1976.

86. Newman AJ, Lee C: Hypothyroidism simulating dermatomyositis. J Pediatr 97:772–774, 1980.

87. Wortmann RL: Metabolic myopathies. Curr Opin Rheumatol 3:925–933, 1991.
88. Editorial: Lipid storage myopathies. Lancet: 1:757–758, 1978.
89. Raifman MA, Bernat M, Lenarsky C: Cold weather and rhabdomyolysis. J Pediatr 93:970–971, 1978.
90. DiMauro S: Metabolic myopathies. In Vinken PJ, Bruyn GW (eds.) Handbook of Clinical Neurology. North-Holland, Amsterdam, 1992, In Press. (Vol 61, #17)
91. Tein I, DiMauro S, Rowland, LP: Myoglobinuria. In Vinken PJ, Bruyn GW (eds.) Handbook of Clinical Neurology. North-Holland, Amsterdam, 1992, In Press. (Vol 61, #17)
92. Fernandez A, Justiniani FR: Massive rhabdomyolysis: a rare presentation of primary vibrio vulnificus septicemia. Am J Med 89:535–536, 1990.
93. Foulkes WD, Sewry C, Calam J, Hodgson HJF: Rhabdomyolysis after intra-muscular iron-dextran in malabsorption. Ann Rheum Dis 50:184–184, 1991.
94. Barnes BE: Dermatomyositis and malignancy. Ann Intern Med 84:68–76, 1976.
95. Singsen BH, Waters KD, Siegel SE, et al.: Lymphocytic leukemia, atypical dermatomyositis, and hyperlipidemia in a 4 year old boy. J Pediatr 90:602–604, 1976.
96. Zundel WS, Tyler FH: The muscular dystrophies. N Engl J Med 273:537–543; 596–601, 1965.
97. Phillips PE, Kassan SS, Kagen LJ: Increased toxoplasma antibodies in idio-pathic inflammatory muscle disease. Arthritis Rheum 22:209–214, 1979.
98. Fernandes L, Swinson DR, Hamilton EDB: Dermatomyositis complicating penicillamine treatment. Ann Rheum Dis 36:94–95, 1977.
99. Kass E, Straume S, Munthe E: Dermatomyositis after BCG vaccination. Lancet 1:722, 1978.
100. Taneja V, Mehra N, Singh YN, et al.: HLA-D region genes and susceptibility to D-penicillamine-induced myositis. Arthritis Rheum 33:1445–1447, 1990.
101. Pierce LR, Wysowski DK, Gross TP: Myopathy and rhabdomyolysis associated with lovastatin-gemfibrozil combination therapy. JAMA 264:71–75, 1990.
102. Doyle DR, McCurley TL, Sergent JS: Fatal polymyositis in D-penicillamine treated rheumatoid arthritis. Ann Intern Med 98:327–330, 1983.
103. Menard DB, Haddad H, Blain JG, et al.: Granulomatous myositis and myopathy associated with Crohn's colitis. N Engl J Med 295:818–819, 1976.
104. Tang TT, Sedmak GV, Siegesmund KA, et al.: Chronic myopathy associated with coxsackie virus type A9. N Engl J Med 292:608–611, 1975.
105. Steinherz R, Chesney RW, Eisentstein B, et al.: Elevated serum calcitriol con-centrations do not fall in response to hyperphosphatemia in familial tumoral calcinosis. Am J Dis Child 139:816–819, 1985.
106. Foster CM, Levin S, Levine M, et al.: Limited dermal ossification: clinical fea-tures and natural history. J Pediatr 109:71–76, 1986.

7

Systemic Vasculitis Syndromes

Vasculitis, inflammation in and around the blood vessels, which is sometimes associated with fibrinoid necrosis, may be seen in many of the conditions discussed in this book. In most rheumatic diseases, vasculitis is only one feature of a well-defined, complex, pathologic process (Fig. 7.1), and the disease (e.g., SLE or dermatomyositis) is best characterized by other distinctive diagnostic clinical and laboratory features. However, in the diverse and perhaps totally unrelated syndromes discussed in this chapter, vasculitis itself is the predominant pathologic process, and the clinical manifestations are primarily a direct result of the damage to the blood vessels (Table 7.1).

The diagnosis of systemic vasculitis is suspected (in the absence of SLE) when (1) several organ systems are mysteriously, simultaneously, or consecutively affected and (2) the clinical manifestations include myalgia, arthralgia/arthritis, rash, abdominal pain, nephritis, hypertension, neurologic manifestations, pulmonary infiltrates, nasal stuffiness, or unusual cardiac manifestations such as pulse deficits, coronary artery disease, or unexplained heart failure (Table 7.2)[1-2] Fever, weight loss, and malaise without apparent cause usually precede or accompany the other manifestations. A variety of classification schemes for the vasculitic syndromes are possible, depending either on the organs predominantly affected; the size of affected vessels, or the location or type of blood vessel damaged; the mechanism of vascular injury; or the characteristics of the cellular response (Table 7.3). For this author, none of the classification schema have any advantage over pattern recognition.

Clinical Presentation

Certain clinical features (patterns) suggest specific vasculitic syndromes (Table 7.4).[1-2] A young infant with unexplained fever, a polymorphous rash,

556

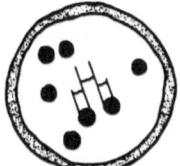

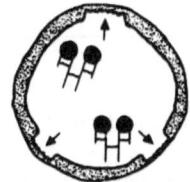

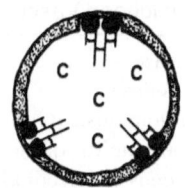

1) Circulating soluble immune complexes in antigen excess.

2) Increased vascular permeability via platelet derived vasoactive amines and IgE mediated reactions.

3) Trapping of immune complexes along basement membrane of vessel wall and activation of complement components (C).

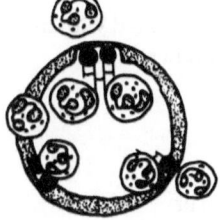

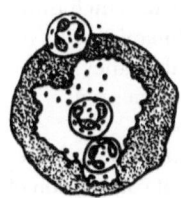

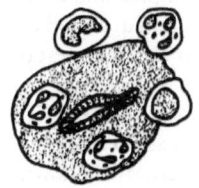

4) Complement derived chemotactic factors (C3a, C5a, C567) cause accumulation of PMNs.

5) PMNs release lysosomal enzymes (collagenase, elastase)

6) Damage and necrosis of vessel wall, thrombosis, occlusion, hemorrhage.

Figure 7.1. Mechanisms of immune-complex-mediated vasculitis. (Reprinted with permission from Fauci A.S., et al., ref. 1.)

and telangiectatic (aneurysmal) dilatation of the conjunctival vessels is suspect for *Kawasaki disease*. An older girl who is not thriving or is having unexplained fevers with vague musculoskeletal complaints, who then suddenly develops seizures, hypertension, and heart failure and is noted to have absent pulses probably has *Takayasu's arteritis*. A young man with glomerulonephritis, a nasal granuloma, and nodular cavitary lesions on chest x-ray has *Wegener's granulomatosis*. A young boy or girl with fever, myalgias, abdominal pain, hypertension, renal disease, and cutaneous and muscular necrotizing vasculitis of small and medium-sized arteries without significant peripheral eosinophilia or granuloma in the respiratory tract has *periarteritis nodosa*. A child with severe asthma, heart failure, eosinophilia, and vasculitic dermal nodules has *allergic granulomatosis*. Angiocentric pulmonary nodules of lymphoid cells with neurologic/psychiatric manifestations suggestive of vasculitis of the brain, in the absence of significant renal disease, suggests *lymphomatoid granulomatosis*. While this sort of syndrome categorization has not yet facilitated elucidation of the pathogenesis of these disorders, it has provided insight into the prognosis and management of each disorder.

Table 7.1. Childhood Vasculitis

Kawasaki disease
Polyarteritis nodosa
Allergic granulomatosis (Churg-Strauss syndrome)
Granulomatous angiitis of the brain
   Steroid-responsive encephalomyelitis (?allergic angiitis of the brain)
Takayasu's arteritis
Wegener's granulomatosis
Lymphomatoid granulomatosis
Hypersensitivity vasculitis
   Serum-sickness-like reactions*
   Henoch-Schönlein purpura*
   Allergic angiitis and overlap syndromes including those associated with hypocom-
      plementemia, mixed cryoglobulinemia, otitis media, and hepatitis[3]
   Vasculitis as a manifestation of malignancy
   Vasculitis as a complication of drug therapy
   Vasculitis associated with drug abuse
   Vasculitis as a feature of inflammatory bowel disease
Mesenteric arteritis following repair of coarctation of the aorta
Cutaneous vasculitis
   Cutaneous periarteritis nodosa
   Segmental hyalinizing vasculitis
   Erythema elevatum diutinum
Behçet's syndrome
Cogan's syndrome
Malignant papulosis (Kohlmeier-Degos disease)
Perivasculitis syndromes with arthritis*
   Mucha-Habermann disease*
   Sweet's syndrome*
"Juvenile temporal arteritis"
Alpha$_1$-antitrypsin deficiency with vasculitis[4]
Generalized venulopathy[5]

* Discussed in Chapter 2.

Table 7.2. Symptoms Suggesting Systemic Vasculitis in Children

*Multiple Organ Systems**	*Symptoms*
Rheumatic	Fever, myalgia, arthritis, abdominal pain, rash, high ESR out of proportion to physical findings
Renal	Nephritis, hypertension
Respiratory	Nasal stuffiness, pulmonary infiltrates, eosinophilia
Neurologic	Multiple neurologic manifestations
Cardiovascular	Pulse deficits, pericarditis, heart failure, coronary artery disease

* Simultaneous or consecutive involvement.

Table 7.3. Classification of Vasculitis by Size and Location of Affected Vessels

Small vessels	Upper dermis: hypersensitivity angiitis; urticaria; Henoch-Schönlein purpura; Mucha-Habermann disease
	Middle and lower dermis: Sweet's syndrome; erythema elevatum diutinum; segmental hyalinizing (livedoid) vasculitis (atrophie blanche); malignant papulosis (Kohlmeier-Degos)
	Panniculus: erythema nodosum; erythema induratum; Weber-Christian disease
Medium-sized vessels	Periarteritis nodosa; allergic granulomatosis; Wegener's granulamatosis; lymphomatoid granulomatosis; Kawasaki disease
Aortitis	Takayasu's disease; spondyloarthritis (ankylosing spondylitis and Reiter's syndrome); Behçet's syndrome; Cogan's syndrome; systemic infections (syphilis, tuberculosis, salmonellosis)

No classification system for the vasculitides is entirely satisfactory. Overlap syndromes are not infrequent. A problem of terminology arises when a child is ill with fever, musculoskeletal complaints, and vasculitic skin lesions but does not have the features of one of the more highly defined syndromes mentioned above. These patients have one of a variety of syndromes that have been called *hypersensitivity vasculitis*, cutaneous periarteritis nodosa, serum-sickness-like reactions, leukocytoclastic vasculitis, overlap vasculitis syndrome, mixed cryoglobulinemia, vasculitis associated with hepatitis B antigen, and vasculitis after serous otitis media. Many children with these vasculitides have features of more than one of these entities, and some seem to defy subclassification. Diagnosis and management seem to be enhanced by avoiding the use of all of these overlapping and confusing terms. Unless the child has one of the well-defined specific vasculitic syndromes named above, it may be best to refer to the process merely as a systemic vasculitis and get on with the care of the patient *using principles of management extrapolated from the closest analogous syndrome.*

Kawasaki Disease

Mucocutaneous lymph-node syndrome, now called Kawasaki disease (KD), is by far the most common systemic vasculitis syndrome of childhood. In the initial report published in Japanese in 1967, Kawasaki was able to gather data on 50 cases. Nationwide surveys have been regularly conducted in Japan since 1970; over 100,000 cases have been recorded in Japan since that

Table 7.4. Clinical Features of the Chronic Vasculitic Syndromes

Syndrome	Diagnostic Procedures
Periarteritis Nodosa Malaise and weight loss, fever Vasculitic skin rash Hypertension Myalgias Abdominal pain Arthralgias/arthritis Mononeuritis multiplex/CNS	Abdominal/CNS arteriography, MRI Skin, muscle, sural-nerve biopsy EMG/nerve-conduction studies ANCA
Allergic Granulomatosis History of asthma Pulmonary infiltrates Eosinophilia Heart failure Dermal nodules Fever	Nodule biopsy ANCA
Wegener's Granulomatosis Nasal stuffiness/granulomas Nodular lesions on chest films Ulcerating skin purpura Nephritis Malaise and weight loss, fever	Nasal lesional biopsy, skin biopsy Renal biopsy ANCA
Malignant Atrophic Papulosis *(Kohlmeier-Degos Disease)* Asymptomatic white skin papules Intestinal infarction, obstruction, perforation Multifocal nervous-system manifestations	Lesional skin biopsy CT scan of brain Cerebral arteriogram
Takayasu's Arteritis Female with failure to thrive and vague musculoskeletal complaints; unexplained fever Hypertension/seizures Heart failure; pulmonary hypertension Absent pulses Tuberculosis (±)	MRI, aortogram, digital venous angiography
Lymphomatous Granulomatosis Multifocal CNS manifestions Angiocentric lymphoblastic pulmonary nodules Dermal nodules Fever	Lung biopsy
Behçet's Syndrome Relapsing genital and oral ulcers Iritis	Skin pathergy test

Table 7.4. (Continued)

Syndrome	Diagnostic Procedures
Arthritis and vasculitis (±) Ulcerative esophagitis and colitis (±)	
Cogan's Syndrome Nerve deafness Interstitial keratitis Arthritis and vasculitis (±)	
Sweet's Syndrome Episodic fever and rash (painful plaques) Arthralgia/arthritis High ESR Also seen after intestinal bypass surgery	Skin biopsy
Mucha-Habermann Disease Episodic chickenpox-like rash with fever Arthralgia/arthritis High ESR	Skin biopsy
Erythema Elevatum Diutinum Chronic recurrent painful plaques or nodules over knees, elbows, hands Arthralgia/arthritis Increased susceptibility to infection	Skin biopsy

Segmental Hyalinizing Vasculitis
Females with chronic recurring infarctive
  ulcers of the lower legs that scar (atrophie
  blanche)
Livedo reticularis
	Skin biopsy

Allergic Angiitis Fever and rheumatic symptoms without major organ manifestations Palpable purpura, hives (leukoclastic angiitis)	Skin biopsy, muscle biopsy

time; 15,519 newly registered cases were reported in one epidemic year. In that year two children out of every 1000 babies under age 1 year developed KD.[6] The true incidence in the United States is unknown. In 1984–1990 the annual reported mean incidence was at least six cases per 100,000 children less than 5 years of age in one large city.[7]

Clinical Presentation (Table 7.5). The illness begins with unexplained fever, often with striking cervical lymphadenopathy. Frequently the adenitis is unilateral and simulates a cervical-gland abscess.[7a] After a few days,

Table 7.5. Clinical Manifestations of Kawasaki Disease

	Characteristics
Fever* (95)	Spiking to 104 Unresponsive to intermittent doses of aspirin Lasts 5–23 days in untreated cases
Rash* (92)	"Polymorphous" = many forms (papular, morbiliform, multiforme, raised plaques, scarlatiniform, vesicular); perineal accentuation; site of BCG vaccination may develop Arthus-like reaction Pruritic Followed by desquamation
Lymphadenopathy* (75)	Mostly cervical (mediastinal has been noted) Single nodes may be very large and simulate abscess May be unilateral Frequently subsides early (but not always)
Conjunctival hyperemia* (88)	Suffused bulbar conjunctivae without exudate
Extremity changes* (94)	Induration of the hands and feet (76) Erythema of the palms and soles (88) Typical desquamation of fingers and toes in the convalescent period (94) Beau's lines (transverse grooves) in nails later in the recovery period in some severe cases
Mouth lesions* (90)	Erythema and fissuring of the lips and oropharynx Strawberry tongue
Associated features	Arthralgia and arthritis Aseptic meningitis Abdominal pain, obstructive jaundice, intestinal perforation, hydrops of the gallbladder Myocarditis, pericarditis, tamponade, cardiac failure, arrhythmia, acute mitral insufficiency, myocardial infarction
Laboratory features	Leukocytosis with shift to left, high ESR, elevations of liver enzymes (and occasionally bilirubin), sterile pyuria, cerbrospinal fluid pleocytosis EKG and 2-D echocardiographic abnormalities Hydrops of gallbladder on ultrasound study Thrombocytosis in the convalescent period**

*Definite diagnosis requires manifestations in five of these six categories in the absence of evidence implicating other well-known diseases. Number in parenthesis indicates percent of diagnosed cases with these manifestations.[11] **KD accounts for only 2% of all cases of thrombocytosis, >900,000 in childhood.[22]

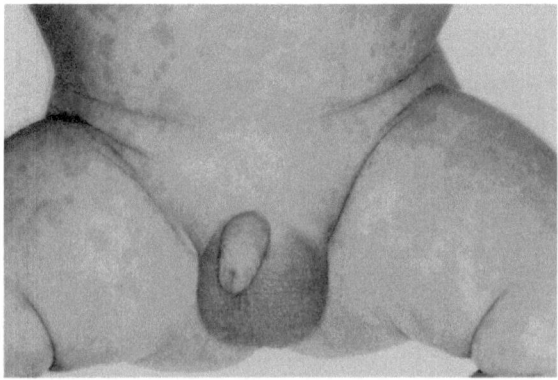

Figure 7.2. Polymorphous rash of KD with diffuse hyperemia in the genital area. (Courtesy of Dr. Kawasaki.)

a polymorphous rash appears all over the body (Fig. 7.2). The ocular conjunctivae become suffused with hyperemic vessels (Fig. 7.3); sometimes aneurysms are grossly visible in these vessels. The oral mucosa and lips are red and the tongue "strawberry"; the lips fissure. Striking indurative edema appears on the dorsums of the hands and feet (Fig. 7.4); the palms and soles become strikingly red, often with a sharp line of color demarcation at the wrists and ankles. Similar redness may be seen about the genitalia; the perineal rash is a useful diagnostic feature.[8] During the recovery period, desquamation occurs in the areas that were previously reddened. The desquamation often begins under the finger- or toenails producing a distinctive appearance (Fig. 7.5).[9–14] In severe cases, transverse grooves or furrows (Beau's lines) are seen in the fingernails 1–2 months after the illness.[15]

Not every patient has every feature, and there is variability in the persistence of each clinical manifestation (Fig. 7.6). Lymphadenopathy may be present only for a day or 2, and the rash on the palms and soles may be disappearing by the time one sees the patient. Physicians who have seen a prior case tend to suspect the diagnosis promptly. Initial reluctance to make the

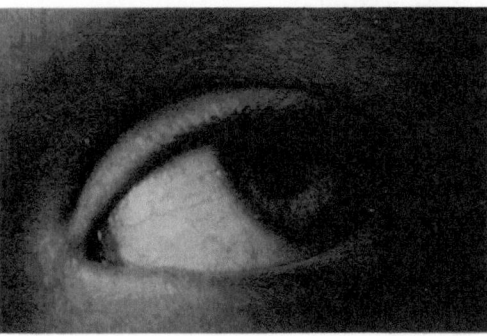

Figure 7.3. Hyperemia of the ocular conjunctiva in KD; aneurysmal dilation of some vessels was grossly visible in this patient and can be seen with magnification in this photograph.

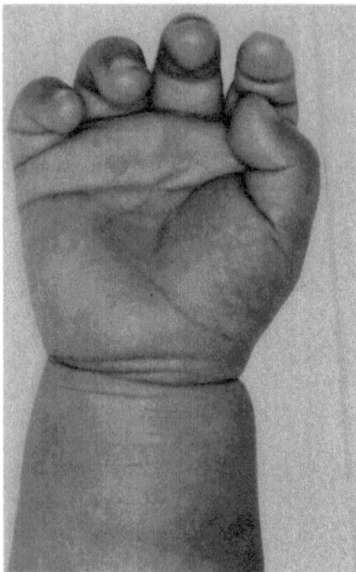

Figure 7.4. Swelling of the hand with erythema of the palm in KD. (Courtesy of Dr. Kawasaki.)

diagnosis seemed to result from a general feeling among American physicians that the disease was Japanese, exotic, rare, inevitably fatal, and couldn't appear unexpectedly "out of the blue" in their office. Physicians who had more experience with measles, infectious mononucleosis, scarlet fever, Rocky Mountain spotted fever (tick typhus), yersinosis,[16] and leptospirosis tended to think first of those diagnoses. The clinical syndrome can resemble all of these disorders, but in the young infant, KD should be the presumptive diagnosis (Table 7.6). Despite some overlapping features, distinction from these disorders and from toxic shock syndrome, drug eruptions,[17] Stevens-

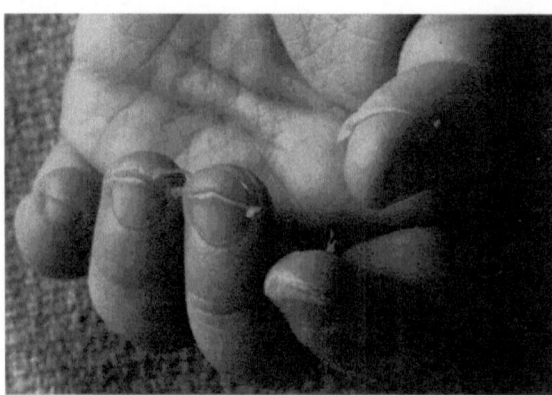

Figure 7.5. Typical desquamation seen during the second week of KD. Although desquamation may occur wherever there was antecedent rash, the pieces of peel protruding from under and around the finger- and toenails is quite specific for KD.

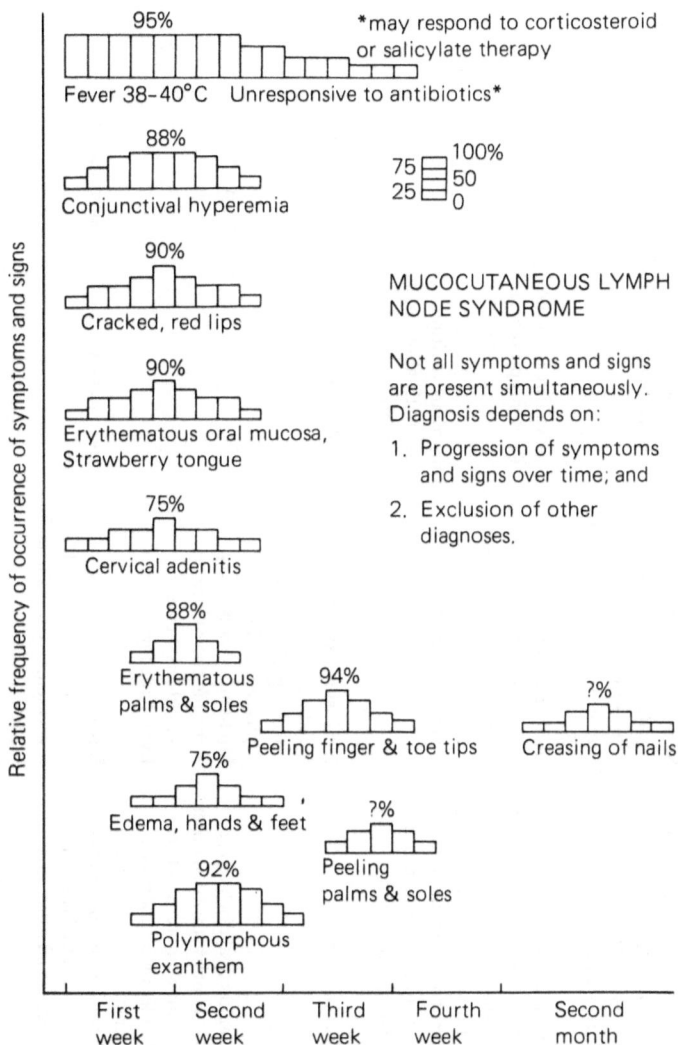

Figure 7.6. Clinical manifestations of KD. (Reprinted with permission from Yanagihara R., Todd J.K.: "Muco-Cutaneous Lymph Node Syndrome." *Am J Dis Child* 134:603–614, 1980; copyright 1980, American Medical Association.) (Percentages from Kawasaki, ref. 11.)

Johnson syndrome, JRA, Reiter's syndrome, toxoplasmosis, and acrodynia is generally not difficult. Diagnostic difficulty primarily results from inexperience and a general physician attitude of skepticism and disbelief. KD is considerably more frequent than most of the disorders in the differential diagnostic list, especially in infancy!

Laboratory Studies. The most useful test has been an ESR, which is often greatly elevated and helps to distinguish this disorder in its early stages from

Table 7.6.   Differential Diagnosis of Exanthems and Mucocutaneous Syndromes That May Be Confused with Kawasaki Disease

			Laboratory Aids	
	Different Characteristics	Absent Findings	Immediate	Late
Erythema multiforme	Rare in infants; conjunctival discharge, aphthouslike mouth ulcers; bullous and iris skin lesions	Significant lymphadenopathy; swelling of the hands and feet; diffuse redness of the hands and feet	Occasional hypocomplementemia	
Scarlet fever	Scarlatiniform rash with Pastia's lines and circumoral pallor; streptococcal sore throat; rare in infants	Conjunctival hyperemia; lip fissures; swelling and redness of the hands and feet	Positive throat culture for β-streptococcus	Rising Ab titers
Toxic shock syndrome	Rapid onset; erythroderma; confusion; shock; rare in young children	Lymphadenopathy	Immediate multiple dramatic abnormalities (see Tables 7.5 and 7.11)	
Leptospirosis	Rare in infants	Lip fissures; swelling and redness of the hands and feet; significant lymphadenopathy	F-A of urine	Agglutination
Reiter's syndrome	Conjunctival discharge; severe polyarthritis at onset; evanescent rash or keratoderma blennorrhagicum; very rare in infants	Lip fissures; strawberry tongue and diffuse mouth erythema; Lymphadenopathy		HLA-B27
Rocky Mountain spotted fever and other tick typhus fevers	Tick exposure, older children; spotted rash on palms and soles; stupor	Lip fissures; strawberry tongue; diffuse mouth erythema, lymphadenopathy	Hyponatremia	Agglutination
Measles	Profuse conjunctival and nasal discharge; cough; Koplik spots; fever precedes rash by 5 days	Lip fissures; swelling and redness of the hands and feet	Leukopenia; low ESR	

the various "viral" illnesses the child is thought to have. Considerable leukocytosis is frequently found (15,000–46,000 in 82% of cases) with a left shift, also suggesting that the child does not have a "simple" viral illness. Central-nervous-system pleocytosis, usually fewer than 50 cells, sometimes with a predominance of polys and sterile pyuria (56%) are also frequently present early in the disease. Elevation of serum transaminases, which tends to disappear in a few days, is also a common early laboratory abnormality. The platelet count is usually normal during the acute phase. However, thrombocytosis is frequent during the recovery phase, and the platelet count in untreated patients may exceed 1 million per millimeter.

Diagnosis. Kawasaki has proposed that patients fulfill five of six criteria, as shown in Table 7.5.[11]

For purposes of gathering data in a uniform manner, physicians have agreed to report as definite cases only patients fulfilling these diagnostic criteria. However, as in all other rheumatic diseases, there are affected individuals who do not fulfill these criteria and who have this illness. They are also at risk of long-term complications from KD.[18–20] Patients with incomplete forms should be identified and treated as KD.[21]

Often, the examiner who does not consider the diagnosis fails to note the presence of some of the typical findings that would enable him to make the diagnosis. Earlier diagnosis can be achieved by a raised awareness that a child seen with fever and ocular hyperemia or lymphadenopathy may have KD or that the diagnosis should be considered in all children with polymorphous rashes. For example, an infant seen in our clinic for unexplained fever was noted to have ocular conjunctival hyperemia without other signs of KD. Because of this, an ESR was obtained and found to be 98 mm/h. The baby was admitted to the hospital and watched overnight as the other diagnostic features of KD became apparent. Treatment was instituted 12h after admission. This experience indicates how greatly heightened diagnostic awareness can facilitate both early diagnosis and consideration of this diagnosis in patients with only some of the clinical features of KD. Diagnosis is especially difficult in tiny infants who are at highest risk of death.[23]

In some cases, using these diagnostic criteria, the diagnosis can only be firmly established during the convalescent period, when typical finger desquamation is observed; this applies especially to patients who do not have other extremity changes during the acute period. It is important, therefore, to advise parents of those children to look for the peeling of the fingers and toes and to advise the physician of its occurrence.

Immunopathology. Histologic examination of the affected ateries in KD reveals a panarteritis.[24–34] At first, the microvessels (arterioles, capillaries, and venules) are affected, but within a few days, small and medium-sized arteries and the main coronary arteries are involved. Although the skin, mucous membranes, and heart are most frequently affected, arteries everywhere may

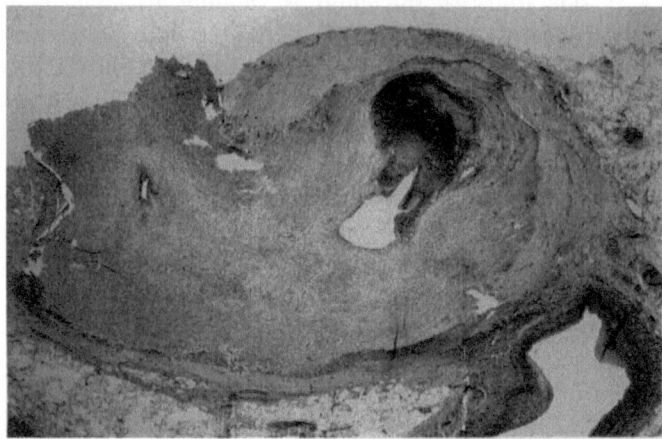

Figure 7.7. Tortuous coronary artery with old and recent thrombosis of an aneurysmal portion. ×22.

have lesions that can result in occlusive or ischemic manifestations, either during the acute phase or at some time later in life.[25]

The origin of the initial angiitis is in the perivascular area. Mononuclear cells predominate and relatively few polymorphs are seen. The inflammation rapidly progresses into the media and intima of the vessels, where palisading may resemble a rheumatoid nodule. Fibrinoid is not prominent but may be seen in the intima and in the internal and external elastic membranes. Severe necrosis of the vessel wall may be associated with aneurysmal dilatation. Acute thrombosis may occur, and in some cases old thrombi are also seen with recanalization (Fig. 7.7).[35]

Superficial large and medium-sized coronary arteries are most affected with relative sparing of small epicardial and myocardial arteries. The aorta is mildly inflamed with intimal thickening; branching medium-sized vessels are often more severely affected. Parenchymal vessels are less severely affected, and infarcts of organs are rare. The vasculitis is not limited to the arterial lesions and is frequently also seen in veins.

Arteritis of the main coronary arteries may lead to myocardial ischemia; intramyocardial small-vessel arteritis may result in focal myocardial necrosis. Thrombosis, stenosis, and rupture of vessels all occur. Invasion of the myocardium and pericardium by inflammatory cells from the periarteritis results in myocarditis and pericarditis. Endomyocardial biopsies performed in 201 Japanese children as research procedures are reported to have shown evidence of myocarditis in all patients.[30] Platelet thrombi occur during the convalescent period. Lesions in all stages of development may be seen in autopsy material.

Lymph nodes biopsied at the beginning of the disease or examined later at

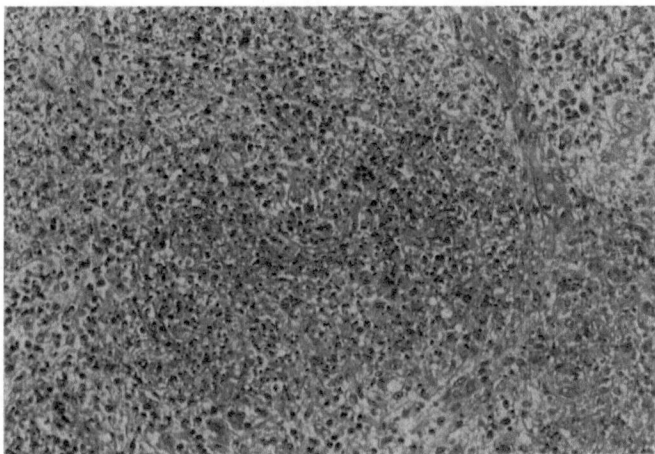

Figure 7.8. Lymph-node biopsy specimen obtained early in the course of KD showing obliteration of the nodal architecture and acute necrotizing and chronic arteritis.

the time of autopsy have generally been reported to show "nonspecific lymphadenitis."[25] However, acute necrotizing obliteration of the nodal architecture with severe fragmentation and acute and chronic arteritis with small foci of fibrinoid material containing nuclear debris have been reported in one case and demonstrated in one of our patients in whom, prior to diagnosis, biopsy was obtained during the acute phase of the illness (Fig. 7.8).[36] These findings resemble those usually found in cat-scratch disease.

Where pathologic material has been obtained in patients with hydrops of the gallbladder, inflammation about the blood vessels of the cystic duct and in the muscularis and serosa of the gallbladder was seen. The inflammatory reaction showed a marked polymorphous infiltrate, including granulocytes, lymphocytes, and eosinophils.

In a review of 20 hearts obtained at autopsy from Japanese children with KD, Fujiwara described differing pathologic findings in children who died at different stages of diseases (Fig. 7.9).[27] Characteristic features of stage I (0–9 days) were acute perivasculitis and vasculitis of microvessels (arterioles, venules, and capillaries), including the three major coronary arteries. Stage II (12–25 days) had similar findings plus the appearance of coronary artery aneurysms, thrombi, stenosis, and obstruction. In children who died during this period, many stages of vasculitis were apparent in each child. These included exudative edema, infiltration, necrosis, granulation, and rupture of aneurysms. These varying lesions were not seen in those who died during the convalescent period (28–31 days). At that stage (III), there was partial or total obliteration of the major coronary arteries due to granulating thrombi; myocarditis and pericarditis were less frequent; and angiitis had disappeared. Deaths during stage IV (40 days to 4 years) were due to cardiac

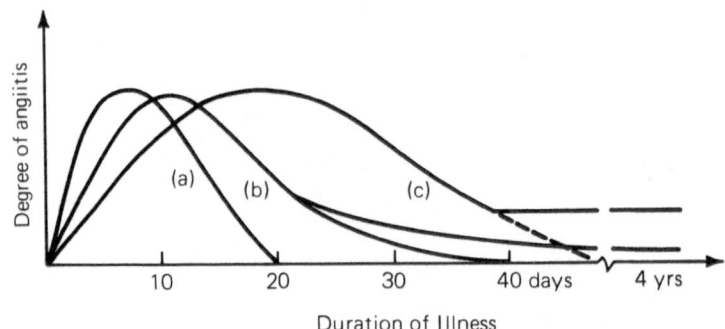

Figure 7.9. Process of angiitis classified by the size of vessels in KD. (a) Microvessels (arterioles, capillaries, and venules). (b) Small arteries. (c) Main coronary arteries. (Reprinted with permission from Fujiwara and Hamashima, ref. 27.)

ischemia associated with scars and calcification of the main coronary arteries. Fibrosis of the myocardium and endocardial fibroelastosis were common. Endocarditis of mitral and tricuspid valves was seen in 20% of the autopsy material. Inflammatory cell infiltrates were seen in the AV node of all patients in whom they were looked for and were sometimes noted in the His bundle and bundle branches.

It is generally agreed that most cases previously reported as infantile periarteritis nodosa had KD.[25-29] Thus, KD is not a new pathologic entity, although the disease does seem to be increasing in frequency throughout the world.

The closest naturally acquired animal model of KD is *equine viral arteritis*. An epidemic occurred in Ohio in 1956. Affected animals had sudden onset of high fever, intense red discoloration of the conjunctivae, edematous swelling of the limbs, arthritis, and enteritis. Most of the animals recovered; a few animals died. In fatal cases, necrotizing arteritis was demonstrated throughout the body; in survivors, the arteritis healed, leaving few scars.[37] Direct invasion of vessel walls by virus is thought to be the pathogenic mechanism of the vasculitis in equine arteritis and may also be involved in the pathogenesis of KD. A mouse model may be created by intraperitoneal injection of nonviable lactobacillus casei cell-wall fragments.[38]

The occurrence of KD after what appears to be a viral prodrome suggests that hypersensitivity or disordered immunologic reactivity may also play a role in the pathogenesis of KD. Elevation of immune globulins, including IgE, does occur. However, circulating immune complexes have only rarely been reported in KD, and we have been unable to demonstrate hypocomplementemia or rheumatoid factors.

In addition to direct invasion of vessel walls and myocardium by virus and hypersensitivity, other theoretical mechanisms of vascular injury that could account for this syndrome include cell-mediated immune hyperreac-

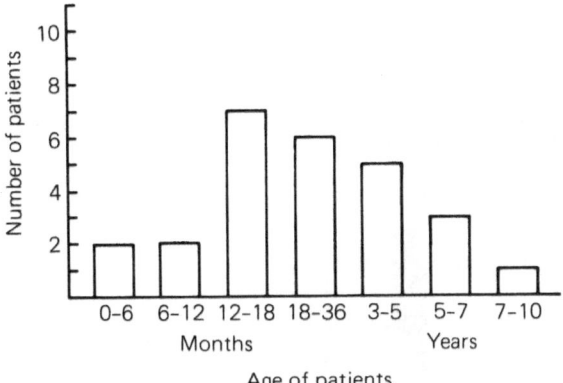

Figure 7.10. Relative frequency of KD at various ages. (Reprinted with permission from Jacobs, ref. 44.)

tivity, production of cross-reacting antibodies that react with blood-vessel walls, and antibody-mediated cellular cytotoxicity against vessel-wall constituents.[39]

Epidemiology. The great frequency of the disease in Japan has suggested genetic susceptibility factors; Hawaiians of Japanese ancestry are reported to be more susceptible than other Hawaiians, and there seems to be an increased incidence among Japanese in the continental United States. The reasons for the apparently greatly increased susceptibility of Japanese remains obscure. Studies of HLA-A and -B types in KD have not resolved the mystery, although they did reveal some increase in HLA-Bw22 antigen, and especially HLA-B22J2, in Japanese patients and in HLA-Bw51 in white patients.[40,41]

Infants age 12–18 months are most susceptible to KD, although the disease may be seen at any age (Fig. 7.10). However, the illness is infrequent in adults, and 80% of patients are under 4 years old. One "congenital" case with symptoms noted at age 3 days has been reported. About 9% of Japanese siblings under age 2 years will develop KD; more than half of these second cases in a family occur within 10 days of the first case.[42] The disease may recur in 4% of cases.

Males are slightly more frequently affected. Poor children are thought to be less susceptible.[43] In our population, all races are affected; there were 15 blacks, 22 whites, 8 with Hispanic surnames, and 4 Orientals among 49 cases.[44] Forty of these cases occurred between October 1, 1977, and April 30, 1978, and were selected for further study with epidemiologists from the U.S. Public Health Service Centers for Disease Control. This study confirmed our report of an epidemic of KD in New York and New Jersey in 1977 (Fig. 7.11). Twenty-six cases occurred in the 3-month period October 1, 1977, to December 31, 1977 (the "epidemic period"). The five counties immediately

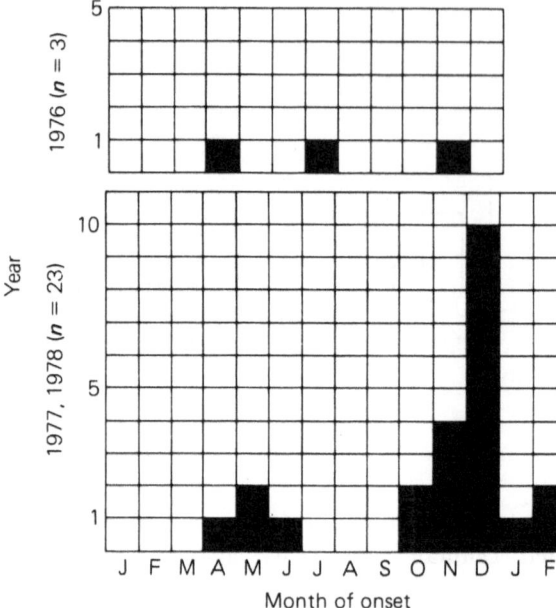

Figure 7.11. Seasonal incidence of KD in New York City. This pattern has continued to be observed throughout the Northern Hemisphere. (Reprinted with permission from Jacobs, ref. 44.)

north and west of Manhattan had a significantly increased incidence of the disease when compared to the incidence in the rest of New York State and New Jersey during the epidemic period or to the incidence in these five counties during the nonepidemic period. The attack rate during the 3-month epidemic period in these five counties was 5 in 100,000 children under age 5 years; in one county, the attack rate was 17 in 100,000 children under age 5 (Fig. 7.12). Affected children were demonstrated to have a significantly increased incidence of mild antecedent respiratory illness when compared to a control population. Many similar outbreaks have since been reported. A history of antecedent respiratory illness was also observed in other outbreaks, but this finding is not consistent and no particular organism could be demonstrated to be etiologically related to KD.[43] Exposure to rug shampoo or residence near a body of water have also been inconsistently noted.[43,45–49]

Manifestations and Course of the Disease. The severity of disease varies from outbreak to outbreak, accounting for different incidences of various manifestations and their severity in different reports. A scoring system has been devised by Asai as an aid to assessing the risk of coronary aneurysms.[50] This system can also be used to compare severity of illness in different groups of patients (Table 7.7).

As might be expected in a systemic vasculitis, many organ systems may be affected. In our experience, essentially all patients have some clinical evidence of cardiac involvement, with tachycardia out of proportion to fever the

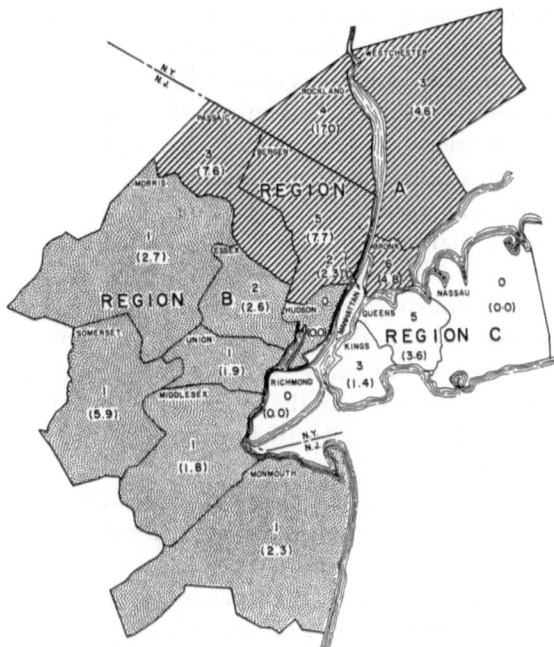

Figure 7.12. KD cases and attack rates (cases per 100,000 population <5 years old) in New York City and vicinity, October 1, 1977–April 30, 1978. The number in parentheses in each county represents the attack rate. (From Anderson et al., unpublished CDC data cited in Bell et al., ref. 49.)

Table 7.7. ASAI Scoring Chart for Assessing Risk of Coronary Changes from Clinical Data[50]

	2 Points	*1 Point*	*0 Point*
Sex		Male	Female
Age		Under 1 yr	Over 1 yr
Duration of fever	16 days+	14–15 days	−14 days
Double-peaked fever	Yes		No
Double-peaked eruption		Yes	No
Hemoglobin < 10 grams		Yes	No
WBC (max)	30,000+	26,000–30,000	−26,000
ESR (max)	Over 100	60–100	−60
CRP/ESR—return to normal	Over 30 days		Under 30 days
Double-peaked ESR/CRP	Yes		No
Cardiomegaly		Yes	No
Arrhythmia		Yes	No
Increased Q (II,III,AVr)	Yes		No
Infarctlike symptoms	Yes		No
Reappearance of the disease		Yes	No

Note: Nakano et al. report the level of CRP to be the best predictor of risk at 4–7 days after onset of illness.[52]

most minimal manifestation. Minor abnormalities of the electrocardiogram are usually seen and probably reflect the myocarditis demonstrable pathologically in all cases.[30,51] Congestive heart failure occurred in 20% of our epidemic patients and in 13% of cases seen in an epidemic in Boston.[53] Sudden cardiac arrhythmia or complications of uncontrolled tamponade and cardiac failure may result in death during the acute phase of the illness. Arrhythmia may occur in children who are thought to be doing well. Later deaths are usually a result of myocardial infarction.

Anemia is common and may contribute to congestive heart failure. In our epidemic evidence of hemolysis was frequently found. The hemolysis was due to a variety of antibodies, most frequently IgG anti-I during the epidemic, but in endemic cases anemia may most commonly be due to cellular fragmentation in which erythrocytes are disrupted as they pass over abnormal surfaces.[54,55] Thrombocytosis is seen in almost all patients during the recovery period; a very few children have developed thrombopenia.[56,57]

Striking hepatomegaly may occur. In some cases, this is associated with hydrops of the gallbladder.[58] Mild jaundice and chemical evidence of hepatitis are frequent during the first week of disease.[58a] Diarrhea is common during the first 2 weeks of disease. Adynamic ileus was an unusual gastrointestinal manifestation during our mini-epidemic in 1977 but is rarely seen in sporadic cases.[59] Intestinal obstruction and ischemic vasculitis with perforation may occur.[60,61] We have seen a patient in whom the diagnosis of KD was first suggested by the finding of mesenteric vasculitis and a perforation in the small intestine. Pancreatitis occurs occasionally.[62]

Arthritis is a very frequent manifestation either as part of the early course of disease when it may be overshadowed by the other features or as a late manifestation in the third week of disease. The early arthritis is mainly in the fingers; knees are the most commonly affected large joints and, together with the ankles, are the joints most frequently affected in the late-onset group. Avascular necrosis of the hip occurred in a 20-month-old child.[63]

Aseptic meningitis is frequently demonstrated if lumbar puncture is performed. Children with KD are very irritable, and parents report great improvement in this CNS manifestation during the recovery period. Facial palsy, hemiplegic stroke, encephalopathy, and sensineural hearing loss occur occasionally.[64] Autopsy series have not provided details of the examination of the CNS. In our only fatality, the CNS was carefully examined and was normal, without evidence of cerebral vasculitis. We are aware of a death associated with contrast-enhanced CT scan; this procedure should be avoided if possible.[65]

Patients may present with uvulitis and supraglottitis.[65a] Cough is usually not prominent but was very prominent during our 1977 epidemic and was associated in 23% of that series of patients with radiographically demonstrable pulmonary infiltrates and atelectasis, not a previously noted feature of KD. Hilar and paratracheal lymphadenopathy is occasionally seen radiographically (Fig. 7.13).

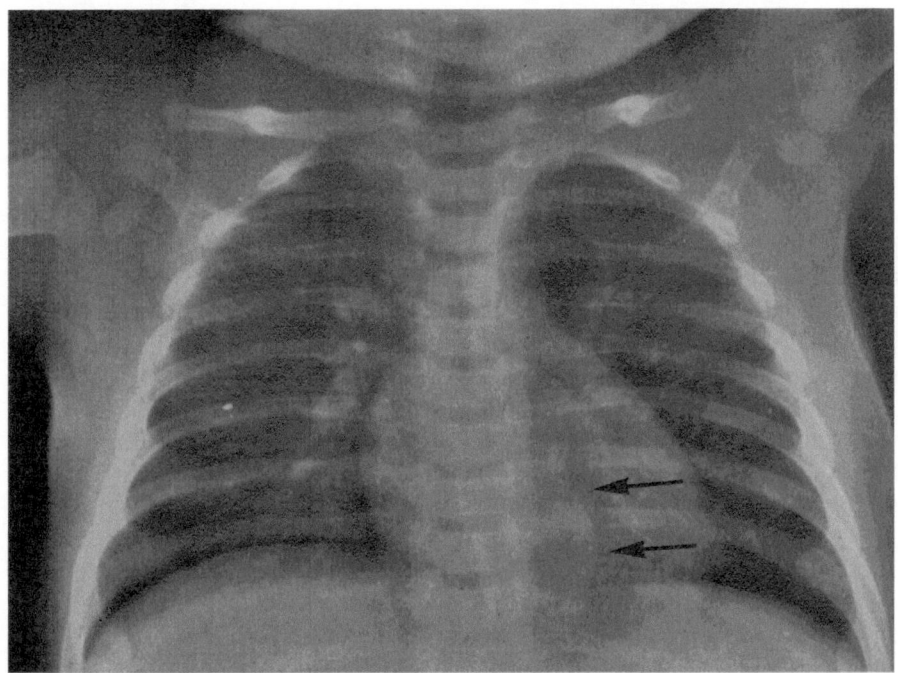

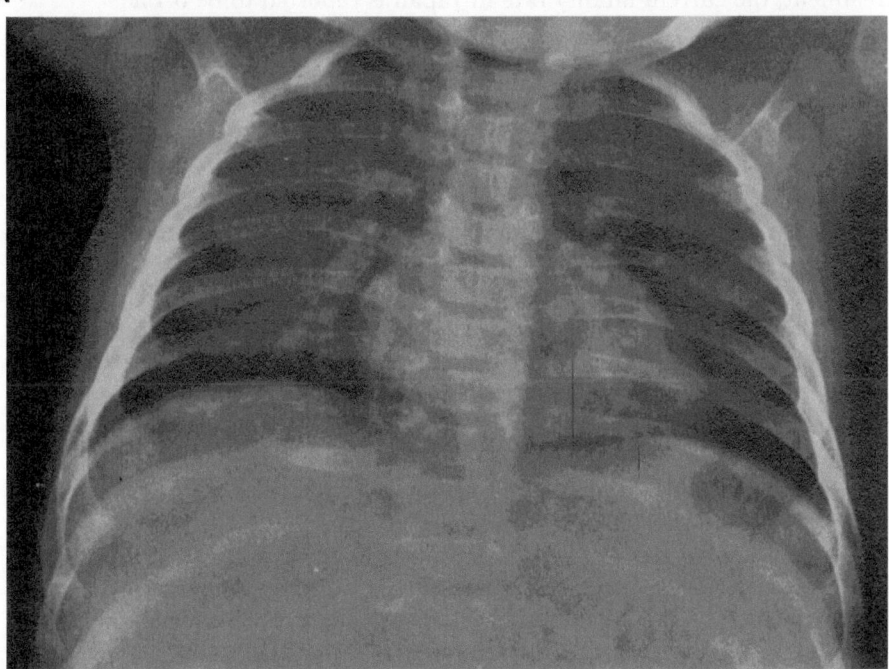

Figure 7.13. (**A**) Large hilar adenopathy *(arrows)* seen in a 2½-month-old baby with KD: patient was referred with a diagnosis of mediastinal tumor, and the other manifestations of KD became apparent only after admission. (**B**) Normal chest film 10 days later.

Urethral discomfort is reported by older children. Sterile pyuria is demonstrable in 53% of patients, and mild transient proteinuria is common. Priapism may occur.[66] Although autopsy series have shown renal-artery stenosis to be a common finding in fatal KD, hypertension is not seen in KD. However, it is possible that some older children who present with hypertension and renal-artery stenosis have had unrecognized KD earlier in life.

Mild anterior uveitis was noted in one of our patients with KD; she was positive for HLA-B27. Several other patients with KD have been noted to have mild uveitis during the acute illness; HLA typing on some of these patients showed an association with DR5.[67-69] Severe peripheral ischemia with threat of digital or distal-extremity gangrene may occur; loss of digits may be prevented by infusing prostaglandin E_1.[31]

Without treatment, fever and other symptoms may continue for several weeks and arthritis may even appear as the patient seems to be improving. Sometimes a recrudescence of symptoms and fever occurs after the patient seemed to be recovering; arthritis may also first appear during this "second hump" of the illness. After a variable period of time, the symptoms gradually subside, and the child recovers, even without treatment. Second attacks of KD may occur in up to 5% of patients. Death is rare even in untreated and severely ill patients. The initial reports included 1–2% deaths in Japan but the death rate has been higher in the United States (2.8%). With aspirin treatment, the current fatality rate in Japan is reported to be 0.1%.[6]

Treatment

Management of the Acute Phase. *Gamma globulin:* Furusho et al.[70] first demonstrated that dilatations of the coronary arteries (defined as a diameter greater than 3 mm) were less frequent in patients treated by the 10th day of illness with intravenous gamma globulin and oral aspirin than with conventional doses of aspirin alone. (No study of gamma globulin alone has been performed.) These findings were eloquently confirmed in a multicenter study in the United States in which the incidence of coronary artery abnormalities was reduced from 7.7% to 3.8% at 8 weeks after onset,[71] even though there was no better effect on ESR, platelet count, platelet activation, acute-phase reactants, AT-III, or fibrinolytic activity.[72] A dose of 400 mg/kg/day for 4 days was required; preliminary data suggested that a single does of 1 gram/kg of gamma globulin infused over 4 h may be well tolerated, equally effective, and result in shorter hospitalization.[73] The current "approved" regimen is 2 grams/kg over 8 h.[74-76] Although gamma-globulin treatment does not totally prevent aneurysms even if promptly administered together with high-dose aspirin, several small studies suggest that the frequency of giant aneurysms (>8 mm) is greatly reduced by gamma-globulin treatment.[77] Most important sequelae of KD aneurysms are in patients with giant aneurysms; therefore, all children with KD should be treated with gamma globulin as well as aspirin.[78] The efficacy of gamma-globulin therapy initi-

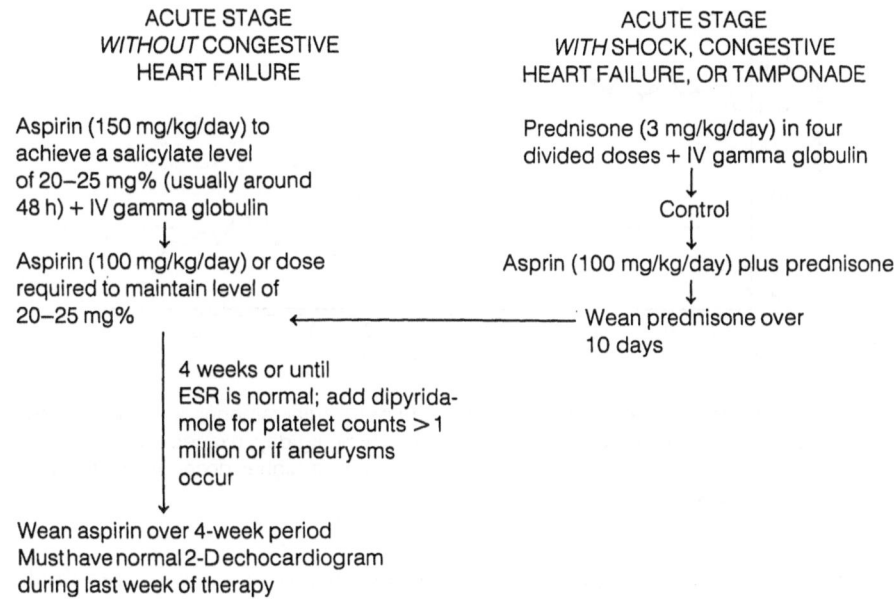

ACUTE STAGE
WITHOUT CONGESTIVE
HEART FAILURE

Aspirin (150 mg/kg/day) to
achieve a salicylate level
of 20–25 mg% (usually around
48 h) + IV gamma globulin
↓
Aspirin (100 mg/kg/day) or dose
required to maintain level of
20–25 mg%

ACUTE STAGE
WITH SHOCK, CONGESTIVE
HEART FAILURE, OR TAMPONADE

Prednisone (3 mg/kg/day) in four
divided doses + IV gamma globulin
↓
Control
↓
Asprin (100 mg/kg/day) plus prednisone
↓
Wean prednisone over
10 days

4 weeks or until
ESR is normal; add dipyridamole for platelet counts > 1
million or if aneurysms
occur
↓
Wean aspirin over 4-week period
Must have normal 2-D echocardiogram
during last week of therapy

CHRONIC STAGE

If ESR or platelet count remains elevated
or coronary aneurysms persist, maintain
aspirin at 30 mg/kg/day (with
dipyridamole for aneurysms)

Figure 7.14. Treatment module for management of KD.

ated after the 10th day of illness or after the coronary arteries have already dilated to a size greater than 3 mm has not been established;[74,75] at the time of this writing we do not generally offer gamma-globulin therapy after the 10th day of illness but we do give it to all children with KD of shorter duration, even if there is coronary artery dilatation.[79]

Gamma globulin may induce anaphylactic reactions, especially in patients with IgA deficiency,[80] and possibly aseptic meningitis[81] and serum sickness with hemolysis and DIC.[81a] The production process, if carried out properly, inactivates all viruses.[82] Gamma-globulin preparations may not all be equally efficacious.[74]

Corticosteroids: Most KD deaths are now a result of acute myocarditis.[82a] Most authors agree that life-threatening myocarditis and/or pericarditis should be treated with prednisone (Fig. 7.14).[83] Oral doses as high as 3 mg/kg/day have been required for control of cardiac symptoms (Fig. 7.15).[44] When corticosteroids must be used, there is evidence that coincident administration of aspirin is associated with a reduced incidence of coronary-artery

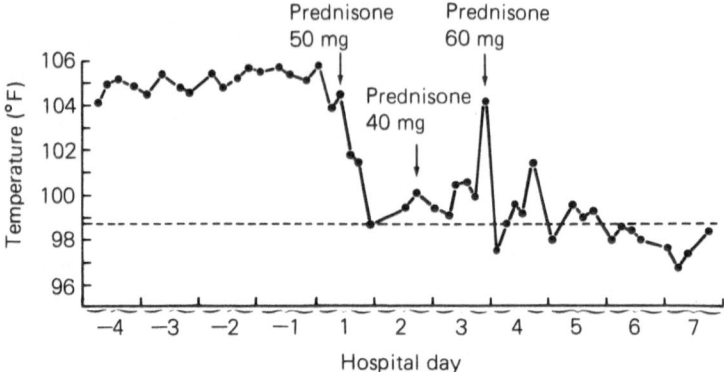

Figure 7.15. Response of a 16-kg boy with KD and pericardial tamponade to prednisone. All symptoms were promptly controlled with a dose of 3 mg/kg/day, exacerbated on reduction to 2 mg/kg/day, and were controlled again by giving a higher dose. (Reprinted with permission from Jacobs, ref. 44.)

aneurysms.[84] For this purpose less than 30 mg/kg/day of aspirin is required. A study that showed increased incidence of coronary-artery aneurysms associated with prednisone treatment is hard to interpret since the angiograms were done soon after abrupt withdrawal of prednisone, allowing for recrudescence of disease and perhaps artificial drug-withdrawal-induced aneurysms.[84] In any case, small doses of aspirin seemed to prevent the

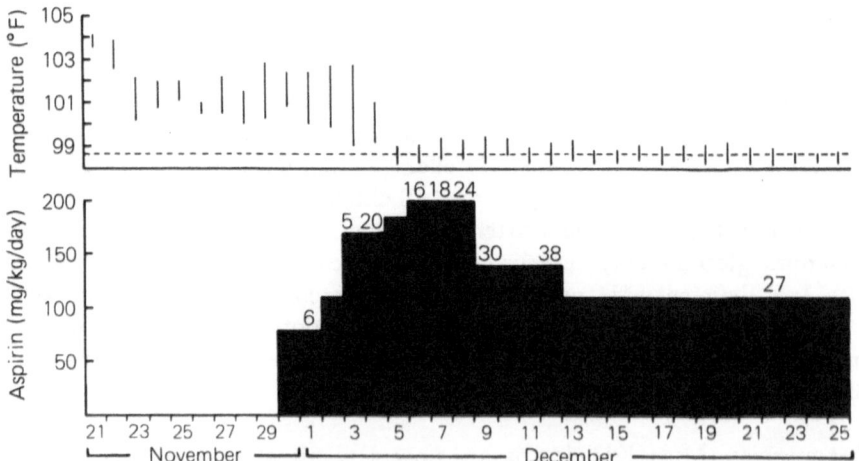

Figure 7.16. Typical response of KD to aspirin, indicating lack of achievement of therapeutic salicylate level (20 mg/dl) until patient received 165 mg/kg/day without buffer and lack of clinical response at lower levels. Numbers at top of bars represent salicylate level in mg/dl on that day. As patient recovered, aspirin dosage had to be reduced to conventional amounts to avoid toxicity. (Reprinted with permission from Jacobs, ref. 44.)

aneurysms and would seem relatively harmless.[84] We have also treated one boy with tamponade with intrapericardial steroids.

Aspirin: Although initially the disease was reported to be unresponsive to aspirin, we were able to demonstrate that the fever and other symptoms respond to adequate salicylate therapy (Fig. 7.16) and that inadequate response is often due to malabsorption of the aspirin (Fig. 7.17).[85-87] As in all other conditions, efficacy of therapy must be determined with monitoring of serum levels. *Prompt control of fever* may be the most important factor in preventing aneurysms.[50,88-90] In our experience, KD is responsive to relatively low serum levels of salicylate (generally 20–25 mg/dl), as contrasted with the systemic form of JRA, which often requires levels around 30 mg/dl but these levels are not achieved quickly with doses of 100 mg/kg/day. At least in part this may be related to decreased protein binding.[91] Our general procedure is to start with unbuffered aspirin, 150 mg/kg/day (maximum 4.5 grams daily) in six divided doses, measure the salicylate level and SGOT/PT each day and obtain a "stat" report of the results, and adjust the dose down to 100 mg/kg/day as soon as an adequate salicylate level is achieved. In clinics in which "stat" salicylate levels and enzyme determinations cannot be obtained, use of such high doses of salicylate would be unsafe. In rare instances, in babies, as much as 200 mg/kg/day has been required initially to achieve a satisfactory level. However, most sporadic cases (as contrasted to our 1977 epidemic) absorb aspirin satisfactorily and achieve therapeutic levels within 24–48 h of the loading dose. High salicylate levels are often not

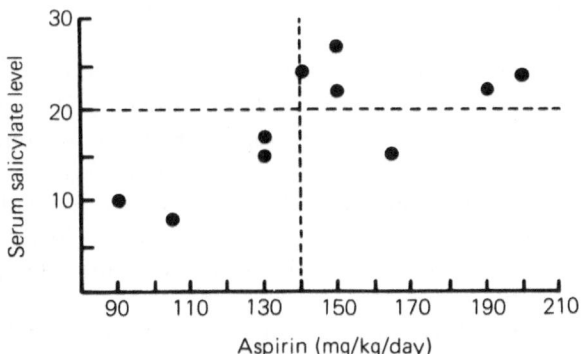

Figure 7.17. Relationship of aspirin dosage (mg/kg/day) to serum salicylate level achieved in 10 patients treated with plain aspirin alone during the acute phase of KD. No patient achieved therapeutic levels (20 mg/dl for this condition) unless given at least 140 mg/kg/day, and two patients of the five who achieved levels of 20 mg/kg/dl or more required a minimum of 190–200 mg/kg/day. These observations were from an epidemic of KD in which salicylate malabsorption was especially frequent. The frequency or extent of salicylate malabsorption in endemic cases or in other epidemics has not been as great as during this particular epidemic. (Reprinted with permission from Jacobs, ref. 44.)

required. For example, in a 45-kg teenager with KD, we started with a dose of 4.5 grams daily and achieved control of symptoms even though the salicylate level was only 15 mg/dl. After 2 weeks, as she recovered more completely and despite weight gain and increased food intake, the salicylate level rose to 27 mg/dl without any increase in dose, indicating that the acute stage had been characterized by malabsorption, which in this instance was of no clinical significance. However, in patients who do malabsorb aspirin during the acute phase, improved absorption and higher levels must be anticipated, and dosage must be adjusted downward during recovery.

Hepatic intolerance to aspirin in seen in some patients. If aspirin cannot be tolerated, newer nonsteroidal anti-inflammatory agents such as naproxen can be used with equally satisfactory results. However, aspirin substitutes that do not have an anticoagulant effect should not be used.

Aside from control of the acute cardiac manifestations threatening immediate death, there is no definite evidence that control of the manifestations with aspirin alters the ultimate prognosis.[92] Nevertheless, it seems likely that control of the manifestations is achieved by reduction of the vasculitis. In other vasculitides, control of the clinical manifestations is associated with improved survival. There seems little reason to take a nihilistic position about this particular vasculitis. Our sole death to date was in an infant, not diagnosed during the first 10 days of illness, who was in shock when we first instituted therapy. We suspect that most early deaths can be prevented by prompt control of the vasculitis and hope that scarring will be avoided or at least reduced. The prevention of late death will be discussed separately below. Our experience with truly high-dose aspirin (prompt achievement of levels >20 mg/dl) and that of Koren[85] suggests that high salicylate levels reduce the incidence of coronary artery lesions in KD.

Management of the Recovery Period. In patients being treated with prednisone, the medication is gradually withdrawn over a 10-day period with replacement, at the time weaning is begun, with aspirin in conventional 100 mg/kg/day dosage. Salicylate levels are monitored, and the dosage is adjusted as necessary. Reduction of prednisone is known to result in increases in serum salicylate levels, and the patient is always closely observed for salicylate toxicity when steroids are reduced in patients taking both aspirin and steroids (see Fig. 3.17).

In patients stabilized with aspirin, after the ESR and platelet count have returned to normal, the aspirin is gradually weaned away over a 4-week period. In some patients, the ESR remains elevated for many months, and small doses of aspirin (8 mg/kg/day) are continued. Our experience with other rheumatic disorders suggests that abrupt withdrawal of medication may produce exacerbations or recrudescences of disease and may be dangerous. Japanese authors suggest that disease with recrudescence may be associated with an increased incidence of coronary artery aneurysms and death (Table 7.7). We have had minor exacerbations in 2–3% of patients during the weaning period. These were controlled by merely increasing the aspirin to the full dose, waiting again until the ESR was normal, and then beginning the 4-week weaning again. This regimen produced control of the disease within 24 h and avoided hospitalization. Some of our milder patients are never hospitalized, and the average length of hospital stay has been reduced to a few days. More frequent outpatient follow-up has been advocated by some authors.

Electrocardiogram, chest radiograph, and two-dimensional echocardiogram are repeated until normal. Two-dimensional echocardiogram is obtained again 1 year later even in asymptomatic patients. Families must be advised of the potential for late cardiac manifestations despite their great rarity. Physicians should be immediately advised of any unusual symptoms, and patients should be promptly evaluated for signs of myocardial ischemia if symptoms appear.[36] Intracoronary or intravenous injection of streptokinase may relieve acute coronary occlusion if it occurs.[93,94]

Studies Aimed at Preventing Late Complications of KD. Twenty percent of an unselected series of children with acute KD subjected to coronary angiography are reported to have abnormalities, usually coronary-artery aneurysms. Where follow-up studies were performed, most of the aneurysms had disappeared spontaneously. Almost all of the children with aneurysms during the acute phase recovered completely and had no further difficulty.[36,95-98] In the absence of persistent symptoms of cardiac disease or persistent electro- or echocardiographic abnormalities, the risk of performing coronary angiograms on all survivors of KD would seem to exceed the potential benefits.[99] Cross-sectional echocardiography is a noninvasive technique that has the potential to reliably demonstrate aneurysms if present and not give false-positive results.[49,99-104] Almost all of the late fatalities in KD have been from inflow or outflow stenosis in large aneurysms of the main coronary arteries, almost always within 10 mm of the coronary ostium.[105-108] Obstruction of the left main and combinations of left anterior descending and right coronary artery obstruction create the worst risk of myocardial infarction.[107] These proximal lesions can be visualized, although lesions farther along the coronary arteries could not be expected to be revealed with two-dimensional echocardiograms. The procedure is without risk. Together with new tests for myocardial ischemia, it holds the greatest promise for monitoring of patients. Aneurysms shown on two-dimensional echocardiogram can be confirmed on coronary arteriography,[109] MRI,[110] or positron emission tomography,[111] but angiography is becoming obsolete. Myocardial ischemia can be documented with stress thallium scanning, and a decision can be made about coronary bypass procedures.[112] If bypass is decided upon, it should be carried out promptly since one child is reported to have died while awaiting scheduled surgery[36] and myocardial infarction may occur in asymptomatic individuals.[113,114] However, the presence of coronary-artery aneurysms within 6 months of KD does not necessarily imply a poor prognosis. Many

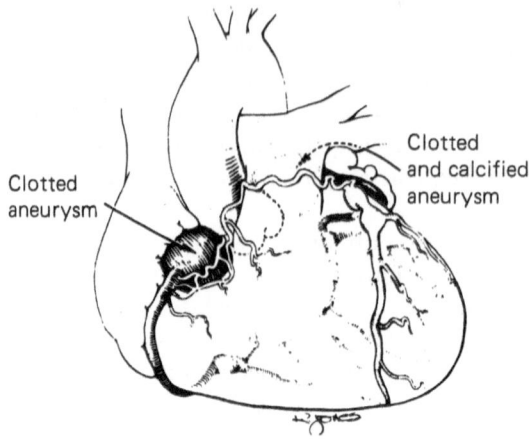

Figure 7.18. Drawing illustrating the coronary artery lesions found at angiogram in a 9-year-old girl. The patient first developed exercise-induced substernal chest pain 3 years after unrecognized KD; the pain was considered "psychological" until an electrocardiogram was obtained during an episode and showed transient ST-segment depression. Cardiac bypass procedures were successful. (Reprinted with permission from Sandiford et al., ref. 118.)

aneurysms present within 6 months of the acute process will disappear.[95–98] The persistence of aneurysms more than 6 months after onset of disease is of special concern, but studies suggest that most asymptomatic aneurysms persisting for many years may ultimately disappear without therapy.[114] Management of patients with symptomatic narrowing of the coronary vessels depends on weighing the risks of surgery and its potential efficacy against the risks of the individual lesion demonstrated.[115–117] Successful coronary-artery bypass has been achieved in symptomatic survivors (Fig. 7.18).[118–121] However, not all coronary lesions that occur as residua of KD are amenable to surgery (Fig. 7.19).[113]

So long as coronary aneurysms are demonstrable or the platelet count or the ESR remains elevated, we continue aspirin therapy. Tiny doses (as little as 8 mg/kg/day) may be sufficient as an anticoagulant; aspirin is administered in this situation for the theoretical benefits of anticoagulation in the presence of coronary aneurysms. We also give dipyridamole 3–5 mg/kg/day.[83,121] While this seems a reasonable approach, it is not of proven value.

Although KD is generally a self-limited syndrome, some late-occurring coronary aneurysms have been observed[28,30,36,118] and unexpected cardiac sequelae including mitral, tricuspid, and aortic regurgitation have been reported in 5% of patients.[114,122,123] While this greatly exceeds the sequelae so far seen in our patients in New York, there seems little harm in doing two-dimensional echocardiograms or stress-thalium tests at infrequent intervals in KD patients as adults, until the late risk is better defined. It is possible that all children with KD sustain some injury to their coronary arteries

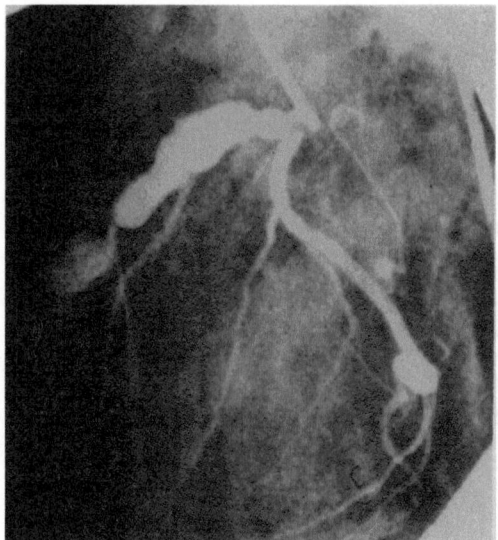

Figure 7.19. Coronary artery angiogram performed in a 15-year-old boy who had undiagnosed KD 4 years earlier and hemobilia secondary to hepatic artery aneurysm rupture 1 year earlier. Patient had no cardiac symptoms at the time of the study, but during the following year had three myocardial infarctions. These diffuse coronary-artery aneurysms have been described only in KD; because they are so diffuse, they are not surgically correctable. (Reprinted with permission from Lipson et al., ref. 113.)

which might predispose them to premature coronary artherosclerosis as adults.[124] One could advocate making a special effort to achieve a healthy diet with monitoring of low-density lipoproteins, and a healthy life-style with exercise and without smoking in this population, whose members could be at a higher risk. At the same time, a conscientious effort must be made to avoid creating psychological cardiac invalidism in children who have had KD.

Extracardiac Sequelae. Coronary-artery stenosis or aneurysms are not the only possible late sequelae of KD (Fig. 7.20).[35] Lipson et al. described a boy with a hepatic artery aneurysm presenting with massive GI bleeding (hemobilia) 3 years after unrecognized KD.[113] Only a proper interpretive history enabled the authors to recognize and report the relationship between the previous mysterious illness and the presence of the new and, at first, seemingly unrelated problem. We wonder whether some children with isolated renal or cerebral artery aneurysm or stenosis, and idiopathic cardiomyopathy, may also represent survivors of previously undiagnosed KD.[30] The full spectrum of KD remains to be determined. At the same time, it is important to reassure families that the natural history of KD is 95–99% total recovery without sequelae.

Polyarteritis Nodosa

We reserve the term *polyarteritis nodosa* (PAN) for a syndrome of necrotizing vasculitis of small and medium-sized muscular arteries in the absence of obvious allergy, significant eosinophilia, or pulmonary lesions (Table 7.4).[1]

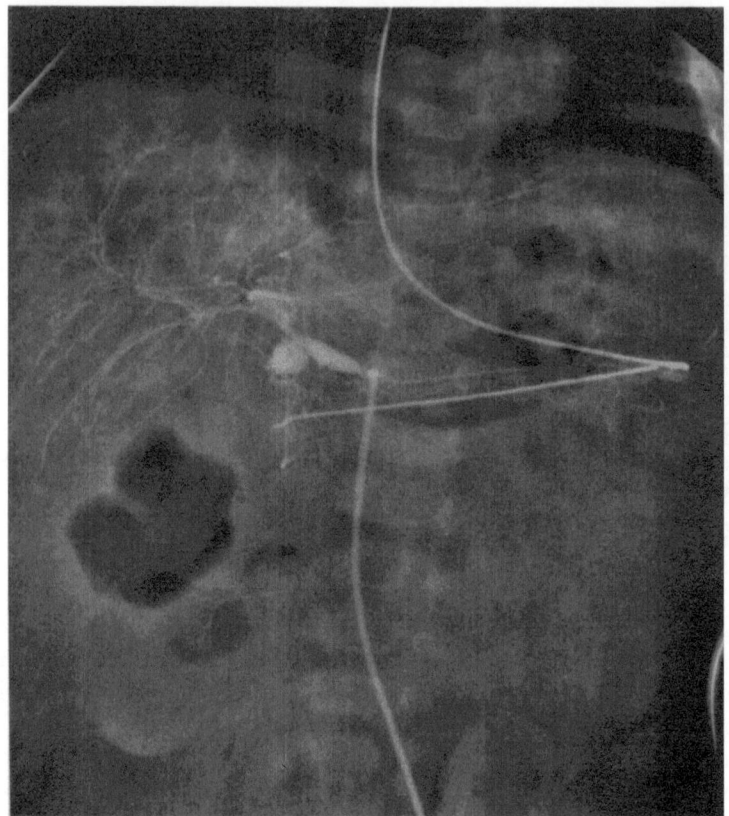

Figure 7.20. Celiac angiogram showing multiple hepatic-artery aneurysms and total obstruction of the splenic artery (catheter cannot pass) in a 2½-month-old boy with KD.

When a systemic vasculitis syndrome includes these latter features, it is considered to represent one of the granulomatous vasculitides rather than PAN (see sections on granulomatous vasculitides below). PAN is characterized by hypertension, renal arteritis, and frequent neurologic involvement.[125] Vasculitis of skin, muscle, testes, and joints is common, and aneurysms may occur in medium-sized renal, visceral (especially hepatic), and cerebral arteries. Males are slightly more frequently affected.

Clinical Presentation. The illness usually begins with unexplained fever, most often associated with arthralgia, abdominal pain, and severe myalgia.[126–129a] In males, testicular pain is often a good diagnostic clue. When present, it is usually an early manifestation, which precedes fever and is often mistaken for torsion of the testis. Some children have obvious vasculitic skin lesions (Fig. 7.21). In a few cases, vasculitis in the extremities is

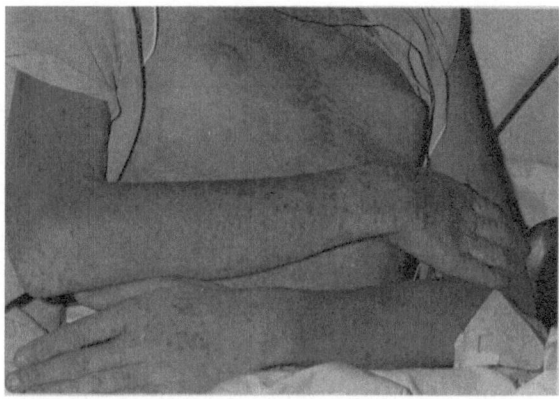

Figure 7.21. Palpable purpuric rash of systemic vasculitis.

severe enough to cause periosteal new-bone formation and exquisite bone tenderness.[130]

While the physician is evaluating the child and trying to form a diagnostic impression of what seems a mysterious process, there is a tendency for sudden deterioration, with involvement of one or another major organ system. Hypertension may occur and may be associated with encephalopathy. Myocarditis and pericarditis may result in congestive heart failure. Occasionally, transient ischemic attacks or strokes are major manifestations. Paresthesias and weakness typical of peripheral neuropathy (mononeuritis multiplex) are common. Renal function may deteriorate rapidly.

Laboratory abnormalities usually include anemia, leukocytosis, and great elevation of the ESR. Proteinuria and hematuria are common. Electrical studies of muscle and nerve conduction are often abnormal.

Precipitating Illnesses. Systemic vasculitis of the polyarteritis type may be associated with persistent hepatitis B antigenemia.[131–133] Only the presence of liver disease, which is often subclinical, differentiates these patients from others without the hepatitis B antigen. This syndrome is most common in areas hyperendemic for hepatitis B.[134]

Necrotizing arteritis has also been reported as a feature of acute poststreptococcal glomerulonephritis,[135] and some children with PAN seem unusually susceptible to nonsuppurative complications of streptococcal illness.[126] Systemic vasculitis may also occur as part of infectious mononucleosis and cytomegalovirus and PARVO-19 infection.[136–138] In adults, Sergent and Christian reported necrotizing vasculitis presenting with sudden loss of hearing.[139] They interpreted this sequence of events as possibly indicating that the vasculitis was an aftermath of a viral illness that also caused serous otitis media. In view of the frequency of otitis media in childhood and the rarity of sudden deafness as a presenting manifestation, it seems at least equally likely that sudden deafness may itself be the presenting manifestation of PAN (see Cogan's syndrome). However, children with PAN often do have a history of an antecedent respiratory infection just prior to the onset of the vasculitic symptoms.[127]

Necrotizing vasculitis has also been seen in the skin, lung, and gastrointestinal tract of older patients with cystic fibrosis of the pancreas, presumably a result of immune-complex formation resulting from repetitive infectious antigenic stimuli.[140,141] While there seems no doubt that in some cases infection may set off or exacerbate vasculitic illness, the infectious agent usually cannot be established, and the associated host factors remain a mystery.

Immunopathology. In PAN, all layers of affected arteries are infiltrated by acute and chronic inflammatory cells, resulting in fibrinoid necrosis, thrombosis, and infarction. Aneurysms form in weakened arterial walls. The lesions are usually segmental, tend to be most apparent at the bifurcations and branchings of small and medium-sized arteries, and are simultaneously seen in all stages of development. Multiple organs are affected. Renal vasculitis is most commonly seen without glomerulitis, but 30% of patients also have proliferative nephritis.

Diagnosis. A presumptive diagnosis of PAN is made in patients with typical clinical manifestations. Positive tests for circulating anti-myeloperoxidase antibodies and antibodies to proteinase 3 (ANCA) may heighten suspicion.[141a,b] Electrophysiologic studies may demonstrate abnormalities in asymptomatic muscle and/or nerve, indicating suitable areas for biopsy confirmation.[142] Muscle or nerve biopsy commonly confirms the diagnosis, especially if specimens are obtained from areas such as the sural nerve when those areas have been demonstrated to have abnormal electrical reactivity (Fig. 7.22).[143] Biopsies of skin nodules or testis may also be diagnostic. In difficult cases, diagnosis may be established by aortogram, showing multiple aneurysms in visceral and renal arteries, or by cerebral angiogram, showing similar lesions in cerebral vessels.[131,144,145] Renal biopsy may show rapidly progressive glomerulonephritis, necrotizing arteritis, or both. Although physicians and families wish biopsy or radiographic confirmation of the clinical diagnosis, it is often unwise to withhold treatment until that confirmation is obtained. Diagnostic studies may be continued after treatment is instituted. Diagnostic parsimony is practiced; unnecessary dangerous procedures are avoided after the diagnosis has been confirmed with the simplest procedure (Table 7.8).[143,146,147]

Treatment. Without prompt treatment, PAN is usually fatal.[126–129] Some patients (50%) respond well to treatment with large doses of prednisone alone (2 mg/kg/day), but some authors currently favor immediate treatment with both prednisone and cyclophosphamide (2 mg/kg/day).[148,149] When renal biopsy demonstrates rapidly progressive glomerulonephritis, immediate

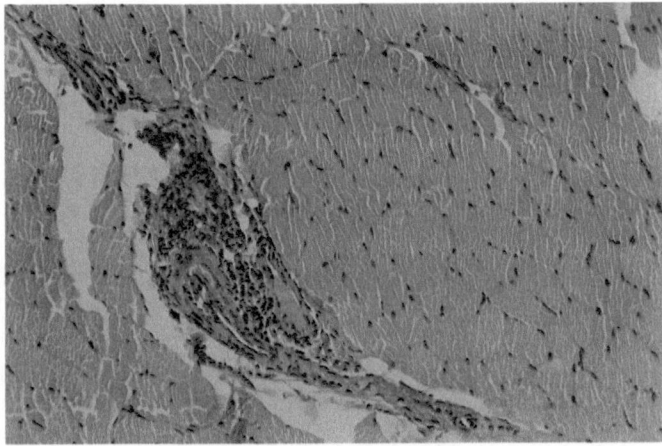

Figure 7.22. Leukocytoclastic perivascular infiltrate affecting a relatively small vessel in the skeletal muscle of a patient with fatal PAN. This pathologic picture may be seen in any systemic vasculitis syndrome ×180.

treatment with heparin may also be beneficial, preventing progression to renal failure.[150] It is tempting to extrapolate the better-documented experience with cyclophosphamide in Wegener's granulomatosis to PAN.[1] A few patients with PAN have been treated successfully with cyclophosphamide alone. While the optimal therapeutic regimen for PAN remains to be determined,[151] certainly patients who are not responding dramatically to prednisone or appear at risk of major organ failure deserve cyclophosphamide therapy. Cyclophosphamide is the treatment of choice for life-threatening necrotizing vasculitis;[152,153] intravenous pulse therapy is required by some severely ill patients.

Prognosis. Recent experience with alternate-day prednisone plus cyclophosphamide in steroid-resistant cases of PAN suggests that long-term clinical remission or cure is possible.[154] Not only could far-advanced, rapidly progressive PAN remit with such aggressive therapy, but the severe

Table 7.8. Diagnostic Procedures in Systemic Vasculitis

Biopsy of dermal vasculitis lesion
Electromyogram and nerve-conduction study
Muscle biopsy; testicular biopsy
Angiography—cerebral for CNS manifestations; aortogram in others*
Sinus films and nasal biopsy for Wegener's granulomatosis
Lung or renal biopsy if these organs and affected and all other diagnostic procedures
  fail

*MRI may replace angiography

aneurysms seen in abdominal vessels could be shown to disappear. Thus, the historically grave prognosis in PAN does not seem appropriate, provided patients are treated aggressively.

Allergic Angiitis and Granulomatosis (Churg-Strauss Syndrome)

Patients with the polyarteritis type of necrotizing vasculitis with predominantly pulmonary manifestations, eosinophilia, and a history of allergy and asthma were initially described by Churg and Strauss; this syndrome is also termed *allergic angiitis and granulomatosis* (AAG).[155–158] McCombs has emphasized the unique characteristics of the lung that might predispose that organ to vasculitis: the enormous complex pulmonary vascular network combined with the obvious opportunity for sensitizing antigens to reach the respiratory tract from the environment.[159] The cause of AAG remains unknown; however, in one recently reported case it may have been due to hyperresponsiveness to ascaris infection.[160]

Clinical Presentation. The usual presentation is the sudden onset of fever, pulmonary infiltrates, vasculitic skin lesions (especially subcutaneous nodules), and pericarditis and congestive heart failure in a child who has had asthma (Table 7.4).[1,155–157,161] Peripheral neuropathy (mononeuritis multiplex) and signs of gastrointestinal vasculitis are common; rarely, there may be granulomatous vasculitis of the CNS. Although there is sometimes clinical overlap with PAN, hypertension and significant renal disease almost never occur.[157,162] Arthralgias and arthritis are noted in approximately 50% of patients. Peripheral eosinophilia is an important diagnostic feature and is generally higher than 1500/mm³.[159]

Immunopathology. In contrast to classic PAN, there is primarily involvement of small vessels, especially capillaries and venules, although fibrinoid necrosis may also be seen in small and medium-sized muscular arteries. The vessels and perivascular tissues are often infiltrated with eosinophils. The extravascular granulomatous nodules consist of central areas of fibrinoid surrounded by large numbers of eosinophils, epithelioid cells, and giant cells (Fig. 7.23).[163] Similar lesions are sometimes seen in the lung, pericardium, and myocardium and in the coronary arteries.

Diagnosis. In this clinical context the diagnosis of AAG is suspected when an asthmatic child with unusual eosinophilia develops a multisystem systemic illness with vasculitis. The diagnosis can usually be confirmed pathologically by biopsy of one of the skin nodules; those nodules are found in about 70% of patients. In patients without skin nodules, testicular or muscle biopsy may sometimes be helpful. When other tissues have not enabled pathologic confirmation of the diagnosis, lung biopsy may be performed. While lung-

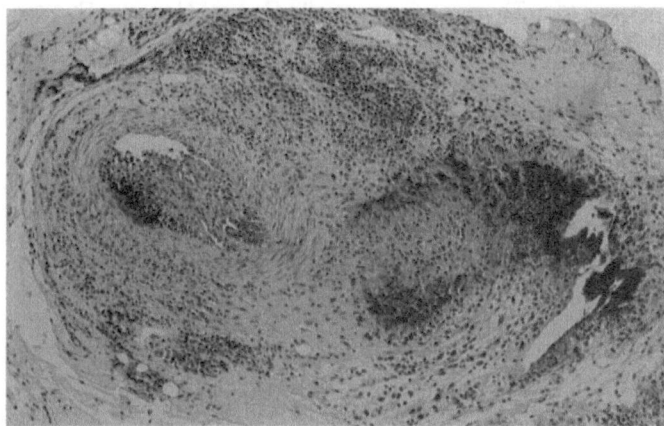

Figure 7.23. Forehead nodule in a 4-year-old boy with severe asthma, eosinophilia, and pericarditis with heart failure shows necrotizing granulomatous vasculitis that is partly calcified and is surrounded by a mixed cellular infiltrate with many plasma cells (allergic granulomatosis—Churg-Strauss vasculitis.) ×90. Only four other children have been reported to have had this syndrome.[161]

biopsy findings may be characteristic of AAG, in some cases granulomas may not be demonstrated, and evidence of vasculitis may be limited to infiltration of eosinophils throughout pulmonary vessels and scarring from prior vasculitis without active destruction of vessel walls. This may be true even when active vasculitis has been demonstrated in other organs.[164] The physician should not hesitate to make the diagnosis based on the clinical findings alone.[157] Tests for ANCA may be positive.[141a,b]

Course and Treatment. Untreated, the disease tends to run a chronic course, often resulting in death.[165] Dramatic relief is generally obtained with corticosteroids, and patients may often be rapidly changed to an alternate-day steroid regimen. However, there is a tendency for symptoms to recur as the dose is reduced, and in some patients steroid side effects have been intolerable. Cytotoxic agents have been used with success in patients who required unacceptable doses of prednisone over a long period of time or who appeared to be steroid-resistant. The prognosis for AAG can also be improved with earlier use of cyclophosphamide, as has been demonstrated for PAN and Wegener's granulomatosis.

Primary Granulomatous Angiitis of the Brain

A few children have been reported with giant-cell vasculitis of the CNS; we suspect that this disorder is much more common than the literature would suggest.[164,166–171] When the CNS vasculitis is part of a systemic vasculitis

Table 7.9. Vasculitides That May Present with Central-Nervous-System Manifestations

Allergic angiitis of the brain ("steroid-responsive encephalomyelitis")
Granulomatous angiitis of the brain and allergic granulomatosis
Periarteritis nodosa
Wegener's granulomatosis
Lymphomatous granulomatosis
Polyangiitis overlap syndromes[172,173]
Malignant atrophic papulosis (Kohlmeier-Degos disease)
Lyme disease

involving other organs, the diagnosis may not be difficult; the danger is recognized, and vigorous treatment is promptly administered. However, when there are no manifestations in other organs and no serologic markers to suggest connective-tissue disease, or only minimal findings such as an elevated ESR and dermal vasculitis,[172] diagnosis seems extraordinarily difficult (Table 7.9). In the past, without treatment most patients have been identified at postmortem examination. Newer studies suggest that vasculitis of the brain can be successfully managed with appropriate drug therapy, analogous to vasculitis elsewhere.[167] It is therefore now more important to consider the diagnosis of cerebral angiitis in patients with bizarre CNS disease even in the absence of any laboratory abnormalities or signs of vasculitis elsewhere. Prompt vigorous treatment should be begun prior to the occurrence of irreversible brain damage.[175]

One case has been reported of CNS vasculitis as the sole manifestation of the X-linked lymphoproliferative syndrome.[176]

Clinical Presentation. Altered mental status and intellectual deterioration may be important initial symptoms. Some children are initially referred for psychiatric care. Headache, nausea, vomiting, blurred or double vision, nystagmus, pupillary abnormalities, and dysarthria are common presenting manifestations. Seizures, hemiparesis, and dysphasia often occur as the disease progresses. Without treatment, all cases presumably progressed and were ultimately fatal. However, until recently, diagnosis was always dependent on autopsy material. Undiagnosed cases may have recovered and not be included in reported series.

Immunopathology. Inflammation of blood vessels may be demonstrated both in the cortex and in the meninges. Perivascular cuffing of the meningeal arteries may sometimes be seen on the operating table with the use of magnifying loupes. The intima of the vessels is greatly thickened and edematous; the media is necrotic and contains giant cells and macrophages. The adventitia is thickened with small lymphocytes. Clinical and experimental evidence suggests that these findings may result either from immune-complex deposition in cerebral blood vessels or from direct invasion by viruses and perhaps also by invasion of mycoplasmal organisms.

Nongranulomatous vasculitis of the brain as the sole manifestation of vasculitic illness has not been well-defined as a clinical entity. However, experience with all systemic vasculitides indicates that any vasculitis may start with CNS manifestations. Therefore, it is a reasonable hypothesis that there exists a group of patients with nongranulomatous angiitis of the nervous system without manifestations of vasculitis elsewhere.

Diagnosis. There are usually cells in the spinal fluid, often increases in CSF protein and pressure, and sometimes decrease in CSF glucose.[172] Computer-assisted tomography and MRI have recently been useful in some cases where microinfarcts were demonstrable. Arteriograms usually show characteristic beading of small vessels with saccular aneurysm formation or nonspecific small-vessel occlusion which may become normal following therapy.[177] Some autopsied cases have shown leptomeningeal involvement, and biopsy of the leptomeninges or brain may be helpful diagnostic procedures.[174,178]

Treatment. Controlled studies have not been done. Anecdotal experience suggests that corticosteroid treatment is often effective and that maintenance therapy with alternate-day regimens may provide long-time control. Immunosuppressive agents arrest the process in patients whose disease does not subside or who require higher-than-tolerable doses of corticosteroids for control.

Lack of control of vasculitis of the brain may result in disastrous permanent impairment or in death. The therapeutic margin for error is less than in other organ systems. Experience extrapolated from patients with CNS manifestations of generalized vasculitic illness such as PAN, Wegener's granulomatosis, Churg-Strauss syndrome, lymphomatoid granulomatosis, and polyangiitis overlap syndromes suggests that a similar aggressive approach may be indicated in some patients with chronic vasculitis that manifests itself solely or primarily in the nervous system. In all of these disorders, survival was poor prior to the institution of aggressive cytotoxic therapy.

Steroid-Responsive Encephalomyelitis (Allergic Angiitis of the Brain)

Pasternak has described a slowly progressive, smoldering neurologic syndrome, characterized by increasing weakness, coma, hemiparesis, and diffuse, severe brainstem manifestations, that is exquisitely steroid-responsive.[179] Some of the patients had documented antecedent viral or leptospiral illness. After initial control of the neurologic symptoms, patients were maintained on an alternate-day steroid regimen for from 3 weeks to 6 months; all achieved complete recovery. It is really this recovery that identifies this syndrome and differentiates it from other unresponsive, mysterious, vasculitic brain syndromes. The characteristics of the illness suggest "allergic cerebral angiitis," although these authors performed no studies to support that hypothesis.[179]

Takayasu's Arteritis

Arteritis resulting in loss of pulses in a young woman was first described by Savory in 1856 and Kussmaul in 1872. In 1908, Takayasu noted the ocular findings: wreathlike arteriovenous anastomoses around the papillae and a peculiar capillary flush. In the discussion of Takayasu's paper, Onishi and Kagoshima established the association between this hypotensive retinal vasculitis and aortic vasculitis.[180,181] Originally, it was thought that the aortic disease was restricted to the arch, but it has more recently been demonstrated that any part of the aorta may be involved and that in some patients there is also involvement of the pulmonary artery.[182–184] The classic eye lesions are often obscured by eye signs of hypertension and are seen in fewer than half the patients. Patients without decreased cerebral blood flow or hypertension have normal fundi and may present with claudication, decreased brachial artery pulse, and bruits over subclavian arteries or the aorta.[185]

Clinical Presentation. Eighty-four percent of patients with Takayasu's arteritis (TA) are female; 80% are between 11 and 30 years of age at the time of diagnosis. Symptoms most commonly begin during the second decade of life, a population increasingly served by pediatricians. Asians, particularly Japanese, are especially susceptible.[180–182]

In our experience, the disease has a chronic onset with anorexia, malaise, fatigue, slowing of linear growth, and failure to gain weight (Table 7.4).[186,187] However, these symptoms may be so mild that they escape prospective attention. Arthralgia, unexplained fever, and brief episodes of arthritis occur in some patients.[188] The only clues to the extent of the process are the finding of a greatly elevated ESR and greatly increased levels of gamma globulin; the increased gamma globulin consists of IgG, M and A, but not D or E. This chronic prepulseless phase may persist for years before an acute exacerbation demands diagnosis, or diagnosis may be accidental, by finding diminished peripheral pulses, a greatly dilated aorta on chest radiograph (Fig. 7.24), or midaortic lesions in children being studied because of hypertension. In those children who have lesions only of the midaorta, peripheral pulses are not affected.

Most frequently, the diagnosis is established following an acute catastrophe, either hypertensive encephalopathy with seizures or profound congestive heart failure. The heart failure is usually a consequence of hypertension due to both renal and systemic arterial occlusion, sometimes combined with aortic valvulitis with aortic insufficiency and pulmonary-artery obstruction. Syncopal spells and sudden episodes of paroxysmal hypertension char-

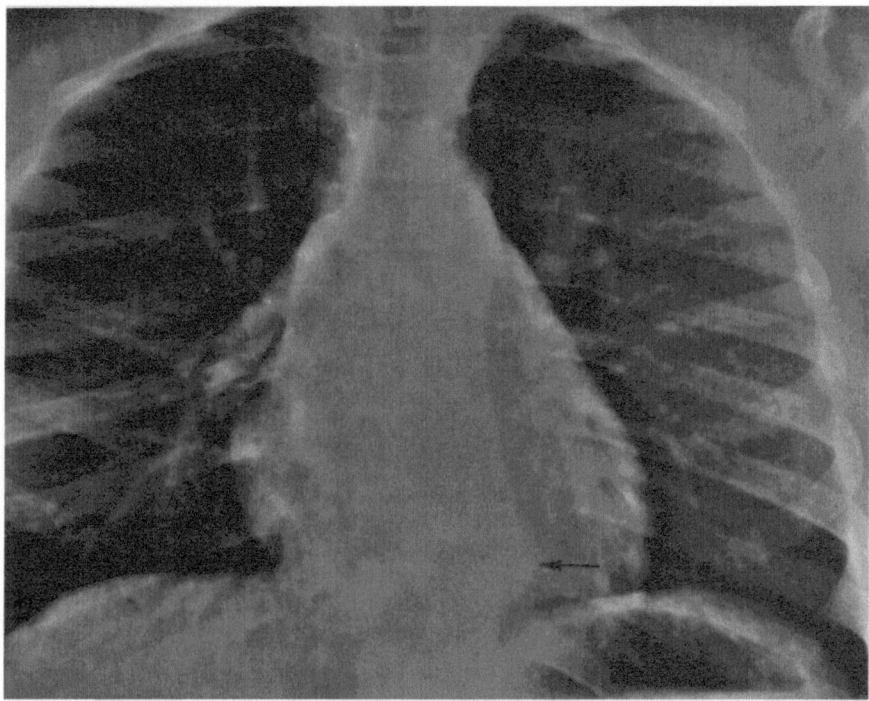

Figure 7.24. Widened aorta *(arrow)* visible on plain chest film of a 10-year-old girl with Takayasu's arteritis. Chest film was obtained at the time of an intercurrent respiratory illness; the child had no clinical complaints at the time of the film but had been ill with fever thought possibly to be systemic JRA 2 years earlier. Radial pulses were absent.

acterized by tachycardia with palpitations, headache, dyspnea, precordial pain, choking sensations, sweating, and flushing of the face may be caused by aortic arch lesions that alter carotid sinus baroreceptor sensitivity.[189] These spells may be set off by sudden changes in posture or by micturition.

Diagnosis. The experienced physician, presented with a girl with these symptoms (heart failure and hypertension/seizures) and noting vascular bruits and the diminution or absence of certain peripheral pulses, makes the correct presumptive diagnosis immediately at the bedside. Diagnosis may be promptly confirmed by MRI or digital venous angiography or aortography that demonstrates irregularity, occlusion, stenosis, poststenotic dilatation, and aneurysms of the proximal portions of branches of the aorta (Fig. 7.25)[190-192a] Takayasu's arteritis has been divided into four subgroups, depending on the pattern of vascular occlusion (Fig. 7.26).[180-182]

Immunopathology. Lesions are limited to the aorta and stem arteries, those larger elastic arteries having a vasa vasorum. Although commonly called

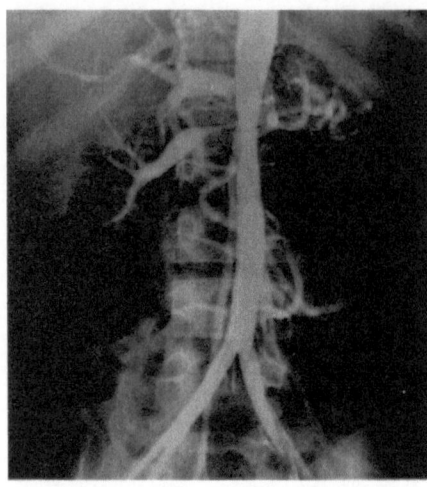

Figure 7.25. Aortogram in an 11-year-old Indian girl with Takayasu's arteritis, showing aortic narrowing with aneurysmal dilatation of the left renal artery and lack of filling of the right renal artery. Patient was admitted with failure to thrive and recent onset of congestive heart failure and hypertension. Radial pulses were diminished.

"aortitis syndrome," Takayasu's is really a truncoarteritis. In long arteries such as the carotids, only the proximal elastic portions are affected; vessels with muscular coats are spared. Microscopic findings include both diffuse productive inflammation in the media of these vessels and granulomata with small necrotic foci, Langhans' giant cells, and foreign-body giant cells that have phagocytized destroyed elastic fibers. In autopsy material, most of these lesions have been replaced by severe fibrosis in the media with degeneration and disappearance of the elastic fibers. In older cases, secondary fibrosis occurs in the adventitia and intima. Granulomatous inflammation with giant cells is frequently found in the vasa vasorum of the aorta and affected vessels, suggesting that the primary lesion might actually be in these vessels. As time

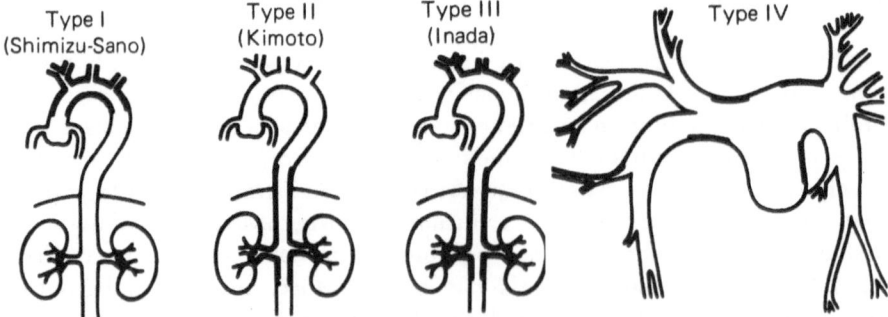

Figure 7.26. Clinical classification of TA as proposed by Ueno and modified by Lupi-Herrera et al. The thicker dash lines represent the areas of involvement. (Reprinted with permission from Lupi-Herrera et al., ref. 182.)

goes on, these granulomatous lesions are also replaced by endothelial proliferation producing an onion-skin-like fibrosis of vessel walls. Overlap syndromes exist between all of the vasculitic syndromes.[193–195]

Tuberculosis and Takayasu's Arteritis. The exact role of tuberculosis in TA remains uncertain, but it is crucially important in some cases. All series of patients seem to contain a greater number of patients with coincident tuberculosis than the authors would expect;[196] this includes our own experience.

In an area such as South Africa, where tuberculosis is almost universal in black children, Takayasu's disease is the single most common cause of renovascular hypertension in black children.[196]

While the mechanism by which tuberculosis might make one more susceptible to TA remains speculative, the practical conclusion is inescapable. The physician must be sensitive to the possibility of coincident tuberculosis in patients with TA and must remain alert to the possibility that new symptoms are a result of tuberculosis. Appropriate antituberculous therapy is frequently necessary in patients with TA.[197]

Course of the Disease and Treatment. After a varying period of either unnoticed or undiagnosable symptoms, acute deterioration with hypertension, congestive heart failure, headaches, and convulsions bring the child to hospital. Ultimately, someone notices the absent pulses, obtains the aortogram or MRI, and makes the correct diagnosis. The hypertension is generally renin-associated as a result of stenosis of the renal artery and from increased baroreceptor sensitivity.[198] In most children, the disease responds to usual doses of prednisone, together with vigorous antihypertensive and cardiotonic therapy.[192a]

Even without corticosteroid treatment, many patients were reported to again enter a chronic phase of the disease and develop collateral circulation, only to subsequently deteriorate and sometimes die either from cardiac failure or from ill-defined catastrophies. In our experience with three girls, after initial control with daily prednisone, all could be adequately maintained relatively symptom-free with alternate-day prednisone therapy aimed at keeping the ESR and immunoglobulins close to normal. Two girls continue to lead normal lives. One year after diagnosis, the other girl complained of severe pain in her leg. She was found in irreversible shock 12 h later. A postmortem examination was not permitted, and the cause of her demise is unknown.

Five-year survival is greatly improved with prednisone therapy. If clinical symptoms are not improved with prednisone, cyclophosphamide should be given in addition to alternate-day prednisone.[186,187] Arterial bypass procedures and cardiac valve replacements are now highly successful techniques in Takayasu's patients. With modern drug therapy for inflammation and hypertension, and modern surgical techniques, 5-year survival is already 94% and will be even better in the next decade.[186,187]

Familial Granulomatous Arteritis

Rotenstein reported a granulomatous arteritis that occurred in three generations of one family, presumably with autosomal-dominant heritability.[199] The illness simulated systemic-onset JRA at onset, but with sarcoid skin lesions; the propositus had iritis. All affected individuals had noncaseating granulomas of skin, liver, and other organs; many of the granulomas were perivascular in location, resulting in large-vessel stenosis and renovascular hypertension. Three similar families have been reported and single cases undoubtedly have been called sarcoidosis. (See Fig. 2.46).

Wegener's Granulomatosis

Wegener's granulomatosis (WG) is a clinical triad consisting of disseminated small-vessel necrotizing vasculitis, focal necrotizing glomerulitis in the kidney, and necrotizing vasculitic granulomas of both the upper and lower respiratory tracts (Table 7.4)[200,201] Most patients have fever, purpuric skin lesions, myositis sinusitis, otitis, nasopharyngeal symptoms, hemoptysis and/or pulmonary infiltrates.[202] Sinusitis may be accompanied by nasal mucosal ulceration and destruction of the bony walls of the sinuses and of the nasal septum. Other patients have severe pulmonary manifestations with impairment of pulmonary function. Pulmonary lesions may sometimes be demonstrated radiographically even in the absence of pulmonary manifestations. Renal disease is the major cause of death but often occurs later than the other symptoms of WG. Prior to the institution of modern therapeutic agents, the average 1-year survival of untreated patients with WG was only 18%; survival after the appearance of clinical renal disease was only 5 months![200,201]

Clinical Presentation. Two-thirds of patients are male. Most present with unexplained fever, anorexia, weight loss, cough, chest pain, pulmonary hemorrhage[200–204] myalgia, and arthritis or arthralgia. Upper-respiratory-tract symptoms include staphylococcal sinusitis, nasal obstruction or mucosal lesions, and serous otitis media. In one of our patients, the nasal obstruction was caused by the formation of nasal eosinophilic casts that she blew out of each nostril every few days (Fig. 7.27). In our experience, the nasal symptoms, although frequently ignored by the physician, are the most important clue to this diagnosis in a child with mysterious multisystem disease. A high level of clinical suspicion in patients with combined respiratory and renal disease in association with biopsy of lesions within the respiratory tract should reduce the delay in establishing the correct diagnosis.[205]

Eye lesions are also common and include lesions of the conjunctiva, cornea, and sclerae as well as uveitis and pseudotumor of the orbit.[205a,205b] Twenty-five percent of patients have hemoptysis, 25% cardiac manifestations of one sort or another, and at least 25% neurologic manifestations. The most common neurologic symptom is mononeuritis multiplex, but occa-

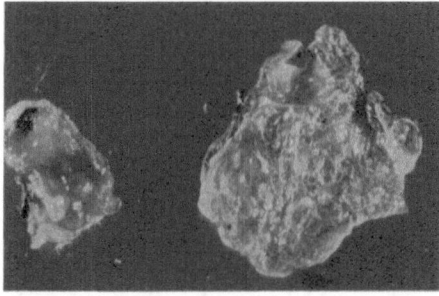

Figure 7.27. Nasal casts blown out of nose by a 9-year-old girl with fever, malaise, weight loss, and recent onset of hematuria and diminished renal function. Nasal symptoms were ignored despite their prominence. Renal biopsy was suggestive of Wegener's granulomatosis.

sionally there are CNS granulomatous lesions. Anemia, leukocytosis, hypergammaglobulinemia, and an elevated ESR are commonly demonstrated.

Immunopathology. The widespread angiitis is indistinguishable from PAN. Diagnosis depends on demonstration of characteristic giant-cell vasculitic granulomas in the upper respiratory tract or lungs.[206–208] Occasional patients have a localized form with respiratory-tract lesions only.

Renal lesions are both focal and segmental and may vary greatly in severity. Subepithelial dense deposits are common; in some cases, IgG and complement deposition suggest that immune-complex deposition triggers the damage. The disease has recurred in a transplanted kidney.[208a]

Diagnosis. The clinical triad suggests the diagnosis that is usually established by biopsy of the respiratory-tract lesions (Fig. 7.28). Biopsy of skin

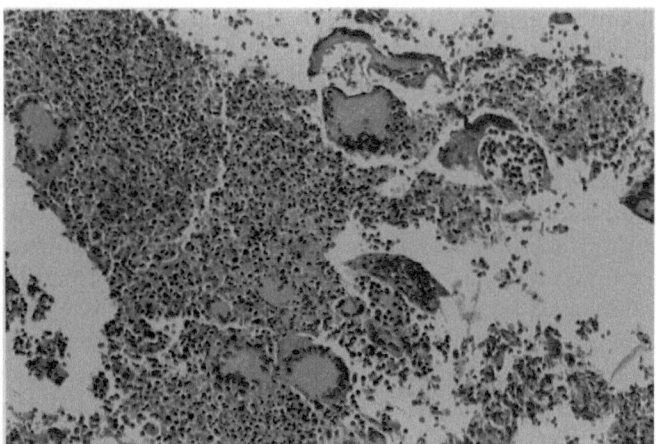

Figure 7.28. Submucosal nasal granuloma, removed from an 11-year-old boy with malaise, fever, and nephritis, is composed of a large number of granulocytes and some histiocytes. Despite the absence of identifiable blood vessels or Langhan's or Touton giant cells sometimes seen in such lesions, this biopsy was sufficient to indicate the diagnosis of Wegener's granulomatosis in this boy, who responded well to treatment with cyclophosphamide. ×180.

lesions or kidney, although of value in confirming the vasculitic nature of the disease, rarely provides a specific diagnosis.[195,205,209,210]

Other disorders, including other vasculitides, are distinguished by the absence of vasculitic granulomas or by their own distinctive clinical features and pathology.

Antineutrophilic cytoplasmic antibodies (ANCA) initially were reported to be diagnostic of WG, with a sensitivity of 97%;[211] these antibodies disappear with treatment and reappear as predictors of exacerbation. The test is technically difficult and further study is required to be certain about its specificity in excluding other vasculitic disorders which may be confused with WG.[141a,141b] At present a cytoplasmic staining pattern (C-ANCA) is said to be typical of WG and distinguishable from the perinuclear (P-ANCA) seen in other types of vasculitis and in necrotizing and crescentic glomerulonephritis.[212,213]

Overlap exists and it remains to be determined if all diseases with these antibodies have a common immunopathogenesis mediated by ANCA-induced neutrophil activation.[214]

Treatment. Corticosteroid treatment of WG has no long-term beneficial effect, although symptoms may be temporarily relieved. The drug of choice has been demonstrated to be cyclophosphamide.[1,215–217] Therapeutic regimens can be adapted to provide remissions of disease without serious side effects. In general, therapy with cyclophosphamide is begun with a dose of 1–2 mg/kg/day. The dose is adjusted to maintain the total leukocyte count above 3000/mm^3 with a total neutrophil count of 1000–1500/mm^3. An additional 25 mg daily is added to the regimen in patients who do not show a prompt, favorable clinical response. An intermittent high-dose itravenous cyclophosphamide regimen analagous to that used in SLE does not have equal beneficial effects.[218]

Children with fulminant disease that is life-threatening or threatens permanent damage to vital organs (cerebral vasculitis, eye involvement, pericarditis, gangrene, severe pulmonary involvement with hypoxemia, rapidly progressive renal failure, or rapidly progressive peripheral neuropathy) require a more aggressive initial approach. There must be no delay (even for a day) in initiation of therapy.[1] The dose of cyclophosphamide, given for the first 3 days, is increased in these children to 4 mg/kg/day, and the medication may be given intravenously, especially if gastrointestinal symptoms are present and absorption is uncertain. Over the next 3 days, the daily dose is reduced to the maintenance 1–2 mg/kg/day. Prednisone, 2 mg/kg/day (maximum 60 mg daily) in four divided doses, is also given in fulminant cases until the effects of cyclophosphamide are seen, usually within 2 weeks. As soon as the child begins to improve, the prednisone is changed to a single morning daily dose and then, within a few days, to an alternate-day regimen of 4–5 mg/kg/dose, which is gradually reduced as tolerated. Steroid treatment can generally be completely withdrawn within a month. In desperate situations, bolus corticosteroids may be used.[219] Cerebritis may occur during therapy with cyclophosphamide and require the addition of corticosteroids.[220]

Modern management of WG has converted an almost invariable fatal disorder into a curable disease provided treatment is begun prior to uncontrollable pulmonary hemorrhage or renal failure.[203,221] After a period of years, all treatment may sometimes be discontinued without exacerbation of symptoms.[1,200,222] Fifty percent of remissions may be followed by one or more relapses. If a patient who is in remission again develops symptoms, retreatment is instituted with the same regimen. Treatment with full doses of cyclophosphamide is continued until the patient has been in remission for 1 year.

Some cases of WG have been reported to be controlled with trimethoprin/sulfa,[223–225] and remissions may be prolonged with continuous antibiotic treatment and prevention of episodes of sinusitis. The prognosis for patients with WG has been transformed by cyclophosphamide, but long-term usage will result in some later deaths from cyclophosphamide-induced malignancy.[226]

Limited Wegener's Granulomatosis

Atypical or limited forms of WG[227] occur primarily in the form of what has been termed "midline granuloma."[228] (Midline granulomas, caused by atypical or limited forms of lymphomatous granulomatosis or by bacteria, fungi, or parasites, must be differentiated histologically from those of WG.) The "limited" form of WG is defined by lesions only in the orbit and respiratory tract (lung, sinuses, and other mucosal surfaces) without involvement of the kidneys or the vascular system. In contrast to the generally rapid progression of generalized WG, the limited forms of disease usually evolve slowly, and diagnosis may be even more difficult. Some patients evolve into "unlimited" WG; although the prognosis is better, half the patients with the limited form require cyclophosphamide treatment.[228] It is important to remember that the diagnosis of WG is not dependent on the finding of vasculitis but rather on the demonstration in biopsy specimens of typical foci of necrosis of the disintegrating and fibrinoid degeneration types, palisading granulomas, and giant cells. Vasculitis may be absent or reflected soley by disruption and segmental disappearance of the elastic laminae, which can be shown only with special elastic-tissue-staining techniques. Limited forms of WG also respond well to treatment with cyclophosphamide. A child we care for has been greatly benefited by trimethaprin-sulfa.

Occasionally the symptom complex of limited WG may be indistinguishable from that of relapsing polychondritis.[229]

Lymphomatoid Granulomatosis

Lymphomatoid granulomatosis (LG) is a disorder that closely resembles WG but is distinguished from it by the presence of pathopneumonic pulmonary nodules made up of lymphocytes and large reticuloendothelial cells that invade and destroy blood vessels (Table 7.4). The highly cellular angiocentric atypical lymphoreticular infiltrates are rich in mitoses, suggestive of a lymphoproliferative disease, and at least 13% of LG patients do eventually evolve into clear-cut lymphomas. Thus, LG has features of both WG and lymphoma, although, as emphasized by Liebow, it does appear to be a distinct clinicopathologic entity.[230-237] Recent studies suggest that angiocentric lymphoma is a T-cell neoplasm.[235-237] Children with Wiskott-Aldrich syndrome may be predisposed to vasculitis and lymphoproliferative malignancy.[238,239]

Clinical Presentation. Most patients with LG present with cough and fever, often associated with vasculitic skin lesions. Central-nervous-system manifestations, similar to those seen in other vasculitis syndromes, are common and may be the sole presenting manifestation; even in patients without pulmonary complaints, multiple, rounded, mass densities can usually be demonstrated on routine chest radiographs and provide the important clue to diagnosis. (Fig. 7.29). In contrast to WG, renal involvement is generally unimpressive, and upper-airway granulomas are less frequently seen in LG. The ESR, always elevated in WG, is often normal in active LG, and patients with LG are frequently anergic.

Immunopathology. Diagnosis depends on biopsy material (most often lung; Fig. 7.30) demonstrating angiocentric polymorphic dense infiltrates of cells belonging to the lymphoid family. The cell population includes mature lymphocytes, stimulated lymphocytes, immunoblasts, histiocytes, and plasma cells. This pathologic appearance has resulted in some authors terming the disorder "polymorphic reticulosis."[232] Single biopsy specimens may be misinterpreted as eosinophilic granuloma, lymphosarcoma, Hodgkin's disease, other granulomas, or even rheumatoid nodules.

   In our own patient (Liebow's case no.19),[230] postmortem examination showed a variety of lesions. Lymph nodes were completely replaced by primitive neoplastic cells (histiocytic lymphoma or reticulum-cell sarcoma). There were plemorphic cellular infiltrates consisting of plasmacytoid elements and lymphocytes with only an occasional neoplastic cell in bone marrow, kidney, spleen, liver, thyroid, tonsils, and salivary glands. Similar lesions in the nervous system were associated with prominent vascular proliferation and cellular invasion of blood-vessel walls with associated tissue breakdown, myelin loss and fragmentation, axonal loss, and reactive gliosis. Lesions were noted in the optic nerve and spinal cord in addition to those in the CNS. Lung biopsy material 7 years before death was typical of LG (Fig. 7.30). A scalp lesion 4 years before death histiologically suggested eosinophilic granuloma.

Course and Therapy. Without drug therapy, LG is usually but not always rapidly fatal.[235] While patients with LG usually have an initial favorable

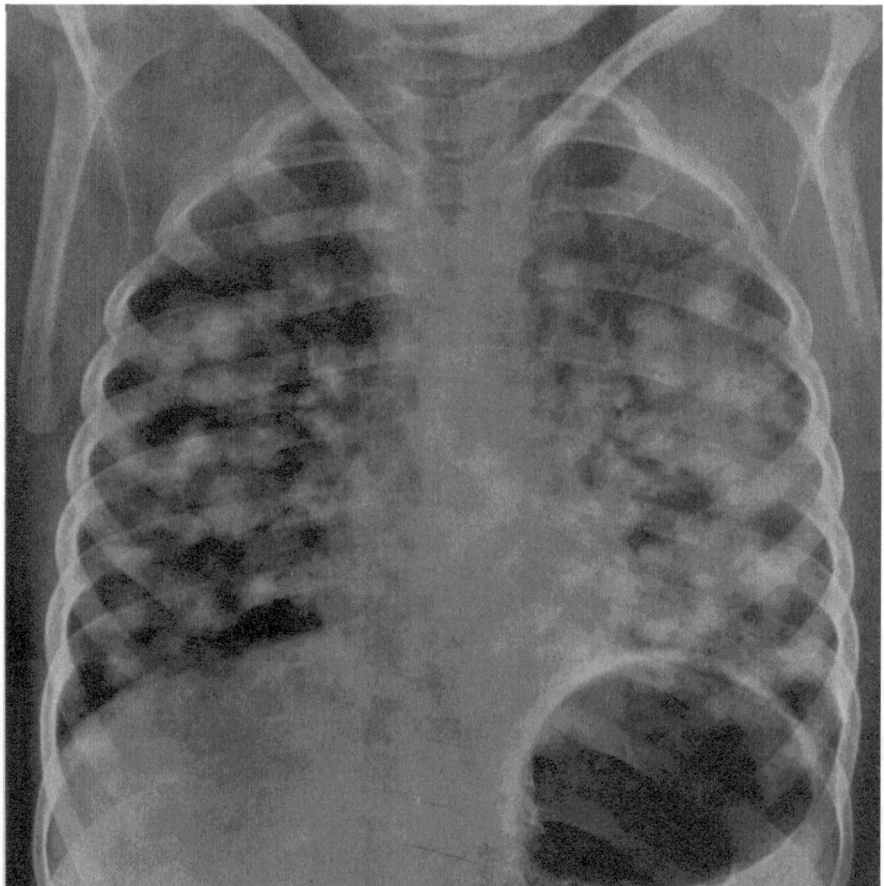

Figure 7.29. Admission (asymptomatic) chest film obtained in an 8-year-old girl who had been hospitalized in a psychiatric institute for several months for behavioral manifestations and now had also developed neurologic symptoms. Biopsy of the lung (Fig. 7.30) revealed lymphomatous granulomatosis.

response to corticosteroid therapy, the improvement tends to be transient. Early aggressive cytotoxic therapy is presently the favored regimen.[234,240]

A limited form of LG, "benign lymphocytic angiitis and granulomatosis" (analogous to "limited Wegener's"), has also been reported. A solitary lesion is limited to the lung and, unlike the lesion in LG, is composed of mature plasma cells, lymphocytes, and histiocytes. These solitary nodules can be surgically removed and do not recur.[231] Similar solitary lesions in the upper airway, "midline granuloma," are radiosensitive, do not require drug therapy or surgical excision, and must be distinguished from those midline granulomas which are manifestations of WG and require treatment with cyclophosphamide.[241]

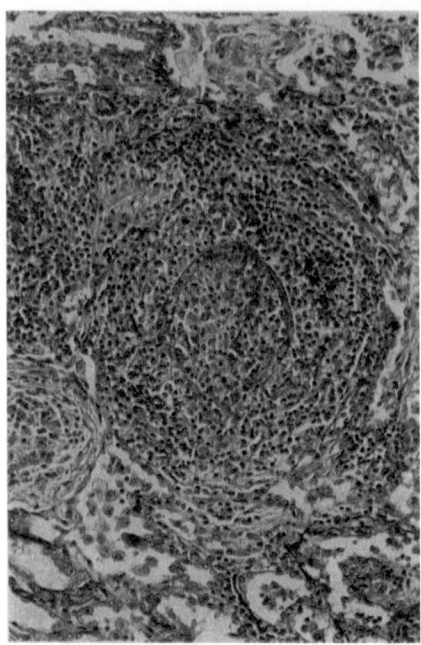

Figure 7.30. Lung biopsy in an 8-year-old girl with lymphomatous granulomatosis shows angiocentric granulomatous inflammation invading and obliterating a pulmonary vessel and leaving the elastica as the only recognizable remnant. ×180.

Hypersensitivity Vasculitis

Henoch-Schönlein (H-S) Purpura. Henoch-Schönlein purpura is a relatively common, self-limited form of generalized leukocytoclastic angiitis with a repetitive pattern of skin, joint, and gastrointestinal manifestations (see Chapter 2).

Allergic Angiitis. Attempts at rigid classification of vasculitic illness often fail,[1] and time spent arguing over such details sometimes serves as a confusing distraction and interferes with appropriate and urgent therapeutic intervention. Allergic angiitis is the diagnostic term applied when the pattern of vasculitic illness does not fit into any of the specific vasculitis syndromes described above (Table 7.4). Some authors report similar cases under the heading Cutaneous Polyarteritis Nodosa.[242,243]

Patients with allergic angiitis have fever, skin rash, and nonspecific rheumatic symptoms, without major organ involvement, that are a result of inflammation in and around small vessels (capillaries, arterioles, and venules).[244] The skin lesions may be painful, itch, or burn. Most cases seem to be reactive to an antigenic stimulus, either an infectious antigen or a drug, and in some cases evidence of immune-complex formation can be demonstrated. The hallmark of this heterogeneous group of vasculitic syndromes is the skin lesion, the purpuric papule (palpable purpura). Recurrent wheals o

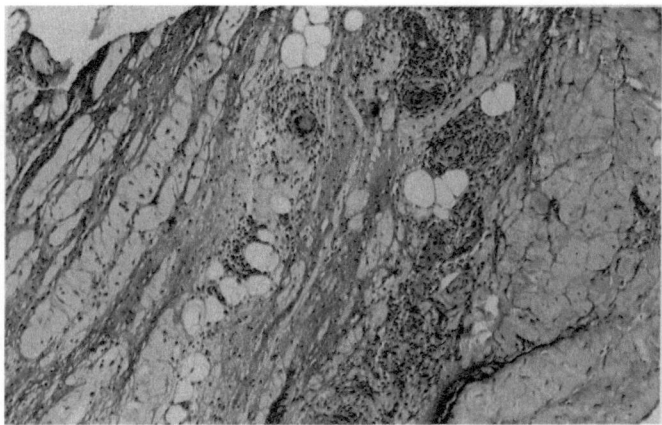

Figure 7.31. Muscle biopsy in a 10-year-old boy with allergic angiitis shows vasculitis and perivasculitis in the fascia, with pleomorphic inflammation in the adjacent fibrofatty tissue. ×90.

hives are less frequent manifestations of cutaneous venulitis. Diagnosis depends on biopsy of the skin lesion (Fig. 7.31).

Clinical Presentation. Almost all patients have fever and vasculitic skin lesions (Fig. 7.32). Arthralgia and myalgia are more common than arthritis, but transient arthritis may be seen, and a few patients present with fever and myositis without skin lesions.[245,246] Clinically apparent involvement of organs other than the skin is not common but may occur in severe cases. Severe systemic necrotizing allergic angiitis is clinically analogous to classic PAN despite the different-size vessels involved and the generally different microscopic pattern of vasculitis.

Immunopathology. Electron microscopy suggests that the initial inflammatory stimulus in allergic angiitis is an immune complex in the blood-vessel wall, which is followed later by the appearance of neutrophils and then by fibrinoid necrosis (Fig. 7.1). Therefore, nuclear debris ("dust") and fibrin may not be seen in very early lesions. A great variety of skin-surface lesions may appear, varying from urticarial papules to nodules, sometimes with vesicles, bullae, pustules, and ulcers. As time goes on, degenerating nuclei (leukocytoclasis) lead to the presence of nuclear debris and to the term "leukoclastic angiitis."

In hypersensitivity angiitis, the vasculitic lesions usually are of the same age and, while necrotizing, tend to be characterized primarily by exudation and hemorrhage rather than by ischemia. These features in the skin lead to the palpable purpuric lesion. Occasionally, digital vasculitis and vasospasm may cause infarction.

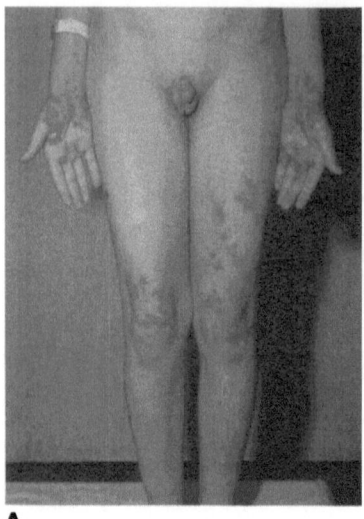
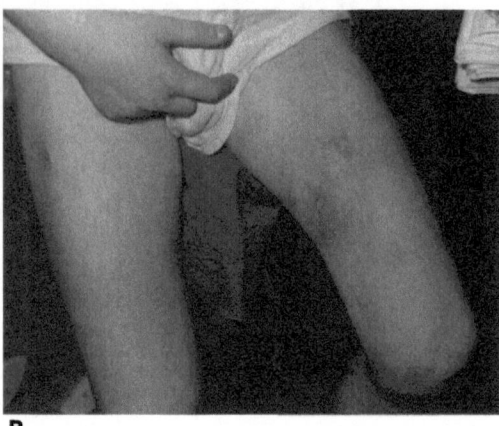

A   **B**

Figure 7.32. (**A**) Vasculitic skin lesions on the hands and legs in a boy with allergic angiitis. The youngster made a complete recovery after several attacks. (**B**) Another young boy with allergic angiitis that resulted in deep necrotic vasculitic ulcers requiring steroid therapy for healing. Healing resulted in atrophic white scars (atrophie blanche). This patient has continued to have episodes of arthralgia/arthritis, fever, and dermal vasculitis for 25 years.

Clinical Course. In most children with allergic angiitis, the disease is self-limited and ultimately will disappear. Sometimes, however, it is recurrent or can become chronic and troublesome for many years or for life. Symptoms may be so severe that normal activities cannot be carried on even with maximum aspirin therapy. Deep ulcers may result from subcutaneous arterial insufficiency (Fig. 7.32B). If hypersensitivity vasculitis involves major organ systems, it may resemble one of the other vasculitic syndromes or represent an overlap syndrome. In such patients, injury to a vital organ may threaten life itself or the quality of life.

Treatment. In general, hypersensitivity vasculitis is responsive to corticosteroid therapy. If fever and arthritis are the major manifestations, aspirin or another NSAID may be useful as an adjunct and for its steroid-sparing effect. Aspirin may also be helpful during weaning of prednisone or to enable an alternate-day steroid regimen to suffice either initially or after control of the disease has been achieved. We most often start patients on aspirin while we are completing our workup. In severe cases, we substitute prednisone 2 mg/kg/day, wean the prednisone down slowly with aspirin "coverage" after complete control has been achieved, or switch to an alternate-day regimen with 5 mg/kg/dose if the clinical situation suggests that steroid treatment cannot be discontinued. At a later time, when remission occurs, the alternate-day steroid can generally be slowly weaned away, often with only minimal aspirin supplement.

The children with hypersensitivity vasculitis constitute such a broad group that no single therapeutic regimen seems appropriate for all patients. However, adequate care requires appropriate study to determine the extent of the vasculitis and clinical experience and judgment to estimate its pace and how threatened the patient is, both in terms of life and future useful function. Where life or vital organ function does not seem threatened immediately but the pace of disease is very active, alternate-day steroids provide a safe and efficient means of controlling the process so that the patient can resume normal activities. In most cases, the child makes a full recovery with no sequelae.

Where the disease is truly chronic or so frequently exacerbates that it interferes with a normal life-style monoclonal antibody therapy may induce remission.[247] Gamma globulin should be tried.

Mixed Cryoglobulinemia. Serum globulins that precipitate on cooling and redissolve on warming are called cryoglobulins.[248] Cryoglobulinemia is now recognized as a physiologic occurrence. which can become pathologic as a result of (1) increased production due to benign or malignant stimulation of B lymphocytes, (2) increased transformation of normal immunoglobulins into cryoglobulins by neuraminidaselike activity generated by invading microorganisms or their products, or (3) impaired removal as a result of liver injury.[248]

Pathologically large amounts of cryoglobulins may be present in some forms of vasculitis and were described by Meltzer and Franklin as associated with a separate syndrome termed essential mixed cryglobulinemia.[249,250] This syndrome is characterized by recurrent episodes of vasculitis of the skin (palpable purpura), weakness, arthralgia, glomerulonephritis, and large quantities of mixed monoclonal and polyclonal immune globulins, the former being IgM, IgG, or IgA-anti-IgG cryoglobulins.[249–252] Most patients have evidence of hepatic dysfunction.[250]

The presence of these immune complexes results in a positive test for rheumatoid factor and in early complement component depletion. Vascular lesions are frequently present in skin and to a lesser extent in kidneys, heart, brain, and pancreas.

The role of cryoglobulins as inducers of disease rather than as reflections of disease activity seems less certain now than in the recent past. Cryoglobulinemia in association with hypocomplementemia has even been reported to occur in rare instances in the absence of clinical disease.[253]

It now seems likely that most instances of essential mixed cryoglobulinemia represent a response to infectious hepatitis B or C antigens and that most or all of the others may be secondary to other, primarily viral, infections.[254–255a] If this syndrome occurs in children, it is rare; so far, we have been unable to demonstrate hepatitis B antigen, significantly positive tests for rheumatoid factor, or significant cryoglobulinemia in any of our childhood patients with systemic vasculitis. One infant with hepatitis-B-associated vasculitis has been reported.[133]

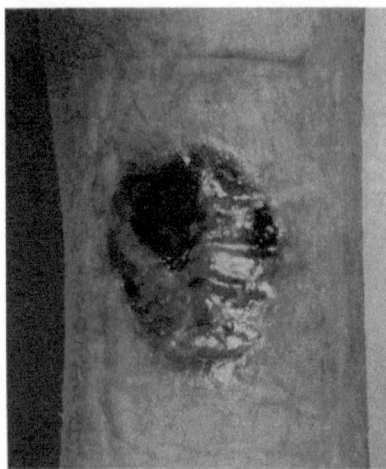

Figure 7.33. Cutaneous vasculitis and lupuslike syndrome induced in a young girl by propylthiouracil. Arthritis or connective-tissue-disease-like reactions occur in 10% of children treated with antithyroid medications.

Hypocomplementemic Vasculitis. Patients with what has been called hypocomplementemic vasculitis have recurrent attacks of hives or leukoclastic angiitis; low levels of serum complement can be demonstrated during the attacks.[256–259] Other manifestations during these acute episodes may include abdominal distress, arthralgias, and increased intracranial pressure (pseudotumor cerebri). Rarely, these patients may develop mild membranoproliferative glomerulonephritis. Fatal hypocomplementemic vasculitis may be seen as a feature of Wiskott-Aldrich syndrome.[238]

Neonatal Vasculitis. One report of simultaneous vasculitis in a mother and newborn infant is of particular interest to pediatricians.[260] The mother had hypersensitivity vasculitis during the pregnancy; the infant developed neonatal gangrene. This syndrome must be differentiated from pheochromocytoma, which can produce a similar clinical picture. (See below for description of determinations required to exclude pheochromocytoma.)

Vasculitis as a Manifestation of Malignancy. Cutaneous vasculitis (palpable purpura), PAN, and granulomatous angiitis of the CNS occasionally occur as a manifestation of malignancy, most often hairy-cell leukemia, lymphoma, or Hodgkin's disease.[261,262] It is presumed that this represents a hypersensitivity reaction to tumor or tumor-related antigens; in some cases, mixed cryoglobulinemia is associated with the vasculitis.

Vasculitis as a Complication of Drug Therapy. Cutaneous vasculitis, PAN, and cerebral vasculitis may occur as complications of drug therapy with pylthiouracil (Fig. 7.33) phenytoin, guanethidine, interferon and methotrexate, and occasionally as an exaggerated type of serum-sickness reaction to other drugs.[263–267a] We have seen a child whose multiple-extremity ischemic

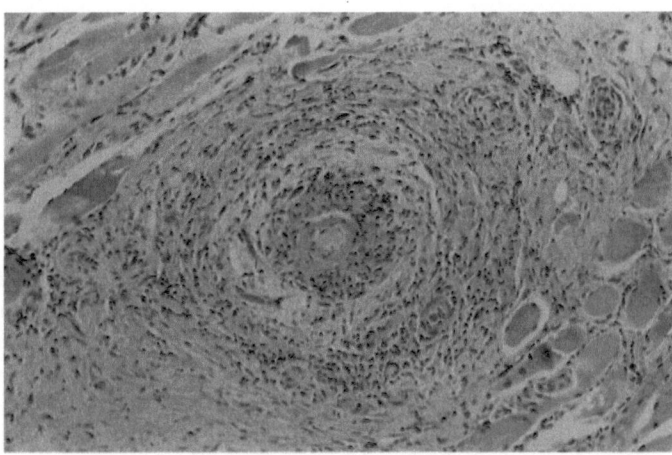

Figure 7.34. Necrotizing vasculitis seen in a gastrocnemius muscle-biopsy performed on an 11-year-old boy with spondyloarthritis and unrecognized Crohn's disease. Patient was thought originally to have PAN, but all musculoskeletal symptoms subsided with control of the Crohn's disease. ×250. (Courtesy of Dr. Adolfo Firpo.)

amputations, resembling vasculitis, were a complication of treatment of hypotension with dopamine, a syndrome described by Golbranson.[268] Phenylpropanolamine, contained in over-the-counter decongestants and diet pills, may cause cerebral vasculitis and hemorrhage.[269]

Vasculitis Associated with Drug Abuse. A syndrome identical to PAN has been identified in drug abusers; intravenous methamphetamine is the most likely causative agent.[270,271] Diseased vessels include medium-sized small arteries in most organs and arterioles in the brain. Some patients with angiographically demonstrated lesions have been asymptomatic. In others, renal failure, hypertension, pulmonary edema, cerebral hemorrhage, and pancreatitis have led to death.

Vasculitis as a Feature of Inflammatory Bowel Disease. Cutaneous angiitis (palpable purpura) is sometimes seen as a manifestation of inflammatory bowel disease (IBD). On rare occasions, necrotizing arteritis or allergic angiitis may be demonstrated in muscle, in mesenteric arteries and veins, in pulmonary arterioles, and in the brain of patients with IBD.[272–274] Occasionally, the history of bowel disease may be hidden or overshadowed by the vasculitic manifestations, resulting in erroneous diagnosis of the basic disorder (Fig. 7.34). We have also seen one child with middle aortic syndrome complicating IBD.

Mesenteric Arteritis Following Repair of Coarctation of the Aorta. A syndrome of mesenteric arteritis with abdominal pain and tenderness, ileus, vomiting, intestinal bleeding, and fever has been reported in children who have developed hypertension following surgical repair of coarctation of the aorta.[275] Bowel necrosis has not occurred and the syndrome subsides with antihypertensive drug treatment.

Cutaneous Vasculitis

Cutaneous PAN. Palpable purpura—the purpuric papula of necrotizing dermal vasculitis—the most typical dermal lesion of all forms of systemic vasculitis, may also occur without systemic manifestations.[276,277] Lesions may come and go over a period of months and years. The only laboratory abnormality is elevation of the ESR. Although this syndrome has been called by Winkelman and others "cutaneous periarteritis nodosa," we find that term confusing. It suggests to some physicians that the patient has a systemic disorder when he doesn't and suggests to others that they may safely presume the disorder is limited to skin even though they have not adequately excluded involvement of more vital organs. What has been called "cutaneous periarteritis nodosa" is actually the mildest form of hypersensitivity vasculitis.

Segmental Hyalinizing Vasculitis. Segmental hyalinizing vasculitis (livedoid vasculitis, atrophie blanche) is a clinically distinctive chronic, segmental, hyalinizing vasculitis of the middle dermal vessels of the lower extremities that occurs almost exclusively in females.[278] By definition, this diagnosis is limited to patients who are otherwise healthy and have no signs of systemic disease, and in whom a diagnosis of primary hyperoxaluria has been excluded.[279] The primary lesion is focal purpura of the lower extremity that proceeds to an infarctive ulcer covered with a dark adherent eschar surrounded by a border of inflammation (Fig. 7.35). Lesions are present in various stages of development. Healing of the ulcers takes months and is followed by the development of a smooth, ivory-white, stellate, atrophic scar (atrophic blanche) surrounded by a hyperpigmented border (Fig. 7.36). Most affected individuals have extensive *livedo reticularis*, a reddish-purple reticulated blotchy pattern on the trunk or extremities. Unlike the normal mottling seen in infants exposed to cold (cutis marmorata), livedo reticularis remains even after the skin has been warmed; histologic examination of longstanding lesions shows endarteritis and endophlebitis.

This disorder is characterized by exacerbations and remissions over a period of many years. Occasionally, the patients improve, and the lesions disappear completely without any specific therapy. A few patients have been reported to respond to treatment with aspirin and dipyridamole, the combination of ethylestranol with fenformin, low-dose heparin, or other fibrinolytic regimens.[2,278,280] A 13-year-old boy with 6 years of disease responded to nifedipine.[281] These lesions do not respond to corticosteroid therapy, un-

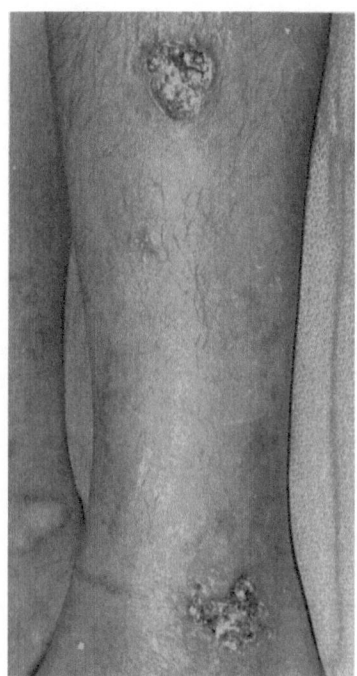

Figure 7.35. Lower legs of a 10-year-old girl with segmental hyalinizing vasculitis (livedoid vasculitis, atrophie blanche), showing livedoid rash, early purpuric lesion that develops into an infarctive ulcer with a dark eschar surrounded by a border of inflammation and multiple ulcers. Healing takes place over a period of months and is followed by the appearance of an ivory-white stellate, atrophic scar (atrophie blanche) that is surrounded by a hyperpigmented border.

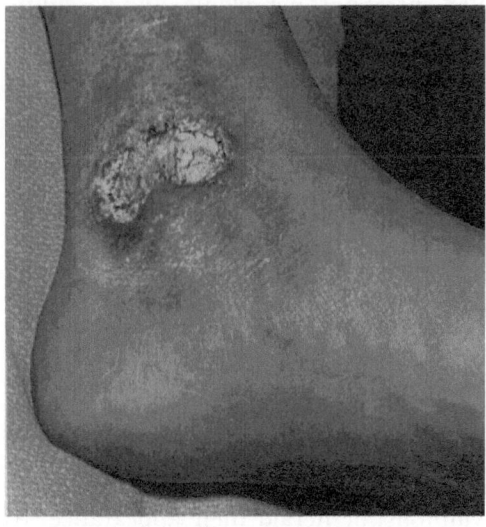

Figure 7.36. Infarctive ankle ulcer, typical of segmental hyalinizing vasculitis (see also Fig. 7.35).

like the livedo and similar lesions that sometimes occur as manifestations of vasculitis in the systemic connective-tissue diseases.

Erythema Elevatum Diutinum. Several children have been reported to have a chronic or recurrent vasculitic rash characterized by painful red, purple, or blue papules, plaques, and nodules over the extensor surfaces of the extremities, especially over the knees, elbows, and hands. The lesions are characterized histopathologically by a dense, mainly neutrophilic, leukoclastic angiitis with fibrinoid necrosis of the upper and mid-dermal vessel walls.[282,283] In some patients, this is associated with chronic infection and an undefined increased susceptibility to infection. Severe arthralgias may accompany the eruption of these lesions. Some authors believe they can distinguish this entity pathologically and have called it erythema elevatum diutinum. Since the lesions suggested the possibility of an Arthus reaction, dapsone, a drug known in experimental animals to inhibit the development of Arthus reactions, was administered, with prompt disappearance of the lesions. However, in most cases the lesions and rheumatic symptoms recurred as soon as the dapsone was stopped.[283] Dapsone has been associated with the development of fatal aplastic anemia and is carcinogenic in some animals.

Behçet's Syndrome

Behçet's syndrome, originally described as recurrent genital and oral ulceration with relapsing iritis, and or conjunctivitis, is included in this chapter because the basic pathologic lesion appears to be a vasculitis.[284–288] In addition to the mucocutaneous-ocular symptom complex, patients with Behçet's syndrome also often develop articular, intestinal, neurologic, and vasculitic manifestations.[287] Children have a lower frequency of ocular disease.[289]

Clinical Presentation. When the disease has its onset in childhood painful recurrent mouth ulcers are generally the only manifestation (Fig. 7.37).[290–295] If arthritis and uveitis occur, these children are generally thought to have JRA. It is only later, when genital ulcers appear, that the syndrome is recognized.

The arthritis of Behçet's syndrome is often a minor manifestation and tends to be primarily in the knees and ankles.[285,296] The mild and recurrent episodes resemble those seen in patients with spondyloarthritis. Radiographic changes are rare, and when sacroiliac changes are demonstrable, they are generally very mild. The most commonly affected upper-extremity joints are the wrists and elbows.

Gastrointestinal complains are common in Behçet's syndrome and resemble those seen in patients with inflammatory bowel disease. Erythema nodosum may accompany the bowel symptoms or herald their appearance. At coloscopy, the findings in these patients are sometimes indistinguishable

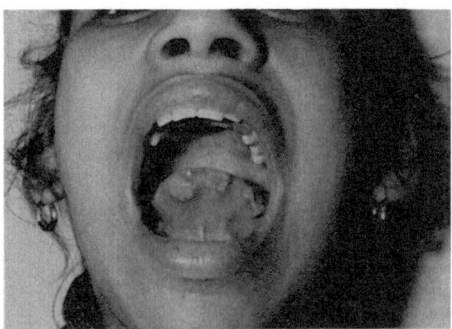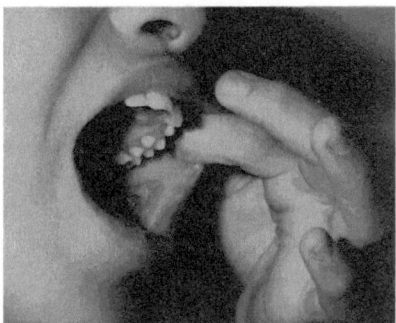

Figure 7.37. Behçet's syndrome; mouth ulcers began in early childhood and were followed in adolescence by genital ulcers and gastrointestinal symptoms (Fig. 7.38).[292]

from granulomatous or ulcerative colitis.[292] However, severe esophageal ulcers are more common in Behçet's syndrome[292–294] (Fig. 7.38), and discrete vesicles and localized ulceration may be demonstrated at various sites within an otherwise-completely-normal gastrointestinal tract. These lesions resemble the aphthous ulcers seen in the mouth and genitals and suggest this diagnosis.

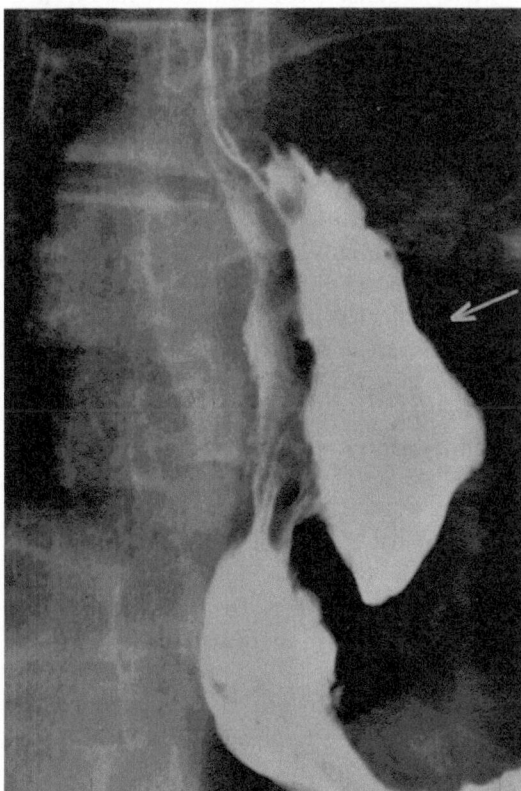

Figure 7.38. Colonic and esophageal ulcers have required surgery. The film shows a huge undermining esophageal ulcer (*arrow*) that looks like a diverticulum. The ulcer was adherent to the aorta but was removed prior to any dissection into the aorta.

Neurologic manifestations occur in about 25% of patients with Behçet's syndrome at some time during the disease and may wax and wane along with the other manifestations.[295,295a] Aseptic meningitis is the most frequent CNS manifestation, but transient ocular palsies, cerebellar ataxia, cerebral venous sinus thrombosis,[298,299] cerebral vasculitis,[297] and corticospinal-tract involvement resulting in hemi- or quadriparesis may occur.

Aortitis, vena caval obstruction from thrombophlebitis, multiple pulmonary artery aneurysms,[300,301] and other arterial aneurysms may occur.[286] Coronary arteritis is rare.[300]

During acute exacerbations of Behçet's synbdrome the skin may show a peculiar hyperreactivity to needle puncture.[285,287,288] Within 24 h, a pustule surrounded by a red halo appears at the site of the puncture. This phenomenon has been reported to be associated with increased random mobility and chemotaxis of polymorphonuclear leukocytes. The unusual response to needle puncture may provide a "diagnostic test" for Behçet's syndrome and has led to therapeutic trials of colchicine, a drug that inhibits white-blood-cell chemotaxis.[302] Erythema nodosum, pyoderma, and dermal vasculitis are other dermatologic manifestations.[303]

Immunopathology. Vascular and perivascular infiltration by polymorphs and lymphocytes has been seen in many organs. These exudative lesions are followed by vascular fibrosis and are often accompanied by nonspecific inflammatory foci in nearby tissues. Small vessels, veins as well as arteries, are affected in all patients. Necrotizing and granulomatous inflammation of the aorta (and occasionally also the pulmonary artery) occurs in a small number of patients but has not been reported in children.

Epidemiology. As with the other vasculitic disorders, there appears to be an increased incidence in Japan. Uveitis associated with Behçet's syndrome is reported to account for 12% of all blindness in Japan. Males are more frequently affected (1.7:1). Studies of large affected families suggest autosomal dominant inheritance with variable penetrance.[291] In Japan, increased susceptibility has been linked to HLA-B5, but this has not been found in the United States, which suggests that the linkage may be racially coincidental rather than a reflection of an abnormality of an immune-response gene linked to HLA-B5.

Course of the Disease. When the disease begins in childhood, the sole manifestation is generally recurrent mouth sores (Fig. 7.37). Genital ulcers appear in the teens and may then be accompanied by the other manifestations of the disease. Occasionally, the entire syndrome may appear in young children. Gastrointestinal manifestations may be most prominent in children, making differentiation from IBD difficult. In one child reported from our clinic, esophageal lesions with perforation and episodes of gastrointestinal obstruction were the most troublesome features.[292] The disease may be associated with many exacerbations and remissions over a long course.

Therapy. Treatment should be individualized; we have one patient who has only required ibuprofen. Our experience with corticosteroid therapy in two childhood patients was generally satisfactory for many years. Exacerbations in one were treated with daily prednisone, and maintenance of a relatively normal life-style was achieved in both with maintenance alternate-day prednisone. The major system being treated was gastrointestinal; the mouth and genital ulcers also promptly responded. Similar results have been reported by others. However, in young adulthood one girl developed a chronic esophageal ulcer impinging on the aorta which required surgical excision (Fig. 7.38). Prior to surgery, there were intractable symptoms of esophagitis and one episode of apparent esophageal perforation. A similar intractable ulcer was removed from the colon at the same time. Thus, the use of prednisone is not wholly satisfactory in this disorder.[292]

It has recently been reported that, in some patients, the ocular lesions of Behçet's syndrome have been prevented by daily administration of colchicine, with a regimen analogous to that used in patients with familial Mediterranean fever (see Chapter 2 under Familial Mediterranean Fever).[304] Genital and oral ulcers were reduced in some patients, but the other manifestations of the disease were generally not benefited as much as the ocular symptoms. Some patients require immunosuppressive therapy; the most effective agent seems to be chlorambucil.[305]

Neonatal Behçet's Syndrome

There is one report of neonatally transmitted disease which was transient but left facial scars.[306]

Cogan's Syndrome

Bilateral nerve deafness and interstitial keratitis (without syphilis) constitute Cogan's syndrome.[307–311] Occasionally, the keratitis is accompanied by iritis. Patients tend to have recurrent attacks resulting in progressive deafness and threatening vision. Primarily young Caucasians are affected.

Twenty-three percent of patients have been reported to have musculoskeletal manifestations, usually arthralgia or mild arthritis. Ten percent of reported cases were associated with life-threatening aortic insufficiency, which sometimes occurred suddenly and unexpectedly.[307–309,311] Pathologic examination in these cases has shown fibrinoid necrosis of the media of the aorta. Necrotizing angiitis may occur in the gastrointestinal tract, spleen, kidneys, and brain and may result in gastrointestinal bleeding or stroke.

Vestibuloauditory symptoms and keratitis may also be features of a number of other vasculitic syndromes. Iritis and sensorineural deafness are seen in relapsing polychondritis; HLA-B27-associated spondyloarthritis;[312] Heerfordt's syndrome (with seventh nerve palsy); Vogt-Koyanagi syndrome (with alopecia, poliosis, and vitiligo); and Harada's syndrome (with cells and protein in spinal fluid). The cause of all of these syndromes is unknown, and they may all be related to one another.

We follow two children with *recurrent* attacks of sensorineural deafness, iritis or keratitis, and arthritis. One patient developed the illness at age 10 years and has permanent auditory impairment. In the other child, the onset was in the first months of life and was accompanied by a vasculitic skin rash (Fig. 2.41). The arthritis in this more severely affected child was radiologically typical of that seen in relapsing polychondritis (Fig. 2.42) and was controlled with an alternate-day steroid regimen; growth and development were inadequate with aspirin treatment alone. Her male sibling has congenital nerve deafness without any other manifestations.

Recent experience suggests that most permanent hearing loss may be prevented by treating single episodes of acute hearing loss in patients with Cogan's syndrome promptly and vigorously with prednisone[310] as illustrated here:

Case Report 1

An 11-year-old boy presented with severe polyarthritis, keratitis, transient hematuria and proteinura, and some hand and foot desquamation 2 weeks after a respiratory illness with otalgia. The arthritis subsided dramatically with naproxen. However, 3 days later he returned with a bulging right tympanic membrane, clouding of the right mastoid, bilateral severe nerve deafness, and severe vertigo. Culture of tympanic fluid revealed mycoplasma pneumoniae. He responded slowly to treatment with prednisome 60 mg daily (1 mg/kg) which was changed to 150 mg QOD. Two months elapsed, and the prednisone was gradually weaned over the next few months. He regained normal vestibular function and speech discrimination but retains 60-dB high-frequency (4000–8000 Hz) sensorineural hearing loss. He is completely well 7 years later.

Case Report 2

A 14-year-old girl developed severe keratoconjunctivitis which persisted for 3 months. Five months later she complained of sore throat and headache and was found to have exudative tonsillitis from which a heavy growth of group A beta-hemolytic streptococcus was documented; urinalysis showed hematuria. She improved with treatment with penicillin but 2 weeks later had a recurrence of identical signs and symptoms. She again responded to antibiotic treatment but then developed severe polyarthritis, bilateral nerve deafness, and severe vertigo. She responded slowly to treatment with prednisone 60 mg daily (1.25 mg/kg); hearing improved but after a month of treatment declined with change of prednisone dosage to 150 mg QOD, did not improve with 300 mg QOD, and finally was controlled with a pulse steroid regimen 1 gram daily for 3 days, followed by 300 mg of prednisone QOD. Prednisone was weaned to 100 mg QOD over a 2-month period with weekly audiologic monitoring but hearing then again deteriorated, requiring three additional 1-gram solumedrol daily pulses as a supplement to the oral alternate-day therapy. Over the next 3 months prednisone was slowly weaned and the patient has remained well for 4 subsequent years. Vestibular function and speech discrimination have returned to normal but bilateral high-frequency (4000–8000 Hz) 75-dB sensorineural hearing loss persists.

Malignant Atrophic Papulosis (Kohlmeier-Degos Disease)

Malignant atrophic papulosis is a lethal intestinal-oculo-neural-cutaneous disorder that is heralded by the appearance of pathognomonic atrophic white skin papules that resemble atrophie blanche.[313,314] At this stage, the lesions, which are most often on the trunk and extremities, generally go unnoticed. After a varying period of time, gastrointestinal or neurologic manifestations appear; either may predominate. The abdominal symptoms usually include intermittent severe infarctive pain and episodes resembling intestinal obstruction and malabsorption. The multifocal central- and peripheral-nervous-system manifestations are suggestive of diffuse vasculitis and may be accompanied by papilledema, optic atrophy, and blindness. Carotid arteriograms in such patients show multiple occlusions in many cerebral vessels; CT scan confirms a loss of brain substance and areas of decreased perfusion.

Death is frequently secondary to intestinal performation as a result of vascular insufficiency but may also result from loss of cerebral function. At autopsy, necrotizing vasculitis is found in the skin, gastrointestinal tract, retina, and brain. The cause of the disorder is unknown. Too few cases have been vigorously treated to allow any statement about the potential for therapeutic response.

Juvenile Temporal Arteritis

In older adults, giant-cell arteritis of the temporal arteries has been associated with a diffuse vasculitis syndrome termed polymyalgia rheumatica. This syndrome has not been reported in children. Occasionally, however, a lump forms over the temporal artery of a youngster. While these lumps are asymptomatic, they may be cosmetically disfiguring, which leads to their surgical removal. Generally, a traumatic aneurysm is seen grossly and on histologic examination, but occasionally a non–giant-cell granulomatous inflammation is reported by the pathologist, and a diagnosis of temporal arteritis is suggested.[315,316]

There have been no instances in which this lesion was a manifestation of systemic arteritis, and no "workup" of these healthy patients is required. "Juvenile temporal arteritis" is a benign, presumably posttraumatic lesion of

Table 7.10. Disorders Simulating Systemic Vasculitis

Left atrial myxoma
Hereditary disorders of amino-acid metabolism
Homocystinuria
Sulfite oxidase deficiency
Primary hyperoxaluria
Pheochromocytoma
Hypercoaguable states (Antithrombin III,
Protein C, Protein S, Heparin cofactor II
deficiencies)
Moyamoya
Hemiplegic migraine
Toxic shock syndrome
Goodpasture's syndrome

only cosmetic import. However, surgeons should be aware of this condition so that when they remove lumps over the temporal artery (often performed as an office procedure), they are prepared to ligate the feeding vessels in order to avoid troublesome intraoperative hemorrhage.

Disorders Simulating Systemic Vasculitis

A number of disorders may mimic the systemic vasculitis syndromes (Table 7.10).

Left Atrial Myxoma

Arthralgia or cramping extremity pain, nonspecific or hemorrhagic and vasculitic rashes, Raynaud's phenomenon, stroke, and signs of systemic illness (fever, weight loss, anemia, elevated ESR, SGOT, CPK, anti-DNA antibodies, lowered serum complement, and hypergammaglobulinemia) may be manifestations of a cardiac myxoma, usually in the left atrium.[1,2,317,318] Systemic embolism of myxomatous tissue or overlying thrombus occurs frequently in these patients and may be found in the brain, gastrointestinal tract, kidney, heart, and extremities. Inflammation about the emboli produces the clinical presentation and suggests a vasculitic multisystem illness. Although at least subtle signs of cardiac disease are probably always present, the clinician may be distracted away from the heart as the primary source of the trouble by the multitude of signs suggestive of connective-tissue disease. Myxomatous material may not be noted on biopsy of an occluded vessel, and necrosis and perivascular inflammation may seem to confirm the diagnosis of a connective-tissue disorder.

Diagnosis is best accomplished by cross-sectional (two-dimensional) echocardiography, now performed in all children with mysterious vasculitis or stroke. It is said that this procedure will eliminate the need for more invasive angiocardiography to demonstrate cardiac tumors. We have misdiagnosed a child with atrial myxoma, and while tumors of the heart are rare, they do occur in children and may be curable. Malignant infiltrative cardiac tumors are very rare in childhood but repetitive 2D echocardiograms may be required for diagnosis.[319]

Hereditary Disorders of Amino-Acid Metabolism Simulating Systemic Vasculitis

Inborn errors of metabolism causing either accumulation of unmetabolized toxic products and/or deficiencies of essential unsynthesizable compounds may result in clinical syndromes characterized by systemic vasculitis and strokes (acute infantile hemiplegia). Two well-described deficiency diseases of this type are homocystinuria and sulfite oxidase deficiency. They should be considered prototypes, and when carotid artery occlusion occurs in childhood in the absence of these disorders, new and undescribed metabolic abnormalities should be sought.

Homocystinuria (Cystathianine Synthase Deficiency). Children with homocystinuria phenotypically look like patients with Marfan's syndrome.[320] Their propensity to intravascular thrombosis (stroke, coronary occlusion, renal artery thrombosis with hypertension, and multiple arterial and venous thrombosis), livedo reticularis, and abnormal nailfold capillaries, features suggestive of other disorders of connective tissue, causes diagnostic confusion. Downward dislocation of the lens (ectopia lentis), generalized skeletal demineralization, striking malar flush, and mental retardation, together with the Marfan habitus, help to suggest the correct diagnosis, which is documented in homozygotes by demonstration of homocystine in urine and increased amounts of homocysteine and methionine in serum. Heterozygotes are also at increased risk of premature peripheral and cerebral occlusive arterial disease and can only be identified by a methionine loading test.[320]

Homocystinuria is the second-most-common inborn error of amino-acid metabolism and is inherited as autosomal-recessive. Although all patients have deficient activity of the enzyme cystathionine synthetase, there is considerable heterogeneity in clinical manifestations. It is thought that the high circulating levels of homocysteine in these patients interfere with the cross-linking of collagen producing the connective-tissue changes. At the molecular level, homocystinuria is probably also a heterogeneous disorder. Some patients have a defect that responds to pyridoxine therapy, while no satisfactory therapy has been found for others. The effectiveness of vitamin B_6 can be tested on cultured skin fibroblasts from the patient and can also be determined by measuring changes in the child's serum levels of homocysteine and methionine and the urinary levels of homocystine following treatment.[320]

Sulfite Oxidase Deficiency. A few children with strokes and ectopia lentis (but without Marfan habitus) have been found to be unable to normally metabolize ingested sulfur to inorganic sulfate and, therefore, to have sulfite and S-sulfocysteine in plasma, and abnormal sulfur-containing metabolites (sulfite, thiosulfite, and S-sulfocysteine) in their urine.[321] No enzymatic activity of sulfite oxidase could be demonstrated in cultured skin fibroblasts. The parents had intermediate levels of enzyme activity, suggesting auto-somal-recessive inheritance.

Screening of children with stroke for this disorder is difficult. Sulfite is unstable in urine, and the urinary amino-acid findings may be missed by one-dimensional chromatographic screening. The best screening methodology involves two-dimensional separation of urinary amino acids and measurement of thiosulfate in relatively fresh urine.

It is not yet known whether early diagnosis and dietary treatment of these patients will prevent the development of symptoms.

Primary Hyperoxaluria[279]

Although the primary manifestations of this rare genetic disorder are oxalate nephrolithiasis and ultimately renal failure, livedo reticularis, peripheral ischemia, and gangrene may result from deposits of oxalate crystals in blood vessels. Diagnosis is established by biopsy showing the crystals with special techniques. Vasculitis has not yet been reported in childhood; the clue to the diagnosis is antecedent renal failure following nephrolithiasis.

Pheochromocytoma

Cool, pale, painful cyanotic extremities with livedo reticularis may suggest systemic vasculitis in patients who have a pheochromocytoma.[322] The symptoms are caused by diffuse arterial spasm caused by tumor-secreted metanephrine. Although vasomotor phenomena are common in pheochromocytoma, they are almost always accompanied by paroxysms of headache, cortical blindness, tachycardia, sweating, pallor, weakness, chest pain, and hypertension. Catecholamines may induce toxic myocarditis/myocardiopathy. Diagnosis is established by demonstration of elevated urine and serum catecholamines and may be confirmed by scintigraphic localization with [131I] meta-iodobenzylguanidine ([131I] MIBG).[323]

Alpha- and beta-adrenergic blockade should be promptly instituted in suspected cases. These agents do not interfere with diagnostic biochemical studies. Following localization and control of blood pressure, the tumor is extirpated.

Hypercoagulable States

Stroke and both venous and arterial thromboembolic disease occur in rheumatic disorders; congenital and acquired hypercoagulable states may lead to disorders simulating rheumatic disease, exist coexistent with them, or be acquired as one manifestation of SLE.[324] The most common of these disorders are antithrombin III and protein C or S deficiency; less frequent heritable disorders include disorders of fibrinogen (abnormal reptilase time), fibrinolytic disorders (defective plasminogen or release of plasminogen activator), and cystathionine beta-synthase deficiency (hypermethioninemia). Periphereal venous emboli may result in stroke as a result of paradoxical embolism through a patent foramen ovale.[325]

The anticardiolipin syndrome is a term used for patients whose propensity to stroke is associated with these antibodies without other signs of rheumatic disease (see Chapter 5). The frequency of these antibodies in association with childhood stroke has not yet been established and how to treat such patients also remains to be determined.[326,327]

When stroke is associated with livedo reticularis the combination, often associated with antiphospholipid antibodies, is termed Snedden's syndrome.[328]

MELAS Syndrome: (Mitochondrial Encephalomyopathy with Lactic Acidosis and Stroke)

Short stature, sensorineural hearing loss, basal-ganglia calcifications on CT scan, episodes of nausea and vomiting with lactic acidosis, gradual decline in cognitive function, and cerebral infarction/stroke–like episodes characterize this familial disorder thought to be due to defects of respiratory enzymes.[329]

Moyamoya

Moyamoya is the term applied to the arteriographic demonstration of multiple stenoses of vessels in and around the circle of Willis, together with the appearance of telangiectasia of collateral vessels.[330] In the few cases examined postmortem, there has been a lack of inflammatory change suggestive of vasculitis.[331] However, thickening of the intima and loss of the elastic membrane have been noted. In one reported case, there was evidence of a systemic vascular abnormality characterized by many years of "chilblains," with gangrene of the fingers and ears.[332] In another fatal case, an elevated ESR and high levels of gamma globulin suggested the possibility of inflammatory vasculitis. The moyamoya angiographic pattern has been demonstrated in a variety of conditions and is probably a secondary reaction to abnormalities in the vessels in and around the circle of Willis. In children with seizures and hemiplegia, therefore, presence of the moyamoya pattern

Table 7.11. Contrasts and Similarities Between Kawasaki Disease (KD) and Toxic Shock Syndrome (TSS)

Clinical Features	KD	TSS
Fever	Precedes other manifestations or accompanies their gradual evolution over 5 days	Accompanied by dramatic illness at onset or within 48 h
Rash	Polymorphous at onset	Diffuse erythroderma at onset; maculopapular rash appears a week later
Extremity changes	Palmar erythema with edema of the hands and feet	Same
Eye findings	Conjunctival hyperemia	Conjunctival hyperemia with brawny edema of the eyelids and face
Mouth lesions	Oropharyngeal hyperemia with strawberry tongue	Same; complaints of sore throat at onset that becomes more severe
	Bleeding cracked lips	Not present
Cervical lymphadenopathy	Often unilateral and severe	Not present
Hypotension	Absent	Present
CNS	Normal/irritable	Severe headache, disoriented or altered consciousness
GI	Diarrhea may occur but usually not present at onset	Vomiting and diarrhea
Sex and age	Rare over age 4 years	Usually young menstruating females
	Most common 12–18 months	
	Males slightly more frequently affected (1:3:1)	
Laboratory Abnormalities		
CPK	Normal	Elevated
Platelet count	Elevated	200,000 (40% 100,000)
Bilirubin	Usually normal	Elevated
Creatinine, BUN, uric acid, lactate	Normal	High
Calcium	Normal	< 7.8 mg/dl
Phosphorus	Normal	< 2.2 mg/dl
Total protein	Normal	< 5.6 mg/dl
Sodium	Normal	< 120 mEq/liter

Calcium, Phosphorus, Total protein, Sodium: in about 50% of case[341]

Table 7.11. (Continued)

Clinical Features	KD	TSS
Urinalysis	Sterile pyuria	Sterile pyuria with casts
CSF	Pleocytosis in those with meningeal signs	Same
SGOT/PT	Occasionally elevated at onset	Usually elevated
Chest x-ray	Usually normal	50% diffuse interstitial infilrates; 25% pleural effusion

on angiogram should not be considered an exclusion to consideration of the possibility of lupus or cerebral vasculitis as the primary disorder.[333]

Hemiplegic Migraine

Alternating hemiplegia in childhood may also be a manifestation of episodic cerebral vasospasm (hemiplegic migraine).[334] In this disorder, the manifestations of cerebral ischemia are a result of spasm rather than inflammation of cerebral vessels. Hemiplegic migraine is usually familial with autosomal-dominant transmission. Differentiation from cerebral vasculitis, even with angiography, may be difficult but must be attempted, since therapy of hemiplegic migraine requires phenytoin and/or propranolol. There is no evidence that hemiplegic migraine responds to corticosteroids or other drugs used in the treatment of vasculitis.[334]

Goodpasture's Syndrome

Pulmonary hemorrhage associated with circulating immune complexes and rapidly progressive glomerulonephritis may occur in PAN, SLE, Wegener's granulomatosis, or as an independent disorder.[204,335,336] Although the diagnosis of Goodpasture's syndrome was initially based solely on the clinical association of glomerulonephritis and pulmonary hemorrhage, it has recently become popular to restrict the term to patients in whom antiglomerular basement-membrane (anti-GBM) antibody can be demonstrated in serum and as linear deposits with complement along glomerular basement membranes. Patients without anti-GBM antibodies but with immune-complex nephritis and pulmonary hemorrhage are considered a separate group.

Patients with either idiopathic immune-complex nephritis with pulmonary hemorrhage or with Goodpasture's syndrome with antiglomerular basement-membrane antibody-induced nephritis do not have clinical, laboratory, or pathologic evidence of systemic vasculitis. They generally present with hemoptysis, radiographic evidence of pulmonary hemorrhage, profound anemia, and rapidly progressive glomerulonephritis without clinical or laboratory evidence of polyarteritis or lupus. The physician must be alert to the pulmonary hemorrhage-nephritis constellation, as these syndromes require immediate dynamic management. All forms of pulmonary capillaritis with hemorrhage are often rapidly fatal—before definitive diagnosis is possible.[204,336,337] We use pheresis, pulse steroids, and cyclophosphamide, without delay, for these emergencies.[338]

Toxic Shock Syndrome

The sudden onset of high fever, headache, shaking chills, vomiting, diarrhea, sore throat, diffuse myalgias, and confusion—often toward the end of a young woman's menstrual period, especially with tampon use—is characteristic of toxic shock syndrome (TSS; Table 7.11).[339-342] The presence of rash, described as diffuse macular erythroderma, and dilated conjunctival blood vessels in a younger child might suggest the possibility of KD. However, *the pattern of presenting manifestations in TSS at any age is much more acute than in KD.* All the symptoms tend to appear at once, and the patient appears very toxic and is often hypotensive when first seen. This acute presentation, as a result of a massive movement of serum proteins, electrolytes, and fluid from the intravascular to the extravascular compartment, characterizes TSS. The onset of KD, in contrast, is generally characterized first by fever alone, and the symptoms evolve over a few days without the initial toxic appearance typical of TSS. Massive cervical lymphadenopathy, often present in KD, is not a feature of TSS. Sore throat, diarrhea, and severe headache are generally present on the first day of TSS, and many patients become disoriented or have an altered state of consciousness by the second day. Familiarity with the appearance of the conjunctiva in children with KD, however, may alert the physician to the early diagnosis of TSS, as the striking conjunctival hyperemia is similar in both disorders.

Laboratory tests help to confirm the diagnosis of TSS. Elevations of BUN, creatinine, uric acid, CPK, bilirubin, SGOT, SGPT, and lactate together with striking reductions in serum calcium, phosphorus, total protein, and albumin are typical of TSS; jaundice is uncommon in KD, and elevations in SGOT/PT are not seen during the first 2 days of illness. Patients with TSS also usually have thrombocytopenia when first seen, whereas 98% of children with KD have normal or elevated platelet counts at the onset of the disease.[57]

The differing age and sex incidence, presenting manifestations, and clinical setting usually make the distinction between KD and TSS apparent even before the laboratory results are known. However, both syndromes may occur at any age and in either sex.[342-345] "Physicians should consider a diagnosis of TSS in all patients with appropriate signs and symptoms, regardless of the patient's age, sex, race, or menstrual status."[342] During the recovery period, skin desquamation may occur in similar fashion in both diseases, but the striking subungual peel that is so typical of KD is not seen in TSS.

Loss of hair and nails occurs in 10% of patients with TSS 2–3 months after the illness.

Treatment of TSS. TSS is usually related to infection with coagulase-positive staphylococci[342] and should be treated promptly with beta-lactamase-resistant antimicrobial agents. Gamma globulin treatment may be effective, just as in KD.[346] All but the most mildly affected individuals require vigorous restoration of the intravascular fluid volume, and many require additional drug therapy to restore and maintain adequate blood pressure. Ventilatory assistance and renal dialysis may also be required.[342] Epidemics caused by other infectious agents may occur.[344,347]

References

1. Fauci AS, Haynes BF, Katz P: The spectrum of vasculitis: Clinical, pathologic immunologic and therapeutic considerations. Ann Intern Med 89 (part 1):660–676, 1978.
1a. LeRoy EC (Ed): Systemic Vasculitis: The Biologic Basis. Marcel Dekker, New York, 1992.
2. Churg A, Churg J (Eds): Systemic Vasculitides. Igaku-Shoin. New York, 1991.
3. Hearth-Holmes M, Zahradka SL, Baethge BA, Wolf RE: Leukocytoclastic vasculitis associated with hepatitis C. Am J Med 90:765–766, 1991.
4. Levy M: Severe deficiency of alpha 1-antitrypsin associated with cutaneous vasculitis, rapidly progressive glomerulonephritis, and colitis. Am J Med 81:363, 1986.
5. Liang MH, Stern S, Fortin PR, et al.: Fatal pulmonary venoocclusive disease secondary to a generalized venulopathy: a new syndrome presenting with facial swelling and pericardial tamponade. Arthritis Rheum 34:228–233, 1991.
6. Yanagawa H, Kawasaki T, Shigematsu I: Nationwide survey on Kawasaki disease in Japan. Pediatrics 80:58–62, 1987.
7. Taubert KA, Rowley AH, Shulman ST: A seven year (1984–1990) U.S. Nationwide hospital survey of Kawasaki disease. Pediatr Research 31 #4 Pt 2:102A, 1992.
7a. Kim JJ, Donalds JS, Corydon KE, Shulman ST: Lymphadenitis as dominant presenting manifestation of Kawasaki disease. Pediatr Research 31 #4 Pt 2:123A, 1992.
8. Friter BS, Lucky AW: The perineal eruption of Kawasaki syndrome. Arch Dermatol 124:1805–1810, 1988.
9. Kawasaki T: Infectious disease (Japan) 7:19–32, 1977; an abstract of the diagnostic guidelines in English and color photographs are available from the Kawasaki Disease Research Information Center; Hosaka Bldg., 1–10 Kanda-Ogawamachi; Chiyoda-ku; Tokyo 101 Japan.
10. Melish ME, Hicks RM, Larson EJ: Mucocutaneous lymph node syndrome in the United States. Am J Dis Child 130:599–607, 1976.
11. Kawasaki T, Kosaki F, Okawa S, et al.: A new infantile acute febrile mucocutaneous lymph node syndrome prevailing in Japan. Pediatrics 54:271–281, 1974.

12. Kawasaki disease—it's official and it's here. Med World News 18 (December 12): 57–69, 1977.
13. A look at mucocutaneous lymph node syndrome. Consultant 18 (March): 60–61, 1978.
14. Fetterman GH, Hashida Y: Mucocutaneous lymph node syndrome: a disease widespread in Japan which demands our attention. Pediatrics 54:268–270, 1974.
15. Bures FA: Beau's lines in mucocutaneous lymph node syndrome. Am J Dis Child 135:383, 1981.
16. Sato K, Ouchi K, Taki M: Yersinia pseudotuberculosis infection in children, resembling Izumi fever and Kawasaki syndrome. Pediatr Infect Dis 2:123–126, 1983 (see also correspondence on p. 494).
17. Hurvitz H, Branski D, Gross-Kieselstein E, et al.: Acetaminophen hypersensitivity resembling Kawasaki disease. Israel J Med Sci 20:145–147, 1984.
18. Burns JC, Wiggin JW Jr, Toews WH, et al.: Clinical spectrum of Kawasaki disease in infants younger than 6 months of age. J Pediatr 109:759–763, 1986.
19. Rowley AH, Gonzalez-Crussi F, Gidding SS, et al.: Incomplete Kawasaki disease with coronary artery involvement. J Pediatr 110:409–413, 1987.
20. McCowen C, Henderson DC: Sudden death in incomplete Kawasaki's disease. Arch Dis Child 63:1254–1271, 1988.
21. Kohr RM: Progressive asymptomatic coronary artery disease as a late fatal sequela of Kawasaki disease. J Pediatr 108:256–259, 1990.
22. Chan KW, Kaikov Y, Wadsworth LD: Thrombocytosis in childhood: A survey of 94 patients. Pediatrics 84:1064–1067, 1989.
23. Byard RW, Edmonds JF, Silverman E, Silver MM: Respiratory distress and fever in a 2-month old infant. J Pediatr 118:306–313, 1991.
24. Kitamura S, Kawashima Y, Kawachi K, et al.: Left ventricular function in patients with coronary arteritis due to acute febrile mucocutaneous lymph node syndrome or related diseases. Am J Cardiol 40:156–164, 1977.
25. Tanaka N, Semimoto K, Fukushima T, et al.: Pathological study of fatal MCLS: relationship with infantile periarteritis nodosa. In Shiokawa Y (ed.). Vascular Lesions of Collagen Diseases and Related Conditions. University Park Press, Baltimore, 1977, pp. 296–307.
26. Landing BH, Larson EJ: Are infantile periarteritis nodosa with coronary artery involvement and fatal, mucocutaneous lymph node syndrome the same? Comparison of 20 patients from North America with patients from Hawaii and Japan. Pediatrics 59:651–662, 1977.
27. Fujiwara H, Hamashima Y: Pathology of the heart in Kawasaki disease. Pediatrics 61:100–107, 1978.
28. Fukushige J, Nihill MR, McNamara DG: Spectrum of cardiovascular lesions in mucocutaneous lymph node syndrome; analysis of eight cases. Am J Cardiol 45:98–107, 1980.
29. Onouchi Z, Tomizawa N, Goto M, et al.: Cardiac involvement and prognosis in acute mucocutaneous lymph node syndrome. Chest 68:297–301, 1975.
30. Yutani C, Go S, Kamiya T, et al.: Cardiac biopsy in Kawasaki disease. Arch Pathol Lab Med 105:470–473, 1981.
31. Westphalen MA, McGrath MA, Kelly W, et al.: Kawasaki disease with severe peripheral ischemia: treatment with prostaglandin E_1 infusion. J Pediatr 112:431–433, 1988.
32. Masuda H, Shozawa T, Naoe S, Tanaka N: The intercostal artery in Kawasaki

disease: a pathologic study of 17 autopsy cases. Arch Pathol Lab Med 110:1136–1142, 1986.

33. Fujiwara T, Fujiwara H, Nakano H: Pathological features of coronary arteries in children with Kawasaki disease in which coronary arterial aneurysm was absent at autopsy. Quantitative Analysis. Circulation 78:345–350, 1988.

34. Tanaka N, Naoe S, Masuda H, Ueno T: Pathological study of sequelae of Kawasaki disease (MCLS) with special reference to the heart and coronary arterial lesions. Acta Pathol Jpn 36:1513–1527, 1986.

35. Sasaguri Y, Kato H: Regression of aneurysms in Kawasaki disease: a pathological study. J Pediatr 100:225–231, 1982.

36. Kegel SM, Dorsey TJ, Rowen M, et al.: Cardiac death in mucocutaneous lymph node syndrome. Am J Cardiol 40:282–286, 1977.

37. Larson EJ: Comparative pathology of vasculitis: natural occurrence in lower animals. In Shiokawa Y (ed.) Vascular Lesions of Collagen Diseases and Related Conditions. University Park Press, Baltimore, 1977, pp. 347–355.

38. Lehman TJA, Warren R, Gietl D, et al.: Variable expression of lactobacillus casei cell wall-induced coronary arteritis: an animal model of Kawasaki's disease in selected inbred mouse strains. Clin Immunol Immunopathol 48:109–118, 1988.

39. Leung DY-M: New developments in Kawasaki disease. Curr Opin Rheum 3:46–55, 1990.

40. Kato S, Kimura M, Tsuji K, et al.: HLA anigens in Kawasaki disease. Pediatrics 61:252–255, 1978.

41. Krensky AM, Berenberg W, Shanley K, et al.: HLA antigens in mucocutaneous lymph node syndrome in New England. Pediatrics 67:741–743, 1981.

42. Fujita Y, Nakamura Y, Sakata K, et al.: Kawasaki disease in families. Pediatrics 84:666–669, 1989.

43. Daniels SR, Specker B: Association of rug shampooing and Kawasaki disease. J Ped 118:485–488, 1991.

44. Jacobs JC: Salicylate treatment of epidemic Kawasaki disease in New York City. Ther Drug Monitor 1:123–130, 1979.

45. Rauch AM, Kaplan SL, Nihill MR, et al.: Kawasaki syndrome clusters in Harris County, Texas, and Eastern North Carolina. A high endemic rate and a new environmental risk factor. Am J Dis Child 142:441–444, 1988.

46. Fatica NS, Ichida F, Engle MA, Lesser ML: Rug shampoo and Kawasaki disease. Pediatrics 84:231–234, 1989.

47. Rauch AM, Glode MP, Wiggins JW Jr., et al.: Outbreak of Kawasaki syndrome in Denver, Colorado: association with rug and carpet cleaning. Pediatrics 87:664–669, 1991.

48. Burns JC, Mason WH, Glode MP, et al.: Clinical and epidemiologic characteristics of patients referred for evaluation of possible Kawasaki disease. J Pediatr 118:680–686, 1991.

49. Bell DM, Brink EW, Nitzkin JL, et al.: Kawasaki syndrome: description of two outbreaks in the United States. N Engl J Med 304:1568–1575, 1981.

50. Jacobs JC: Asai score system. J Thorac Cardiovasc Surg 87:149, 1984.

51. Ichida F, Fatica NS, O'Loughlin JE, et al.: Correlation of electrocardiographic and echocardiographic changes in Kawasaki syndrome. Am Heart J 116:812, 1988.

52. Nakano H, Ueda K, Saito A, et al.: Scoring method for identifying patients with Kawasaki disease at high risk of coronary artery aneurysms. Am J Cardiol

58:739–742, 1986.

53. Chung KJ, Rinaldi RE, Fulton DR, et al.: Cardiac involvement with Kawasaki disease in children from New England, abstracted. Am J Cardiol 47:457, 1981.

54. Chusid MJ, Tang TT: Fever, diarrhea, anemia, rash, and acrocyanosis in a 2-month-old girl. J Pediatr 93:1052–1057, 1978.

55. Diller L, Newburger JW, Burns JC: Characterization of the anemia in Kawasaki disease (KD) patients (Pts). Pediatr Res 25S:177A, 1989.

56. Ishiguro N, Takahashi Y: Kawasaki disease associated with idiopathic thrombocytopenic purpura. Eur J Pediatr 148:379, 1989.

57. Hara T, Mizuno Y, Akeda H, et al.: Thrombocytopenia: a complication of Kawasaki disease. Eur J Pediatr 147:51–53, 1988.

58. Magilavy DB, Speert DP, Silver TM, et al.: Mucocutaneous lymph node syndrome: report of two cases complicated by gallbladder hydrops and diagnosed by ultrasound. Pediatrics 61:699–702, 1978.

58a. Bader-Meunier B, Hadchouel M, Fabre M, et al.: Intrahepatic bile duct damage in children with Kawasaki disease. J Pediatr 120:750–752, 1992.

59. Franken EA Jr, Kleiman MB, Norins AL, et al.: Intestinal pseudo-obstruction in mucocutaneous lymph-node syndrome. Radiology 130:649–651, 1979.

60. Mercer S, Carpenter B: Surgical complications of Kawasaki disease. J Pediatr Surg 16:444–448, 1981.

61. Murphy DJ Jr, Morrow R, Harberg FJ, Hawkins EP: Small bowel obstruction as a complication of Kawasaki disease. Clin Pediatr 26:193–195, 1987.

62. Stoler J, Biller JA, Grand RJ: Pancreatitis in Kawasaki disease. Am J Dis Child 141:306–308, 1987.

63. Yanagitani Y, Fujita M: Avascular necrosis of the femoral head associated with mucocutaneous lymph node syndrome. J Ped Orthop 6:107–109, 1986.

64. Sundel RP, Newburger JW, McGill T, et al.: Sensorineural hearing loss associated with Kawasaki disease. J Pediatr 117:371–377, 1990.

65. Haslam RHA, Cochrane D, Amundson GM, et al.: Neurotoxic complications of contrast computed tomography in children. J Pediatr 111:837–840, 1987.

65a. Kazi A, Gauthier M, Lebel MH, et al.: Uvulitis and supraglottitis: Early manifestations of Kawasaki disease. J Pediatr 120:564–567, 1992.

66. Waring N-P, Ortenberg J, Galen WK, et al.: Priapism in Kawasaki disease. JAMA 261:1730–1731, 1989.

67. Germain BF, Moroney JD, Guggino GS, et al.: Anterior uveitis in Kawasaki disease. J Pediatr 97:780–781, 1980.

68. Rennebohm, MJ, Burke, MJ, Crowe, W, et al.: Anterior uveitis in Kawasaki disease, abstracted. Arthritis Rheum. 24 (Suppl).:88, 1981.

69. Courtecuisse V, Decary F: Kawasaki disease: association with uveitis in seven patients. Pediatrics 69:376–378, 1982.

70. Furusho K, Kamiya T, Nakano H, et al.: High-dose intravenous gammaglobulin for Kawasaki disease. Lancet 2:1055–1058, 1984.

71. Newburger JW, Takahashi M, Burns JC, et al.: The treatment of Kawasaki syndrome with intravenous gamma globulin. N Engl J Med 315:341–347, 1986.

72. Glode MP, Joffe LS, Wiggins J Jr., et al.: Effect of intravenous immune globulin on the coagulopathy of Kawasaki syndrome. J Pediatr 115:469–473, 1989.

73. Barron KS, Murphy DJ Jr.: Kawasaki syndrome: still a fascinating enigma. Hosp Pract pp. 51–60, October 15, 1989.

74. Current therapy for acute Kawasaki syndrome. J Pediatr 118:987–991, 1991.

75. Schackleford PG, Strauss AW: Kawasaki syndrome. N Engl J Med 324:1664–

1666, 1991.

76. Newburger JW, Takahashi M, Beiser AS, et al.: A single intravenous infusion of gamma globulin as compared with four infusions in the treatment of acute Kawasaki syndrome. N Engl J Med 324:1633–1639, 1991.

77. Rowley AH, Duffy CE, Shulman ST: Prevention of giant coronary artery aneurysms in Kawasaki disease by intravenous gamma globulin therapy. J Pediatr 113:290–294, 1988.

78. American Academy of Pediatrics: Committee on Infectious Diseases. Intravenous globulin use in children with Kawasaki disease. Pediatrics 82:122, 1988.

79. Nakamura Y, Fujita Y, Nagai M, et al.: Cardiac sequelae of Kawasaki Disease in Japan: Statsitical Analysis. Pediatrics 88:1144–1147, 1991.

80. Burks AW, Sampson HA, Buckley RH: Anaphylactic reactions after gamma globulin administration in patients with hypogammaglobulinemia. Detection of IgE antibodies to IgA. N Engl J Med 314:560–564, 1986.

81. Kato E, Shindo S, Eto Y, et al.: Administration of immune globulin associated with aseptic meningitis. JAMA 259:3269–3272, 1988.

81a. Comentzo RL, Malachowski ME, Meissner HC, et al.: Immune hemolysis, disseminated intravascular coagulation, and serum sickness after large doses of immune globulin given intravenously for Kawasaki disease. J Pediatr 120:926–928, 1992.

82. White WB, Ryan RW, Staley DD, Ballow M: Passive transfer of antibodies to human T-cell lymphotropic virus type III in patients receiving high-dose intravenous immunoglobulin. JAMA 255:2602–2603, 1986.

82a. Nakamura Y, Yanagawa H, Kawasaki T: Mortality among children with Kawasaki disease in Japan. N Eng J Med 326:1246–1249, 1992.

83. Bierman FZ, Gersony WM: Kawasaki disease: clinical perspective. J Pediatr 111:789–792, 1987 (see also correspondence pp. 1116–1117).

84. Kato H, Koike S, Yokoyama T: Kawasaki disease: effect of treatment on coronary artery involvement Pediatrics 63:175–179, 1979.

85. Koren G, Rose V, Lavi S, Rowe R: Probable efficacy of high dose salicylate in reducing coronary involvement in Kawasaki disease. JAMA 254:767–769, 1985.

86. Koren G, Schaffer F, Silverman E, et al.: Determinants of low serum concentrations of salicylates in patients with Kawasaki disease. J Pediatr 112:663–667, 1988.

87. Koren G, Macloed SM: Difficulty in achieving therapeutic serum concentrations of salicylate in Kawasaki disease. J Pediatr 105:991–995, 1984 (see also correspondence 106:858–860, 1985).

88. Koren G, Lavi S, Rose V, Rowe R: Kawasaki disease: review of risk factors for coronary aneurysms. J Pediatr 108:388–392, 1986.

89. Daniels SR, Specker B, Capannari TE, et al.: Correlates of coronary artery aneurysm formation in patients with Kawasaki disease. Am J Dis Child 141:2057, 1987.

90. Nagashima M, Matsushima M, Matsuoka H, et al.: High-dose gammaglobulin therapy for Kawasaki disease. J Pediatr 110:710–712, 1987.

91. Koren G, Silverman E, Sundel R, et al.: Decreased protein binding of salicylates in Kawasaki disease. J Pediatr 118:456–459, 1991.

92. Melish ME: Kawasaki syndrome (mucocutaneous lymph node syndrome). Pediatr Rev 2:107–114, 1980.

93. Burtt DM, Pollack P, Bianco JA: Intravenous streptokinase in an infant with

Kawasaki's disease complicated by acute myocardial infarcation. Pediatr Cardiol 6:307–311, 1986.

94. Terai M, Ogaata M, Sugimoto K, et al.: Coronary arterial thrombi in Kawasaki disease. J Pediatr 106:76–78, 1985.

95. Kato H, Koike S, Yamamoto M, et al.: Coronary aneurysms in infants and young children with acute mucocutaneous lymph node syndrome. J Pediatr 86:892–898, 1975.

96. Glanz S, Bittner SJ, Berman MA, et al.: Regression of coronary artery aneurysms in infantile polyarteritis nodosa. N Engl J Med 294:939–941, 1976.

97. Kato H: Natural history of Kawasaki disease. In Shiokawa Y (ed.) Vascular Lesions of Collagen Diseases and Related Conditions. University Park Press, Baltimore, 1977, pp. 282–295.

98. Nakano H, Ueda K, Saito A, Nojima K: Repeated quantitative angiograms in coronary arterial aneursym in Kawasaki disease. Am J Cardiol 56:846–851, 1985.

99. Kato H, Inoue O, Akagi T: Kawasaki disease: cardiac problems and management. Pediatr Rev 9:209–217, 1988.

100. Yoshikawa J, Yanagihara K, Owaki T, et al.: Cross-sectional echocardiographic diagnosis of coronary artery aneurysms in patients with the mucocutaneous lymph node syndrome. Circulation 59:133–139, 1979.

101. Hiraishi S, Yashiro K, Kusano S: Noninvasive visualization of coronary arterial aneurysm in infants and young children with mucocutaneous lymph node syndrome with two-dimensional echocardiography. Am J Cardiol 43:1225–1233, 1979.

102. Yoshida H, Funabashi T, Nakaya S, et al.: Mucocutaneous lymph node syndrome: a cross sectional echocardiographic diagnosis of coronary aneurysms. Am J Dis Child 133:1244–1247, 1979.

103. Neches WH: Mucocutaneous lymph node syndrome: coronary artery disease and cross-sectional echocardiography. Am J Dis Child 133:1233–1235, 1979.

104. Capannari TE, Daniels SR, Meyer RA, et al.: Sensitivity, specificity and predictive value of two-dimensional echocardiography in detecting coronary artery aneurysms in patients with Kawasaki disease. J Am Coll Cardiol 7:355–360, 1986.

105. Tatara K, Kusakawa S: Long-term prognosis of giant coronary aneurysm in Kawasaki disease: an angiographic study. J Pediatr 111:705–710, 1987.

106. Akiba T, Sato T, Yoshikawa M, et al.: Prognostic significance of the size of coronary artery aneurysms in Kawasaki disease. Acta Paediatr Jpn 31:7–11, 1989.

107. Nakanishi T, Takao A, Nakazawa M, et al.: Mucocutaneous lymph node syndrome: clinical, hemodynamic and angiographic features of coronary obstructive disease. Am J Cardiol 55:662–668, 1985.

108. Nakano H, Ueda K, Saito A, Nojima K: Repeated quantitative angiograms in coronary arterial aneurysm in Kawasaki disease. Am J Cardiol 56:846–851, 1985.

109. Suzuki A, Kamiya T, Ono Y, et al.: Follow-up study of coronary artery lesions due to Kawasaki disease by serial selective coronary arteriography in 200 patients. Heart Vessels 3:159–165, 1987.

110. Bisset GS III, Strife JL, McCloskey J: MR Imaging of coronary artery aneurysms in a child with Kawasaki disease. AJR 805–807, 1989.

111. Demer LL, et al.: Assessment of coronary artery disease severity by positron emission tomography: comparison with quantitative arteriography in 193 patients. Circulation 79:825–835, 1989.

112. Kato H, Ichinose E, Kawasaki T: Myocardial infarction in Kawasaki disease: clinical analyses in 195 cases. J Pediatr 108:923–927, 1986.

113. Lipson MH, Ament ME, Fonkalsrud EW: Ruptured hepatic artery aneurysm and coronary artery aneurysms with myocardial infarction in a 14-year-old boy: new manifestations of mucocutaneous lymph node syndrome. J Pediatr 98:933–936, 1981.

114. Hicks RV, Melish ME, Paik Y, et al.: Kawasaki syndrome (KS) 2 to 10 years later, abstracted. Arthritis Rheum 25 (Suppl): 125, 1981.

115. Spielmann RP, Nienaber CA, Hausdorf G, Montz R: Tomographic myocardial perfusion scintigraphy in children with Kawasaki disease. J Nucl Med 28:1839–1843, 1987.

116. Nienaber CA, Spielmann RP, Hausdorf G: Dipyridamole-thallium-201 tomography documenting improved myocardial perfusion with therapy in Kawasaki disease. Am Heart J 116:1575, 1988.

117. Paridon SM, Ross RD, Kuhns LR, Pinsky WW: Myocardial performance and perfusion during exercise in patients with coronary artery disease caused by Kawasaki disease. J Pediatr 116:52–56, 1990.

118. Sandiford FM, Vargo TA, Shih JY, et al.: Successful triple coronary artery bypass in a child with multiple coronary aneurysms due to Kawasaki's disease. J Thorac Cardiovasc Surg 79:283–287, 1980.

119. Suzuki A, Kamiya T, Ono Y, et al.: Myocardial ischemia in Kawasaki disease: follow-up study by cardiac catheterization and coronary angiography. Pediatr Cardiol 9:1–5, 1988.

120. Suzuki A, Kamiya T, Ono Y, et al.: Aortocoronary bypass surgery for coronary arterial lesions resulting from Kawasaki disease. J Pediatr 116:567–573, 1990.

121. FitzGerald GA: Dipyridamole. N Engl J Med 316:1247–1256, 1987 (see also correspondence pp. 1734–1736).

122. Nakano H, Ueda K, Saito A, Tsuchitani Y: Doppler detection of tricuspid regurgitation following Kawasaki's disease. Pediatr Radiol 16:123–125, 1990.

123. Nakano H, Nojima K, Saito A, Ueda K: High incidence of aortic regurgitation following Kawasaki disease. J Pediatr 59–63, 1985.

124. Kurisu Y, Azumi T, Sugahara T, et al.: Variation in coronary arterial dimension (distensible abnormality) after disappearing aneurysm in Kawasaki disease. Am Heart J 114:532–538, 1987.

125. Lightfoot RW Jr., Michel BA, Bloch DA, et al.: The American College of Rheumatology 1990 Criteria For The Classification of Polyarteritis Nodosa. Arthritis Rheum 33:1088–1093, 1990.

126. Blau EB, Morris RF, Yunis EJ: Polyarteritis nodosa in older children. Pediatrics 60:227–234, 1977.

127. Reimold EW, Weinberg AG, Fink CW, et al.: Polyarteritis in children. Am J Dis Child 130:534–541, 1976.

128. Magilavy DB, Petty RE, Cassidy JT, et al.: A syndrome of childhood polyarteritis. J Pediatr 91:25–30, 1977.

129. Ettlinger RE, Nelson AM, Burke EC, et al.: Polyarteritis nodosa in childhood, a clinical pathologic study. Arthritis Rheum 22:820–825, 1979.

129a. Ozen S, Besbas N, Saatci U, Bakkaloglu A: Diagnostic criteria for polyarteritis nodosa in children. J Pediatr 120:206–209, 1992.

130. Woodward AH, Andreini PH: Periosteal new bone formation in polyarteritis nodosa. Arthritis Rheum 17:1017–1025, 1974.

131. Sergent JS, Lochshin MD, Christian CL, et al.: Vasculitis with hepatitis B antigenemia. Medicine 55:1–18, 1976.

132. Duffy J, Lidsky MD, Sharp JT, et al.: Polyarthritis, polyarteritis and hepatitis B. Medicine 55:19–37, 1976.

133. Reznik VM, Mendoza SA, Self TW, et al.: Hepatitis B-associated vasculitis in an infant. J Pediatr 98:252–254, 1981.

134. McMahon BJ, Bender TR, Templin DW, et al.: Vasculitis in Eskimos living in an area hyperendemic for hepatitis B. JAMA 244:2180–2182, 1980.

135. Ingelfinger, JR, McCluskey RT, Schneeberger EE: Necrotizing arteritis in acute poststreptococcal glomerulonephritis. J Pediatr 91:228–232, 1977.

136. Bamji A, Salisbury, R: Cytomegalovirus and vasculitis. Br Med J 1:623–624, 1978.

137. Hoffman GS, Franck WA: Infectious mononucleosis, autoimmunity and vasculitis. A case report. JAMA 241:2735–2736, 1979.

138. Finkel TH, Gelfand EW, Harbeck R, et al.: Chronic parvovirus infection presenting as juvenile polyarteritis nodosum. Arthritis Rheum 33:S132, 1990.

139. Sergent JS, Christian CL: Necrotizing vasculitis after acute serous otitis media. Ann Intern Med 81:195–199, 1974.

140. Soter NA, Mihm MC, Colten HR: Cutaneous necrotizing venulitis in patients with cystic fibrosis. J Pediatr 95:197–201, 1979.

141. Berdischewsky M, Pollack M, Young LS, et al.: Circulating immune complexes in cystic fibrosis. J Pediatr Res 14:830–833, 1980.

141a. Case Records of the Massachusetts General Hospital. Case 18-1992. N Engl J Med 326:1204–1212, 1992.

141b. Jennette JC, Falk RJ. Disease associations and pathogenic role of antineutrophil cytoplasmic autoantibodies in vasculitis. Current Opinion in Rheumatology 4:9–15, 1992.

142. Wees SJ, Oh SJ: Sural nerve biopsies in systemic vasculitis, abstracted. Arthritis Rheum 24 (Suppl.): 88, 1981.

143. Albert DA, Rimon D, Silverstein MD, et al.: The diagnosis of polyarteritis nodosa. Arthritis Rheum 31:1117–1134, 1988.

144. Bron KM, Strott CA, Shapiro AP: The diagnostic value of angiographic observations in polyarteritis nodosa. Arch Intern Med 116:450–454, 1965.

145. Hilal SK, Solomon GE, Gold A, et al.: Primary cerebral arterial occlusive disease in children. Radiology 99:71–86, 1971.

146. Mason RA, Arbeit LA, Giron F: Renal dysfunction after arteriography. JAMA 253:1001–1004, 1985 (see also correspondence 254:233–234, 1985).

147. Dahlberg PJ, Lockhart JM, Overholt EL: Diagnostic studies for systemic necrotizing vasculitis: sensitivity, specificity, and predictive value in patients with multisystem disease. Arch Intern Med 149:161–165, 1989.

148. Fauci AS, Katz P, Haynes BF, et al.: Cyclophosphamide therapy of severe systemic necrotizing vasculitis. N Engl J Med 301:235–238, 1979.

149. Guillevin L, Fain O, Lhote F, et al: Lack of superiority of steroids plus plasma exchange to steroids alone in the treatment of polyarteritis nodosa and Churg-Strauss syndrome. A prospective, randomized trial in 78 patients. Arthritis Rheum 35:208–215, 1992.

150. Cunningham RJ III, Gilfoil M, Cavallo T, et al.: Rapidly progressive glomeru-

lonephritis in children: a report of thirteen cases and a review of the literature. Pediatr Res 14:128–132, 1980.

151. McCune WJ, Friedman AW. Immunosuppressive drug therapy for rheumatic disease. Current Opinion in Rheumatology 4:314–321, 1992.

152. Scott DGI, Bacon PA: Intravenous cyclophosphamide plus methylprednisolone in treatment of systemic rheumatoid vasculitis. Am J Med 76:377–384, 1984.

153. Fort JG, Abruzzo JL: Reversal of progressive necrotizing vasculitis with intravenous pulse cyclophosphamide and methylprednisolone. Arthritis Rheum 31:1194–1198, 1988.

154. Fauci AS, Doppman JL, Wolff SM: Cyclophosphamide-induced remissions in advanced polyarteritis nodosa. Am J Med 64:890–894, 1978.

155. Chumbley LC, Harrison EG, Jr, DeRemee RA: Allergic granulomatosis and angiitis (Churg-Strauss syndrome). Report and analysis of 30 cases. Mayo Clin Proc 52:477–484, 1977.

156. Farooki ZQ, Brough AJ, Green EW: Necrotizing arteritis. Am J Dis Child 128:837–840, 1974.

157. Lanham JG, Elkon KB, Pusey CD, Hughes GR: Systemic vasculitis with asthma and eosinophilia: a clinical approach to the Churg-Strauss syndrome. Medicine 63:65–81, 1984.

158. Masi AT, Hunder GG, Lie JT, et al.: The American College of Rheumatology 1990 Criteria For The Classification of Churg-Strauss Syndrome (Allergic Granulomatosis and Angiitis). Arthritis Rheum 33:1094–1100, 1990.

159. McCombs RP: Diseases due to immunologic reactions in the lung. N Engl J Med 286:1186–1194, 1972.

160. Chauhan A, Scott DGI, Neuberger J, et al.: Churg-Strauss vasculitis and ascaris infection. Ann Rheum Dis 49:320–322, 1990.

161. Frayha RA: Churg-Strauss syndrome in a child. J Rheumatol 9:807–809, 1982 (Letters).

162. Fischer TJ, Daughtery C, Gushurst C, et al.: Systemic vasculitis associated with eosinophilia and marked degranulation of tissue eosinophils. Pediatrics 82:69–75, 1988.

163. Finan MC, Winkelmann RK: The cutaneous extravascular necrotizing granuloma (Churg-Strauss granuloma) and systemic disease: a review of 27 cases. Medicine 62:142–158, 1983.

164. Case records of the Massachusetts General Hospital: Case 46-1980. N Engl J Med 303:1218–1225, 1980.

165. Case records of the Massachusetts General Hospital. Case 18-1987. N Engl J Med 316:1139–1147, 1987.

166. Vincent FM: Granulomatous angiitis. N Engl J Med 296:452. 1977.

167. Sandhu R, Alexander WS, Hornabrook RW, et al.: Granulomatous angiitis of the central nervous system. Arch Neurol 36:433–435, 1979.

168. Allen GL, Nelson AM, Gomez MR: Isolated central nervous system (CNS) vasculitis in childhood–a report of five cases with long term followup, Mayo Clinic. Personal communication.

169. Calabrese LH, Furlan AJ, Gragg LA, Ropos TJ. Primary angiitis of the central nervous system: Diagnostic criteria and clinical approach. Cleve Clin J Med 59:293–306, 1992.

170. Lie JT: Angiitis of the central nervous system. Curr Opin Rheumatol 3:36–45, 1991.

171. Crane R, Kerr LD, Spiera H: Clinical analysis of isolated angiitis of the central

nervous system. A report of 11 cases. Arch Intern Med 151:2290–2294, 1991.

172. Case records of the Massachusetts General Hospital. Case 16-1986. N Engl J Med 315:1143–1154, 1986.

173. Leavitt RY, Fauci AS: Polyangiitis overlap syndrome: classification and prospective clinical experience. Am J Med 81:79–85, 1986.

174. Case Records of the Massachusetts General Hospital. Case 8-1989. N Engl J Med 320:514–524, 1989.

175. Sigal LH: The neurologic presentation of vasculitic and rheumatologic syndromes: a review. Medicine 66:157–180, 1987.

176. Loeffel S, Chang CH, Heyn R, et al.: Necrotizing lymphoid vasculitis in X-linked lymphoproliferative syndrome. Arch Pathol Lab Med 109:546–550, 1985.

177. Stein RL, Martino CR, Weinert DM, et al.: Cerebral angiography as a guide for therapy in isolated central nervous system vasculitis. JAMA 257:2193–2196, 1987.

178. Rush PJ, Inman R, Bernstein M, et al.: Isolated vasculitis of the central nervous system in a patient with celiac disease. Am J Med 81:1092–1094, 1986.

179. Pasternak JF, DeVivo DC, Prensky AL: Steroid-responsive encephalomyelitis in childhood. Neurology 30:481–486, 1980.

180. Nakao K, Ikeda M, Shin-ichi K, et al.: Takayasu's arteritis: clinical report of eighty-four cases and immunological studies of seven cases. Circulation 35:1141–1155, 1967.

181. Bonventre MV: Takayasu's disease revisited. NY State J Med 74:1960–1967, 1974.

182. Lupi-Herrera E, Sanchez-Torres G, Marcushamer J, et al.: Takayasu's arteritis. Clinical study of 107 cases. Am Heart J 93:94–103, 1977.

183. Haas A, Stiehm ER: Takayasu's arteritis presenting as pulmonary hypertension. Am J Dis Child 140:372–374, 1986.

184. Lande A, Berkmen YM, McAllister HA Jr (eds.): Aortitis: Clinical, Pathologic and Radiographic Aspects. Raven Press, New York, 278 pp., 1986, illustrated.

185. Arend WP, Michel BA, Bloch DA, et al.: The American College of Rheumatology 1990 Criteria For The Classification of Takayasu Arteritis. Arthritis Rheum 33:1129–1134, 1990.

186. Hall S, Barr W, Lie JT, et al.: Takayasu arteritis: a study of 32 North American patients. Medicine 64:89–99, 1985.

187. Shelhamer JH, Volkman DJ, Parrillo JE, et al.: Takayasu's Arteritis and its therapy. Ann Intern Med 103:121–126, 1985.

188. Wu YJ J, Martin B, Ong K, et al.: Takayasu's arteritis as a cause of fever of unknown origin. Am J Med 87:476, 1989.

189. Tanaka N, Tanaka H, Toyama Y, et al.: Paroxysmal hypertension in aortitis syndrome. Am Heart J 90:369–375, 1975.

190. Lande A, Rossi P: The value of total aortography in the diagnosis of Takayasu's arteritis. Radiology 114:287–297, 1975.

191. Lande A, Bard R, Rossi P, et al.: Takayasu's arteritis. NY State J Med 76:1474–1482, 1976.

192. Lacombe P, Frija G, Boucher D, et al.: Maladie de Takayasu: Interet de l'angiographie numerique intraveineuse: 44 observations. Presse Med 15:1179–1182, 1986. (Takayasu's Arteritis: Usefulness of Digital Intravenous Angiography: 44 Cases.)

192a. Tanigawa K, Eguchi K, Kitamura Y, et al.: Magnetic resonance imaging detection of aortic and pulmonary artery wall thickening in the acute stage of Takayasu arteritis. Improvement of clinical and radiologic findings after steroid therapy. Arthritis Rheum 35:476–480, 1992.

193. Hellmann DB, Hardy K, Lindenfeld S, Ring E: Takayasu's arteritis associated with crescentic glomerulonephritis. Arthritis Rheum 451–454, 1987.

194. Cajigas JC, Amigo MC, Pineda C, et al.: Association between Takayasu's arteritis and cutaneous polyarteritis nodosa. Am J Med 82:382–384, 1987.

195. Perniciaro C, Winkelmann RK: Cutaneous extravascular necrotizing granuloma in a patient with Takayasu's aortitis. Arch Dermatol 122:201, 1986.

196. Wiggelinkhuizen J, Cremin BJ: Takayusu arteritis and renovascular hypertension in childhood. Pediatrics 62:209–217, 1978.

197. Pantell RH, Goodman BW Jr: Takayasu's arteritis: The relationship with tuberculosis. Pediatrics 67:84–88, 1981.

198. Abe K, Miyazaki S, Kusaka T, et al.: Elevated plasma renin activity in aortitis syndrome. Jap Heart J 17:1–11, 1976.

199. Rotenstein D, Gibbas DL, Majmudar B, et al.: Familial granulomatous arteritis associated with polyarthritis of juvenile onset. N Engl J Med 306:86–90, 1982.

200. Hoffman GS, Kerr GS, Leavitt RY, et al.: Wegener granulomatosis: An analysis of 158 patients. Ann Int Med 116:488–498, 1992.

201. Hall SL, Miller LC, Duggan E, et al.: Wegener's granulomatosis in pediatric patients. J Pediatr 106:739–744, 1985.

202. Leavitt RY, Fauci AS, Bloch DA, et al.: The American College of Rheumatology 1990 Criteria for the Classification of Wegener's Granulomatosis. Arthritis Rheum 33:1101–1107, 1990.

203. Case Records of the Massachusetts General Hospital: Case 12-1986. N Engl J Med 31:834–844, 1986.

204. Myers JL, Katzenstein A-L A: Wegener's granulomatosis presenting with massive pulmonary hemorrhage and capillaritis. Am J Surg Pathol 11:895–898, 1987.

205. Appel GB, Gee B, Kashgarian M, et al.: Wegener's granulomatosis—clinical-pathologic correlations and long-term course. Am J Kidney Dis 1:27–37, 1981.

205a. Charles SJ, Meyer PAR, Watson PG: Diagnosis and management of systemic Wegener's granulomatosis presenting with anterior ocular inflammatory disease. Br J Opthalmol 75:201–207, 1991.

205b. Sacks RD, Stock EL, Crawford SE, et al.: Scleritis and Wegener's granulomatosis in children. Am J Opthalmol 111:430–433, 1991.

206. Yoshikawa Y, Watanabe T: Pulmonary lesions in Wegener's granulomatosis: A clinicopathologic study of 22 autopsy cases. Hum Pathol 17:401–410, 1986.

207. Leavitt RY, Fauci AS: Pulmonary vasculitis. Am Rev Respir Dis 134:149–166, 1986.

208. Mark EJ, Matsubara O, Tan-Liu NS, Fienberg R: The pulmonary biopsy in the early diagnosis of Wegener's (pathergic) granulomatosis: a study based on 35 open lung biopsies. Human Pathol 19:1065–1071, 1988.

208a. Lowance DC, Vosataka K, Whelchel J, et al.: Recurrent Wegener's granulomatosis. Am J Med 92:573–575, 1992.

209. Norris MJ, Tomecki KJ, Bergfeld WF, Wilke WS: Cutaneous Wegener's granulomatosis: report of a case and review of the literature. Clev Clin J Med 55:181–184, 1988.

210. Case Records of the Massachusetts General Hospital: Case 17-1986. N Engl J Med 314:1170–1184, 1986.
211. Cohen Tervaert JW, van der Woude FJ, Fauci AS, et al.: Association between active Wegener's granulomatosis and anticytoplasmic antibodies. Arch Intern Med 149:2461–2465, 1989 (see also pp. 2401–2402).
212. Maclsaac AI, Davies DJ, Moran JE, et al.: Correspondence: antineutrophilic cytoplasmic antibodies in systemic vasculitis. Mayo Clin Proc 65:124–125, 1990.
213. Jennette JC, Wilkman AS, Falk RJ: Anti-neutrophil cytoplasmic autoantibody-associated glomerulonephritis and vasculitis. A J Pathol 135:921–930, 1989.
214. Falk FJ, Hogan S, Caey TS, et al.: Clinical course of anti-neutrophil cytoplasmic autoantibody-associated glomerulonephritis and systemic vasculitis. Ann Intern Med 113:656–663, 1990.
215. Moorthy AV, Chesney RW, Segar WE, et al.: Wegener's granulomatosis in childhood: prolonged survival following cytotoxic therapy. J Pediatr 91:616–618, 1977.
216. Orlowski JP, Clough JD, and Dyment PG: Wegener's granulomatosis in the pediatric age group. Pediatrics 61:83–90, 1978.
217. Baliga R, Chang CH, Bidani AK, et al.: A case of generalized Wegener's granulomatosis in childhood: successful therapy with cyclophosphamide. Pediatrics 61:286–290, 1978.
218. Hoffman GS, Leavitt RY, Fleisher TA, et al.: Treatment of Wegener's granulomatosis with intermittent high-dose intravenous cyclophosphamide. Am J Med 89:403–410, 1990 (see also Editorial pp. 399–402).
219. Harrison HL, Linshaw MA, Lindsley CB, et al.: Bolus corticosteroids and cyclophosphamide for initial treatment of Wegener's granulomatosis. JAMA 244:1599–1600, 1980.
220. Kroneman OC, Pevzner M: Failure of cyclophosphamide to prevent cerebritis in Wegener's granulomatosis. Am J Med 80:526–527, 1986.
221. Pinching AJ, Lockwood CM, Pussell BA, et al.: Wegener's granulomatosis: observations on 18 patients with severe renal disease. Q J Med 208:435–460, 1983.
222. Rottem M, Fauci AS, Hallahan CW, et al.: A long term study of Wegener granulomatosis in 23 children and adolescents: Clinical presentation and outcome. J Pediatr In Press, 1993.
223. DeRemee RA: The treatment of Wegener's granulomatosis with trimethoprim/sulfamethoxazole: illusion or vision? Arthritis Rheum 31:1068–1072, 1988 (see also 32:1051–1052, 1989).
224. Israel HL: Sulfamethoxazole-trimethoprim therapy for Wegener's granulomatosis. Arch Intern Med 148:2293–2295, 1988 (see also correspondence 149:1469, 1471).
225. Valeriano-Marcet J, Spiera H: Treatment of Wegener's granulomatosis with sulfamethoxazole-trimethoprim. Arch Intern Med 151:1649–1652, 1991.
226. Ambrus JL Jr, Fauci AS: Diffuse histiocyctic lymphoma in a patient treated with cyclophosphamide for Wagener's granulomatosis. Am J Med 76:745–747, 1984.
227. Case records of the Massachusetts General Hospital, Case no. 43-1981. N Engl J Med 305:999–1008, 1981.
228. Lugmani RA, Adu D, Michael J: Limited Wegener's granulomatosis: mild disease or distinct entity? Arthritis Rheum 33:S132, 1990.

229. Case Records of the Massachusetts General Hospital: Case 26-1985. N Engl J Med 312:1695–1703, 1985.

230. Liebow AA, Carrington CRB, Friedman PJ: Lymphomatoid granulomatosis. Hum Pathol 3:457–558, 1972.

231. Gracey DR, DeRemee RA, Colby TV, et al.: Benign lymphocytic angiitis and granulomatosis: experience with three cases. Mayo Clin Proc 63:323–331, 1988.

232. Pisani RJ, DeRemee RA: Clinical implications of the histopathologic diagnosis of pulmonary lymphomatoid granulomatosis. Mayo Clin Proc 65:151–163, 1990.

233. Katzenstein AL, Carrington CB, Liebow AA: Lymphomatoid granulomatosis; A clinicopathologic study of 152 cases. Cancer 43:360–373, 1979.

234. Lipford EH Jr, Margolick JB, Longo DL, et al.: Angiocentric immunoproliferative lesions: a clinicopathologic spectrum of post-thymic T-cell proliferations. Blood 72:1674–1681, 1988.

235. Case Records of the Massachusetts General Hospital: Case 40-1987. N Engl J Med 317:879–890, 1987.

236. Foley JF, Linder J, Koh J, et al.: Cutaneous necrotizing granulomatous vasculitis with evolution to T cell lymphoma. Am J Med 82:839–844, 1987.

237. Myers JL: Editorial: lymphomatoid granulomatosis: past, present, . . . future? Mayo Clin Proc 65:274–278, 1990.

238. Fillipovich AH, Krivit W, Kersey JH, Burke BA: Fatal arteritis as a complication of Wiskott-Aldrich syndrome. J Pediatr 95:742–744, 1979.

239. Ilowite NT, Fligner CL, Ochs HD, et al.: Pulmonary angiitis with atypical lymphoreticular infiltrates in Wiskott-Aldrich syndrome: possible relationship of lymphomatoid granulomatosis and EBV infection. Clin Immunol Immunopathol 41:479–484, 1986.

240. Letendre L: Treatment of lymphomatoid granulomatosis: old and new perspectives. Semin Respir Med 10:178–181, 1989.

241. Fauci AS, Johnson RE, Wolff SM: Radiation therapy of midline granuloma. Ann Intern Med 84:140–147, 1976.

242. Jones SK, Lane AT, Golitz LE, Weston WL: Cutaneous periarteritis nodosa in a child. Am J Dis Child 139:920–922, 1985.

243. Moreland LW, Ball GV: Cutaneous polyarteritis nodosa. Am J Med 88:426–430, 1990.

244. Calabrese LH, Michel BA, Bloch DA, et al.: The American College of Rheumatology 1990 Criteria For The Classification of Hypersensitivity Vasculitis. Arthritis Rheum 33:1108–1113, 1990.

245. Meredith GS, Mitnick HJ, Burstin HE, Zimmerman SS: Polyarteritis nodosa presenting with migratory soft tissue swelling. NYS J Med 87:402–403, 1987.

246. Ferreiro JE, Saldana MJ, Azevedo SJ: Polyarteritis manifesting as calf myositis and fever. Am J Med 80:312–315, 1986.

247. Mathieson PW, Cobbold SP, Hale G, et al.: Monoclonal-antibody therapy in systemic vasculitis. N Engl J Med 323:250–254, 1990.

248. Levo Y: Nature of cryoglobulinemia. Lancet 1:285–287, 1980.

249. Meltzer M, Franklin EC: Cryoglobulinemia—a study of 29 patients. Am J Med 40:828–836, 1966.

250. Gorevic PD, Kassab HJ, Levo Y, et al.: Mixed cryoglobulinemia: Clinical aspects and long-term follow-up of 40 patients. Am J Med 69:287–308, 1980.

251. Reza MJ, Roth BE, Pops MA, et al.: Intestinal vasculitis in essential, mixed cryoglobulinemia. Ann Intern Med 81:632–634, 1974.

252. Gamble CN, Ruggles SW: The immunopathogenesis of glomerulonephritis associated with mixed cryoglobulinemia. N Engl J Med 299:81–84, 1978.
253. Waterman JR, Winkelstein JA, Berzofsky RN, et al.: Early complement component depletion and mixed cryoglobulinemia in a "healthy" family. Arthritis Rheum 22:1006–1012, 1979.
254. Farivar M, Wands JR, Benson GD, et al.: Cryoprotein complexes and peripheral neuropathy in a patient with chronic active hepatitis. Gastroenterology 71:490–492, 1976.
255. Cosgriff TM, Arnold WJ: Digital vasospasm and infarction associated with hepatitis B antigenemia. JAMA 235:1362–1363, 1976.
255a. Knox TA, Hillyer CD, Kaplan MM, Berkman EM. Mixed cryoglobulinemia responsive to interferon-α. Am J Med 91:554–555, 1991. (See also 93:115–116, 1992.)
256. McDuffie FC, Sams WM Jr, Maldonado JE, et al.: Hypocomplementemia with cutaneous vasculitis and arthritis. Mayo Clin Proc 48:340–347, 1973.
257. Feig PU, Soter NA, Yager HM, et al.: Vasculitis with urticaria, hypocomplementemia, and multiple system involvement. JAMA 236:2065–2068, 1976.
258. Ludivico CL, Myers AR, Maurer K: Hypocomplementemic urticarial vasculitis with glomerulonephritis and pseudotumor cerebri. Arthritis Rheum 22:1024–1028, 1979.
259. Lieberman J, Gephardt G, Calabrese LH: Urticaria, nephritis, and pseudotumor cerebri. Cleve Clin J Med 57:197–201, 1990.
260. Miller JJ, Fries JF: Simultaneous vasculitis in a mother and newborn infant. J Pediatr 87:443–445, 1975.
261. Elkon KB, Hughes GRV, Catovsky D, et al.: Hairy-cell leukemia with polyarteritis nodosa. Lancet 2:280–282, 1979.
262. Longley S, Caldwell JR, Panush RS: Paraneoplastic vasculitis: unique syndrome of cutaneous angiitis and arthritis associated with myeloproliferative disorders. Am J Med 80:1027–1030, 1986.
263. Vasily DB, Tyler WB: Propylthiouracil-induced cutaneous vasculitis. JAMA 243:458–461, 1980.
264. Lanzkowsky P, Jayabose SJ, Shende R, et al.: Vasculitis as a complication of high-dose methotrexate in the treatment of acute leukemia. Am J Dis Child 130:675, 1976.
265. Dewar HA, Peaston MJT. Three cases resembling polyarteritis nodosa arising during treatment with guanethidine. Br Med J 12:609, 1964.
266. Cassorla FO, Finegold DN, Parks JS, et al.: Vasculitis, pulmonary cavitation, and anemia during antithyroid drug therapy. Am J Dis Child 137:118–122, 1983.
267. Gaffey CM, Chun B, Harvey JC, Manz HJ: Phenytoin-induced systemic granulomatous vasculitis. Arch Pathol Lab Med 110:131–135, 1986.
267a. Reid TJ III, Lombardo FA, Redmond J III, et al.: Digital vasculitis associated with interferon therapy. Am J Med 92:702–703, 1992.
268. Golbranson FL, Lurie L, Vance RM, et al.: Multiple extremity amputations in hypotensive patients treated with dopamine. JAMA 243:1145–1146, 1980.
269. Forman HP, Levin S, Stewart B: Cerebral vasculitis and hemorrhage in an adolescent taking diet pills containing phenylpropanolamine: case report and review of literature. Pediatrics 83:737–741, 1989.
270. Citron BP, Halpern M, McCarron M, et al.: Necrotizing angiitis associated with drug abuse. N Engl J Med 283:1003–1011, 1970.

271. Halper M, Citron BP: Necrotizing angiitis associated with drug abuse. Am J Roentgenol Radium Ther Nucl Med 3:663–671, 1971.
272. Wacker FJ, Tytojat GN, Vreeken J: Necrotizing vasculitis and ulcerative colitis. Br Med J 4:83–84, 1974.
273. Forrest JA, Shearman DJ: Pulmonary vasculitis and ulcerative colitis. Am J Dig Dis 20:482–486, 1975.
274. Edwards KR: Hemorrhagic complications of cerebral arteritis. Arch Neurol 34:549–552, 1977.
275. Ho EC, Moss AJ: The syndrome of "mesenteric arteritis" following surgical repair of aortic coarctation. Pediatrics 49:40–45, 1972.
276. Diaz-Perez JL, Winkelmann RK: Cutaneous periarteritis nodosa. Arch Dermatol 110:407–414, 1974.
277. Cherubin CE: So-called cutaneous polyarteritis nodosa. NY State J Med 66:1673–1678, 1966.
278. Milstone LM, Braverman IM, Lucky P, Fleckman P: Classification and therapy of atrophie blanche. Arch Dermatol 119:963–969, 1983.
279. Baethge BA, Sanusi ID, Landreneau MD, et al.: Livedo reticularis and peripheral gangrene associated with primary hyperoxaluria. Arthritis Rheum 31:1199–1203, 1988.
280. Heine KG: Idiopathic atrophie blanche: treatment with low-dose heparin. Arch Dermatol 122:855–856, 1986.
281. Purcell SM, Hayes TJ: Nifedipine treatment of idiopathic atrophie blanche. J Am Acad Dermatol 14:851–854, 1986.
282. Katz SI, Gallin JI, Hertz KC, et al.: Erythema elevatum diutinum: Skin and systemic manifestations, immunologic studies, and successful treatment with dapsone. Medicine 56:443–455, 1977.
283. McNeely MC, Jorizzo JL, Solomon AR, Peltier FA: Erythema elevatum diutinum. Clin Rheumatol Pract, pp. 17–20, January/February 1985.
284. Rakover Y, Adar H, Tal I, et al.: Behcet disease: long-term follow-up of three children and review of the literature. Pediatrics 83:986–992, 1989.
285. Plotkin GR, Calabro JJ, O'Duffy JD (eds.) Behcet's Disease: A Contemporary Synopsis. Futura Publishing Company, Mount Kisco, NY, 1988.
286. Bartlett ST, McCarthy WJ, Palmer AS: Multiple aneurysms in Behcet's disease. Arch Surg 123:1004–1008, 1988.
287. Fukuda Y, Sakuma Y, Sumita M: Pathologic studies of vascular changes in Behcet's disease. In Shiokawa, Y (ed.) Vascular Lesions of Collagen Diseases and Related Conditions. University Park Press, Baltimore, 1977, pp. 212–225.
288. Murakami T: Pathologic changes in the large blood vessels caused by Behcet's disease, especially by neuro-Behcet's disease. Bull Rheum Dis: S29:229–235, 1978.
289. Lang BA, Laxer RM, Thorner P, et al.: Pediatric onset of Behcet's syndrome with myositis: case report and literature review illustrating unusual features. Arthritis Rheum 33:418–425, 1990. (see also correspondence 34:791, 1991).
290. Ammann AJ, Johnson A, Fyfe GA, et al.: Behcet's syndrome. J Pediatr 107:41–43, 1985.
291. Hamuryudan V, Yurdakul S, Ozbakir F: Monozygotic twins concordant for Behcet's syndrome. Arthritis Rheum 34:1071–1072, 1991.
292. Lebwohl O, Forde KA, Berdon WE, et al.: Ulcerative esophagitis and colitis in a pediatric patient with Behcet's syndrome: Response to steroid therapy. Am J Gastroenterol 68:550–555, 1977.

293. Vlymen WJ, Moskowitz PS: Roentgenographic manifestations of esophageal and intestinal involvement in Behcet's disease in children. Pediatr Radiol 10:193–196, 1981.
294. Mori S, Yoshihira A, Kawamura H, et al.: Esophageal involvement in Behcet's Disease. Am J Gastroenterol 78:548–553, 1983.
295. Kataora S, Hirose G, Tsukada K: Brain stem type neuro-Behcet's syndrome: Correlation of enhanced CT scans and MRI during the acute and chronic stage of the illness. Neuroradiology 31:258–262, 1989.
295a. Al-Kawi MS, Bohlega S, Banna M: MRI findings in neuro-Behcet's disease. Neurology 41:405–408, 1991.
296. Yurdakul S, Yazici H, Tuzun Y, et al.: The arthritis of Behcet's disease: a prospective study. Ann Rheum Dis 42:505–515, 1983.
297. Zelenski JD, Capraro JA, Holden D, Calabrese LH: Central nervous system vasculitis in Behcet's syndrome: angiographic improvement after therapy cytotoxic agents. Arthritis Rheum 32:217–220, 1989.
298. Harper CM, O'Neill BP, O'Duffy JD, Forbes GS: Intracranial hypertension in Behcet's disease: demonstration of sinus occlusion with use of digital subtraction angiography. Mayo Clin Proc 60:419–422, 1985.
299. Weschsler B, Bousser MG, Huong Du LT, et al.: Cerebral venous sinus thrombosis in Behcet's disease. Mayo Clin Proc 60:891–892, 1985.
300. Bowles CA, Nelson AM, Hammill SC, O'Duffy JD: Cardiac involvement in Behcet's disease. Arthritis Rheum 28:345–348, 1985.
301. Stricker H, Malinverni R: Multiple, large aneurysms of pulmonary arteries in Behcet's disease: clinical remission and radiologic resolution after corticosteriod therapy. Arch Intern Med 149:925–927, 1989.
302. Mizushima Y, Matsumura N: Chemotaxis of leukocytes and colchicine treatment in Behcet's disease. J Rheumatol 6:108–110, 1979.
303. Jorlzzo JL, Solomon AR, Zanolli MD, Leshin B: Neutrophilic vascular reactions. J Am Acad Dermatol 19:983–1005, 1988.
304. Tafi L, Matucci-Cerinic M, Falcini F, et al.: Colchicine treatment of Behcet's disease in children. Arthritis Rheum 30:1435, 1987.
305. O'Duffy JD: Behcet's Syndrome. N Engl J Med 322:326–328, 1990.
306. Fam AG, Siminovitch KA, Carette S, From L: Case report: neonatal Behcet's syndrome in an infant of a mother with the disease. Ann Rheum Dis 40:509–512, 1981.
307. Cheson BD, Bluming AZ, Alroy J: Cogan's syndrome: A systemic vasculitis. Am J Med 60:549–555, 1976.
308. Kundell SP, Ochs HD: Cogan's syndrome in childhood. J Pediatr 97:96–98, 1980.
309. Haynes BF, Kaiser-Kupfer MI, Mason P, et al.: Cogan's syndrome: studies in thirteen patients, long-term follow-up, and a review of the literature. Medicine 59:426–441, 1980.
310. Haynes BF, Pikus A, Kaiser-Kupfer M, et al.: Successful treatment of sudden hearing loss in Cogan's syndrome with corticosteroids. Arthritis Rheum 24:501–503, 1981.
311. Allen NB, Cox C, Cobo M, et al.: Use of immunosuppressive agents in the treatment of severe ocular and vascular manifestations of Cogan's syndrome. Am J Med 88:296–301, 1990.
312. Jacobs JC: Arthritis as a manifestation of connective tissue disease. In Moore

TD (ed.) Arthritis in Childhood: Report of the Eightieth Ross Conference on Pediatric Research. Ross Laboratories Columbus, Ohio, 1981, pp. 18–23.

313. Case Reports of the Massachusetts General Hospital. Case no. 44-1980. N Engl J Med 303:1103–1111, 1980.

314. Su WP, Schroeter AL, Lee DA, et al.: Clinical and histologic findings in Degos syndrome (malignant atrophic papulosis). Cutis 35:131–138, 1985.

315. Lie JT, Gordon LP, Titus JL: Juvenile temporal arteritis. JAMA 234:496–499, 1975.

316. Golden GT, Fox JW, Williams GS, et al.: Traumatic aneurysm of the superficial temporal artery. JAMA 234:517–518, 1975.

317. Huston KA, Combs JJ, Lie JT, Giuliani ER: Left atrial myxoma simulating peripheral vasculitis. Mayo Clin Proc 53:752–756, 1978.

318. Byrd WE, Matthews OP, Hunt RE: Left atrial myxoma presenting as a systemic vasculitis. Arthritis Rheum 23:240–243, 1980.

319. Fitzpatrick AP, Lanham JG, Doyle DV: Cardiac tumours simulating collagen vascular disease. Br Heart J 55:592–595, 1986.

320. Boers GHJ, Smals AGH, Trijbels FJM, et al.: Heterozygosity for homocystinuria in premature peripheral and cerebral occlusive areterial disease. N Engl J Med 313:709–715, 1985.

321. Shih VE, Abroms IF, Johnson JL, et al.: Sulfite oxidase deficiency. N Engl J Med 297:1022–1028, 1977.

322. Radtke WE, Kazmier FJ, Rutherford BD: Cardiovascular complications of pheochromocytoma crisis. Am J Cardiol 35:701–705, 1975.

323. Sisson JC, Frager MS, Valk TW, et al.: Scintigraphic localization of pheochromocytoma. N Engl J Med 305:12–17, 1981.

324. Ambruso DR, Jacobson LJ, Hathaway WE: Inherited antithrombin-III deficiency and cerebral thrombosis in a child. Pediatrics 65:125–131, 1980.

325. Lechat PH, Mas JL, Lascault G, et al.: Prevalence of patient foramen ovale in patients with stroke. New Engl J Med 318:1148–1152, 1988.

326. Olsen ML, O'Connor S, Arnett FC, et al.: Autoantibodies and rheumatic disorders in a neurology inpatient population: a prospective study. Am J Med 90:479–488, 1991.

327. Roddy SM, Giang DW: Antiphospholipid antibodies and stroke in an infant. Pediatrics 87:933–935, 1991.

328. Case records of the Massachusetts General Hospital. Case 37-1988. N Engl J Med 319:699–712, 1988.

329. Driscoll PF, Larsen PD, Gruber AB: MELAS syndrome involving a mother and two children. Arch Neurol 44:971–973, 1987.

330. Ohtoh T, Iwasaki Y, Namiki T, et al.: Hemodynamic characteristics of the vertebrobasilar system in moyamoya disease. Hum Pathol 19:465–470, 1988.

331. Carlson CB, Harvey FH, Loop J: Progressive alternating hemiplegia in early childhood with basal artery stenosis and telangiectasia (Moyamoya syndrome). Neurology 23:734–744, 1973.

332. Goldberg HJ: Moyamoya associated with peripheral vascular occlusive disease. Arch Dis Child 49:964–966, 1974.

333. Provost TT, Moses H, Morris EL, et al.: Cerebral vasculopathy associated with collateralization resembling Moya Moya phenomenon and with anti-Ro/SS-A and anti-La/SS-B antibodies. Arthritis Rheum 34:1052–1055, 1991.

334. Goldie W: Headache, hemiparesis, and hemianopsia in a five-year-old. Hosp

Pract 17:200–201, 1982.

335. Loughlin GM, Taussig LM, Murphy SA, et al.: Immune-complex-mediated glomerulonephritis and pulmonary hemorrhage simulating Goodpasture's syndrome. J Pediatr 93:181–184, 1978.

336. Mark EJ, Ramirez JF: Pulmonary capillaritis and hemorrhage in patients with systemic vasulitis. Arch Pathol Lab Med 109:413–418, 1985.

337. Myers JL, Katzenstein A-LA: Microangiitis in lupus-induced pulmonary hemorrhage. Am J Clin Pathol 85:552, 1986.

338. Urizar RE, McGoldrick MD, Cerda J: Pulmonary-renal syndrome. Its Clinico-pathologic approach in 1991. NYS J Med 91:212–221, 1991.

339. Davis JP, Chesney PJ, Wand PJ, et al.: Toxic-shock syndrome. Epidemiologic features, recurrence, risk factors, and prevention. N Engl J Med 303:1429–1435, 1980.

340. Shands KN, Schmid MD, Dan BB, et al.: Toxic-shock syndrome in menstruating women. Association with tampon use and *Staphylococcus aureus* and clinical features in 52 cases. N Engl J Med 303:1436–1442, 1980.

341. Chesney PJ, Davis JP, Purdy WK, et al.: Clinical manifestations of toxic shock syndrome. JAMA 246:741–748, 1981.

342. Reingold AL, Shands KN, Dan BB, et al.: Toxic-shock syndrome not associated with menstruation. A review of 54 cases. Lancet 1:1–4, 1982.

343. Buchdahl R, Levin M, Wilkins B, et al.: Toxic shock syndrome. Arch Dis Child 60:563–567, 1985.

344. MacDonald KL, Osterholm MT, Hedberg CW, et al.: Toxic shock syndrome. A newly recognized complication of influenza and influenzalike illness. JAMA 257:1053–1058, 1987.

345. Resnick SD: Toxic shock syndrome: recent developments in pathogenesis. J Pediatr 116:321–328, 1990.

346. Barry W, Hudgins L, Donta ST, Pesanti EL: Intravenous immunoglobulin therapy for toxic shock syndrome. JAMA 267:3315–3316, 1992.

347. Stevens DL, Tanner MH, Winship J, et al.: Severe group a streptococcal infections associated with a toxic shock-like syndrome and scarlet fever toxin A. N Engl J Med 321:1–7, 1989.

8

Scleroderma

The hallmark of the heterogeneous but related group of disorders called *sclero-derma* is an area of hard, tight, inelastic (hide-bound) skin and subcutaneous tissue (Fig. 8.1).[1,2] Fewer than 200 affected children have been reported on in the more than 130 years since the disorder was first described. The paucity of case reports does not reflect great rarity; one pediatric rheumatology clinic alone has reported 48 cases.[3] It does reflect physician frustration: this disorder has been difficult to categorize; pathogenesis has defied understanding; treatment has been unsatisfactory.

Clinical Presentation

The term *scleroderma* is used to refer to two distinctly different syndromes: (1) localized scleroderma and (2) progressive systemic sclerosis (SSc) (Fig. 8.2). These disorders are distinguishable one from the other by their different modes of onset. *Localized scleroderma*, the childhood form, usually begins with one or more oval plaques called *morphea* (Figs. 8.1 and 8.3), a bandlike sclero-tic lesion called *linear scleroderma* (Figs. 8.4 and 8.5), or a combination of these lesions. In 10% of children, localized scleroderma begins with arthritis alone, a clinical presentation indistinguishable from JRA, and the diagnostic skin lesions first appear months or years later.[4] Localized scleroderma does not develop into progressive systemic sclerosis,[5] but in rare cases may be a fea-ture of MCTD or other more generalized disease.[6]

SSC occasionally occurs in childhood.[5,7,8] In our clinic, 15% of childhood scleroderma is systemic sclerosis, but the actual relative frequency is no doubt lower since many cases of localized scleroderma are not referred to the rheumatology service. The initial symptom of SSc is almost always Raynaud's phenomenon, which is followed after a period of months or years by diffuse thickening of the skin of the fingers and hands. The diagnosis is

641

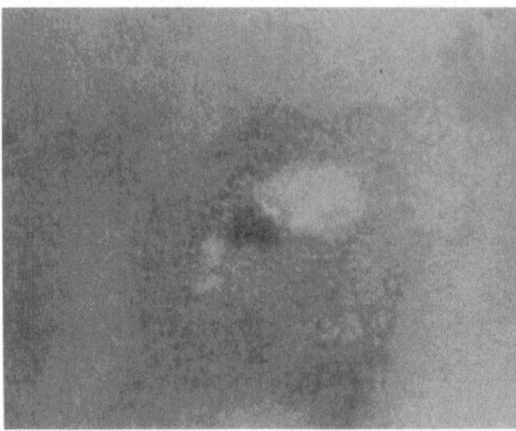

Figure 8.1. Early lesions of morphea start with erythema and evolve into firm, waxy, shiny white lesions with slightly violaceous borders.

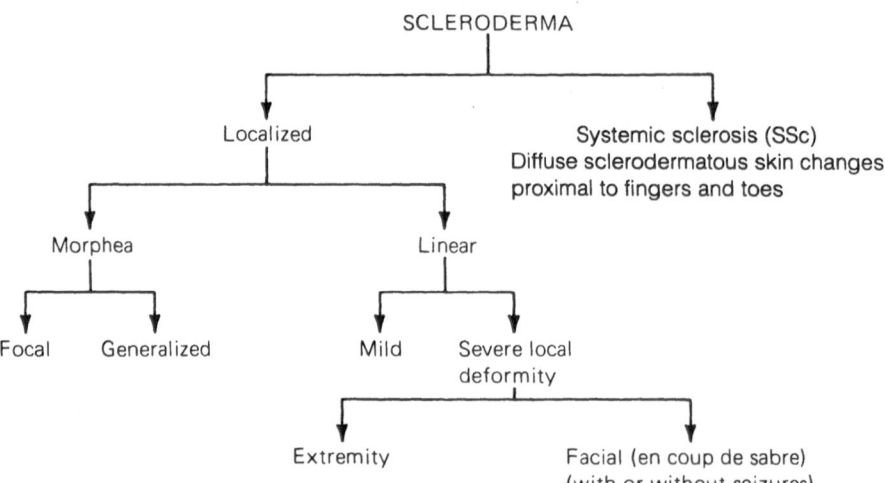

Figure 8.2. Types of scleroderma in childhood.

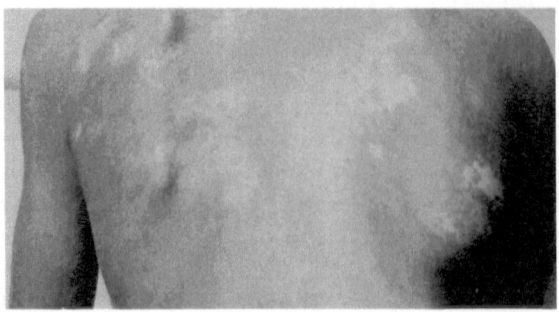

Figure 8.3. Diffuse morphea lesions in a young child.

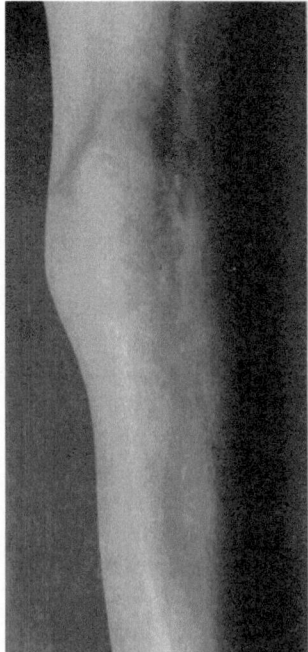

Figure 8.4. Linear scleroderma crossing the knee.

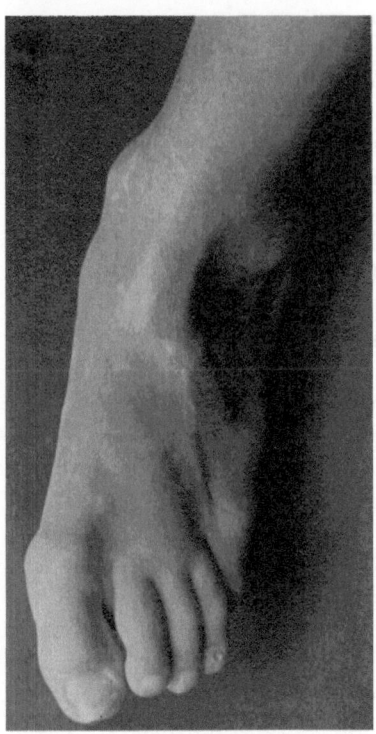

Figure 8.5. Band of linear scleroderma on the foot, with growth disturbance.

established when this generalized skin thickening becomes apparent proximal to the metacarpo- or metatarsophalangeal joints. This presentation distinguishes PSS from localized scleroderma. The presence of anti-topoisomerase (Scl 70) autoantibodies is a bad prognostic finding.[8]

Immunopathology

The earliest histologic change in sclerodermatous skin is reported to be a neutrophilic vasculitis involving small to medium-sized arteries in the subcutaneous fat.[9] No vasculitis is seen in dermal blood vessels of these early specimens, but every small vessel in the fat contains a dense neutrophilic infiltrate within the thickened vessel wall. Interstitial and perivascular lymphocytic infiltrate is soon seen in the dermis and in the thickened fibrous septa. This is followed by an invasion of histiocytes, plasma cells, and eosinophils. Fat necrosis then occurs, with replacement by sclerotic collagen. The dermis ultimately becomes filled with thick collagen obliterating the adnexal structures and some dermal and subcutaneous arterioles. Some of these skin capillary abnormalities may be visualized by placing the patient's fingers under a wide-field microscope and examining the nailfold capillary bed. Large dilated capillary loops are seen in the ungual areas in 90% of patients with scleroderma and dermatomyositis (see Fig. 6.5). These ungual telangiectasias may be grossly visible to the trained examiner.

In SSc, the microvasculature of the internal organs, including the heart, lungs, gastrointestinal tract, and kidneys, may be similarly affected. Subendothelial myxomatous changes may be seen in the large muscular arteries. The small arteries and arterioles of all of these vital organs may be diffusely involved by both intimal proliferation and muscular hypertrophy. Fibrosis follows in the lungs, heart, and gastrointestinal tract. Inflammatory cells are frequently seen in the synovium and also in the other organs.

Although scleroderma shares a number of clinical and morphologic features with disorders thought to be caused by abnormalities of cellular or humoral immune function such as SLE, dermatomyositis, and RA, and all of these disorders also share a number of laboratory markers (hypergammaglobulinemia, rheumatoid factor, and antinuclear antibodies),[1] there is relatively little evidence of either cellular or humoral immune dysfunction in scleroderma.[10-11a] Recent studies have demonstrated a diversity of antinuclear antibodies; those to nucleoli, centromere, and SCl-70 antigen are relatively specific for scleroderma (see Table 5.3).[7-10] Lymphocytes from some patients with scleroderma can be shown to be sensitized to human collagen, which might result in enhanced collagen production. The clinical manifestations of scleroderma, however, do not suggest immunologic dysfunction as the primary cause of the disease.

As might be expected, scleroderma fibroblasts isolated from skin lesions make collagen at many times the rate of normal skin fibroblasts.[10-13] These cells seem to be permanently altered, as this effect continues in tissue culture even after many subcultures. However, the factors that control collagen synthesis and regulate collagen metabolism are not understood, and the ultimate cause of the overgrowth of connective tissue in scleroderma remains a mystery. LeRoy has suggested that endothelial-cell damage rather than immunologic dysfunction is the primary pathogenic mechanism in scleroderma and has provided a hypothetical model that explains how the various disease manifestations may all result from endothelial cell injury. In support of this hypothesis, some sera from patients with Raynaud's phenomenon and from scleroderma patients have been found to contain a fraction that is cytotoxic to endothelial cells.[14] This material is not found in patients with other rheumatic diseases. At the present time, the endothelial-cell injury hypothesis best explains the initiation of all of the clinical features of scleroderma. Nonimmune cellular and humoral immune mechanisms involving fibroblasts, endothelial cells, platelets, monocytes, lymphocytes, mast cells, transforming growth factor B, platelet-derived growth factor, and tumor necrosis factor may all play a role in a complex fashion both in the initiation of the endothelial injury and in its perpetuation in scleroderma.[10-13] Some cases of morphea may be due to chronic skin infection with *borrelia*.[14a]

Diagnosis

Cutaneous scleroderma is generally easily recognized, and a skin biopsy is frequently unnecessary. Characteristic histologic findings of scleroderma include atrophy of the dermal appendages; flattening of rete pegs; and thickening, condensation, and/or homogenization of dermal collagen. Similar findings can sometimes be seen in the other connective-tissue diseases.[2]

The diagnosis of systemic sclerosis is generally made on the basis of generalized bilateral symmetrical scleroderma present proximal to the metacarpophalangeal joints or metatarsophalangeal joints (i.e., scleroderma of the fingers and toes alone is insufficient for diagnosis). This single criterion in a large American Rheumatism Association study had 91% sensitivity and greater than 99% specificity.[2] Sensitivity can be improved to 97% with loss of only 1% specificity by permitting the diagnosis in patients without proximal sclerodermatous changes who have two out of the following three other findings: (1) sclerodatyly, (2) digital pitting scars of fingertips or loss of substance of the finger pad (Figs. 8.6 and 8.7), and (3) bibasilar pulmonary fibrosis (Table 8.1).

Absence of antibodies to DNA, Ro, La, Sm and RNP antigens helps to differentiate systemic sclerosis from SLE and MCTD.[15,16,17] Anticentromere and antitopoisomerase antibodies were not studied by the ARA group and so are not included in the criteria; they appear to be highly specific for systemic sclerosis and may be of diagnostic help in the future. Some overlap syndromes occur.[15,16]

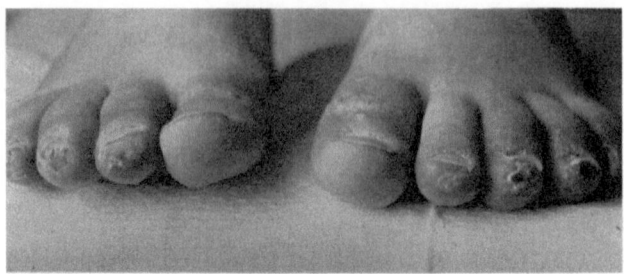

Figure 8.6. Digital pitting scars of toes and loss of substance of the toe pads (SSc). Healing of such lesions has recently been reported with the use of recombinant tissue plasminogen activator (rt-PA).[18]

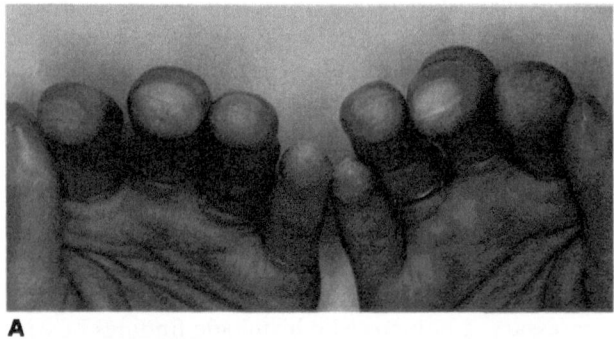

A

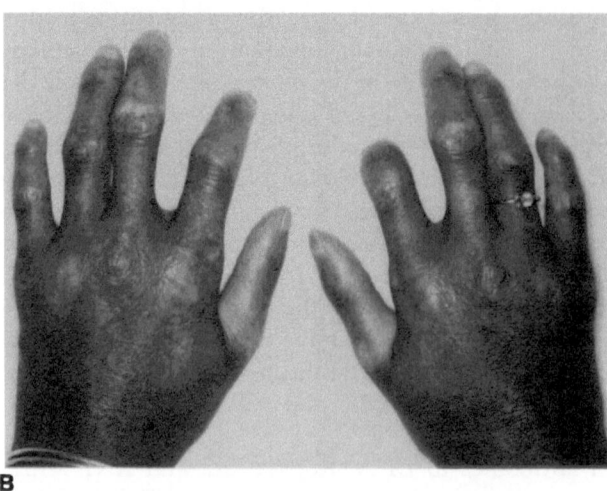

B

Figure 8.7. Loss of finger substance, pathognomonic of SSc, occurred by age 9 (A) in a child whose disease began at age 6 (see Case Report 1). (B) At age 21 (same patient as Fig. 8.15). Presence of anticentromere antibody increases the risk of digital ischemic loss.[16a]

Table 8.1. Manifestations of Progressive Systemic Sclerosis in Children

Raynaud's phenomenon
Generalized diffuse scleroderma of the skin*
Sclerodactyly†
Digital pitting scars of fingertips; and/or loss of substance of finger pad†
Esophageal dysfunction
Dilatation of the duodenum and jejunum
Sacculations of the small bowel and colon
Fibrosing alveolitis (interstitial pneumonia); pulmonary fibrosis†
Malignant hypertension
Renal failure
Pericarditis, pulmonary artery hypertension, cardiomyopathy due to myocardial
   fibrosis

---

*Scleroderma present proximal to the metacarpo- or metatarsophalangeal joints is sufficient by itself for diagnosis (91% sensitivity, 99% specificity).
†In the absence of diffuse scleroderma, diagnosis may be made in the presence of any two of these three items (97% sensitivity, 98% specificity).

Epidemiology

At least two-thirds of affected children are girls. The incidence of affected adult women to men during the childbearing age is reported to be 15:1, strikingly higher than in the premenarchial pediatric population.[3,4] Familial cases are rare, but among the small number of children in the literature, there are one pair of sisters and one mother-son occurrence.[19] We have recently reported a father-daughter occurrence[20] with a grand-daughter with Raynaud's phenomenon and pulmonary hypertension; and a pair of sibs, one with linear scleroderma and the other with pulmonary hypertension and Raynaud's phenomenon.[21] Occasional families of index cases have an increased incidence of hypergammaglobulinemia, antinuclear antibodies, or other rheumatic diseases in close relatives and there is one report of husband and wife developing SSc within a 3-year period.[22] There has been no consistent deviation from the normal population in the incidence of the major HLA-A or B histocompatibility antigens, but recent studies suggest some linkage of DR5 in SSc with Scl 70 autoantibodies. No significant racial differences have been demonstrated.

Classification

Patients may be divided into two major groups, those with localized scleroderma and those with systemic sclerosis (Fig. 8.2). Only children with diffuse scleroderma have developed systemic sclerosis. There are two different types of localized skin lesions: morphea and linear scleroderma; in addition,

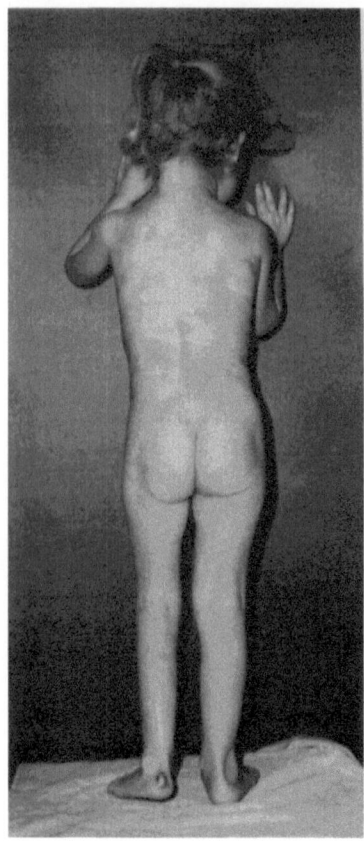

Figure 8.8. Localized scleroderma, at age 3 years, soon after onset. Generalized morphea lesions are visible on trunk. The linear lesions pictured 7 years later in Fig. 8.5 are just beginning in the left leg, foot, and hand. Differential growth of the extremities, pictured 7 years later in Figs 8.12 and 8.13, is just beginning at age 3.

patients with linear scleroderma often have some morphea lesions (Fig. 8.8).[3] The location and depth of lesions determine cosmetic and functional loss. While the classification may seem intricate and confusing at first, it is essential in determining prognosis and therapy. One may choose not to use a dangerous experimental agent in a child whose life and bodily function are not threatened. On the other hand, a child with linear scleroderma who is threatened with such severe deformity of a leg that amputation may have to be considered may be a suitable candidate for a trial of a new agent.

Clinical Features

Raynaud's Phenomenon (see Fig. 5.20). Intermittent symmetric spasm of the small cutaneous arterioles causing intermittent changes in color of the fingers and toes (rarely the ears, nose, and lips) is common is systemic sclerosis, occurring in up to 75% of patients.[4] Raynaud's phenomenon includes three phases: pallor (complete spasm of the vessel), cyanosis (partial spasm), and hyperemia (reactive dilatation), but the hyperemic phase is frequently not seen. Not only skin vessels are affected; 38% of individuals may have decreased vital capacity, especially when exposed to cold.[23]

Raynaud's phenomenon is rare in young children, common in teenage girls, and said to occur in 1.9–4.6% of the population. Many experts have tried to establish criteria for distinguishing Raynaud's sufferers (i.e., those in whom a diagnosis of connective-tissue diseases [CTD] cannot be established) from those who are at increased risk of later-developing scleroderma or other connective-tissue diseases.[24–28] The presence of ANA, and especially anticentromere antibodies, and antitopoisomerase[29] or of nailfold capillary abnormalities, has consistently identified a population at increased risk; digital tip pitting (ulcerations) or scars, decreased eosphageal motility, and decreased pulmonary diffusing capacity identify a subset of Raynaud's patients at higher than usual risk for development of CREST syndrome. An analysis of many studies suggests that the risk of a teenager with Raynaud's and normal physical examination later developing CTD is probably about 3%; in the presence of physical findings or laboratory markers of increased risk, still only 25% of teenagers, at most, later develop diagnosable CTD.[30] One case of paraneoplastic Raynaud's has been reported in a child.[30a]

Skin Lesions. Flesh-colored erythematous edematous plaques that evolve into firm, waxy ivory, or yellow-white shiny lesions, sometimes with a violaceous border, are called morphea (Fig. 8.1).[31] Lesions may be single or multiple or may coalesce (Figs. 8.3 and 8.8).

Linear scleroderma lesions sometimes resemble morphea at onset but have a linear configuration which appears as a broad band, often running along an entire extremity (Figs. 8.4 and 8.5). The initial inflammatory phase may be accompanied by more generalized edema. A particular localized form of this lesion termed "coup de sabre" appears in the forehead and scalp (Fig. 8.9) and may extend down into the face (Fig. 8.10) and be accompanied by morphea lesions. Coup de sabre and linear scleroderma are not limited to the skin. Involvement of the underlying fat, muscle, fascia, and sometimes bone may result in severe growth deformities or mutilation (Figs. 8.11–8.14). Scalp and facial lesions may be accompanied by uveitis and epileptic seizures.[32,33] Facial hemiatrophy (Parry-Romberg syndrome), a rare congenital or acquired disorder, may be difficult to distinguish from linear scleroderma (coup de sabre) (Fig. 8.27).[33]

Generalized scleroderma often begins with an edematous inflammatory phase. There may be striking edematous swelling of the fingers that lasts for several weeks before it is replaced by thick, tight, unpliable skin that becomes increasingly taut, shiny, and atrophied. The face becomes pinched, immobile, and expressionless; the mouth cannot be opened properly (tobacco-pouch mouth; Fig. 8.15).

In all forms of scleroderma, pigmentary changes are often striking with areas of hypo- and hyperpigmentation and, in some cases, telangiectasia

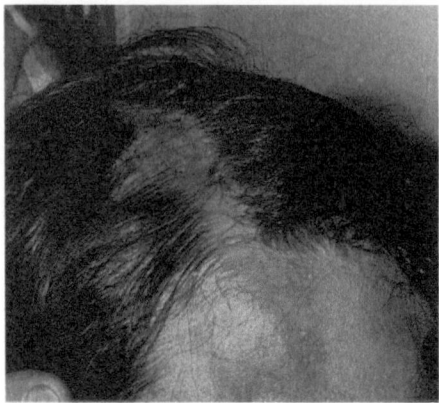

Figure 8.9. Coup-de-sabre lesions of scalp and forehead in a 13-year-old boy.

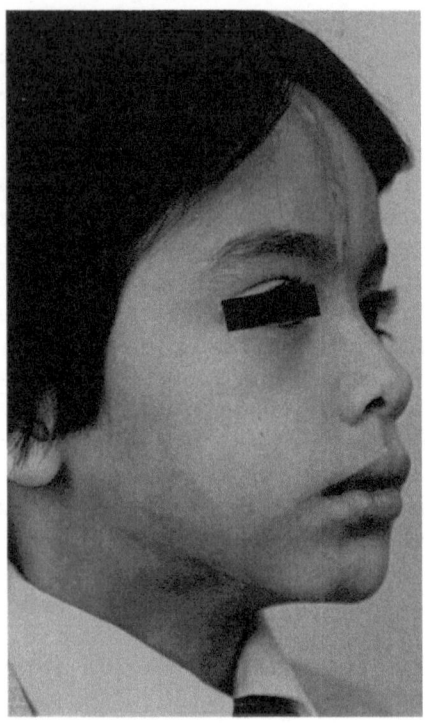

Figure 8.10. Coup-de-sabre linear lesion in a 10-year-old boy carries down from the scalp across the nose and mouth and on to the chin. Morphea lesions are apparent on the lower right side of the face and neck.

(Fig. 8.12). Capillary blood flow is diminished, especially with cooling.[34] Ulcers may appear in thin areas overlying joints or on the fingertips. Secondary infections of these areas may be disastrous. Subcutaneous calcifications may be seen, especially in the fingers and at the elbows (Fig. 8.16) and distal bone erosion and osteolysis may occur in the tips of the phalanges in systemic

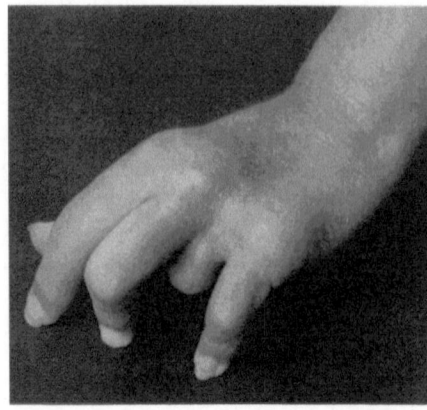

Figure 8.11. The lesion seen just beginning in the hand of the patient pictured in Fig. 8.8 has progressed, by age 10, to produce a significant deformity that will require surgery.

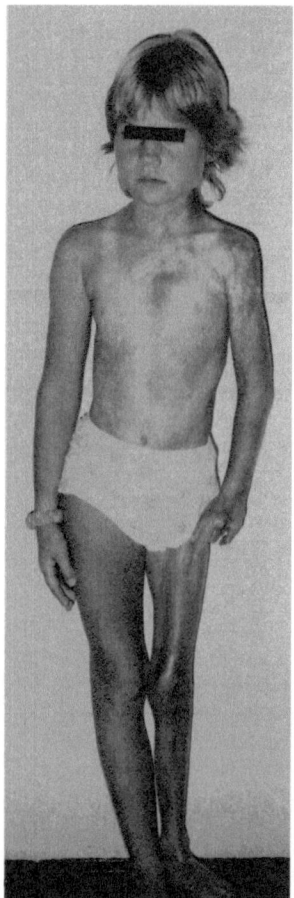

Figure 8.12. Striking shortening of the left lower extremity (3 inches at age 10) ultimately required above-knee amputation as growth difference accelerated during adolescence. The left hip will require rotational osteotomy. The left arm is also considerably shorter than the right, and the left hand is dwarfed and deformed.

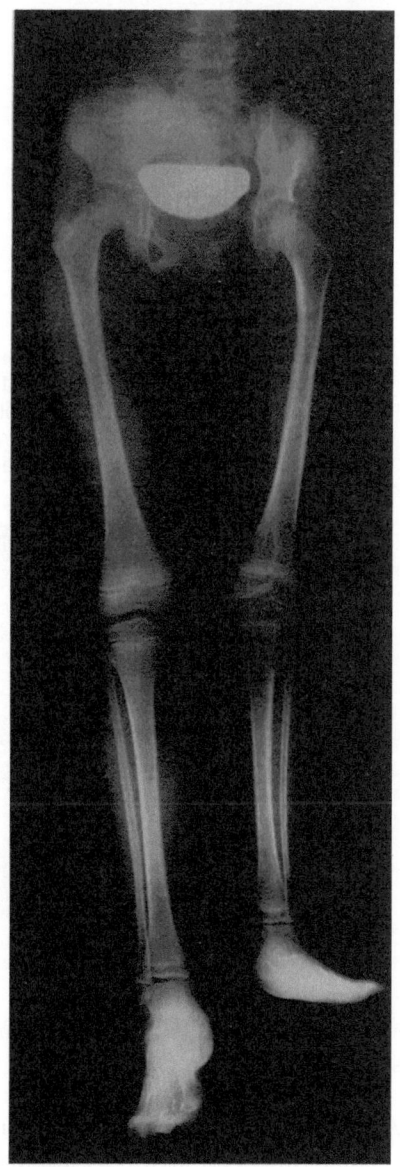

Figure 8.13. Radiograph of patient shown in Fig. 8.12, showing leg-length discrepancy and joint deformities at hip and knee.

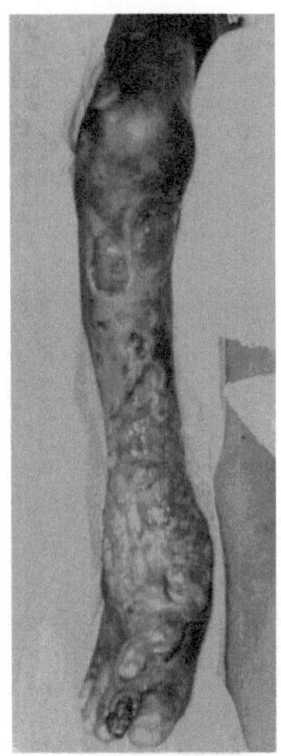

Figure 8.14. Linear scleroderma/morphea with secondary osteomyelitis. (**A**) Patient referred from Guatemala. (**B**) Following amputation no new lesions developed in 10 subsequent years.

A

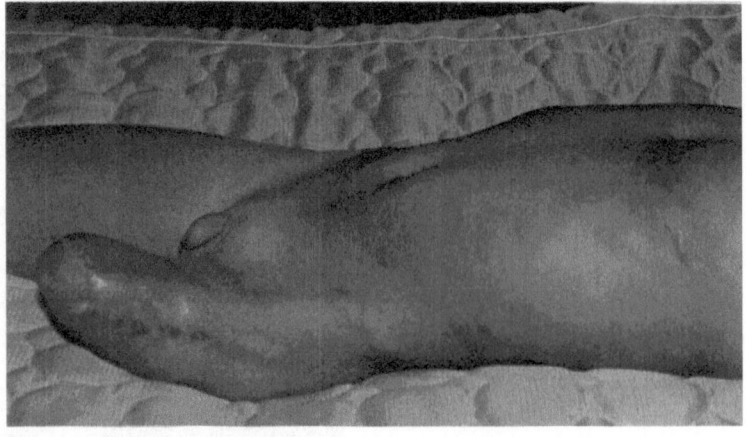

B

sclerosis (Fig. 8.7). Nailfold capillary abnormalities are not seen in localized scleroderma.[35]

Arthritis. Joints may be limited and symptomatic as a result of overlying scleroderma (Fig. 8.12). Occasional patients may have polyarthritis resem-

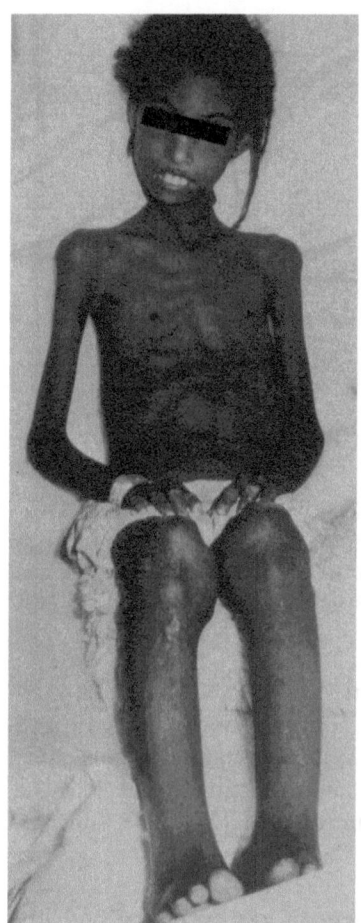

Figure 8.15. Progressive systemic sclerosis at age 9 (onset, age 6; same patient as shown in Figs. 8.7, 8.16, 8.18). Note pinched, immobile, expressionless "mask" face and "tobacco-pouch" mouth.

bling JRA as part of their disease. Brief episodes of monarticular inflammation occur in some children.[3] Myositis resembling that seen in dermatomyositis is also seen in some patients with scleroderma, and when present seems to be associated with an increased frequency of myocarditis.[36,37]

Esophageal Dysfunction. Twenty percent of children with localized scleroderma have been reported to have radiographic evidence of esophageal dysmotility; the changes are not necessarily permanent and do not imply systemic sclerosis. In some cases, repeat studies on the same patients were normal. Abnormal esophageal motility due to smooth-muscle atrophy and fibrosis occurs in almost all patients with systemic sclerosis, may be manifested by chest pain,[38] and may cause acid esophagitis and stricture.[39] Dry mouth and Sjögren's syndrome may also contribute to swallowing difficulties.

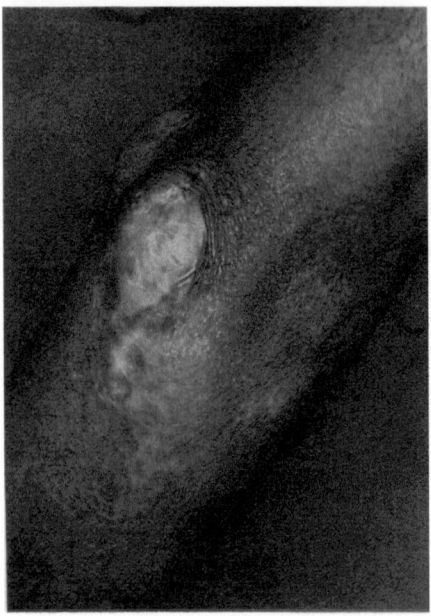

Figure 8.16. Calcinosis and scars of lesions that have discharged calcium at the elbow.

Other Systemic Manifestations. Children with localized scleroderma may have arthritis, esophageal dysfunction, and coup-de-sabre-induced CNS manifestations, but they do not have the other systemic manifestations characteristic of SSc. The lungs, heart, kidney, and intestinal tract may be affected in (Table 8.1) mixed connective-tissue disease (MCTD) and SSc overlap syndromes.[40]

Lungs. Most children with SSc have impairment of gas exchange and impaired vital capacity as a result of pulmonary fibrosis.[4,41] Dyspnea becomes a prominent symptom, although the child may be unaware of it having already restricted her activities greatly. Dyspnea may be accentuated on exposure to cold as a result of pulmonary vasoconstriction. Severe pulmonary vascular hypertension may result from involvement of the pulmonary vascular bed, even in the absence of pulmonary fibrosis. Pulmonary hypertension often presents with syncopal episodes.

Heart. At postmorten examination there may be extensive loss of myocardial fibers and replacement with severe interstitial myocardial fibrosis; as would be expected in the presence of such pathology, arrhythmias, pericarditis, and congestive heart failure from cardiomyopathy are common.[3,4,42] Myocarditis and pericarditis may be early manifestations. Abnormalities of myocardial perfusion are common.[43,44] Pulmonary vascular hypertension may accentuate the cardiac difficulties. As the disease progresses, if enough of the pulmonary vascular bed becomes fibrosed, there may be some relief of pulmonary hypertension. Cardiac decompensation has been the most common cause of death in children with PSS. In at least some of these children, malignant hypertension and renal failure were important contributors to cardiac failure. It is not known whether idiopathic pulmonary hypertension in children is an isolated scleroderma manifestation in some cases.[44a]

Kidneys. Devastating renal disease has accounted for up to 15% of deaths in children with PSS.[3] Renal failure may be slowly progressive, or there may be sudden onset of highly malignant hypertension and rapidly progressive renal failure.[45–48] This may occur at any time but is more frequent within the first few years of disease and in pregnancy.[47] Recent studies indicate that the malignant renal failure is a result of excessive production of renin and angiotension II.[1,48] There is little evidence that the renal disease is immunologically mediated. The primary renal lesion appears to be ischemic cortical necrosis, a result of obstructing intimal lesions in interlobular and arcuate arteries and functional vasoconstriction—the same primary pathogenetic mechanisms seen in other organs in this disease.[49] Patients with scleroderma without hypertension have recently been shown to have increased renin secretion in response to standing or cold stress.[48] A subset of patients with scleroderma renal crisis are normotensive; these patients frequently have microangiopathic hemolytic anemia, thrombocytopenia, and pulmonary hemorrhage.[50]

Continous ambulatory peritoneal dialysis (CAPD) may be the optimal form of dialytic therapy for SSc patients as renal function sometimes improves months after an episode of scleroderma renal crisis.[51]

Intestinal Tract.   Dilatation of the duodenum as a result of striking hypomotility of the small intestine may lead to severe malabsorption and wasting. Patients often have bloating, abdominal cramps, diarrhea, or severe constipation. All of these symptoms may be relieved by the administration of tetracycline, which helps avoid ileus (Fig. 8.17), misdiagnosis of mechanical obstruction, and unnecessary, often fatal, surgery. Barium meal examination sometimes shows localized areas of dilatation and hypersegmentation throughout the small bowel; striking dilatation of the jejunum with "closed accordion" sign; and wide-mouthed diverticuli (sacculations) in the small bowel and colon, a radiographic finding specific for PSS that results from patchy atrophy of the muscularis as the disease progresses. Central venous hyperalimentation may be necessary.[52]

Course of the Disease

All authors agree that localized forms of scleroderma may progress for a period of a few years and then may improve, with a decrease in the shiny appearance and pigmentary change. The progression, if it continues, tends to

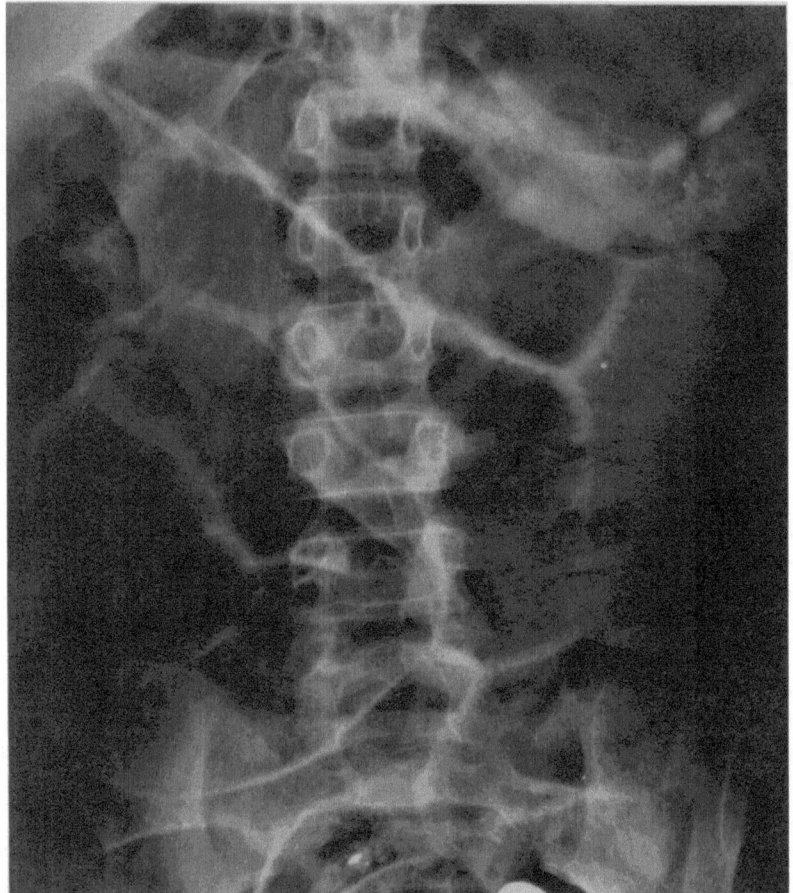

Figure 8.17. Psuedointestinal obstruction with giant scybala in 10-year-old girl with systemic sclerosis.

be at a slower pace. The major problems with linear scleroderma are disfigurement (especially facial), functional impairment or disfigurement in a dominant hand or a lower extremity,[3] and neurologic damage with coup-de-sabre lesions.

The prognosis for SSc is quite variable in children, but in our experience is generally unpleasant. However, even a child who resembles a mummy at age 9 (Fig. 8.15) may improve and function well as a college student (Fig. 8.18) (see Case Report 1). In the past, 20–45% of children with SSc died within 10 years of onset, primarily of cardiac disease.[3,4] With modern management, these figures are no longer applicable. LeRoy and others have identified a subset with an especially bad prognosis, characterized by rapid progression within weeks from Raynaud's to edematous skin changes to the hidebound

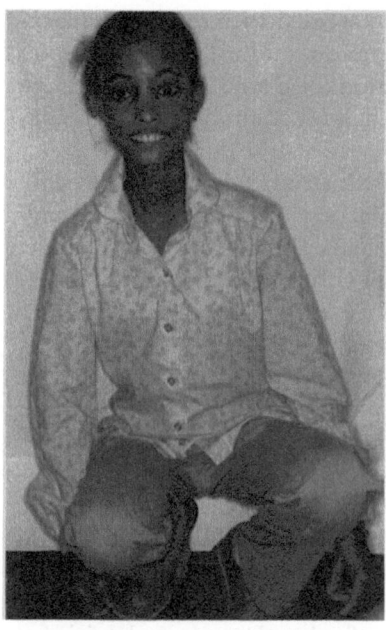

Figure 8.18. Patient shown in Figure 8.15, at age 21 in college. Mobility and muscle strength had greatly improved, as shown in this pose.

state, including trunchal skin.[1,53] These patients often have antitopoisomerase antibodies.

Treatment

So far, there is no cure for scleroderma. Unlike the other connective-tissue diseases, there is no drug that provides good control of the disease. While physiotherapy is advocated to prevent deformity, this author knows of no evidence that deformity can be prevented or even lessened. Nevertheless, patients with this disorder can be helped by a knowledgeable physician who applies specific therapeutic maneuvers in individual circumstances:

1. In the early inflammatory phase of scleroderma, if there is considerable myositis or if the inflammatory skin, cardiac, or lung manifestations are predominant, prednisone may be helpful.[1] This is especially important when inflammation in heart or lungs is immediately life-threatening, but early steroid treatment in this situation may also contribute to the prevention of irreversible scarring in the heart and lungs.[1] The myositis often responds adequately to relatively small alternate-day doses of prednisone.

2. Malabsorption and intestinal hypomotility may be treated with metoclopramide octreotide,[54] and erythromycin or tetracycline, which may prevent inanition and avoid inappropriate life-threatening surgery for intestinal obstruction.[55] Acid esophagitis is treated with antacids, H_2 blockers, and

bethanechol.[56] Esophageal stricture may be treated with recurrent dilatation. Insofar as possible newer surgical techniques for relief of esophageal stricture are avoided because of the potential for excessive postoperative scar formation, but they are occasionally helpful. Liquid dietary supplements may be helpful.

3. Raynaud's phenomenon may be treated with strong advice to take every precaution against exposure to cold. Protection of hands and feet with thermal gloves and socks is important. Patients are instructed to keep the core of the body warm to avoid peripheral vasoconstriction with further compromise of peripheral circulation. Nifedipine is generally accepted as the drug of choice, which may produce healing of digital ulcers and may also benefit other manifestations of SSc.[57–59] In patients unresponsive to or intolerant of nifedipine control may be achieved with reserpine, guanethidine, diltiazem, prazosin, alpha-methyldopa, phenoxybenzamine, and a variety of other agents. The topical application of 1% glyceryl trinitrate ointment may be a helpful adjunct to a basic regimen of oral sympatholytic agents.[60,61] In desperate situations, prostaglandin E_1[62] or plasmapheresis[63] may save digits. Biofeedback techniques, which have no adverse side effects, have been reported to help some children.[64]

4. The first reports of successful treatment of scleroderma renal crisis required nephrectomy and renal dialysis and/or transplant. Further study supported the hypothesis that excessive renin activity and the resulting excess of angiotension II were important in the pathogenesis of malignant scleroderma renal disease. An oral angiotensin-converting enzyme inhibitor (captopril) has been successfully used in the treatment of scleroderma renal crisis.[65] In addition to improvement and control of the renal disease, healing of the fingertip ulcers was achieved. Other new antihypertensive drugs have also prevented death in scleroderma renal crisis without the need for nephrectomy; patients so treated improved in other parameters as well.[66] One teenager whose life was preserved by such treatment has only minimal scleroderma in other sites and now leads an almost normal life.[67]

5. Although early reports of successful treatment of adult scleroderma with penicillamine seem now to have been overenthusiastic, penicillamine may be useful in the treatment of some children with scleroderma.[68,69] In some patients with a great deal of inflammation in the skin, subcutaneous tissues, and systemic organs, penicillamine may be steroid-sparing (see Case Report 2). We have not had much success with penicillamine as a treatment for linear scleroderma despite reports by others of success. Several studies suggests that long-term administration of penicillamine reduces skin thickness, has a beneficial effect on interstitial lung disease, and increases long-term survival of adults with SSc.[70–71a] Further trials may be indicated. POTABA, DMSO, EDTA, colchicine, chlorambucil, recombinant tissue plasminogen activator,[18] and other agents have been reported to be helpful on occasion.[1,10] Cyclosporine, methotrexate, and

photochemotherapy may be the best agents for early aggressive disease.[18,72–75] Methotrexate is also now being tried in linear scleroderma.

In the past 5 years, there has been an increased interest in scleroderma and an increased intensity of productive research. Death has now been averted in some young patients. Recent studies suggest that an increased understanding of this depressing illness may soon be forthcoming. Physicians with an optimistic attitude can help prevent debilitating depression in these children and their families.

Case Report 1: Systemic Sclerosis

At age 6 years, this black girl developed Raynaud's phenomenon and hardening of the skin of her hands followed by painless ulcers on her digits. Over a period of 3 years, the disease progressed to involve all of the skin of the extremities and face, producing marked shininess and tightening with areas of depigmentation (Fig. 8.15). Ulcerations appeared over all the fingertips, some toes, the elbows, and the medial malleoli (Fig. 8.7). X-rays showed atrophy of the soft tissues and destruction and resorption of the distal finger tufts. Chest x-rays showed a diffuse fibrotic process and EKG a shifting pacemaker. At age 11, she developed dysphagia, and esophageal dysmotility was demonstrated radiographically. One year later she was admitted to the hospital with intestinal obstruction (Fig. 8.17). Chest x-ray showed bilateral pleural thickening with early fibrosis bilaterally. An EKG showed sinus bradycardia with a rate of 55. Oxygen saturation was 85–92%. The child had a respiratory arrest associated with manipulation of the Miller-Abbott tube, following which she developed pericarditis, pleural effusion, and congestive heart failure. When all of this was controlled, the abdomen was explored because of persistent intestinal obstruction, and the left colon was disimpacted of massive amounts of "concrete" scabellae.

With daily enemas and mineral oil, she did relatively well, requiring hospitalization only once, at age 15, again for intestinal obstruction, which was relieved with a Miller-Abbott tube. With tetracycline and mineral oil as needed, there were no further episodes of intestinal obstruction. No specific treatment was given. Her overall condition improved (Fig 8.18) and she graduated from high school and college. However, over the text few years inanition and cardiopulmonary progression led to death at age 26.

Disorders Resembling Scleroderma (Table 8.2)[76]

A subset of scleroderma patients has been referred to as the CREST syndrome. Disease in these patients is characterized by prominent calcinosis (C), Raynaud's phenomenon (R), esophageal dysmotility (E), sclerodactyly (S), and telangiectasia (T). Severe pulmonary artery hypertension (without pulmonary fibrosis) and biliary cirrhosis, both unusual features of PSS, are not rare manifestations in CREST syndrome. Anticentromere ANA, thought

Table 8.2. Disorders Resembling Scleroderma

Scleredema
Subcutaneous lipogranulomatosis (Rothmann Makai syndrome)
Eosinophilic fasciitis
Toxic oil syndrome and eosinophilic myalgia syndrome induced by "toxic"
   L-tryptophan
Special connective-tissue syndromes
   Mixed connective-tissue disease
   CREST syndrome
Iatrogenic fibrous myopathy
Chronic cutaneous graft-versus-host reaction
Human adjuvant disease
Chemical and drug-induced sclerodermalike conditions
   Bleomycin
   Pentazocine
   Isoniazid
   L-5-Hydroxytryptophan and carbidopa
   Vinyl chloride
Systemic disorders associated with induration or atrophy of skin and subcutaneous
   tissues: phenylketonuria, porphyria cutanea tarda, acromegaly, amyloid, carci-
   noid
Premature aging: scleromyxedema, progeria, Werner's and Rothmund's syndromes
Parry-Romberg syndrome

to be specific to this syndrome have not yet been reported in childhood but may appear later in adults whose disease began in childhood.[7] CREST syndrome patients tend to have a slower, more indolent course than others with scleroderma,[77] but after many years the disease may suddenly become very aggressive and is then indistinguishable from PSS.

Children with MCTD may have Raynaud's phenomenon, esophageal dysmotility, myositis, scleroderma, and features of systemic lupus (see Chapter 5). Thick skin may also be seen as a feature of certain indurative diseases (phenylketonuria, porphyria cutanea tarda, acromegaly, amyloid, and carcinoid) and of disorders that are associated with atrophy of skin or subcutaneous tissues (progeria and Werner's and Rothmund's syndromes).[78] Other sclerodermalike syndromes include the following:

Scleredema (The China-Doll Syndrome)[79–81]

This syndrome is characterized by the sudden development of indurative edema of the neck, shoulder girdle, face, and sometimes the trunk and proximal (but not distal) extremities. The onset is dramatic, and the edema appears all at one time. Unlike scleroderma where the disease usually begins in the hands and feet and progresses centrally, the hands and feet are rarely affected at all in scleredema, a feature which helps in differentiation from eosinophilic fasciitis as well as from scleroderma. True sclerodermatous patches do not occur in scleredema, and there is complete recovery without atrophy, pigmentation, or telangiectasia. This disorder was previously called scleredema adultorum of Buschke; the name was changed when it was recognized that most cases occurred in childhood. Girls are more frequently affected. While the disease has an acute onset, it does not disappear quickly. The average course lasts 12–18 months. Eye involvement may be severe.[81]

Cardiac manifestations indistinguishable from those of acute rheumatic fever occasionally accompany scleredema. At least in these patients, it seems likely that scleredema is another nonsuppurative sequelae of an antecedent streptococcal sore throat. Most patients with scleredema give a history of an antecedent respiratory illness 1–6 weeks before the onset of edema, and in many cases the illness was due to group-A beta-hemolytic streptococci. Various components of the *Streptococcus* have been shown to disrupt collagen in experimental models, and it is possible that this is the mechanism by which this disorder occurs. Skin biopsies in scleredema show abnormalities only in the subcutaneous tissues, where swelling of collagen fibers, edema, acid mucopolysaccharide deposition, and occasional lymphocytic perivascular cuffing may be seen. The epidermis is normal.

No treatment is usually given for scleredema since the patients are relatively asymptomatic despite their "china-doll" appearance and the disease is self-limited. There is some evidence that corticosteroids may shorten the course of the illness, although corticosteroid treatment does not prevent the appearance of the syndrome and may not control corneal exposure sufficiently to avoid the need for temporary tarsorrhaphies.[81]

Subcutaneous Lipogranulomatosis (Rothmann-Makai Syndrome)[82]

In 1894 and 1928, Rothmann and Makai described a distinctive syndrome of circumscribed panniculitis ("lipogranulomatosis subcutanea") in children. Four patients with this rarely recognized syndrome have been followed by us, one for 28 years (Fig. 8.19). During the acute phase, the skin of the lower extremities may feel tight and hard and the subcutaneous tissue woody. Multiple painless lumps appear throughout the muscle and subcutaneous tissues. Patches of overlying skin simulate morphea or linear scleroderma; the nodules may be confused with erythema nodosum, erythema induratum, or nodular vasculitis. New lesions continue to appear over a period of 6–12 months and then subside, leaving extensive permanent atrophic depressions in the lower extremities and occasionally also in the arms. The patients are not systemically ill. The only laboratory abnormalities are increased immunoglobulins and a high ESR.

Microscopic examination of biopsy specimens of both lesions and normal-

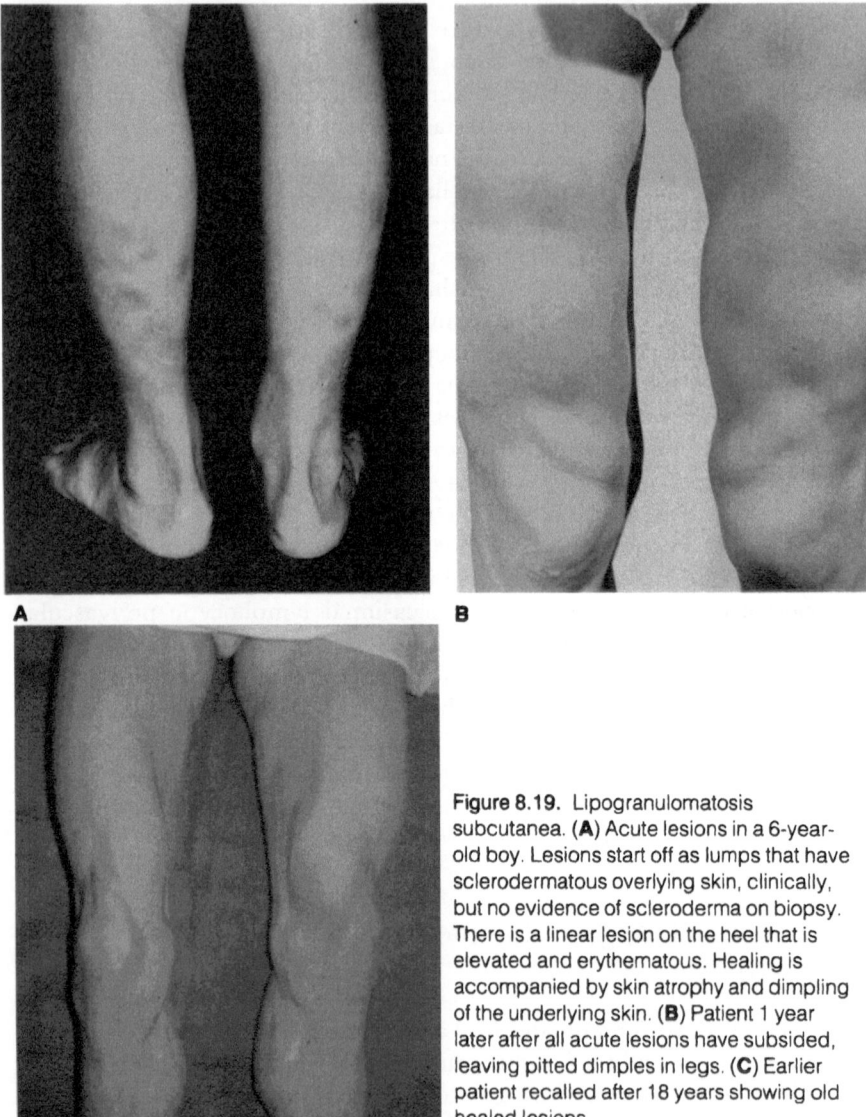

Figure 8.19. Lipogranulomatosis subcutanea. (**A**) Acute lesions in a 6-year-old boy. Lesions start off as lumps that have sclerodermatous overlying skin, clinically, but no evidence of scleroderma on biopsy. There is a linear lesion on the heel that is elevated and erythematous. Healing is accompanied by skin atrophy and dimpling of the underlying skin. (**B**) Patient 1 year later after all acute lesions have subsided, leaving pitted dimples in legs. (**C**) Earlier patient recalled after 18 years showing old healed lesions.

appearing adjacent areas show granulomatous necrosis of subcutaneous fat with foamy histiocytic giant cells, microcyst formation, and in some cases panarteritis with fibrinoid necrosis (Figs. 8.20 and 8.21). Corticosteroid treatment reduces inflammation but does not prevent new lesions or seem to alter the course of the self-limited disease.

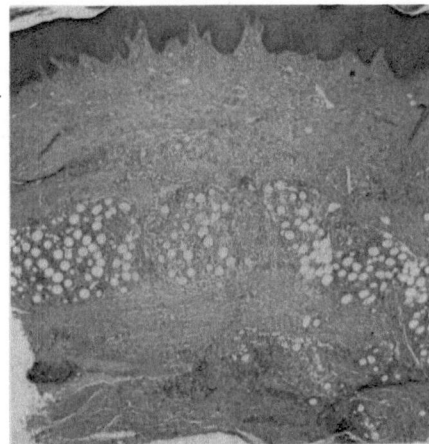

Figure 8.20. Histologic section showing normal skin with lipogranulomatous inflammation in the panniculus. ×25.

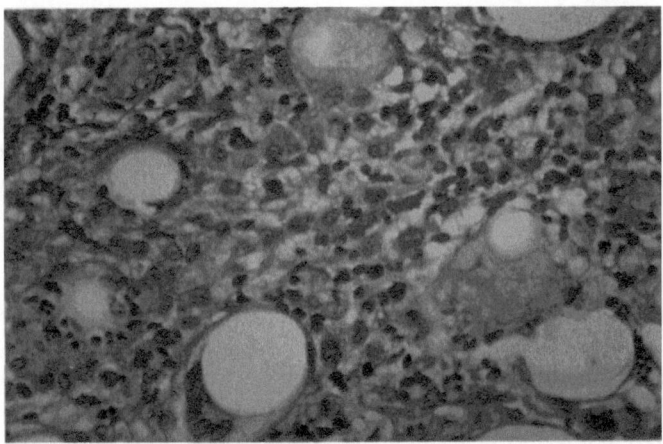

Figure 8.21. Higher-power view of the inflammation in the panniculus, showing collections of multinucleated giant cells, histiocytes, and a few neutrophils. ×250.

Eosinophilic Fasciitis[83–89]

In 1974, Shulman described a new syndrome characterized by painful generalized indurated sclerodermalike swelling of the hands and feet following exercise. The progressive swelling of the extremities is so dramatic that pitting edema is often demonstrable (Fig. 8.22). Our patients rapidly developed extensive flexion contractures. In some cases, the face and trunk are also involved. In Shulman's cases, there were no visceral manifestations, and esophageal dysmotility could not be demonstrated. Biopsies of affected areas

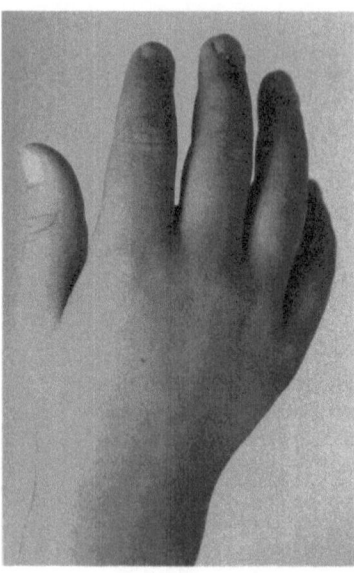

Figure 8.22. Diffuse edema and rapidly developing flexion contracture of the wrist and hand in a 6-year-old girl with eosinophilic fasciitis.

revealed severe inflammation of the panniculus and deep fascia. The inflammatory reaction was characterized by lymphocytes, plasma cells, and histiocytes and only rarely contained eosinophils (Fig. 8.23). However, there was impressive eosinophilia in the peripheral white blood cell count (8–29% of the differential count), which provided the syndrome with its original (more accurate) name "fasciitis with eosinophilia" (Fig. 8.24). The erythrocyte sedimentation rate is elevated and hypergammaglobulinemia is usually present.

Many cases of eosinophilic fasciitis have now being reported in childhood, and we have seen three children with this disorder. Most of the children have had localized scleroderma lesions (morphea and/or linear scleroderma) in addition to diffuse fasciitis.[89] In our limited series, the syndrome in childhood consists of (1) localized scleroderma (Fig. 8.25); (2) superimposed, rapidly developing diffuse fasciitis with binding down of the grossly edematous skin to underlying structures and rapid development of severe flexion contractures of the wrists, elbows, shoulders, ankles, knees, and hips; and (3) eosinophilia in blood, bone marrow, and sometimes in fascia. This triad, once identified by Shulman, was distinguishable from the slowly progressive diffuse scleroderma of systemic sclerosis, from scleredema, and from other children who had localized scleroderma alone. However, one of our patients had a slower-onset, visceral manifestations, and a later period of destructive arthritis. Patients may present with arthritis, or develop late arthritis, lupus, or scleroderma.[90,91] (see Case Report 2). The clinical pattern of eosinophilic fasciitis is evolving and must be considered to be in a state of flux. Unfortunately, several adult patients with this syndrome have now developed

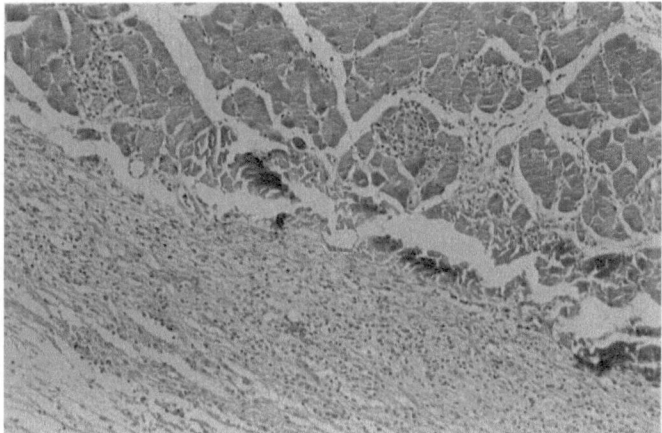

Figure 8.23. Muscle and fascia showing a diffuse mononuclear inflammatory infiltrate present in muscle and strikingly severe in underlying fascia. Eosinophils are present in slightly greater frequency than expected. ×180.

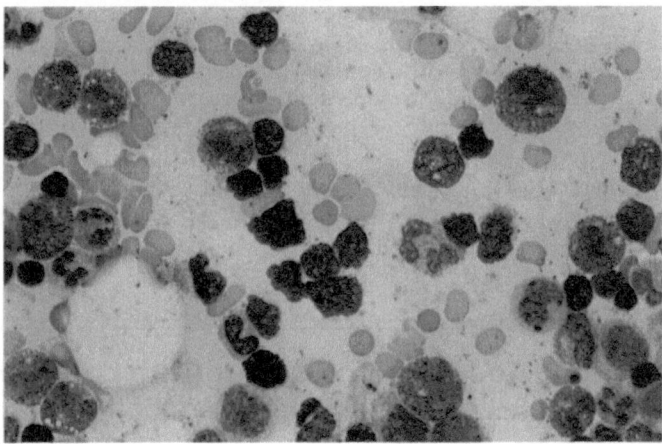

Figure 8.24. Bone marrow from patient with fasciitis (Fig. 8.23) showing striking hyperplasia of eosinophilic leukocytes. (Wright's stain) ×1218.

antibody-mediated aplastic anemia, suggesting that in some cases fasciitis with eosinophilia can be a manifestation of an underlying lymphoproliferative disorder.[84] This has not yet been reported in children.

Patients with this disorder respond dramatically to corticosteroids, which can usually be discontinued without exacerbation after a variable period of time. Our most recent patient responded well to an alternate-day prednisone regimen as initial therapy. Penicillamine and hydroxychloroquine may also

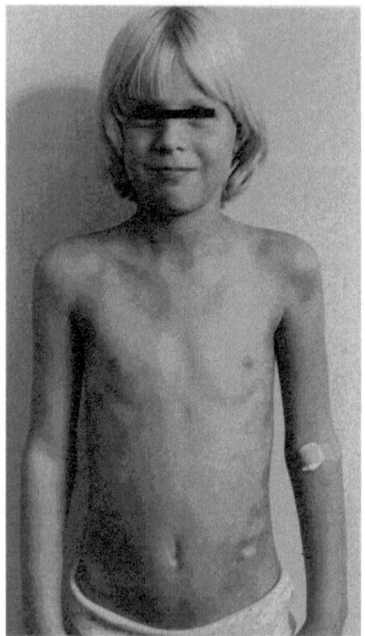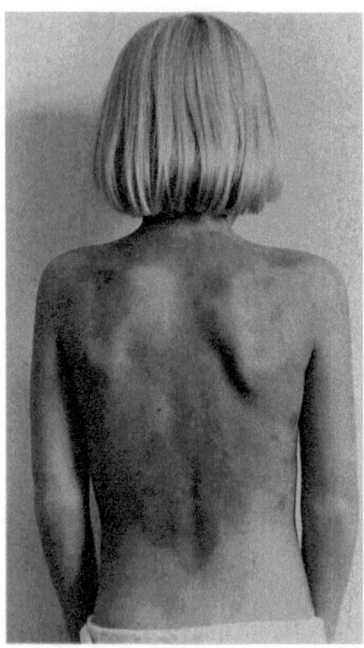

A   **B**

Figure 8.25. (**A** and **B**) Patient with eosinophilic fasciitis; antecedent morphea was present for 1 year prior to sudden onset of fasciitis. Ten years later patient is well off all medication. Residual flexion contractures persist in the fingers, wrists, elbows, ankles, and hips.

be helpful.[90] Some features of this illness suggest that it may at least in some cases be induced by a toxin, analogous to eosinophilia myalgia/toxic oil syndrome.[91a]

Case Report 2: Eosinophilic Fasciitis (with Localized Scleroderma and Recurrent Myopericarditis)

This 4-year-old, previously healthy white girl developed fever and a sore throat, irritable behavior, hepatosplenomegaly, and lymphadenopathy in August 1974, at a time when her brother had heterophile-positive infectious mononucleosis. Over a period of months, although her heterophil remained negative, a rise in titer against Epstein-Barr virus to 1:40 was documented. However, during this time, she had become hypergammaglobulinemic and was shown to have high antibody titers to many antigens. She remained irritable, complained of pain in her extremities, and gradually developed a doughy consistency of her muscles. There were no skin changes. Peripheral white blood counts ranged from 10,000 to 25,200 between September 1974 and March 1975; peripheral blood eosinophilia between 15 and 25% was demonstrated with total eosinophil counts varying from 1500 to 3325. In January, a cardiac gallop was heard without other cardiac abnormalities, and the child was started on prednisone, 2 mg/kg/day. This improved her symptoms, but during the next month typical sclerodermatous patches appeared on her chest, dorsum of both feet, and left flank.

Biopsy of skin and muscle showed inflammation in the dermis and an intense inflammatory reaction of the interstitial and supporting structures of striated muscle; that is, a fasciitis with some degenerative changes in the muscle fibers associated with perivasculitis of arterioles and venules (Fig. 8.23). The inflammation consisted primarily of lymphocytes and plasma cells with only rare eosinophils. However, marked eosinophilia was demonstrated in a bone-marrow aspirant (Fig. 8.24). A lymph-node biopsy showed reticuloendothelial hyperplasia with increased plasma cells. CPK and EMG were normal; ANA and ENA were negative.

When first seen here in March 1975, all of the skin and muscles felt indurated and tight. This was accentuated proximally. There were discrete patches of morphea and linear scleroderma on the left ankle, foot, and abdomen. She was weak but reported to be getting stronger. In April, the prednisone was changed to 75 mg on alternate mornings. She continued to improve with softening of the skin. However, some new patches of morphea appeared, and there continued to be some mild flexion contractures at the wrists, elbows, shoulders, and ankles. Prednisone was gradually reduced and discontinued in October 1975. In January 1976, she had a recurrence of all of the earlier manifestations, including carditis with pericarditis. This responded immediately to reinstitution of prednisone. Penicillamine (gradually increased to 500 mg daily) was introduced and prednisone changed to alternate-day without adverse effect. By January 1977, it was possible to discontinue the prednisone. Penicillamine was then gradually reduced. In June 1977, objective arthritis became troublesome in the previously affected joints and in the hips, although she was still taking 350 mg of penicillamine daily. Aspirin therapy was instituted, and penicillamine was reduced further; however, the arthritis persisted, and penicillamine was again increased to 250 mg daily. During 1978, the arthritis improved, and the aspirin was discontinued; further improvement was noted in 1979, and the penicillamine was discontinued in 1980. However, when examined in 1987 at age 17, although she said she had felt well for many years but now had symptoms of esophagitis, documented on endoscopy, which responded to Ranitidine, the major finding on examination was severe destructive arthritis with flexion contractures at the wrists ($-90°$) (Fig. 8.26), PIP joints, elbows ($-10°$), shoulders ($-50°$), ankles ($-10°$), knees ($-4°$), and hips ($-40°$). The arthritis has not progressed and she remains well in 1992.

Toxic Oil Syndrome and Eosinophilia-Myalgia Syndrome Induced by "Toxic" L-Tryptophan

In May and June, 1981, ingestion of contaminated rapeseed oil in northern Spain resulted in an epidemic (17,000 cases) of a new hypereosinophilic syndrome characterized by excrutiating fever, myalgia, polymorphous rashes, hepatitis, and interstitial pneumonia resulting in early pulmonary death in 1% of cases.[92] Corticosteroids improved the symptoms.

Convalescence was often protracted and 6 weeks later, after the pneumo-

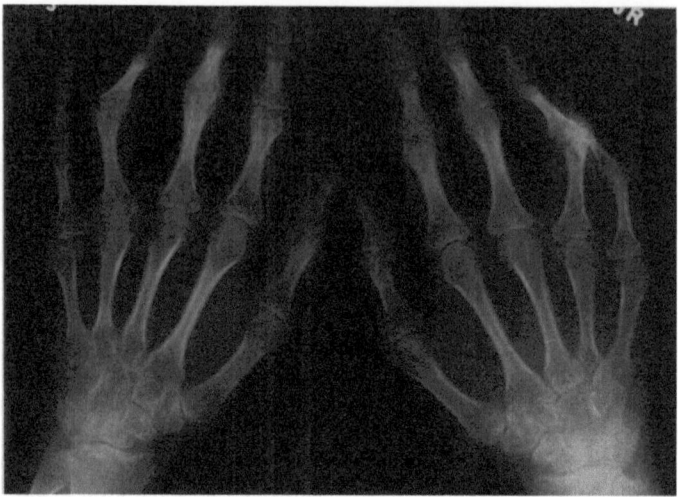

Figure 8.26. Arthritis following eosinophilic fasciitis (see Case Report).

nia cleared, many patients developed severe muscle pains; neurologic signs
and symptoms including sensory loss, hyporeflexia, and paresthesias; nonpitting edema of the face, hands, and feet; and sometimes thrombopenia,
thrombo-embolism, and pulmonary hypertension/cor-pulmonale. Terminal
axonal death and denervation muscle atrophy resulted in a need for mechanical ventilation and caused some additional deaths. In the third month of
illness some patients developed sclerodermalike skin lesions,[93] dysphagia,
Raynaud's phenomenon, and Sjögren's syndrome. Fifteen percent of patients
died and at autopsy all had severe vasculitis with an initial endothelial proliferative lesion which progressed to infiltrate the vessel wall and later caused
obliterative fibrosis of the intima. Ten percent of patients ultimately fulfilled
the diagnostic criteria for PSS. The prognosis was somewhat better in the 170
cases reported in children: two died and three were crippled but after 1
year, 64% were completely well.[94] No new cases have been seen since July
1981.

In October 1989, physicians in New Mexico recognized that three patients
with a new hypereosinophilic syndrome—characterized by fever; incapacitating myalgia; arthralgia; shortness of breath, cough, dyspnea, interstitial
pneumonia; polymorphous rashes; and swelling of the extremities with pitting or nonpitting edema of the hands and feet, resembling the toxic oil
syndrome—had ingested L-tryptophan, an amino acid, as a food additive.
By July 1990, 1531 cases of this syndrome had been reported to the Centers
for Disease Control; 32% required hospitalization; fewer than 1% died.[95–97]
The course, following cessation of L-tryptophan and, in severe cases, institution of steroid therapy, is often prolonged, resembling that seen in the toxic
oil syndrome.[98,99] It is likely this syndrome is due to a contaminant.[100,101]

Different contaminants may have caused the similar eosinophilic fasciitis patients we have described above; our patients were not exposed to toxic oil or L-tryptophan but these syndromes are only defined in epidemics. Methotrexate may be the most efficacious medication.[102]

Iatrogenic Fibrous Myopathy[76]

Repeated injection of medication (antibiotics, corticosteroids, pentazocine) into muscle may result in the creation of a fibrous scar in the body of the muscle. When severe, a marked depression of the overlying skin is apparent, and a fibrous band can be palpated in the underlying muscle. Because the condition is slowly progressive for a few years, the injections may have been forgotten; occasionally, no history of such trauma can be elicited. The deltoid and quadriceps muscles, usually used for intramuscular injections, are most commonly affected. Abduction contractures of the shoulders and hips may result and may require surgical release of the bands.

Drug-Chemical-Induced Sclerodermalike Disease[76]

Bleomycin, used in cancer therapy, may induce plaques of thickened skin. Histologic examination shows dense collagen bundles in the dermis. Patients may develop thickened skin with Raynaud's phenomenon and pulmonary fibrosis.

A small number of workers with vinyl chloride have developed sore fingers, synovial thickening of the PIP joints, pulmonary fibrosis, hepatic fibrosis, Raynaud's phenomenon, and acro-osteolysis. Capillary microscopy of ungual telangiectasia resembles that of scleroderma, and digital angiography has shown severe narrowing of the lumina of digital arteries. There is an excess of new collagen production just as in scleroderma. The skin manifestations regress following discontinuation of exposure to vinyl chloride. We think we have seen a young child with Raynaud's induced by vinyl chloride gas given off from a vinyl chloride bedsheet prescribed for mold allergy.

Drugs and disorders associated with high plasma serotonin and elevated kynurenine may also induce a generalized reversible sclerodermalike syndrome. These agents include isoniazid and the combination of L-5-hydroxytryptophan and carbidopa, used for treatment of certain neurologic disorders.[103]

Sclerodermalike Syndrome as Part of Chronic Cutaneous Graft-Versus-Host Reaction[104]

Increasing numbers of human allogeneic bone-marrow transplants are being performed as part of the treatment for aplastic anemia, leukemia, and combined immunodeficiency. Ten percent of these patients have graft-versus-

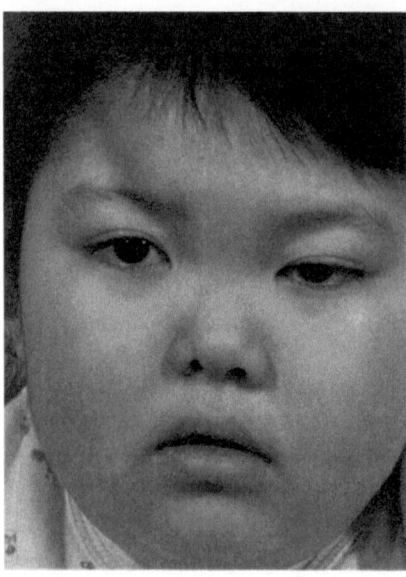

Figure 8.27. Parry-Romberg Syndrome (facial hemiatrophy, left) with coup-de-sabre-like indentation of the right side of the face without sclerodermatous features. Patient had cerebral vasculitis with recurrent episodes of hemiparesis and progressive calcifications in the right temporal and frontal areas. Spirochete forms compatible with borrelia were shown in the brain biopsy.

host reactions; in 90% of these, sclerodermalike syndromes develop. Dermal induration is followed by the skin becoming firm, inelastic, and hide-bound to deep fascial structures. These dermal manifestations may be accompanied by other connective-tissue-disease-like findings including Sjögren's syndrome, polymyositis, panniculitis, fibrosis of the gut wall, and chronic aggressive hepatitis. Similar graft-versus-host reactions may occur following renal transplantation.

Scleroderma Syndromes as Part of Human Adjuvant Disease[105]

The term *human adjuvant disease* has been adopted to indicate the development of connective-tissue-disease-like manifestations after plastic surgery with implantation of foreign material (paraffin-silicone and related substances). Twenty-five to fifty percent of patients had a history of tuberculosis, possibly important in the adjuvant reaction. These women developed PSS or morphea. An increased incidence of scleroderma has been reported in men exposed to silica (stonemasons and coal miners), where similar foreign-body granulomas can be demonstrated.

Scleromyxedema[106]

This is a rare fibromucinous disorder, seen primarily in adults with monoclonal gammopathies, characterized by waxy skin papules with marked sclerosis and induration of the skin of the hands, arms, and face.

Parry-Romberg Syndrome (PRS)

Progressive facial hemiatrophy without linear scleroderma has been called PRS;[107] the one patient we have seen (Fig. 8.27) had left facial hemiatrophy, a coup-de-sabre-like indentation on the right side of the face without sclerodermatous features, and calcifying cerebral vasculitis associated with borrelia spirochetes in the brain biopsy.[108] Lyme disease has been previously associated with morphea and linear scleroderma and with PRS.[109,110]

References

1. LeRoy EC, Lomeo R: The spectrum of scleroderma. Hosp Pract pp. 33–42, October 30, 1989; The spectrum of scleroderma (II). Hosp Pract pp. 65–84, November 15, 1989.
2. Masi AT, Rodnan GP, Medsger TA, et al.: Preliminary criteria for the classification of systemic sclerosis (scleroderma). Bull Rheum Dis 31:1–6, 1981; Arthritis Rheum 23:581–590, 1980.
3. Kornreich HK, King KK, Bernstein, BH, et al.: Scleroderma in childhood. Arthritis Rheum 20:343–350, 1977.
4. Cassidy JT, Sullivan DB, Dabich L, et al.: Scleroderma in children. Arthritis Rheum 20:351–354, 1977.
5. Burge SM, Ryan TJ, Dawber RPR: Case reports: juvenile onset systemic sclerosis. J R Soc Med 77:793–794, 1984.
6. Woo TY, Rasmussen JE: Juvenile linear scleroderma associated with serologic abnormalities. Arch Dermatol 12:1403–1405, 1985.
7. Helfrich DJ, Londino AV, Steen VD, Medsger TA Jr: Systemic sclerosis with onset in chilhood. Arthritis Rheum 33:S144, 1990.
8. Suarez-Almazor ME, Catoggio LJ, Maldonado-Cocco JA, et al.: Juvenile progressive systemic sclerosis: clinical and serologic findings. Arthritis Rheum 28:699–702, 1985.
9. Ackerman AB: Histologic Diagnosis of Inflammatory Skin Diseases. Lea and Febiger, Philadelphia, 1978.
10. LeRoy EC, Smith EA, Kahaleh MB, et al.: A strategy for determining the pathogenesis of systemic sclerosis: is transforming growth factor B the answer? Arthritis Rheum 32:817–825, 1989.
11. Jayson MIV, Black CM (eds.) Systemic Sclerosis: Scleroderma. John Wiley & Sons, Chicester, pp. 1–350, 1988.
11a. Kantor TV, Whiteside TL, Friberg D, et al.: Lymphokine-activated killer cells and natural killer cell activities in patients with systemic sclerosis. Arthritis Rheum 35:694–699, 1992.
12. Korn JH: Immunologic aspects of scleroderma. Curr Opin Rheumatol 3:947–952, 1991.

13. Claman HN: On scleroderma: mast cells, endothelial cells, and fibroblasts. JAMA 262:1206–1209, 1989.
14. Kahaleh MB, Sherber GK, LeRoy EC: Endothelial injury in scleroderma. J Exp Med 149:1326–1335, 1979.
14a. Duray P, Zhang L, Cheng J, Bayer M, et al.: Improved accuracy of identifying and implicating Lyme infection in skin and soft tissue samples in humans. V International Conference on Lyme Borreliosis May 30–June 2, 1992, Arlington, Virginia, U.S.A.
15. Bennett RM: Scleroderma overlap syndromes. Rheum Dis Clin North Am 16:185–199, 1990.
16. Reimer G, Steen VD, Penning CA, et al.: Correlates between autoantibodies to nucleolar antigens and clinical features in patients with systemic sclerosis (scleroderma). Arthritis Rheum 31:525–532, 1988.
16a. Wigley FM, Wise RA, Miller R et. al.: Anticentromere antibody as a predictor of digital ischemic loss in patients with systemic sclerosis. Arthritis Rheum 35:688–693, 1992.
17. Bell S, Krieg T, Meurer M: Antibodies to Ro/SSA detected by ELISA: correlation with clinical features in systemic scleroderma. Br J Dermatol 121:35–41, 1989.
18. Fritzler MJ, Hart DA: Prolonged improvement of Raynaud's phenomenon and scleroderma after recombinant tissue plasminogen activator therapy. Arthritis Rheum 33:274–276, 1990.
19. Gray RG, Altman RD: Progressive systemic sclerosis in a family. Arthritis Rheum 20:35–41, 1977.
20. Morse JH, Barst RJ, Whitman H III, et al.: Isolated pulmonary hypertension in the grandchild of a kindred with scleroderma (systemic sclerosis): "neonatal scleroderma?". J Rheumatol 16:1536–1541, 1989.
21. Barst RJ, Jacobs JC, Gersony WM: Childhood primary pulmonary hypertension and maternal connective tissue disease. Pediatr Res 25:520A, 1989.
22. Christy WC, Rodnan GP: Conjugal progressive systemic sclerosis (scleroderma): report of the disease in husband and wife. Arthritis Rheum 27:1180–1182, 1984.
23. Groen H, Wichers G, Ter Borg EJ, et al.: Pulmonary diffusing capacity disturbances are related to nailfold capillary changes in patients with Raynaud's phenomenon with and without an underlying connective tissue disease. Am J Med 89:34–41, 1990.
24. Gerbracht DD, Steen VD, Ziegler GL, et al.: Evolution of primary Raynaud's phenomenon (Raynaud's disease) to connective tissue disease. Arthritis Rheum 28:87–92, 1985.
25. Priollet P, Vayssairat M, Housset E: How to classify Raynaud's phenomenon. Am J Med 83:494–498, 1987.
26. Duffy CM, Laxer RM, Lee P, et al.: Raynaud syndrome in childhood. J Pediatr 114:73–78, 1989.
27. Fitzgerald O, Hess EV, O'Connor G, Spencer-Green G: Prospective evolution of Raynaud's phenomenon. Am J Med 84:718–726, 1988.
28. Sarkozi J, Bookman AAM, Lee P, et al.: Significance of anticentromere antibody in idiopathic Raynaud's syndrome. Am J Med 83:893–898, 1987.
29. Weiner ES, Hildebrandt S, Senecal J-L, et al.: Prognostic significance of anticentromere antibodies and anti-topoisomerase I antibodies in Raynaud's disease. A prospective study. Arthritis Rheum 34:68–77, 1991.

30. Burns EC, Dunger DB, Dillon MJ: Raynaud's disease. Arch Dis Child 60:537–541, 1985.

30a. DeCross AJ, Sahasrabudhe DM. Paraneoplastic Raynaud's phenomenon. Am J Med 92:571–572, 1992.

31. Braverman IM: Skin Signs of Systemic Disease. Saunders, Philadelphia, 1981.

32. Lehman TJA, Passo M, Siampoulou-Mavridou A, et al.: Neurologic and ophthalmologic complications of linear scleroderma en coup de sabre. Arthritis Rheum 33:S145, 1990.

33. Goldstein-Schainberg C, Rodrigues Pereira RM, Gusukuma MC, et al.: Childhood linear scleroderma "en coup de sabre" with uveitis. J Pediatr 117:581–584, 1990.

34. LeRoy EC, Downey JA, Cannon PJ: Skin capillary blood flow in scleroderma. J Clin Invest 50:930–939, 1971.

35. Spencer-Green G, Schlesinger M, Bove KE, et al.: Nailfold capillary abnormalities in childhood rheumatic disease. J Pediatr 102:341–346, 1983.

36. West SG, Killian PJ, Lawless OJ: Association of myositis and myocarditis in progressive systemic sclerosis. Arthritis Rheum 24:662–667, 1981.

37. Ringel RA, Brick JE, Brick JF, et al.: Muscle involvement in the scleroderma syndromes. Arch Intern Med 150:2550–2552, 1990.

38. Goyal RK, Crist JR: Chest pain of esophageal etiology. Hosp Pract pp. 15–20, September 30, 1988.

39. Flick JA, Boyle JT, Tuchman DN, et al.: Esophageal motor abnormalities in children and adolescents with scleroderma and mixed connective tissue disease. Pediatrics 82:107–111, 1988.

40. Asherson RA, Angus H, Matthews JA, et al.: The progressive systemic sclerosis/systemic lupus overlap: an unusual clinical progression. Ann Rheum Dis 50:323–327, 1991.

41. Garty Ben-Zion, Athreya BH, Wilmott R, et al.: Pulmonary functions in children with progressive systemic sclerosis. Pediatrics 88:1161–1167, 1991.

42. Smith JW, Clements PJ, Levisman J, et al.: Echocardiographic features of progressive systemic sclerosis (PSS). Correlation with hemodynamic and postmortem studies. Am J Med 66:28–33, 1979.

43. Follansbee WP, Curtiss EI, Medsger TA, et al.: Physiologic abnormalities of cardiac function in progressive systemic sclerosis: review of a 25-year experience with 68 cases. Medicine 62:335–352, 1983. (See also: N Engl J Med 310:142–148, 1984.)

44. LeRoy EC: The heart in systemic sclerosis. N Engl J Med 310:188–190, 1984.

44a. Barst RJ, Flaster ER, Menon A, et al.: Evidence for the association of unexplained pulmonary hypertension in children with the major histocompatibility complex. Circulation 85:249–258. (See also: Editorial pp. 380–381), 1992.

45. Traub YM, Shapiro AP, Rodnan GP, et al.: Hypertension and renal failure (scleroderma renal crisis) in progressive systemic sclerosis: review of a 25-year experience with 68 cases. Medicine 62:335–352, 1983.

46. D'Agati VD, Cannon PJ: Scleroderma (progressive systemic sclerosis). In: Tischer CC, Brenner BM (eds.) Renal Pathology, J.B. Lippincott Co., Philadelphia, pp. 994–1020, 1989.

47. Steen VD, Conte C, Day N, et al.: Pregnancy in women with systemic sclerosis. Arthritis Rheum 30:643–650, 1987.

48. Cannon PJ: Medical management of renal scleroderma. N Engl J Med 299:886–

887, 1978.

49. Cannon PJ, Hassar M, Case DB, et al.: The relationship of hypertension and renal failure in scleroderma (PSS) to structural and functional abnormalities of the renal cortical circulation. Medicine 53:1–46, 1974.

50. Helfrich DJ, Banner B, Steen VD, Medsger TA: Normotensive renal failure in systemic sclerosis. Arthritis Rheum 32:1128–1134, 1989.

51. Cantaluppi A: CAPD and systemic diseases. Clin Nephrol 30: Suppl. No. 1— 1988. (pp. S8–S12).

52. Ng SC, Clements PJ, Berquist WE, et al.: Home central venous hyperalimentation in fifteen patients with severe scleroderma bowel disease. Arthritis Rheum 32:212–216, 1989.

53. Clements PJ, Lachenbruch PA, Ng SC, et al.: Skin score. A semiquantitative measure of cutaneous involvement that improves prediction of prognosis in systemic sclerosis. Arthritis Rheum 33:1256–1263, 1990.

54. Soudah HC, Haslep WL, Owyang C: Effect of octreotide on intestinal motility and bacterial overgrowth in scleroderma. N Engl J Med 325:1461–1467, 1991. (See also: Editorial pp. 1508–1509).

55. Dull JS, Raufman J-P, Zakai D, et al.: Successful treatment of gastroparesis with erythromycin in a patient with progressive systemic sclerosis. Am J Med 89:528–530, 1990.

56. Thanik KD, Chey WY, Shah AN, et al.: Reflux esophagitis: effects of oral bethanechol on symptoms and endoscopic findings. Ann Intern Med 93:805–808, 1980.

57. Duboc D, Kahan A, Maziere B, et al.: The effect of nifedipine on myocardial perfusion and metabolism in systemic sclerosis. A positron emission tomographic study. Arthritis Rheum 84:198–203, 1991.

58. Sfikakis PP, Kyriakidis MK, Vergos CG, et al.: Cardiopulmonary hemodynamics in systemic sclerosis and response to nifedipine and captopril. Am J Med 90:541–546, 1991.

59. LeRoy EC: Pulmonary hypertension: the bete noire of the diffuse connective tissue disease. Am J Med 90:539–540, 1991.

60. Franks AG Jr.: Topical glyceryl trinitrate as adjunctive treatment in Raynaud's disease. Lancet 1:76–77, 1982.

61. Coffman JD: Symptomatic therapy for Raynaud's phenomenon. Drug Ther pp. 95–104, June 1989.

62. Langevitz P, Buskila D, Lee P, Urowitz MB: Treatment of refractory ischemic skin ulcers in patients with Raynaud's phenomenon with PGE₁ infusions. J Rheumatol 16:1433–1435, 1989.

63. O'Reilly MJG, Talpos G, Roberts VG, et al.: Controlled trial of plasma exchange in treatment of Raynaud's syndrome. Br Med J 1:1113–1115, 1979.

64. Gordon RS (ed.) From the NIH: research findings of potential value to the practitioner: biofeedback for patients with Raynaud's phenomenon. JAMA 242:509–510, 1979.

65. Lopez-Ovejero JA, Saal SD, D'Angelo WA, et al. Reversal of vascular and renal crises of scleroderma by oral angiotensin-converting-enzyme blockade. N Engl J Med 300:1417–1419, 1979.

66. Mitnick PD, Feig PU: Control of hypertension and reversal of vascular and renal failure in scleroderma. N Engl J Med 299:871–872, 1978.

67. Wasner C, Cooke CR, Fries JF: Successful medical treatment of scleroderma

renal crisis. N Engl J Med 299:873–875, 1978.

68. Moynahan EJ: Penicillamine in the treatment of morphea and keloid in children. Postgrad Med J 50(Suppl. 2):39–40, 1974.

69. Falange V, Medsger TA Jr: d-Penicillamine in the treatment of localized scleroderma. Arch Dermatol 126:609–612, 1990.

70. Steen VD, Medsger TA, Rodnan GP: d-Pencillamine therapy in progressive sytemic sclerosis (scleroderma): a retrospective analysis. Ann Intern Med 97:652–659, 1982.

71. De Clerck LS, Dequeker J, Francx L, Demedts M: D-penicillamine therapy and interstitial lung disease in scleroderma: a long-term followup study. Arthritis Rheum 30:643–650, 1987.

71a. Jiminez SA, Sigal SH: A 15 year perspective study of treatment of rapidly progressive systemic sclerosis with D-Penicillamine. J Rheumatol 18:1496–1503, 1991.

72. Bode BY, Yocum DE, Gall EP, et al.: Methotrexate (MTX) in scleroderma: experience in ten patients. Arthritis Rheum 33:S66, 1990.

73. Appelboom T, Itzkowitch D: Cyclosporine in successful control of rapidly progressive scleroderma. Letters to the Editor. Am J Med 82:866–867, 1987.

74. Clements PJ, Paulus HE, Sterz M, Ng S-C: A preliminary report of cyclosporin A (CSA) in systemic sclerosis (SSc). Arthritis Rheum 33:S66, 1990.

75. Freundlich B, Rook AH, Edelson R, et al.: Extracorporeal photochemotherapy in the treatment of systemic sclerosis. Arthritis Rheum 33:S35, 1990.

76. Rodnan GP: When is scleroderma not scleroderma: the differential diagnosis of progressive systemic sclerosis. Bull Rheum Dis 31:7–10, 1981.

77. Follansbee WP, Curtiss EI, Medsger TA, et al.: Myocardial function and perfusion in the CREST syndrome variant of progressive systemic sclerosis: exercise radionuclide evaluation and comparison with diffuse scleroderma. Am J Med 77:489–496, 1984.

78. Escalante A, Beardmore TD, Kaufman RL: Musculoskeletal manifestations of Werner's syndrome. Semin Arthritis Rheum 19:1–8, 1990.

79. Greenberg LM, Geppert C, Worthen HG, et al.: Scleredema "adultorum" in children. Pediatrics 32:1044–1054, 1963.

80. Yogman M, Echeverria P: Scleredema and carditis: report of a case and review of the literature. Pediatrics 54:108–110, 1974.

81. Burke MJ, Seguin J, Bove KE: Scleroderma: an unusual presentation with edema limited to scalp, upper face and orbits. J Pediatr 101:960–963, 1982.

82. Laymon CW, Peterson WC Jr: Lipogranulomatosis subcutanea (Rothmann-Makai). Arch Dermatol 90:288–292, 1964.

83. Shulman LE: Diffuse fasciitis with eosinophilia: A new syndrome? Trans Assoc Am Physicians 88:70–86, 1975.

84. Hoffman R, Dainiak N, Sibrack L, et al.: Antibody-mediated aplastic anemia and diffuse fasciitis. N Engl J Med 300:718–721, 1979.

85. Britt WJ, Duray PH, Dahl MV, et al.: Diffuse fasciitis with eosinophilia: a steroid-responsive variant of scleroderma. J Pediatr 97:432–434, 1980.

86. Lakhapal S, Ginsburg WW, Michet CJ, et al.: Eosinophilic fasciitis: clinical spectrum and therapeutic response in 52 cases. Semin Arthritis Rheum 17:221–231, 1988.

87. Ansell BM, Nasseh GA, Bywaters, EGL: Scleroderma in childhood. Ann Rheum Dis 35:189–197, 1976.

88. Grisanti MW, Moore TL, Osborn TG, Haber PL: Eosinophilic fasciitis in children. Semin Arthritis Rheum 19:151–157, 1989.

89. Jimenez SA, Varga J: The eosinophilia-myalgia syndrome and eosinophilic fasciitis. Curr Opin Rheumatol 3:986–994, 1991.

90. Olson NY, Lindsley CB, Kepes JJ: Eosinophilic fascilitis presenting as inflammatory polyarthritis. Pediatrics 78:512–514, 1990.

91. Sills EM: Systemic lupus erythematosus in a patient diagnosed as having Shulman disease. Arthritis Rheum 31:694–695, 1981.

91a. Hibbs JR, Mittleman B, Hill P, Medsger TA Jr.: L-tryptophan-associated eosinophilic fasciitis prior to the 1989 eosinophilia-myalgia syndrome outbreak. Arthritis Rheum 35:299–303, 1992.

92. Noriega AR, Gomez-Reino J, Lopez-Encuentra A, et al.: Ocassional survey: toxic epidemic syndrome, Spain, 1981. Lancet 2:697–702, 1982.

93. Winkelmann RK, Connolly SM, Quimby SR, et al.: Histopathologic features of the L-tryptophan-related eosinophilia-myalgia (fasciitis) syndrome. Mayo Clin Proc 66:457–463, 1991.

94. Casado de Frias E, Andujar PH, Oliete F, et al.: Intoxication caused by ingestion of rape oil denatured with aniline. Am J Dis Child 37:988–991, 1983.

95. Swyert LA, Maes EF, Sewell LE, et al.: Eosinophilia-myalgia syndrome. Results of national surveillance. JAMA 264:1698–1693, 1990 (see also 266:195–196, 1991).

96. Shulman LE: The eosinophilia-myalgia syndrome associated with ingestion of L-tryptophan. Arthritis Rheum 33:913–917, 1990.

97. Medsger TA: Tryptophan-induced eosinophilia-myalgia syndrome. N Engl J Med 322:926–928, 1990.

98. Duffy J: The lessons of eosinophilia-myalgia syndrome. Hospital Practice April 30, 1992; pp. 65–90.

99. Strongwater SL, Woda BA, Yood RA, et al.: Eosinophilia-myalgia syndrome associated with L-tryptophan ingestion. Analysis of four patients and implications for differential diagnosis and pathogenesis. Arch Intern Med 150:2178–2186, 1990.

100. Slutsker L, Hoesly FC, Mller L, et al.: Eosinophilia-myalgia syndrome associated with exposure to tryptophan from a single manufacturer. JAMA 264:213–217, 1990.

101. Belongia EA, Hedberg CW, Gleich GJ, et al.: An investigation of the cause of the eosinophilia-myalgia syndrome associated with trytophan use. N Engl J Med 323:357–365, 1990.

102. Martinez-Osuna P, Espinoza LR: On the treatment of the eosinophilia-myalgia syndrome. Arch Intern Med 151:1239, 1991.

103. Sternberg EM, VanWoert MH, Young SN, et al.: Development of a scleroderma-like illness during therapy with L-5-hydroxytryptophan and carbidopa. N Engl J Med 303:782–787, 1980.

104. Shulman HM, Sale GE, Lerner KG, et al.: Chronic graft-versus-host disease in man. Am J Pathol 91:545–570, 1978.

105. Kumagai Y, Abe C, Shiokawa Y: Scleroderma after cosmetic surgery. Arthritis Rheum 22:532–537, 1979.

106. Gabriel SE, Perry HO, Oleson GB, et al.: Scleromyxedema: a scleroderma-like disorder with systemic manifestations. Medicine 67:58–65, 1988.

107. Miller MT, Sloane H, Goldberg MF, et al.: Progressive hemifacial atrophy (Parry-Romberg disease). J Pediatr Ophthalmol Strabismus 24:27–36, 1987.
108. Jacobs JC, Gold AP, Duray P, et al.: Parry-Romberg syndrome with cerebral vasculitis associated with borrelia spirochetes in the brain biopsy. Pediatr Res 31 #4 Pt 2: 349a, 1992.
109. Aberer E, Kollegger H, Kristoferitsch W, Stanek G: Neuroborreliosis in morphea and lichen sclerosus et atrophicus. J Am Acad Dermatol 19:820–825, 1988.
110. Abele DC, Bedingfield RB, Chandler FW, Given KS: Progressive facial hemiatrophy (Parry-Romberg syndrome) and borreliosis. J Am Acad Dermatol 22: 531–533, 1990.

9

The Power of Positive Thinking

The credit belongs to the man who is actually in the arena, whose face is marred with sweat and dust and blood; who strives valiantly; who errs and comes short again and again; who knows the great enthusiasms, the great devotions, and spends himself in a worthy cause; who, if he wins, knows the triumph of high achievement; and who, if he fails at least fails while daring greatly, so that his place shall never be with those cold and timid souls who know neither victory nor defeat.[1] (Fig. 9.1)

In Greek, the root for the words *pain* and *punishment* is the same. It is no surprise that humans look upon pain as punishment. Guilty feelings induced by pain lead to penitence, atonement, self-denial, and self-deprecation.

Painful sickness is a discouraging business for patients and their families, interfering with developing independence and self-esteem and creating anxiety, fear, and anger.[2] Pessimism and gloom lead to increasing defeat and humiliation (Fig. 9.2).[3] Not all symptoms are relieved by drugs. Healing is psychological, spiritual, emotional, and social, too.

With support, encouragement, and expert technical care, the patient can make the best of an unenviable situation.[4–8] The traditional goal of cure is replaced with that of control and maintenance of function. By being a partner with the physician and the therapeutic team and with the support of other family members, friends, and professionals, the sick child and his family can achieve some sense of control over the disease, avoiding depression and further loss of esteem. Many physicians forget the depression, guilt, shame, and anger they themselves suffer when faced with merely a clinical problem over which they have no control. Our childhood patients are threatened with disfigurement, impaired mobility or crippling, loss of vision, and a limited future. They may be subjected to teasing, ridicule, and rejec-

678

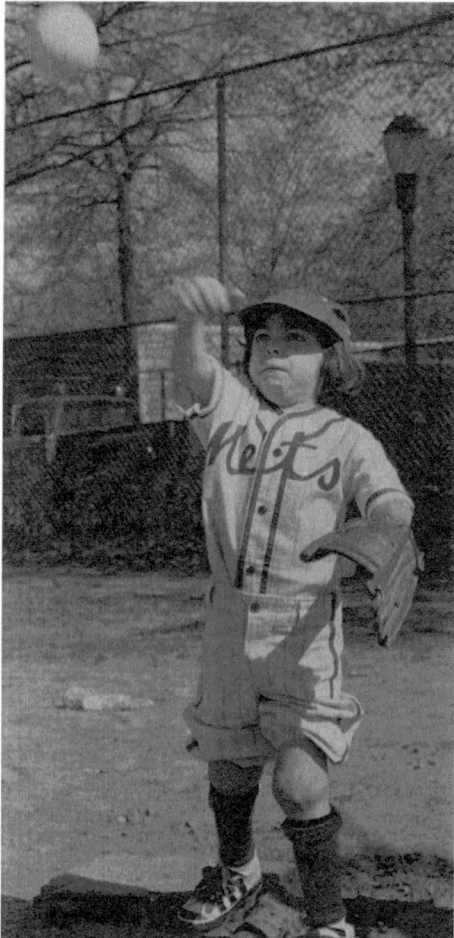

Figure 9.1. *(left)* "The credit belongs to the man who is actually in the arena, whose face is marred with sweat and dust. . . . " At age 13, ball playing, even with large effusions of the knees, ankles, wrists, and elbows, can be important.

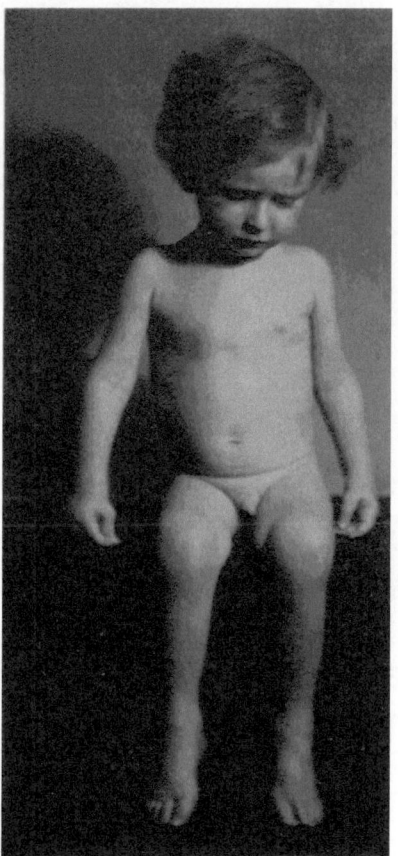

Figure 9.2. *(right)* Early descriptions of arthritic children emphasized their gloomy affect and immobile posture (see also Figs. 3.3 and 9.9). Pessimism and gloom lead to increasing defeat and humiliation.

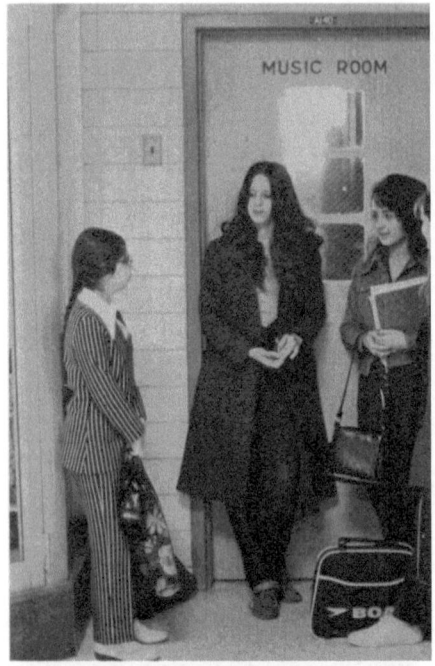

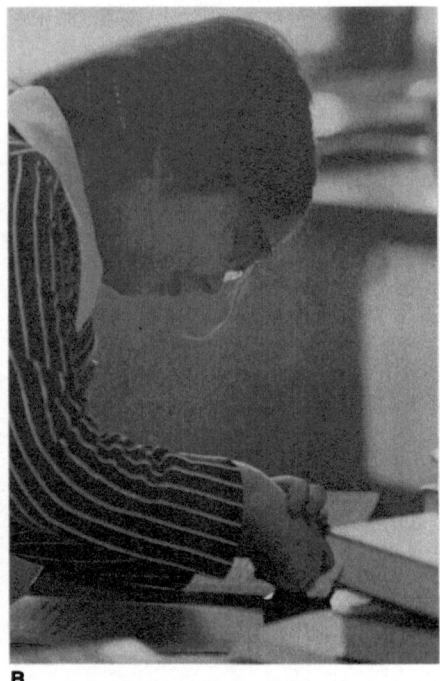

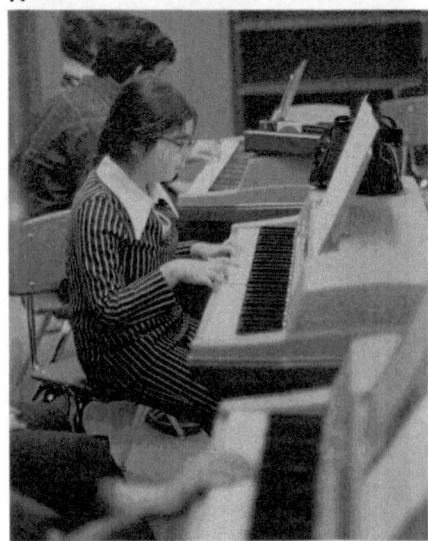

Figure 9.3. (**A**, **B**, and **C**) Although our patients may stand out among their peers, what with their stunted growth, crippled fingers, small mandibles, and visual handicaps, they can achieve success and participate in all activities in school. We had to overcome great resistance from school guidance personnel to get this child accepted in regular school; it's easy to see the importance of her being in the "mainstream." Regular school is an essential part of our therapeutic program. We often have to combat old-fashioned attitudes such as: "What is *this* child doing here?", "What if there's a fire?", "We don't have time." These photographs show the rewards of such combat.

tion by their peers (Fig. 9.3). All of this just when they are establishing their body image and sense of self! A positive attitude, a sense of hope, a fighting spirit, and a feeling of strength may be associated with an improved prognosis.[9–12] Gloom is self-fulfilling.[13]

Table 9.1. Mechanisms for Coping with Chronic Sickness

Intellectualization
Constructive denial
Displacement
Compensation

From Hofmann, ref. 14.

Coping with Chronic Illness

One may ask, how does the severely ill or crippled child cope adaptively with illness (Table 9.1)? How can depression, which seems natural enough, be avoided? One method used by both adolescents and the parents of sick children is to intellectualize: they process information about the disease in rational, abstract terms dissociated from the emotional impact of the information.[14] Intellectualization and reasonable denial of the situation may help the child and family gradually adapt to the problems of illness without withdrawal, fantasy, and overwhelming loss of esteem. The child and the family compromise, giving up the wish for the way things were or could have been, without giving up completely (Fig. 9.4).

As has been observed by a psychologist with an embryonal-cell carcinoma of the testis and pulmonary metastases, "Rather than conclude that I had

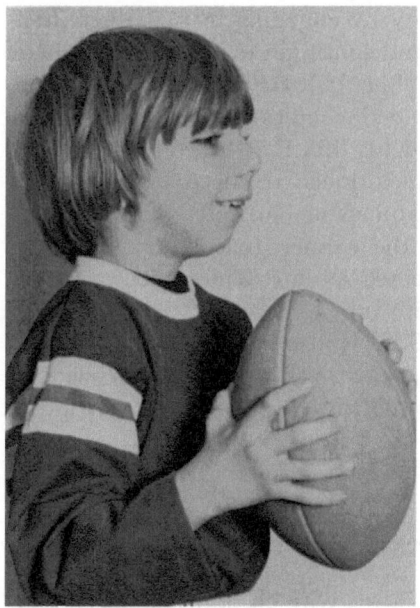

Figure 9.4. Throwing a football is fun despite a tiny mandible and flexion contractures in all joints in this 6-year-old.

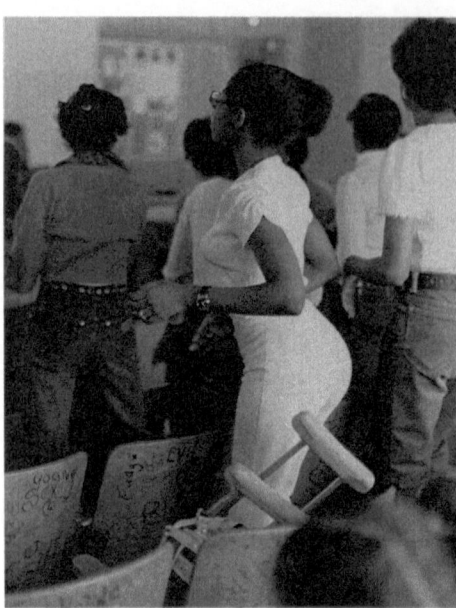

Figure 9.5. These kids "are into rhythm"; our patient holds her own among her peers and capitalizes on her assets.

suddenly become totally unhealthy, I reasoned that 99% of me was healthy and with the help of powerful drugs capable of holding back that crazy 1% that was cancerous." Effective therapy must treat the healthy portion of the patient as well as combat the disease.[9]

When a child compensates for disability by engaging in social activities within his capacity, he attracts his peers and continues to interact with them and to grow with them toward adulthood (Fig. 9.5). Helplessness means that one cannot help oneself. Depression is avoided when the patient is convinced he has some control over his disease and his life, that he can achieve the gratification he requires (albeit less than he formerly required)—that is, that he is an effective human being.[15,16] The youngster must settle for doing his best; the "good try" may replace being the winner; reasonably successful completion of what is attempted is accepted as fine achievement and becomes ego-restoring. This interaction with other youngsters is essential to growth, dignity, and independence (Fig 9.6). It also helps to avoid neurotic interaction with a parent at home. Patients have every reason to take pride in getting on despite their handicap; they are positively rewarded by their peers for doing so.

Helping the Family Cope with Sickness

Studies of parental stress in families of children with chronic disease emphasize the drains on finances, time, and energy that interfere with leisure and

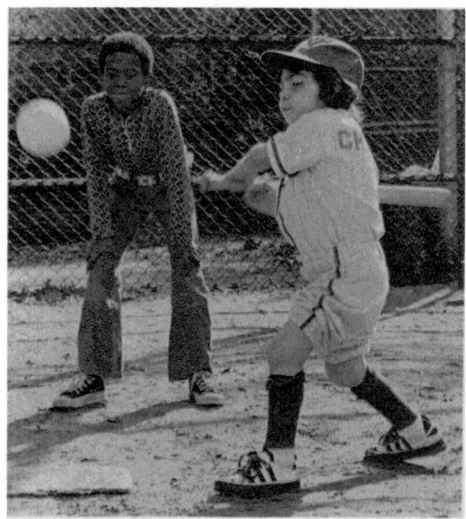

Figure 9.6. With the right attitude, it's amazing what a kid can do with a hemoglobin of 6 grams and active arthritis everywhere.

the personal needs of the other family members.[17-23] Family strain increases with weariness. Inevitably, fatigue, anxiety, and depression reduce the frequency and/or the quality of marital and sexual gratification. Marital discord is common.

Parents of sick children feel inadequate. They, too, suffer from fear and a sense of loss of control, which is sometimes reflected by anger directed against the sick child, his siblings, the spouse, or the physician who is unable to make the child well. These negative feelings, whether directed inward and hidden or openly displayed hostility, all interfere with optimal care of the chronically ill child.

Siblings of chronically sick children often suffer either from displaced anger, or from relative neglect by exhausted parents, or from being made to assume the role of surrogate parent.[24] Years ago, a neurotic attachment of mother to the handicapped child was quite common.[25] The mother often isolated herself and the child, neither of whom had any meaningful life outside of themselves. Marital disruption, already at an all-time high, was almost universal in such situations. There was no opportunity for the child to grow into an independent self-sustaining adult. We rarely see this problem with handicapped children today. Physicians and parents have joined together to avoid this misery. Positive attitudes of physicians, community resources, improved educational attitudes, and general education of the public about such psychological mechanisms have greatly reduced this phenomenon (Tables 9.2 and 9.3).

When the marriage is a good one, and the extended family is optimal, grandparents and other relatives unite in the care of the child and the preservation of family relationships. The problem is accepted and dealt with. The family capitalizes on its strengths, and while I do not believe that illness

Table 9.2. Helping Chronically Sick Youngsters to Cope

Provide for the growing need for independence and self-determination in the patient's own care

Reassure sense of body image

Provide for participation in mastery and control of the disease

Encourage peer activities and socialization

Encourage personal interests

Respect dignity and privacy

Show respect and affection for patient as a person and admire courage and determination in the face of adversity

Provide vocational and educational counseling and opportunity

Acknowledge and encourage sexuality

ever makes a positive net contribution to family life, the family can gain strength from being able to deal with it successfully as a united group.[26] In such optimal situations, the illness is only one feature of a family's life, not the only feature.

When family resources are limited, the physician must be especially careful to conserve the energies of the parents. Clinic appointments are kept to a minimum, and the "team" effort is coordinated. Vacations are encouraged; a simple statement that the physician will be in town and available to the babysitter while the parents are away can go a long way toward encouraging the parents to take this vacation. Such a statement also implies that the physician is accustomed to this role—other parents of sick children get away for a few days.

On the whole, the job of the physician is to help the sick child and his family to reorder their priorities and make every moment count, to enjoy every opportunity for pleasure, and not to waste time on depression. It is in man's nature to cope successfully with adversity. There is a sense of power and control achieved by making the best of an undesirable situation, integrating it into family life, with some positive enhancement of the quality of life. If a family can cope successfully with sickness, they can cope with anything in life.[27]

The Importance of Motor Activity in the Personality Development of Children

Restraint of muscular movement in infants has been observed to produce a picture of increased dullness and apathy.[27] On the other hand, pride in motor abilities in Erikson's studies of ego development results in autonomy overcoming doubt.[28] Children given the opportunity and freedom to initiate motor play such as running, bike riding, sliding, skating, tussling, and wrestling have their sense of initiative reinforced. Praise and reward for industry

Table 9.3. Sources of Help for the Disabled and Sources of Information for the Handicapped

1. American Juvenile Arthritis Organization (AJAO)
   Arthritis Foundation (AF)*
   3400 Peachtree Road NE
   Atlanta, GA 30326
   (1-800-283-7800)

2. National Arthritis and Musculoskeletal and Skin
   Diseases Information Clearinghouse
   Box NAMSIC, 9000 Rockville Pike
   Bethesda, MD 20892

3. Council on the Handicapped
   (202) 526-2976
   1709 3 Street NE
   Washington, D.C. 20004

4. Mainstream Inc.
   (202) 898-0202
   1030 15 St. NW
   Suite 1010
   Washington, D.C. 20005

5. National Easter Seal Society
   (312) 726-6200
   70 East Lake Street
   Chicago, IL 60601

6. National Rehabilitation information Center
   Catholic University of America
   4407 Eighth Street NE
   Washington, D.C. 20017

7. President's Committee on the Employment of the Handicapped
   1111 20 Street NW
   Washington, D.C. 20036
   (All states have governors' committees and all large cities mayors' committees.)

8. The Council for Exceptional Children
   (703) 620-3660
   1920 Association Drive
   Reston, VA 22091

9. Rehabilitation Services Administration
   Office of Human Development, DHHS
   330 "C" Street SW
   Washington, D.C. 20201

10. HEATH Resource Center
    (Higher Education and the Handicapped
    American Council on Education)
    (202) 939-9300
    1 Dupont Circle NW
    Suite 800
    Washington, D.C. 20036

* Provides addresses for American Lupus Society, Ankylosing Spondylitis Association, Ehlers-Danlos National Foundation, Lupus Foundation of America, Lyme Borreliosis Foundation, National Psoriasis Foundation, Reflex Sympathetic Dystrophy Syndome Association, Scleroderma Federation, Sjögren's Syndrome Foundation, United Scleroderma Foundation and others

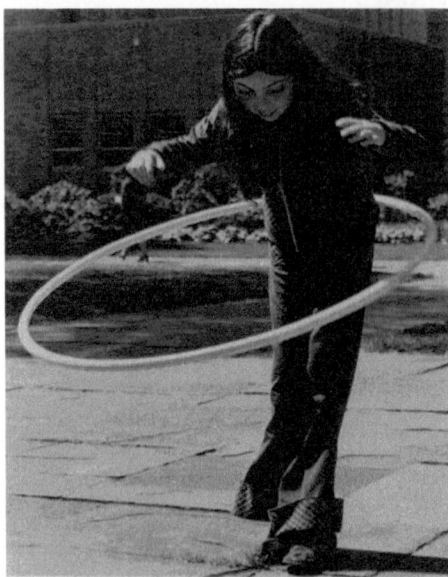

Figure 9.7. Hula-hooping is not our favorite sport (it can result in destructive arthritis of the spine), but for this youngster it's what makes her a star on her block (aside from arthritis).

encourage rejection of feelings of inferiority. Avoidance of feelings of mistrust, shame, doubt, guilt, and inferiority enables our patients to develop an integrated psychosocial identity rather than sink into isolation and despair.[29]

The Importance of Physician Attitudes in the Care of the Chronically Ill

The physician encourages healthy adaptation by his attitudes. He educates and assures, promotes awareness of the complex reality, and gives steady guidance in dealing with it. His basic philosophy is always positive, always geared to what the child can do, not to what cannot be accomplished. Fiore has emphasized the suggestibility of the sick and the importance of positive statements.[9] No restrictions are placed on the child; he is allowed to do whatever he wishes (Fig. 9.7). If he does not succeed, he is complimented for the "good try." In time, such attempts help the child achieve a realistic acceptance of his situation. We do not worry that a tiny bit of extra damage may be done to joints by physical activity; the damage to the whole human being imposed by endless infantilization is much more dangerous.[29-31] No physical or occupational therapy program can compare with being busy with the activities of life. Depression is associated with decreased muscular movement and resultant increased joint contractures.

The ability to be responsible for oneself is ego-rewarding. Dependency is debilitating. Thus, we allow the child to take as much responsibility as he can for his own medications, exercises, and activities. Intelligent patients and their families want an opportunity to participate actively and to bear some responsibility for their own care and thus to have a sense of control over the disease. Ancillary personnel and the team approach encourage the family and patient in this regard.

Long-term prognoses in rheumatic disease should generally be avoided since they are often erroneous and do not encourage function. Unless the acceptance of statistics enchances the quality of life, we fight to beat the statistics.[9] Most arthritic children get well and have normal lives. With proper care, most children with vasculitis make a full recovery. Almost 100% of children with SLE now live for 10 years. It seems reasonable to expect SLE to be a curable disease within the lifetime of children now developing the disease. Almost all children with dermatomyositis get well and lead normal lives. Even the prognosis for systemic sclerosis in childhood is for a long and useful life, and certainly one can expect the prognosis for each disease to be improved in the future.

What has to be dealt with is today. Each day should be well-spent. The sick child is certainly entitled to make the best of every day. It is not only the responsibility of the physician for sick children but a rewarding pleasure to enhance their quality of life and the life-style of their families. He does this not only with technical skill but also by providing hope, love, comfort, protection, and understanding.

Society's Attitudes Toward the Crippled

It is not natural for people to love the sick, the crippled, and disabled.[32,33] Society adopts a superficially charitable attitude toward the handicapped but then degrades, humiliates, and punishes them further. "If parents treated their children the way society treats the helpless, they would be cited for neglect and child abuse."[33]

If we want the disabled to be self-sustaining, we will have to stop using a visible handicap to symbolize evil in human nature and stop projecting upon the disabled our devaluation of the handicapped.[34] We are all handicapped to one extent or another; no one has only assets, strengths, and beauty. Society's self-interest (if not compassion) demands that we capitalize on assets and not accentuate liabilities.

It is not their handicap that the disabled find insurmountable: it is the normal individual's perception of the handicapped (Fig. 9.8). One reason we who care for the handicapped favor mainstreaming is so that the next generation of normal adults can be accustomed to interacting with the handicapped in healthy fashion. The only way to change the view of the healthy toward the handicapped is to see that the healthy interact with the handicapped from childhood on. Any physician who has witnessed the interaction between healthy sibs and a handicapped sib in a large, well-adapted family realizes the potential for improved life of handicapped adults in an accepting society.

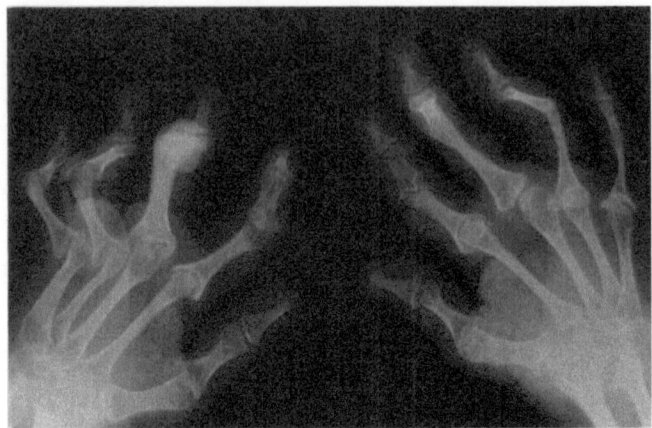

A

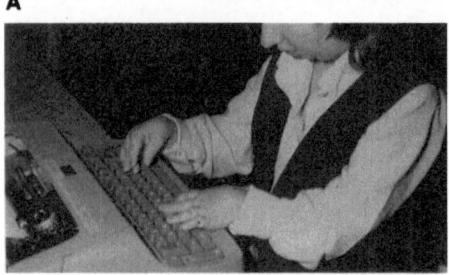

B

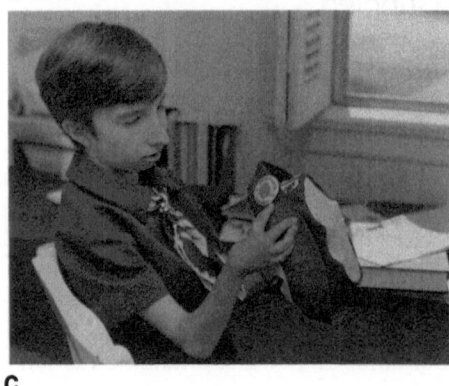

C

Figure 9.8. Fingers that look like these (**A**) can still type rapidly enough to win the typing prize at graduation (**B**). This girl went on to college where she was a cheerleader (**C**).

Efforts to indoctrinate youth in beneficial attitudes toward the handicapped have not met with any more success than other efforts at preventing behavior detrimental to health. With the stimulus of mainstreaming, there is an opportunity for development of a peer leadership curriculum to strengthen students' commitment to the handicapped. Peer leaders have been found useful in other situations in which undesirable behavior of children was so embedded in the social milieu that ordinary forms of instruction had no beneficial effect.[35] It is hoped that schools will adopt such innovative programs.

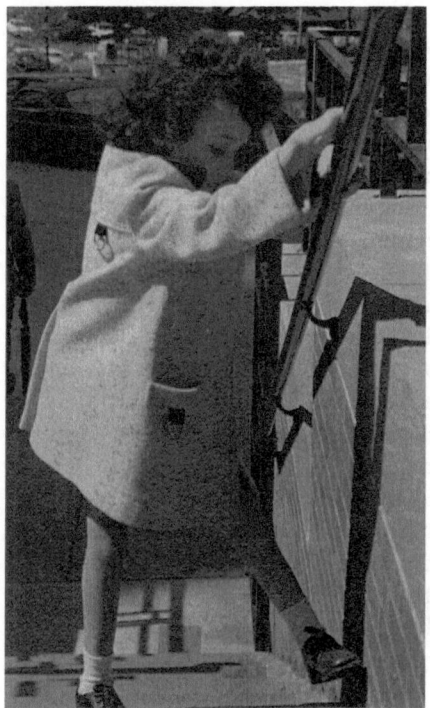

Figure 9.9. Climbing stairs is tough but a necessity in school. This patient has graduated from high school now and has a healthy baby. Also, note her picture at age 3 (Fig. 3.3).

Physicians and others who care for crippled youngsters will all benefit from reading Rose Marie MacElman's discussion of her own childhood problems with crippling illness.[36] No summary could do this magnificent piece justice. Ms. MacElman describes the social isolation, rejection, embarrassment, annoying questioning, stares, unsolicited prayer offerings, and smothering unnecessarily and harmfully projected onto the handicapped. At the same time, she shows how handicapped young people can cope, provided they are offered kind and compassionate understanding and help in accomplishing what they are capable of accomplishing. "They look for my personality rather than my handicap. . . . Most of my friends have problems of their own. My best friends enjoy my company and want me to go places with them and participate in activities that they enjoy. . . . Handicapped individuals must not give in to the negative stereotypes and negative expectations of others. They must maintain positive self-esteem."

School and the Crippled Child

School is an important part of a child's society, just as work is an important part of adult life (Fig. 9.9).[37–42] If the child is to grow into a useful, productive, and self-sustaining adult, he must learn to do so in school. In the short term, mainstreaming is costly; without the appropriation of extra funds, mainstreaming will result in decreased services to the healthy. In the final analysis, mainstreaming is cost-effective for society. Enabling the crippled to become self-sufficient prevents a lifetime of dependency on society. However, if mainstreaming is not accompanied by adequate funds, services are inadequate, teachers are frustrated, and hostility toward the handicapped is increased. Physicians for the handicapped must serve as advocates for their patients in school and in school budget committees.[43,44]

Schools offer the greatest opportunity for our children to develop their full potential and to fulfill adult roles in the most satisfying and constructive ways. Adequate adolescent emotional development depends on success in school. Failure in school leads to loss of self-esteem, depression and withdrawal, antisocial acting-out behavior, family dysfunction, and ultimately to unemployment and lack of self-sufficiency in adult life.

Another problem for our youngsters in school is their medication. We are proud of our patients who are taught to take the responsibility for taking their own medications in school.[31] The chronic sick are degraded by schools that force them to go to the nurse for medications, resulting in infantilization, noncompliance, and inability to get their medicine when the nurse is absent.[45,46] Arguments that the school must give the medication to our patients have no more validity than arguments that the parent must give the medicine to children who can bear that responsibility themselves. The schools seem to confuse drug abuse with the fine example set by those youngsters who can assume the responsibility for taking medications in accordance with the needs imposed by their physical illness.

Skillful care for chronically ill children must be based on an understanding of the importance of the developmental needs of children and adolescents and must encourage resiliency and adaptation to the demands and disappointments of chronic illness rather than further handicap such adaptation or impose additional burdens on the child and family. If teenagers are not given appropriate ways for participation in their own care, they may see no alternative except resistance to therapy as a method of exercising control over their disease. When patients are given the opportunity for responsibility, they are more likely to cooperate. These observations are not limited to the care of the sick since industrial psychologists have demonstrated that authoritarian leaders get short-term obedience at the subsequent cost of sabotage and increased sick leave or quitting.[9] Increased productivity is enhanced by employee exuberance, independence, responsibility, and participation in decision-making.

Sex and the Disabled

Pediatricians are now caring for more teenagers with rheumatic disease and so have increased opportunity to contribute to the development of healthy sexuality in handicapped youth. Sex is just as important for the handicapped as for the rest of us, providing in addition to genital release an opportunity for kissing, holding, touching, stroking, fondling, caressing, reassuring body contact, and an opportunity to get cuddled, nurtured, cared for, and loved.[47] Sexuality is a powerful tool for pleasure and for increasing self-esteem. When sexual gratification is thwarted or frustrated, it creates incredible unhappiness that spreads beyond our own lives into the lives of those around us.

The physician must be careful to reject his own stereotype of what is attractive as being universal. Our patients need our help to see themselves as beautiful and sexy despite their crippled limbs. As is true in so many areas, if they see themselves that way, the world may also see them so—another self-fulfilling prophecy. That the doctor sees them as beautiful and sexy may be extremely important in their development into healthy adults. The skillful physician, comfortable with sexual topics, takes advantage of his opportunity to demonstrate his acceptance and encouragement of sexuality in the crippled, to provide these youngsters with an opportunity to "rap" about their problems, and to help them overcome negative or self-defeating attitudes.[48]

Psychosocial Concepts in the Etiology of RA

Arthritic patients have been observed to be self-sacrificing, masochistic, rigid, hostile but unable to show overt anger, moralistic, comforming, self-conscious, shy, inhibited, perfectionistic, and interested in activity.[49,50] The mothers of arthritic children have been shown to be pathologically possessive and the children overly dependent, withdrawn, depressed, and listless.[25] Several authors have reported life changes as etiologic factors in JRA.[51–53] All of these studies tend to be anecdotal and/or retrospective. Most reviewers find the weight of evidence to support the view that any chronic disease may induce undesirable personality and psychosocial constellations but that these personality traits are not present in particular prior to the onset of disease and do not predispose to chronic disease or to RA in particular.[49,52,53] That depression, as a result of altered endocrine or immunologic function, favors the development of disease, including JRA, seems a real possibility.[54,55]

The public press, meddlesome neighbors, and some physicians tend to overvalue studies of the predisposing psychodeterminants of disease. "Psychological theories of illness are a powerful means of placing blame on the ill. Patients who are instructed that they have, unwittingly, caused their disease are also made to feel that they have deserved it."[32] Thus, the normal feelings of helplessness, grief, shame, and anger induced by illness may be accentuated by projected guilt. Little wonder that the sick may be enraged by and at those around them who imply that they got what they deserved!

Physician attitudes may result in increased psychosomatic symptomatology and are a critical determinant of current function and of later-life disability.[56–59] Psychological factors in all studies do seem to affect outcome, measured in terms of function, and so document the power of positive thinking in chronic disease. However, there are major methodologic problems involved in studying whether "fighting back" actually prevents or ameliorates organic diseases. Theoretically, it should be possible to set up randomized controlled studies of adjuvant psychological support, but such studies seem impractical, at least at present. However, while one may doubt that a positive attitude prolongs life in cancer patients or reduces destruction in arthritic joints or avoids destruction of the kidney in SLE, it certainly seems certain that by one mechanism or another absence of hope may shorten life, and certainly absence of the ability to fight back against illness vitiates the quality of life for the sick.[60]

Psychotherapy in the Care of Chronically Ill Children

Psychological studies of arthritic children reveal areas in which we can improve our care. Studies of the psychological adjustment of chronically ill children and also of the siblings of chronically ill children have shown a surprising inverse correlation between the severity of the disease and the severity of the psychopathology in both patients and their siblings.[24,61] Children who have fully recovered from arthritis have been found to continue to lead restricted lives for reasons other than arthritis.[17,61] It appears as if the unexpected finding that mildly affected children and their siblings have more psychopathology than those more severely affected may be a reflection of a family's ability to adapt to the reality of a significant illness but that the special problems introduced by very mild arthritis may result in a lack of psychological adaptation or an increased incidence of familial maladaptation.

The appropriate preventive action would be to do one's best to render the care to mildly arthritic children in a way that maintains a normal life-style and does not impose "psychological crippling" upon the family. While the studies reported are relatively small and it may be unwise to generalize from them, they at least provide an opportunity for focusing discussion of management on the potential that certain techniques of management of mild disease may yield net harm to a family; the treatment may do more harm than good when weighed in the context of the total child or total family. Considerable harm may be done by unnecessary limitations, surgery, hospitalizations, and procedures. In rheumatology and perhaps in all of medicine, it is generally best to provide only those prescriptions and instructions that are essential and to recognize that there is a potential negative effect in every direction given to the patient.

Sickness is a shameless intruder into the lives of our patients and their families. No one can predict the reaction of each individual and how he will cope with the stress of sickness. We recognize that individuals subjected to certain stresses in life (i.e., hostages and prisoners of war) are at special risk and should be afforded an opportunity for "preventive" psychiatric care. While we recognize that children who are sick and crippled are at special risk, we have not committed the resources of society to provide "preventive" psychiatric care for them. I think there is little doubt in the minds of those who care for these youngsters that this is a proper and cost-effective goal for our society.[62]

With the help of a thoughtful physician, parents can be oriented to be flexible, to verbalize their feeling, to feel less responsible for the disease in their children and less guilty about it, and to look after their own needs so that they have adequate satisfactions from life. They can be helped to feel good about their child and help the child to feel good about himself. Parents can take pride in their ability to deal with the stress of the sick child and, despite their natural sadness, to make the best of things and reap the rewards of having made the best of a situation no one desires.

Insofar as is possible, the pediatrician should be helped in the care of his patients by a pediatric psychiatrist. Psychiatrists, like other physicians, can usually be of more help to the least severely ill. Unfortunately, we tend to call on them for help only in the most hopeless cases and then to belabor their failures.

Group Psychotherapy for Sick Children and Their Parents

Psychotherapeutic efforts on behalf of sick children at Babies Hospital have included group sessions for parents of children with arthritis and leukemia.[63] Parents have been enthusiastic about participating in such groups, which have been led by an experienced pediatric psychiatrist with the assistance of a physician from the subspecialty group and a social worker assigned to that group. It is helpful for both the children and their parents to "rap," to know they are not alone, and to see how others are coping.

One of the most valuable resources for children with chronic disease in the Babies Hospital is our pediatric psychiatric nurse practitioner. She is available to all children with life-threatening or chronic disease and is supervised and counseled by a child psychiatrist who has become expert in the care of these children. The same team has worked together for 20 years. The children have a chance to explore their feelings with a trained person, who is also able to work with families having difficulty adapting to the child's illness.[63]

Group sessions for children on our urology service have been led by a social worker; parallel sessions were held with the parents and led by a child psychiatrist.[64] Group sessions were well accepted by parents who opposed individual psychotherapy. In this example of group therapy for inpatients, the group continued to offer a supportive relationship to both parents and children on the ward after the psychiatric session was over.[64]

In our experience, group sessions are best led by those with psychiatric training. We are not equally enthusiastic about parent and patient groups that meet without trained personnel to lead the discussions. While lay groups without any professional leader may provide an element of convivial support, there may be instances in which inadvertent harm is done. The needs of one parent or patient may be met at the expense of another, perhaps less able to afford any further loss of esteem.

Consumer-oriented groups have achieved great improvement in attitudes and services to the handicapped, however, and have done so more effectively than physicians. We encourage such groups, since their achievements have been in the interests of our patients, and they no doubt reduce the frequency of patients resorting to unconventional remedies.[65]

Vocational Education for the Handicapped

Our patients are entitled to find the work they would like to do—and can do, with training. In the recent past, many handicapped young adults could not get work or were forced to accept jobs below their potential. Recent federal legislation recognizes that the handicapped require greater services than others to qualify them for jobs. Special programs are being developed to teach the handicapped skills required for getting and keeping a job. Handicapped teenagers should register with their state office of vocational rehabilitation, an agency funded with both state and federal monies that provides a counselor who can get to know the youngster and who is an expert in job development. Testing and guidance are provided, and scholarships are available to provide college or vocational school tuition for needy qualified youngsters.

Funds available under the Supplemental Social Security Act for the support of families with crippled children can be very helpful to economically eligible families with handicapped children under age 18. Families are encouraged to apply for these grants since sick children consume a large part of a family's income and any additional monies are useful in the care of the children. We do not refer those over 18 for social security disability since each young person who can be self-supporting should be encouraged to learn a trade and make his own way. Dependency on the state is no more ego-rewarding than dependency on a parent.

There are common-sense ways of adapting one's home or place of work to the needs of disability, and there are thousands of self-help devices that are simple but ingenious and enable handicapped individuals to be self-sufficient. Glorya Hale, in her fine *Source Book for the Disabled* (Paddington, 1980), illustrates many ways to make life easier for the handicapped. Agencies that provide additional information for the handicapped are listed in Table 9.3.

Staying in the Mainstream*

Not long ago, half of all arthritic children were on home instruction or in special health classes. Major interruptions of schooling with protracted absences at home or in hospital were routine for all arthritic children, and gloom, anxiety, withdrawal, and dependent passivity were the rule.[66] Now, arthritis-related absences in children cared for in large centers average only 3.6 days per year.[43] Recent studies confirm that chronically ill children afforded the support of a hopeful positive attitude from health professionals remain psychologically healthy.[67,68] The principles and observations discussed in this chapter may be translated into management policies that keep the sick child in the mainstream.[31]

1. Adequate drug therapy is defined as an amount or combination sufficient to allow attendance in normal school and play activities insofar as is possible. No child is placed on home instruction or in a special class for the handicapped. Activities are limited only by the child, not by the parent, physician, or teacher. Play and school and the dynamics of family life are recognized as essential for growth into a well-functioning adult.
2. Children are cared for by a pediatric rheumatologist who can convey an atmosphere of expert knowledge developed through years of long-term relationships with arthritic children and their families. The confidence secured by this relationship transmits itself to the child and family so that they develop an increasingly mature sense of control over the disease. Decision-making increasingly involves the participation of the child and family.
3. Although rapport is initially established with stress on the possibilities for full recovery, function is emphasized as the major goal. The child is allowed to experience disappointment in attempting tasks beyond his abilities so that he is ready to accept lower goals more confidently. The staff expresses admiration not only for successful accomplishments but for "a good try," an attitude that communicates that we never give up prematurely without exhausting all possibilities and makes lower goals seem appropriate and respectable.
4. The parents of these children, once having accepted the reality of the disease, become self-confident about its management and are our greatest allies in educating the public to avoid creating unnecessary barriers, both physical and emotional, for the handicapped. Stilted and stereotyped behavior by school personnel is discouraged. For example, the child is allowed to take his own medicine in school without having to go to the

---

*This subject is beautifully portrayed in a 30-minute movie, *I'm Krista, I Have Arthritis*, available free on loan for parent, teacher, and physician groups from local chapters of the Arthritis Foundation.

nurse's office. Anxieties engendered in the healthy when they encounter the disabled are combated. The stigma of disability is shunted to the periphery of the relationship between the child and surrounding adults; thus, the example is set for the other children.

5. Visits to the office are limited to a minimum so as to avoid interfering with both the child's normal activities and the parents'. Physiotherapy is done at home, and insofar as possible, visits to the hospital are coordinated so that eye doctor, physiatrist, and rheumatologist are all seen on one trip, if required. Unnecessary hospitalizations and procedures of doubtful therapeutic value are avoided.[69]

6. Support from the physician is always available via telephone, a time being set aside each day when he or she can be reached directly for any questions. The difficulty for the parents in managing the administration of medicine and doing the exercises and the fatigue engendered by the added responsibility and its effects on family life are frequently openly discussed. The importance of vacations, rest, recreation, and sexual gratification to the health of the family is emphasized. When problems arise, the parents, knowing that such subjects are openly and willingly discussed, feel free to verbalize them. It is acknowledged that if the mother's and father's needs are not met, ultimately the child's needs will also not be met.[70]

References

1. Roosevelt T: Speech given at the Sorbonne, Paris, April 23, 1910. Works of Theodore Roosevelt. Memorial Edition, Vol. 15. Scribners, New York, p. 354.
2. Krupp NE: Psychiatric implications of chronic and crippling illness. Psychosomatics 9:109–113, 1968.
3. Engle EW, Callahan LF, Pincus T, Hochberg MC: Learned helplessness in systemic lupus erythematosus: analysis using the rheumatology attitudes index. Arthritis Rheum 33:281–285, 1990.
4. Blum RW, Leonard B (eds.) Conference on Youth with Disability: The Transition Years. J Adolesc Health Care 6:77–184, 1985.
5. Adams JA, Weaver SJ: Self-esteem and perceived stress in young adolescents with chronic disease. Unexpected findings. J Adolesc Health Care 7:173–177, 1986.
6. King K, Hanson V: Psychosocial aspects of juvenile rheumatoid arthritis. Pediatr Clin North Am 33:1221–1237, 1986.
7. Billings AG, Moos RH, Miller JJ III, Gottlieb JE: Psychosocial adaptation in juvenile rheumatic disease: a controlled evaluation. Health Psychol 6:343–359, 1987.
8. Ungerer JA, Horgan B, Chaitow J, Champion GD: Psychosocial functioning in children and young adults with juvenile arthritis. Pediatrics 87:195–202, 1988.
9. Fiore N: Fighting cancer—one patient's perspective. N Engl J Med 300:284–289, 1979.
10. Greer S, Morris T, Pettingale KW: Psychological response to breast cancer: Effect on outcome. Lancet 2:785–787, 1979.

11. Cousins N: Anatomy of an illness (as perceived by the patient). N Engl J Med 295:1458–1463, 1976.
12. Walco GA, Varni JW, Ilowite NT. Cognitive-behavioral pain management in children with juvenile rheumatoid arthritis. Pediatrics 89:1075–1079, 1992.
13. Wells KB, Stewart A, Hays RD, et al.: The functioning and well-being of depressed patients. Results from the medical outcomes study. JAMA 262:914–919, 1989.
14. Hofmann AD: The impact of illness in adolescence and coping behavior. Acta Paediatr Scand [Suppl.] 256:29–38, 1975.
15. Seligman ME: Helplessness: On Depression, Development and Death. Freeman, San Francisco, 1975.
16. Pelletier KR: Mind as Healer, Mind as Slayer: A Holistic Approach to Preventing Stress Disorders. Delacorte Press, New York, 1977.
17. Kroll F: Children with Juvenile Rheumatoid Arthritis, Social and Developmental Problems. New York State Chapter, Arthritis and Rheumatism Foundation, New York, 1958.
18. Turk J: Impact of cystic fibrosis on family functioning. Pediatrics 34:67–71, 1964.
19. Lawler RH, Nakielny W, et al.: Psychological implications of cystic fibrosis. Can Med Assoc J 94:1034–1046, 1966.
20. McCollum AT, Gibson LE: Family adaptation to the child with cystic fibrosis. J Pediatr 77:571–578, 1970.
21. McCormick MC, Stemmler MM, Athreya BH: The impact of childhood rheumatic diseases on the family. Arthritis Rheum 29:872–879, 1986.
22. Tropauer A, Franz MN, et al.: Psychological aspects of care of children with cystic fibrosis. Am J Dis Child 199:424–432, 1970.
23. Driscoll CB, Lubin AH: Conferences with parents of children with cystic fibrosis. Social Casework 53:140–146, 1972.
24. Lavigne JV, Ryan M: Psychologic adjustment of siblings of children with chronic illness. Pediatrics 63:616–627, 1979.
25. Blom GE, Nicholls G: Emotional factors in children with rheumatoid arthritis. Am J Orthopsychiatry 24:588–601, 1954.
26. Daniels D, Miller JJ III, Billings AG, Moos RH: Psychosocial functioning of siblings of children with rheumatic disease. J Pediatr 109:379–383, 1986.
27. Burlingham D: Notes on problems of motor restraint during illness. In Lowenstein RM (ed.) Drives, Affects, Behavior. International Universities Press, New York, 1953.
28. Erikson EH: Childhood and Society, 2nd ed. Norton, New York, 1963, pp. 247–274.
29. McDermott JF Jr., Akina E: Understanding and improving the personality development of children with physical handicaps. Clin Pediatr 11:130–134, 1972.
30. Baretz RM, Stephenson GR: Unrealistic patient. NY State J Med 76:54–57, 1976.
31. Jacobs JC: The arthritic child and the family: Staying in the mainstream. Arthritis Rheum 20:595–597, 1977.
32. Sontag S: Illness as Metaphor. Doubleday, New York, 1978.
33. Gaylin W, Glasser I, Marcus S, Rothman DJ: Doing Good, the Limits of Benevolence. Pantheon Books, New York, 1978.
34. Preston RP: The Dilemmas of Care: Social and Nursing Adaptations to the Deformed, the Disabled, and the Aged. Elsevier Press, New York, 1979.

35. McAlister AL, Perry C, Maccoby N: Adolescent smoking: onset and prevention. Pediatrics 63:650–658, 1979.
36. MacElman RM: Society vs the wheelchair. Pediatrics 63:576–579, 1979.
37. Klerman LV, Weitzman M, Alpert JJ, et al.: Why adolescents do not attend school. The views of students and parents. J Adolesc Health Care, 8:425–430, 1987.
38. Taylor J, Passo MH, Champion VL: School problems and teacher responsibilities in juvenile rheumatoid arthritis. J School Health 57:186–190, 1987.
39. Weitzman M, Alpert JJ, Klerman LV, et al.: High-risk youth and health: the case of excessive school absence. Pediatrics 78:313–322, 1986.
40. Weitzman M: School absence rates as outcome measures in studies of children with chronic illness. J Chron Dis 39:799–808, 1986.
41. Weitzman M, Klerman LV, Lamb GA, et al.: Demographic and educational characteristics of inner city middle school problem absence students. Amer J Orthopsychiat 53:378–383, 1985.
42. Weitzman M, Klerman LV, Lamb G, et al.: School absence: a problem for the pediatrician. Pediatrics 69:739–746, 1982.
43. Whitehouse R, Shope JT, Sullivan DB, Kulik C-L: Children with juvenile rheumatoid arthritis at School. Functional problems, participation in physical education. The Implementation of Public Law 94-192. Clin Ped 28:509–514, 1989.
44. Brewer EJ Jr, McPherson M, Magrab PR, Hutchins VL: Family-centered, coordinated care for children with special health care needs. Pediatrics 83:1055–1060, 1989.
45. Stern RC, Boat TF: Taking medications in school: Committee report challenged. Pediatrics 63:348–350, 1979. See also: American Academy of Pediatrics; Committee on school health: Administration of medication in school. Pediatrics 74:433(1984).
46. Lovell DJ, Athreya B, Emery HM, et al.: School attendance and patterns, special services and special needs in pediatric patients with rheumatic diseases. Results of a multicenter study. Arthritis Care and Research 3:196–203, 1990.
47. Rosenbaum M-B: Sexuality and the physically disabled: the role of the professional. Bull NY Acad Med 54:501–509, 1978.
48. Hill RH, Herstein A, Walters K: Juvenile rheumatoid arthritis: followup into adulthood—medical, sexual and social status. CMA J 114:790–796, 1976.
49. Wolff BB: Current psychosocial concepts in rheumatoid arthritis. Bull Rheum Dis 22:656–661, 1972.
50. Cleveland SE, Reitman EE, Brewer EJ, et al.: Psychological factors in juvenile rheumatoid arthritis. Arthritis Rheum 8:1152–1158, 1965.
51. Henoch MJ, Batson JW, Baum J: Emotional factors in children with rheumatoid arthritis. Arthritis Rheum 21:229–233, 1978.
52. Singsen BH, Johnson MA, Bernstein BA: Psychodynamics of juvenile rheumatoid arthritis. In Miller JJ III (ed.) Juvenile Rheumatoid Arthritis. PSG, Littleton, MA, 1979, pp. 249–265.
53. Figley BA, Ziebell B: Psychological and sexual health in rheumatic diseases. In Kelley WN, Harris Ed, Ruddy S, Sledge CB, et al. (eds.) Textbook of Rheumatology. Saunders, Philadelphia, 1989, 3rd ed. pp. 497–510.
54. Seyle H: The Stress of Life (Revised). McGraw-Hill, New York, 1976.

55. Achterberg OC, Simonton S, Matthews-Simonton S (eds.). Stress, Psychological Factors and Cancer: An Annotated Collection of Readings From the Professional Literature. New Medicine Press, Fort Worth, Texas, 1976.

56. Bardach JL: Psychological assessment procedures as indicators of patients' abilities to meet tasks in rehabilitation. J Counsel Psychol 15:471–475, 1968.

57. Morse J: Aspiration and achievement, a study of one hundred patients with juvenile rheumatoid arthritis. Rehabil Lit 33:290–303, 1972.

58. Caplan LR: Mutliple sclerosis and hysteria: lessons learned from their association. JAMA 243:2418–2421, 1980.

59. Shulman R: Psychogenic illness with physical manifestations and the other side of the coin. A practical approach. Lancet 1:524–526, 1977.

60. Editorial: Mind and cancer. Lancet 1:706–707, 1979.

61. McAnarney ER, Pless IB, Satterwhite MA et al.: Psychological problems of children with chronic juvenile arthritis. Pediatrics 53:523–528, 1974.

62. Pless B, Roghmann K, Haggerty RJ: Chronic illness, family functioning, and psychological adjustment: a model for the allocation of preventive mental health services. Int J Epidemiol 1:271–277, 1972.

63. Gilder R, Buschman P: Approaches to the dying child. In Bemporad J (ed.) Child Development in Normality and Psychopathology. Brunner/Mazel, New York, 1980.

64. Beck L, Lattimer JK, Braun E: Group psychotherapy on a children's urology service. Soc Work Health Care 4:275–285, 1979.

65. Southwood TR, Malleson PN, Roberts-Thompson PJ, Mahy M: Unconventional remedies used for patients with Juvenile Arthritis. Pediatrics 85:150–154, 1990.

66. Manheimer RH, Greene KRC, Kroll F: Juvenile rheumatoid arthritis in New York City. Arch Pediatr 76:173–184, 1959.

67. Kellerman J, Zelter L, Ellenberg L, et al.: Psychologic effects of illness in adolescence. I. Anxiety, self-esteem, and perception of control. J Pediatr 97:126–131, 1980.

68. Zelter L, Kellerman J, Ellenberg L, et al.: Psychologic effects of illness in adolescence. II. Impact of illness in adolescents—crucial issues and coping styles. J Pediatr 97:132–138, 1980.

69. Allaire SH, DeNardo BS, Szer IS, et al.: Economic impacts of juvenile rheumatoid arthritis (JRA). Arthritis Rheum 34:S82, 1991.

70. Brewer EJ Jr, Angel KC: Parenting a child with arthritis. Lowell House, Los Angeles, 1992.

Index